NOVEL ASPECTS OF
PAIN MANAGEMENT

NOVEL ASPECTS OF PAIN MANAGEMENT
Opioids and Beyond

Edited by

JANA SAWYNOK
Department of Pharmacology
Dalhousie University
Nova Scotia, Canada

ALAN COWAN
Department of Pharmacology
Temple University
Philadelphia, Pennsylvania

WILEY-LISS

A JOHN WILEY & SONS, INC., PUBLICATION

New York • Chichester • Weinheim • Brisbane • Singapore • Toronto

This book is printed on acid-free paper. ∞

Copyright © 1999 by Wiley-Liss, Inc. All rights reserved.

Published simultaneously in Canada.

While the authors, editors, and publisher believe that drug selection and dosage and the specification and usage of equipment and devices, as set forth in this book, are in accord with current recommendations and practice at the time of publication, they accept no legal responsibility for any errors or omissions, and make no warranty, expressed or implied, with respect to material contained herein. In view of ongoing research, equipment modifications, changes in governmental regulations, and the constant flow of information relating to drug therapy, drug reactions, and the use of equipment and devices, the reader is urged to review and evaluate the information provided in the package insert or instructions for each drug, piece of equipment, or device for, among other things, any changes in the instructions or indication of dosage or usage and for added warnings and precautions.

No part of this publication may be reproduced, stored in a retrieval system or transmitted in any form or by any means, electronic, mechanical, photocopying, recording, scanning or otherwise, except as permitted under Section 107 or 108 of the 1976 United States Copyright Act, without either the prior written permission of the Publisher, or authorization through payment of the appropriate per-copy fee to the Copyright Clearance Center, 222 Rosewood Drive, Danvers, MA 01923, (978) 750-8400, fax (978) 750-4744. Requests to the Publisher for permission should be addressed to the Permissions Department, John Wiley & Sons, Inc., 605 Third Avenue, New York, NY 10158-0012, (212) 850-6011, fax (212) 850-6008, E-Mail: PERMREQ@WILEY.COM.

For ordering and customer service, call 1-800-CALL-WILEY.

Library of Congress Cataloging-in-Publication Data:

Novel aspects of pain management : opioids and beyond / edited by Jana
   Sawynok and Alan Cowan.
      p. cm.
   Includes index.
   ISBN 0-471-18017-3 (alk. paper)
   1. Analgesics. 2. Analgesia. 3. Pain. 4. Chronic pain.
I. Sawynok, Jana, 1950–   . II. Cowan, Alan, 1942–   .
   [DNLM: 1. Analgesics—therapeutic use. 2. Pain—drug therapy.
QV 95 N937 1999]
RM319.N68   1999
615'.783—dc21

DNLM/DLC
for Library of Congress   98-32316

Printed in the United States of America.

10 9 8 7 6 5 4 3 2 1

CONTENTS

Preface		vii
Contributors		ix
1	**NEUROPHYSIOLOGY OF ACUTE AND CHRONIC PAIN** Anthony Dickenson and Alison Reeve	1
2	**ANIMAL MODELS OF PAIN** Alan Cowan	21
3	**RECENT ADVANCES IN THE PHARMACOLOGY OF OPIOIDS** Michael H. Ossipov, Josephine Lai, T. Philip Malan, Jr., and Frank Porreca	49
4	**SOME NEW INSIGHTS INTO THE PHARMACOLOGY OF NONSTEROIDAL ANTI-INFLAMMATORY DRUGS** Keith McCormack	73
5	**PERIPHERALLY ACTING ANALGESIC AGENTS** Humphrey P. Rang, Stuart J. Bevan, and Martin N. Perkins	95
6	**VANILLOIDS AS ANALGESICS** Andy Dray	117
7	**NEUROKININ ANTAGONISTS** Nadia M. J. Rupniak and Raymond G. Hill	135
8	**EXCITATORY AMINO ACID ANTAGONISTS: POTENTIAL ANALGESICS FOR PERSISTENT PAIN** Terence J. Coderre	157

9	ALPHA-2 ADRENERGIC AGONISTS AS ANALGESICS	179
	Tony L. Yaksh	
10	SEROTONIN AND ITS RECEPTORS IN PAIN CONTROL	203
	Michel Hamon and Sylvie Bourgoin	
11	PURINES: POTENTIAL FOR DEVELOPMENT AS ANALGESIC AGENTS	229
	Jana Sawynok and Anthony Poon	
12	γ-AMINOBUTYRIC ACID AND PAIN	249
	Norman G. Bowery and Marzia Malcangio	
13	CHOLINERGIC AGONISTS AS ANALGESICS	265
	Edgar T. Iwamoto	
14	DOPAMINERGIC DRUGS AS ANALGESICS	287
	Keith B. J. Franklin	
15	TRICYCLIC AND OTHER ANTIDEPRESSANTS AS ANALGESICS	303
	A. Eschalier, D. Ardid and C. Dubray	
16	VOLTAGE-GATED ION CHANNEL MODULATORS	321
	John C. Hunter	
17	SPINAL DRUG INTERACTIONS	345
	James C. Eisenach and G. F. Gebhart	
Index		363

PREFACE

The past 30 years have witnessed a number of significant advances in our understanding of the means by which pain signaling and pain suppression occur. In 1965, the Gate Control Theory of pain was published, and this stimulated a great deal of research in terms of understanding endogenous pain suppressing mechanisms. The 1970s saw the discovery of three families of endogenous opioid peptides, and the development of receptor binding techniques that enabled multiple opioid receptors to be characterized. Since that time, two additional advances have occurred. The first is an appreciation of the role of central sensitization in both inflammatory and neuropathic pain states. The second is a growing awareness of the multiplicity of neurochemical mediators that can influence pain signaling at peripheral sites where pain originates, within the dorsal spinal cord where pain information first enters the central nervous system, and at supraspinal sites where pain is processed. Although opioids and nonsteroidal anti-inflammatory drugs are still the mainstays of analgesic therapy, there has been a growing willingness to consider and experiment with alternative strategies for the relief of pain. This may be useful not only in optimizing pain relief, but also in developing novel medications for poorly treated clinical conditions (e.g., neuropathic pain). In this book, properties of the many chemicals that influence pain processing are reviewed in a comprehensive and systematic manner. We solicited the expertise of an international cohort of scientists who are experienced pain researchers and scholars. Each author was asked to provide a historical perspective on the class of agents being considered and then assess its potential for therapeutic development. The panoramic scope of the book should appeal to a wide range of professionals, particularly academic scientists, clinicians who are interested in potential new therapies for pain control, and scientists developing novel analgesics in the pharmaceutical industry.

We wish to thank the authors for sharing their formidable collective knowledge, Michael Williams for suggesting the topic, Fiona Stevens and Joe Ingram at Wiley for their assistance in many aspects of this endeavor, and Allison Reid for her most able editorial assistance throughout the entire project.

JANA SAWYNOK
ALAN COWAN

CONTRIBUTORS

D. ARDID, Equipe NPPUA, Laboratoire de Pharmacologie Médicale, Faculté de Médecine, Université d'Auvergne, 63001 Clermont-Ferrand Cedex 1, France

STUART D. BEVAN, Novartis Institute for Medical Sciences, 5 Gower Place, London WC1E 6BN, United Kingdom

SYLVIE BOURGOIN, INSERM U288, NeuroPsychoPharmacologie, Moléculaire, Cellulaire et Fonctionnelle, Faculté de Médecine Pitié-Salpêtrière, 91 Boulevard de l'Hôpital, 75634 Paris Cedex 13, France

NORMAN BOWERY, Department of Pharmacology, The Medical School, University of Birmingham, Edgbaston, Birmingham B15 2TT, United Kingdom

TERENCE J. CODERRE, Pain Mechanisms Laboratory, Clinical Research Institute of Montreal, McGill University, 110 Pine Avenue West, Montreal, Quebec H2W 1R7, Canada

ALAN COWAN, Department of Pharmacology, Temple University School of Medicine, 3420 N. Broad St., Philadelphia, Pennsylvania 19140

ANTHONY DICKENSON, Departments of Pharmacology and Anesthesiology, University College London, Gower Street, London WC1E 6BT, United Kingdom

ANDY DRAY, Astra Research Centre Montreal, 7171 Frederick Banting Street, Montreal, Quebec H4S 1Z9, Canada

C. DUBRAY, Equipe NPPUA, Laboratoire de Pharmacologie Médicale, Faculté de Médecine, Université d'Auvergne, 63001 Clermont-Ferrand Cedex 1, France

JAMES C. EISENACH, Department of Anesthesiology, Wake Forest University School of Medicine, 300 S. Hawthorne Rd., Winston-Salem, North Carolina 27103

A. ESCHALIER, Equipe NPPUA, Laboratoire de Pharmacologie Médicale, Faculté de Médecine, Université d'Auvergne, 63001 Clermont-Ferrand Cedex 1, France

KEITH B. J. FRANKLIN, Department of Psychology, McGill University, 1205 Dr. Penfield Ave., Montreal, Quebec H3A 1B1, Canada

G. F. GEBHART, Department of Pharmacology, University of Iowa College of Medicine, Iowa City, Iowa 52242-1109

MICHEL HAMON, INSERM U288, NeuroPsychoPharmacologie, Moléculaire, Cellulaire et Fonctionnelle, Faculté de Médecine Pitié-Salpêtrière, 91 Boulevard de l'Hôpital, 75634 Paris Cedex 13, France

RAYMOND G. HILL, Merck Sharp and Dohme Research Laboratories, Neuroscience Research Centre, Terlings Park, Harlow, Essex CM20 2QR, United Kingdom

JOHN C. HUNTER, Department of Analgesia, Neurobiology Unit, Roche Bioscience, Palo Alto, California 94304

EDGAR T. IWAMOTO, Department of Pharmacology, University of Kentucky College of Medicine, Lexington, Kentucky 40536

JOSEPHINE LAI, Department of Pharmacology, University of Arizona Health Sciences Center, Tucson, Arizona 85724

T. PHILIP MALAN, JR., Departments of Anesthesiology and Pharmacology, University of Arizona Health Sciences Center, Tucson, Arizona 85724

MARZIA MALCANGIO, Department of Pharmacology, UMDS, St. Thomas's Campus, London, United Kingdom

KEITH MCCORMACK, Drug Research Group, McCormack Limited, Church House, Church Square, Leighton Buzzard, Bedfordshire LU7 7AE, United Kingdom

MICHAEL H. OSSIPOV, Department of Pharmacology, University of Arizona Health Sciences Center, Tucson, Arizona 85724

MARTIN N. PERKINS, Novartis Institute for Medical Sciences, 5 Gower Place, London WC1E 6BN, United Kingdom

ANTHONY POON, Department of Pharmacology, Dalhousie University, Halifax, Nova Scotia B3H 4H7, Canada

FRANK PORRECA, Departments of Pharmacology and Anesthesiology, University of Arizona Health Sciences Center, Tucson, Arizona 85724

HUMPHREY P. RANG, Novartis Institute for Medical Sciences, 5 Gower Place, London WC1E 6BN, United Kingdom

ALISON REEVE, Department of Pharmacology, University College London, Gower Street, London WC1E 6BT, United Kingdom

NADIA M. J. RUPNIAK, Merck Sharp and Dohme Research Laboratories, Neuroscience Research Centre, Terlings Park, Harlow, Essex CM20 2QR, United Kingdom

JANA SAWYNOK, Department of Pharmacology, Dalhousie University, Halifax, Nova Scotia B3H 4H7, Canada

TONY L. YAKSH, Department of Anesthesiology, University of California, San Diego, 9500 Gilman Drive, La Jolla, California 92093-0818

CHAPTER 1

NEUROPHYSIOLOGY OF ACUTE AND CHRONIC PAIN

ANTHONY DICKENSON and ALISON REEVE
University College London
London, United Kingdom

"Pain" is not a simple process, in that the stimulus received is not always the same as the stimulus perceived. The reasons for this involve changes in physiological and pharmacological systems caused by different pain states. The aim of this chapter is to describe the neurophysiology of acute and chronic pain, with emphasis on neuronal and nerve fiber responses in different pain states.

PERIPHERAL RECEPTOR SIGNALING

Receptors throughout the body convey external stimuli into common electrical signals. The appropriate, adequate stimulus can produce changes in the membrane potential of a sensory receptor by converting the energy of the stimulus to a change in the receptor permeability to ions, thus causing an action potential. The information this action potential conveys is determined by the type of receptor that has been activated as well as by the frequency and strength of the signal.

Sensory Receptors

These receptors include mechano-, chemo-, and thermoreceptors. A "receptor" is usually thought of as a protein structure embedded in a cell membrane. However, the terminology describing "receptors" for transmission of somatosensory information can incorporate the fiber type they are innervating, the proposed transduction mechanism, and the adequate stimulus that activates them; often the term "unit" is used to encompass this. Generally, there are

---

Novel Aspects of Pain Management: Opioids and Beyond, Edited by Jana Sawynok and Alan Cowan
ISBN 0-471-180173 Copyright © 1999 by Wiley-Liss, Inc.

"units" that respond to nonpainful, low-threshold stimulation, and these are conveyed by the Aβ fibers and associated endings. Aδ fibers can be nociceptive or non-nociceptive. The nociceptors associated with C fibers are often termed polymodal because they can respond to a variety of adequate stimuli. The transduction mechanism associated with the free endings of these latter fibers has still to be ascertained. Some C fibers, however, also convey low-threshold information. Aδ fibers have also been shown to behave as polymodal receptors in their own right as well as Aδ mechanoreceptors behaving like C-polymodal afferents after sensitization. Often the situation (e.g., inflammation) has an effect on the transmission of information.

Mechanoreceptors

Mechanoreceptors respond to mechanical changes in the skin such as indentation and displacement and may be activated by stimuli in the non-noxious range or respond to noxious mechanical stimuli (Burgess and Perl, 1967). The non-noxious activated mechanoreceptors may be divided into two groups, the slowly adapting and rapidly adapting mechanical receptors. They consist of a specially adapted end-organ associated with an afferent nerve fiber terminal.

The slowly adapting receptors can be further categorized into slowly adapting I (SAI) and slowly adapting II (SAII). The SAI receptors respond to skin deflection and displacement and are associated with Merkel's disk and tactile domes in the epidermis of the skin (see Gebhart, 1995). The SAII receptors respond to indentation and stretch of the skin, associated with the activation of the Ruffini endings in the dermis. SAI tend to have small receptive fields in comparison to the SAII. Both classes of receptor continue to discharge as long as the stimulus is maintained. The fast-adapting receptors respond to skin indentation but they signal only the velocity of the stimulus, responding to tapping and vibration but not to sustained pressure on the skin. They respond only briefly when the stimulus is applied and in some cases when it is removed (see Willis and Coggeshall, 1991). The sensory end-organs associated with these stimuli are the Meissner's corpuscles in glabrous (nonhairy) skin and the Pacinian corpuscles in both the subdermal glabrous and hairy skin.

The sense organs described above all respond to stimuli in the non-noxious range and are associated with Aβ-myelinated afferents. However, under certain circumstances Aβ-fiber evoked activity causes enhanced responses, usually associated with C-fiber driven activity, and so may be responsible for allodynia (Woolf, 1991). A recent study has shown that the Aβ-fibers have the capacity to change their phenotype under certain conditions (Neumann et al., 1996).

There are also mechanoreceptors that respond to noxious stimuli. These are the C mechanoreceptors associated with unmyelinated afferent fibers; they represent 10% of mechanically activated receptors (Bessou and Perl, 1969; Georgopoulos, 1976). The majority of noxious mechanoreceptors are associated with myelinated afferents, the Aδ high-threshold mechanoreceptors (HTM) (Burgess and Perl, 1967; Georgopoulos, 1976; Lynn and Shakhanbeh, 1988). These do not respond to non-noxious mechanical stimuli or to noxious stimuli other than mechanical (Burgess and Perl, 1967; Campbell et al., 1979; Lynn and Shakhanbeh, 1988) although there are receptors that respond to both noxious mechanical and thermal stimulation (Beck et al., 1974; Georgopoulos, 1976; Lynn and Shakhanbeh, 1988). The C fiber-associated and the Aδ fiber mechanoreceptors have similar thresholds (Georgopoulos, 1976); after sensitization the Aδ mechanoreceptor can also respond like a C-polymodal receptor (Fitzgerald and Lynn, 1977).

Thermoreceptors

There are receptors that convey information on cold and warm temperatures in the non-noxious range as well as noci-thermoreceptors that respond to temperatures in the noxious range (Georgopoulos, 1976; see Willis and Coggeshall, 1991). In the rat, only C-fibers are responsible for conveying noxious temperature (Lynn and Shakhanbeh, 1988), whereas in other species, high-threshold mechanical Aδ fibers can convey this information under certain conditions (Georgopoulos, 1976; Fitzgerald and Lynn, 1977). There are also Aδ fibers that are sensitive to lower thresholds for heat compared to the Aδ mechanothermal fibers (Beck et al., 1974; Georgopoulos, 1976). The basis for cold allodynia after nerve damage remains unclear.

Nociceptors

There are two main categories of cutaneous nociceptor, the Aδ mechanical and C polymodal (Bessou and Perl, 1969). Along with these receptors present in the skin, which are available for activation at all times, there is also a group of nociceptors that for the majority of the time are not available for recruitment, known as "silent" nociceptors (Lynn and Carpenter, 1992). It is believed that this population of receptors must first become sensitized before they can be activated, such as may occur after inflammation, and their activity appears to be associated with hyperalgesia (Reeh et al., 1987).

The Aδ mechanoreceptors are believed not to have free endings in that their fine endings are covered by Schwann cells. Their endings are located in the epidermis of the skin and are activated by mechanical stimuli in most instances (Burgess and Perl, 1967; Georgopoulos, 1976; Handwerker et al., 1987; Lynn and Shakhanbeh, 1988). Application of noxious heat to these receptors sensitizes them to heat (Fitzgerald and Lynn, 1977; Campbell et al., 1979). This characteristic is also thought to play a role in hyperalgesia. Repeated application of intense mechanical stimuli can decrease the responsiveness of this receptor to mechanical stimuli and abolish it in some instances (Lynn and Carpenter, 1992). Some Aδ nociceptors respond to mechanical, thermal, and chemical noxious stimuli without having to be sensitized first and are known as Aδ polymodal nociceptors (Adriaensen et al., 1980).

The C-polymodal nociceptor is associated with the unmyelinated C fiber. As the name suggests, these receptors respond to a variety of adequate noxious stimuli (see Bessou and Perl, 1969; Croze et al., 1976). Their receptive fields are smaller than the Aδ nociceptors, although often the receptive fields of these fibers overlap. Polymodal nociceptors show both adaptation and fatigue, where the response to a repetitive stimulus to the same area can diminish. There are also nociceptors activated by stimuli in the non-noxious range; these progressively respond as the stimulus intensity is increased (Van Hees and Gybels, 1972; Torebjork and Hallin, 1974).

There are also receptors responding to noxious stimuli found in skeletal muscle, joints, and visceral tissue, along with receptors that respond to non-noxious stimuli and convey position, movement, and mechanical forces (Clark and Burgess, 1975).

In skeletal muscle there are pressure-pain endings that are associated with unmyelinated and thinly myelinated afferents as well as a few associated with the larger myelinated afferents (see Willis and Coggeshall, 1991). In joints, there are receptors associated with both Aδ and C fibers that respond to movement of a joint beyond its usual range and mechanical stimulation (Schaible and Schmidt, 1983). A proportion of these are silent, especially those associated with C-fibers, and are activated only when a joint has become inflamed, especially becoming sensitive to mechanical stimulation (Coggeshall et al., 1983). The visceral organs, such as the heart, reproductive organs, respiratory system, and gastrointestinal tract have also been shown to be innervated by nociceptors (see Meller and Gebhart, 1992; Meyer et al., 1994). Unlike receptors in the skin, which give a very precise location of the stimulus, pain arising from activation of deep visceral nociceptors is often very diffuse and poorly localized (Cervero, 1991).

Chemicals Contributing to the Activation of Nociceptors

The peripheral terminals of small diameter neurons, especially in conditions of inflammation, may be excited by a number of endogenous chemical mediators (see Rang et al., 1991). These can be released from non-neuronal cells, the afferent fibers themselves, and products triggered by activation of the body's defense mechanisms. These produce primary hyperalgesia due to peripheral sensitization of nociceptors so that afferent activity to a given stimulus is increased by the presence of inflammation.

Bradykinin is cleaved from kininogens in response to tissue injury and can cause vasodilation and edema and mobilize arachidonic acid metabolites. There are two receptors for bradykinin. Bradykinin receptors have been shown in the dorsal root ganglia (DRG) as well as peripheral to the DRG cells (Steranka et al., 1988). The B_1 receptor is constitutively expressed less than the B_2 receptor, but in chronic inflammation, it is upregulated (Hall, 1992; Perkins et al., 1993). Pain may arise via the activation of the B_2 receptor, abundant in most tissues, which can activate C-polymodal units and to a lesser extent, heat-insensitive units (Rang et al., 1991; Steranka et al., 1988). The response to bradykinin can be enhanced by prostaglandin E_2, heat, and serotonin (Lang et al., 1990).

Protons increase in inflammation and ischemia and may activate nociceptors directly as well as sensitizing them to mechanical stimulation (Steen et al., 1992). Protons cause a brief depolarization in many neuronal cells (Krishtal and Pidoplichko, 1980) as well as causing a sustained depolarization in sensory neurons, which are sensitive to capsaicin (Bevan and Yeats, 1991). The proton site is believed to be similar to the one activated by capsaicin (Rang et al., 1991).

Serotonin, 5-hydroxytryptamine (5HT), is released from non-neuronal cells such as platelets, mast cells, and specialized cells within the digestive tract. Serotonin can cause excitation of nociceptive afferents via the activation of its own membrane-bound receptors, for example, $5HT_{1A}$, $5HT_2$, and $5HT_3$ (Dray, 1997), as well as sensitizing nociceptors, especially to bradykinin (Lang et al., 1990; see Rang et al., 1991). Serotonin may play a prominent role in the pain associated with migraine (Moskowitz, 1994).

Mast cells, as well as releasing 5-HT, can also release histamine, which causes vasodilation, edema, and itch (Simone et al., 1991). Adenosine, via the A_3-receptor, can also cause mast cells to degranulate, and is thus pro-inflammatory under these conditions (Sawynok et al., 1997). Substance P released from the peripheral terminals of primary afferents (via axon reflex) can also cause the mast cells to degranulate. Histamine can act at the H_1 receptor to activate afferent fibers by increasing the calcium permeability of the membranes (see Rang et al., 1991).

An important component in inflammation is the release of arachidonic acid metabolites. Arachidonic acid, a component of cell membranes, is liberated by phospholipase A_2 and is subsequently metabolized by two main pathways controlled by two enzymes, cyclooxygenase (COX) and lipoxygenase (Flower and Vane, 1974). This metabolism gives rise to the the eicosanoids, (leukotrienes, thromboxanes, prostacyclins, and prostaglandins). They do not activate nociceptors directly but sensitize them to other mediators and stimuli. Steroids and the nonsteroidal anti-inflammatory (NSAIDs) group of drugs, which attenuate the conversion of arachidonic acid to these mediators, can only prevent further conversion and can not halt the effects of mediators that have already been released. Importantly, a second inducible form of COX, COX 2, has been described. Because inhibition of the constitutive enzyme COX-1 results in the gastric and renal side effects of NSAIDs, there is hope that selective COX-2 inhibitors may have improved therapeutic profiles. Several novel agents with this latter profile have been reported to be effective in inflammatory pain models (see Appleton, 1997).

The afferent fibers themselves can also release mediators. These can be peptides, such as substance P, calcitonin gene-related peptide (CGRP), and adenosine triphosphate (ATP). The peptides cause a number of effects including vasodilation, plasma extravasation, and mast cell degranulation, and ATP causes direct nociceptor activation (Dray, 1997).

The consequences of ATP release from peripheral terminals is complex. ATP release can excite P2 receptors, which can activate the sensory neurons themselves via a mono- and divalent sensitive ion channel (Krishtal et al., 1983). ATP receptors are also present on macrophages and may result in the release of cytokines. ATP can also be converted to adenosine via ectoenzymes, which can activate the P1 receptors. The P1 receptors may be pronociceptive (A_2), pro-inflammatory (A_3), or antinociceptive (A_1) (see Burnstock and Wood, 1996). The role of peripheral adenosine will then depend on the local distribution of specific receptors and levels of adenosine.

PERIPHERAL NERVE SIGNALING MECHANISMS

Whatever the mechanism of activation and transduction, the activation of the peripheral terminals of the afferent fibers results in the generation of an action potential. The propagation of action potentials relays the electrical signal to the central terminal of the afferent fiber, where neurotransmitters are released into the dorsal horn of the spinal cord. The use of different types of peripheral stimulation can be employed to study the consequences of activation of these fiber types on the dorsal horn of the spinal cord. Acute peripheral electrical stimulation can be used to observe the different fiber evoked responses before and after pharmacological manipulation. Because electrical stimulation activates the nerve axons directly there is no sensitization of transduction mechanisms, as can occur with repetitive physiological stimulation. Models of inflammation (e.g., carrageenan and formalin) can also be used to observe the changes that occur in the periphery and at the spinal cord level after inflammation, and nerve injury provides a means of examining changes that occur in neuropathic states.

Afferent Nerves

The nerve fibers associated with the relay of non-noxious information are the Aβ fibers. These fibers innervate various receptors in the dermis and are myelinated by Schwann cells so that these fibers have a rapid conduction velocity, between 30 and 100 m/s. The Aδ fibers are thinly myelinated and therefore their conduction velocities (4–30 m/s) are slower than the Aβ fiber responses (Kruger et al., 1981). These fibers have the capacity to convey both non-noxious and noxious information. The C fibers are not myelinated so their conduction velocity is the slowest of these three fiber types, < 2.5 m/s, and in most cases are activated by high-threshold stimuli. There are also afferent fibers innervating muscle and joints. There are three classes of myelinated axons: group I, conduction velocity of 72–120 m/s; group II, 24–71 m/s; and group III, 6–23 m/s. There are also unmyelinated axons associated with these tissues with conduction velocities of less than 2.5 m/s, known as group IV axons. Group I includes the muscle spindle afferents, group II corresponds to the Aβ fibers and groups III and IV to the Aδ- and C-fibers, respectively. There are few large myelinated axons associated with the viscerae, and the Aδ and C fibers convey information from these tissues (Gebhart, 1995).

Peripheral Changes Occuring In Neuropathy

Following damage to peripheral nerves, a number of changes can be produced. The recent advent of a number of animal models of neuropathic pain states has facilitated understanding of the peripheral mechanisms involved. Damaged nerves may start to produce ectopic activity due to clustering of sodium channels around the damaged axons and also mechanoreceptors become highly sensitive to natural stimuli. The activity can spread rapidly to the dorsal root ganglia. In addition, sympathetic efferents become able to activate sensory afferents via alpha-adrenergic receptors. There is also evidence for interactions between adjacent sensory nerve axons and between ganglion cells so that excitation can spread between neural structures. These peripheral ectopic impulses can cause spontaneous pain and prime the spinal cord to exhibit enhanced evoked responses to stimuli, which themselves have greater effects due to increased sensitivity of the peripheral nerves. This area has recently been reviewed by Devor (1996).

DORSAL ROOT GANGLIA

The cell bodies in the dorsal root ganglia synthesise cell proteins, such as enzymes and receptors. Once synthesized, these substances can be transported to both the peripheral and the central terminals of the cell. Under normal conditions, opioid receptors are expressed but nonfunctional at the peripheral terminal. However, after inflammation, the perineurium surrounding the free endings is broken down, making the opioid receptors accessible (see Stein, 1993).

Cells in the DRG can be separated on the basis of size. The large-diameter axons tend to have large cell bodies and make up the Aβ fibers, group I and II from muscles and joints. The smaller fibers have smaller cell bodies and make up Aδ, C fibers as well as group III and IV afferents. These cell bodies can be further subdivided depending on which peptides and enzymes they are positive for. All the cell bodies stain for the excitatory amino acid glutamate. Many cells contain calcitonin gene-related peptide (CGRP), vasopressin, and oxytocin (30%), with 10–30% staining for substance P (SP) (see Willis and Coggeshall, 1991). A smaller percentage (10%) stain for somatostatin (SOM), cholecystokinin (CCK), bombesin (BOM), vasoactive intestinal polypeptide (VIP), galanin (GAL), dynorphin (DYN), endorphin (END), enkephalin (ENK), and corticotrophin-releasing factor (CRF). Co-localization of these peptides can occur (Lundberg and Hokfelt 1986). Immunocytochemical studies have demonstrated that substance P can co-localize with CGRP (Wiesenfeld-Hallin et al., 1984). Substance P is nearly always associated with CGRP in small type cells, whereas CGRP can be located without SP (Wiesenfeld-Hallin et al., 1984). SP also co-localizes with CCK, SOM, BOM, VIP, and DYN or ENK (see Willis and Coggeshall, 1991).

The precise function of these transmitters is open to debate. Many of the small fibers stain predominantly for these peptides compared to the larger fibers. This suggests that the transmission of noxious information is subject to considerable fine tuning, if all of these substances can act as neurotransmitters or neuromodulators. A clear definition of the role of these transmitters relies on the use of selective antagonists; these are available for only some of the receptors at present.

After the induction of peripheral inflammation, there is an upregulation of the major peptide transmitters so that for a given stimulus, there will be increased transmitter released into the spinal cord. Together with peripheral sensitization, this provides a basis for increased central excitability, central hypersensitivity, in the presence of inflammation (see Dickenson, 1997). After nerve damage, the situation is different in that substance P and CGRP are lost and are replaced by novel peptides such as neuropeptide Y and galanin (see Hokfelt et al., 1994). The consequences of this are unclear at present.

CENTRAL SPINAL CORD SIGNALING MECHANISMS

It is generally thought that there is a functional separation between the dorsal and ventral roots, in that the dorsal roots contain afferent sensory fibers and the ventral roots contain efferent motor fibers. However, a variety of studies have shown that this separation is not absolute. A small proportion of the afferent fibers, predominantly small in diameter, enter not by the dorsal roots but via the ventral root and terminate in the marginal zone and substantia gelatinosa (Light and Metz, 1978).

Large sensory fibers enter via the dorsal columns, and smaller fibers via a bundle known as Lissauer's tract (Molander et al., 1984). Lissauer's tract also contains axons of cells originating in the dorsal horn, from marginal cells as well as substantia gelatinosa neurons. Both large and small fiber types split into two, and may project both rostrally and caudally to the dorsal root before entering the spinal cord.

Spinal Cord Neuronal Organization

The spinal cord white matter contains axons and the gray matter is further divided into 10 laminae, first described in the cat by Rexed (1952) and subsequently by others in the rat (Wall, 1967; Molander et al., 1984). The laminae can be seen as layers of functionally distinct cells that form columns of functionally related cells extending the length of the cord. The different laminae contain different intrinsic cells, and receive different inputs and outputs to the ventral horn and to the brain.

Spinal laminae are not separated by distinct borders. Lamina I forms a rim around the most dorsal part of the gray matter and white matter. This lamina contains large horizontal neurones known as the marginal cells of Waldeyer and historically has been called the marginal zone. These cells have long dendrites that mainly pass over the surface of the dorsal horn, occasionally entering the substantia gelatinosa and forming a vague boundary between the white and gray matter. The dendrites, as well as covering the outer surface of the dorsal horn, also join Lissauer's tract for up to five or six segments where they join the gray matter again (Cervero and Iggo, 1980). There are also more smaller neurons located here that may make up the more dorsally located substantia gelatinosa cells. These cells are more prolific in number than the marginal cells. As well as these intrinsic, propriospinal cells, the various laminae also receive afferent inputs. The marginal plexus contains the processes of afferent neurons, superficial neurons, and the processes of deeper cells.

Aδ fibers terminate in lamina I entering via this marginal plexus (Light and Perl, 1979). Some of the visceral inputs terminate here as well as in laminae II, V, and X. Visceral inputs, only 10% of the afferent input into the spinal cord although with a greater rostro-caudal distribution than afferents from the skin, usually synapse onto the same cells that concurrently receive inputs from the skin and muscle. This is known as convergence, because a variety of inputs project to the same neuron and may be one of the reasons why visceral pain is often diffuse.

Lamina II of the spinal cord is also known as the substantia gelatinosa and historically has been called Rolandi substance (see Rexed, 1952; Cervero and Iggo, 1980). The substantia gelatinosa is composed of lamina II outer (which is more dorsal and contains densely packed cells) and lamina II inner, which is less compact and more ventrally located. Intrinsic cells in this region are predominantly stalk and islet cells but there are also arboreal cells, border cells, and spiny cells. The stalk cells have classically been called limiting cells, with cell bodies in II outer with dendrites extending toward the ventral horn. The stalk cells relay transmission from the superficial lamina to deeper laminae, and are presumed to be mainly excitatory, although the presence of enkephalin has been shown in some of these cells (Bennett et al., 1980). The islet cells have their cell bodies in II outer and inner and their dendrites extend in a rostro-caudal plane. The islet cells are inhibitory cells and play an important role in the control of the presynaptic terminals of afferent inputs, via axo-axonic connections as well as a postsynaptic inhibitory control via axo-dendritic connections. It is presumably activation of these cells by the collaterals of the large-diameter fibers that control the inputs of predominantly the Aδ-fiber terminals and to a lesser extent the C-fiber terminals and underlies the Gate Theory of Melzack and Wall (1965).

Hair follicle afferents are the only large-diameter afferents to terminate in lamina II inner (Molander et al., 1984). The innocuous C fibers terminate in lamina IIi and the noxious C-fiber terminals are in lamina II outer. However, although C fibers do not terminate in deeper lamina, cells located in laminae

V and VI can receive C-fiber inputs onto their dendrites, which extend into more superficial laminae (Fitzgerald and Wall, 1980). Afferent terminals from Aδ fibers are few in this lamina, although some have been shown to terminate in lamina II outer (Molander et al., 1984).

Laminae III–VI make up the deep dorsal horn. Cells located here have dendrites extending into deeper laminae or into superficial laminae. Inputs arising from cutaneous mechano- and proprioceptors terminate in laminae III and IV (SAI mechano, fast-adapting I and II, and hair follicle afferents). Lamina IV forms the base of the head of the dorsal horn. The cells found here are diffusely arranged, are large, and have dendrites that extend into more superficial laminae so they can receive inputs from afferents terminating more dorsally as well as direct inputs. There are no fine afferents terminating in this lamina. Muscle stretch receptors, joint receptors, and SAII terminate in laminae IV–VII and IX. Lamina V forms the neck of the dorsal horn and lamina VI forms the base of the dorsal horn; both receive inputs from thick myelinated fibers. More ventral laminae (VII–IX) have mainly efferents of visceral and somatic motor neurones. Lamina X is located close to the central canal.

The clear distinction between large- and small-fiber termination zones is disrupted after peripheral nerve damage and inflammation, in that the large Aβ fibers are able to sprout into previously exclusive C-fiber terminal zones, because these fibers can also now produce substance P; the combination of changes could contribute to the genesis of allodynia (Neumann et al., 1996).

Cells within the spinal cord can send projections to other areas of the spinal cord (propriospinal connections) or out of the spinal cord to areas of the brain (projection neurons). The large fibers, as well as sending collaterals into the dorsal horn at their point of entry, ascend ipsilaterally in the dorsal columns to terminate on second-order neurons in the medullary dorsal column nuclei. They then cross over to the contralateral side to the thalamus and cortex. The small fibers may project both rostrally and caudally along the dorsal root before entering the spinal cord where they terminate in the dorsal horn of the spinal cord in superficial laminae. These afferents synapse with interneurons that relay their information to deeper projection neurons, to dendrites of more ventrally located projection neurons, or back to spinothalamic neurons in lamina I. Projection neurons from laminae I, III, and IV transmit noxious and thermal sensations to the brain in the anterolateral white matter. This includes the spinoreticular, spino-mesencephalon, and spinothalamic tracts. These project to the reticular formation of the brain stem (spinoreticular) or the parabrachial area in the midbrain (spinomesencephalic), then on to the thalamus and cortical systems.

Spinal Cord Neuronal Responses

It has been demonstrated in a variety of species that cells within the dorsal horn can be divided into categories depending on their adequate stimulus. Cells that respond to non-noxious stimuli only have been categorized as class 1 cells (Menetrey et al., 1977). If electrical stimulation is used the subsequent responses have a short latency and duration of response. Increasing the stimulation intensity does not give rise to an increase in response. Cells can also respond to noxious and non-noxious stimuli (Mendell, 1966; Menetrey et al., 1977; Fitzgerald and Wall, 1980; Schouenborg and Sjolund, 1983). If search techniques involve natural stimuli of both non-noxious as well as noxious intensity, touch and pinch, respectively, the cells selected for recording appear to correspond to class 2A described in the rat (Menetrey et al., 1977). These cells have been shown to display a prolonged discharge to noxious pinch, and with electrical stimulation a response to Aβ-, Aδ-, and C-fiber components (Menetrey et al., 1977; Schouenborg and Sjolund, 1983). Class 2 neurons have projections to supraspinal sites via the spinocervical and spinothalamic tracts (Mendell, 1966; Hongo et al., 1968). Convergent neurons are located in the marginal zone (lamina I) as well as in a wide area throughout the middle of the dorsal horn. The substantia contains intrinsic cells, many of which are inhibitory (Woolf and Fitzgerald 1981).

The evoked responses of spinal neurons to transcutaneous electrical stimulation can be separated based on threshold and latency. The Aβ-fiber-evoked responses have a short latency, because their axons are myelinated and have a rapid conduction velocity, between 30 and 100 m/s, and so appear early after peripheral stimulation. The Aβ-fiber-evoked responses are the first to be evoked with electrical stimulation of low intensity; as the intensity is increased the response to Aδ-fiber-evoked responses now is apparent at a later latency band. The C-fiber-evoked responses appear in response to high-threshold stimulation and have the slowest conduction velocity because their axons are unmyelinated. These evoked responses appear after the Aδ-fiber responses in the latest latency bands. The responses recorded have latencies in the same range as that shown by direct sural nerve activation to be attributed to C-fibers and give comparable latencies of the "late component" of transcutaneous electrical stimulation (Mendell, 1966; Menetrey et al., 1977; Schouenborg and Sjolund, 1983).

Repetitive stimulation results in the appearance of post-discharges at a latency beyond that produced by C-fibers and an increase in the entire neuronal response. This is indicative of "wind-up," first observed and termed by Mendell (1966). Single unit recordings of spinocervical tract neurons in the anesthetized cat showed enhanced activity to a volley of unmyelinated fiber stimulation occurring after the C-fiber-evoked activity (Mendell, 1966). Wind-up is driven by the activity of centrally located cells, for there was no change in the size of the C-fiber volley with a repetitive stimulus, even though the central effects increased (Mendell, 1966). This increase in activity has subsequently been shown to be due to the activation of the *N*-methyl-D-aspartate (NMDA) receptor, which results in increased excitation (Davies and Lodge, 1987; Dickenson and Sullivan, 1987). The enhanced response to a constant stimulus reaches a plateau toward the end of the train of stimuli.

Pharmacology of the Spinal Cord

The stimulation of afferents causes the excitation of intrinsic dorsal horn cells. Neurotransmitters released from afferents have been characterized by their ability to produce excitatory postsynaptic potentials (EPSPs) in second-order neurons. These EPSPs may be fast and of a short duration or slow and longer lasting. The fast EPSPs result from the effects of the amino acid glutamate (Jessell et al., 1986) and the slow EPSPs from peptides (Murase et al., 1989).

Glutamate is the main neurotransmitter in the central nervous system (Watkins and Evans, 1981) including the primary afferents in the dorsal horn of the spinal cord, regardless of whether they are small or large diameter. The excitatory effects of amino acids were first demonstrated in the dorsal horn of the cat (Curtis et al., 1959). Once released, glutamate has an excitatory effect on the postsynaptic cell, causing a depolarization via three distinct receptor subclasses, the ionotrophic α-amino-3-hydroxy 5-methyl-4-isoxazolepropionic acid (AMPA) and NMDA receptors and the G-protein-linked metabotropic group of receptors (see Chapter 8).

Amino acids are released in response to acute and more sustained noxious inputs (Skilling et al., 1988; Kangrga and Randic, 1991). AMPA-receptor activation is responsible for components of acute and tonic noxious inputs, as well as tactile transmission (Jessell et al., 1986). However, during repetitive high-frequency stimulation of noxious inputs there is an enhanced response of convergent neurons, or wind-up, as discussed (Mendell, 1966). This enhanced activity has been attributed to the recruitment and activation of another class of excitatory amino acid receptors, the NMDA receptors (Davies and Lodge, 1987; Dickenson and Sullivan, 1987), and underlies hyperalgesia in more persistent pain states including inflammation and neuropathic conditions (see Yaksh, 1989; Ren et al., 1992; Dickenson, 1994a).

During circumstances of acute noxious inputs (low-frequency) activation of the NMDA receptor is not possible, because under normal physiological conditions the ion channel of this receptor is blocked by Mg^{2+} (Mayer et al., 1984). The NMDA-receptor channel is ligand gated but it is unique in that the Mg^{2+} plug also means that it requires concurrent membrane depolarization to become activated. There is an upregulation of peptide production and an increase in spinal peptide release, predominantly substance P and CGRP during inflammation (Noguchi et al., 1988). This peptide release is responsible for the slow EPSPs in postsynaptic neurons (Randic and Miletic, 1977; Urban and Randic, 1984; Murase et al., 1989) and has been shown to enhance the responses of excitatory amino acids (Murase et al., 1989; Randic et al., 1990). Increased dorsal horn excitability is blocked by NMDA receptors that have no effect on underlying basal transmission (Dickenson and Sullivan, 1987; Haley et al., 1990; Yamamoto and Yaksh, 1992). The slow EPSPs caused by peptides allows these enhanced responses, because as the membrane potential moves away from a hyperpolarized state to a more positive transmembrane potential, the affinity of Mg^{2+} for the ion channel of the NMDA receptor is reduced and the Mg^{2+} block is removed (MacDonald and Nowak, 1990).

There are a number of peptides located in dense core vesicles in the primary afferent terminals (Hokfelt, 1991) which include the tachykinins (substance P, neurokinin A and B, acting on neurokinin 1, 2, and 3 receptors respectively), CGRP, bombesin, somatostatin, and VIP. Substance P is released in response to noxious stimulation (Kuraishi et al., 1985; Duggan et al., 1987; Go and Yaksh, 1987). The effect of substance P is to provide a longer lasting depolarization by inactivating K^+ currents (Nowak and MacDonald, 1982) or by increasing Na^+ or Ca^{2+} currents (Murase et al., 1989). Neurokinin 1-receptor antagonists have been shown to block the initiation of wind-up and enhanced spinal responses (DeKoninck and Henry 1989; Yamamoto and Yaksh, 1991). There are high basal levels of neurokinin A throughout the dorsal horn in the absence of stimulation (Duggan et al., 1990). However, neurokinin A is also released in response to noxious stimulation (Duggan et al., 1990) and neurokinin-2 receptor antagonists have been shown to attenuate the effects of noxious inputs (Fleetwood-Walker et al., 1990). Neurokinin A has been shown to spread more diffusely after release (volume transmission), even being present in the white matter (Duggan et al., 1990). Neurokinin B is practically absent from dorsal roots and appears to be derived from intrinsic cells (Ogawa et al., 1985). CGRP immunoreactivity in the dorsal horn is reduced by dorsal rhizotomies (Gibson et al., 1984) whereas in monoarthritic animals, CGRP increases in the DRG (Smith et al., 1992). CGRP can interact with substance P by attenuating the breakdown of substance P, thereby enhancing its effects (Wiesenfeld-Hallin et al., 1984). CGRP causes a slow depolarization of postsynaptic cells, which may also contribute to the enhanced responses of these cells to further stimulation (Ryu et al., 1988).

Opioids, especially those acting at μ and δ receptors, are capable of producing antinociception (see Yaksh, 1993; Dickenson, 1994b) and have little if any effect on non-noxious inputs (Duggan and North, 1984; Dickenson and Sullivan, 1986). The μ receptors are predominantly located in the substantia gelatinosa, especially on primary afferent terminals with a smaller portion on interneurons (see LaMotte et al., 1976; Yaksh, 1993). Spinal application of opioid-receptor agonists produces a decrease in substance P and glutamate release from primary afferent terminals (see Dickenson, 1994b). Peripheral nerve damage results in a decrease in opioid receptors (LaMotte et al., 1976); any loss of receptors may be partly responsible for the reduced opioid sensitivity of neuropathic states.

Glycine and γ-aminobutyric acid (GABA) are found in intrinsic cells in the spinal cord and have an important role in the control of sensory inputs (Game and Lodge, 1975). GABA has been shown to be located in the superficial laminae of the spinal cord, especially in the islet cells in lamina II_0 together with glycine (Todd et al., 1996). The GABAergic neurons make axo-axonic as well as axo-dendritic connections (Baba et al., 1994), implying that GABA can control both primary afferent terminals and intrinsic neurons. The receptors ($GABA_A$, $GABA_B$, and glycine) for these inhibitory agents are known to be on primary afferent terminals and interneurons (Bowery et al., 1987).

Spinal application of both GABA and glycine receptor antagonists produce both cardiovascular changes and behaviors indicative of noxious stimulation in response to low-threshold stimulation (allodynia) (Roberts et al., 1986; Yaksh, 1989; Sherman and Loomis, 1994). Electrophysiological experiments have also demonstrated that there are changes in the patterns of neuronal firing, such as increased responses in the presence of antagonists of these receptors (Game and Lodge, 1975; Duggan et al., 1981; Sivilotti and Woolf, 1994). Damage to small, possibly GABAergic, interneurons has been described after peripheral nerve damage; this loss of central inhibition could be a factor in central hypersensitivity and miscoding of afferent impulses leading to aberrent pain signals (Sugimoto et al., 1990).

CONCLUSIONS

It is difficult to define the relative importance of changes in peripheral versus central neurophysiological mechanisms that occur in persistent inflammatory or neuropathic pain, for changes in both pain states occur at both sites. In inflammation, the major peripheral change induced is nociceptor sensitization, whereas in neuropathic pain, ectopic activity and other changes occur in the nerve fibers thenselves and dorsal root ganglion. The final result of enhanced transmission in the spinal cord appears to involve less disparate final mechanisms. The plasticity that occurs at many levels in different pain states may allow selective therapy to be produced for specific pain syndromes.

REFERENCES

Adriaensen H, Gybels J, Handwerker HO, Van Hees J (1980): Latencies of chemically evoked discharges in human cutaneous nociceptors and of the concurrent subjective sensations. Neurosci Lett 20:55–60.

Appleton I (1997): Non-steroidal anti-inflammatory drugs and pain. In Dickenson AH, Besson JM (eds): *The Pharmacology of Pain*, Vol. 130 of *Handbook of Experimental Pharmacology*. Springer-Verlag, Berlin, pp. 43–60.

Baba H, Yoshimura M, Nishi S, Shimoji K (1994): Synaptic responses of substantia gelatinosa neurones to dorsal column stimulation in rat spinal cord in vitro. J Physiol 478:87–99.

Beck PW, Handwerker HO, Zimmermann M (1974): Nervous outflow from the cat's foot during noxious radiant heat stimulation. Brain Res 67:373–386.

Bennett GJ, Abdelmoumene M, Hayashi H (1980): Physiology and morphology of substantia gelatinosa neurons intracellularly stained with horseradish peroxidase. J Comp Neurol 194:809–827.

Bessou P, Perl ER (1969): Response of cutaneous sensory units with unmyelinated fibres to noxious stimuli. J Neurophys 32:1025–1043.

Bevan S, Yeats J (1991): Protons activate a cation conductance in a sub-population of rat dorsal root ganglion neurones. J Physiol 433:145–161.

Bowery NG, Hudson AL, Price GW (1987): GABA$_A$ and GABA$_B$ receptor site distribution in the rat central nervous system. Neuroscience 20:365–383.

Burgess PR, Perl ER (1967): Myelinated afferent fibres responding specifically to noxious stimulation of the skin. J Physiol 190:541–562.

Burnstock G, Wood J (1996): Purinergic receptors: their role in nociception and primary afferent transmission. Curr Opinion Neurobiol 6:526–532.

Campbell JN, Meyer RA, LaMotte RH (1979): Sensitization of myelinated nociceptive afferents that innervate monkey hand. J Neurophys 42:1669–1679.

Cervero F (1991) Mechanisms of acute visceral pain. In Wells JCD, Woolf CJ (eds): *British Medical Bulletin*, Vol. 47. Edinburgh: Churchill Livingstone, pp. 549–560.

Cervero F, Iggo A (1980): The substantia gelatinosa of the spinal cord. Brain 103: 717–772.

Clark FJ, Burgess PR (1975): Slowly adapting receptors in cat knee joint: can they signal joint angle? J Neurophys 38:1448–1463.

Coggeshall RE, Hong KAP, Langford LA, Schaible H-G, Schmidt RF (1983): Discharge characteristics of fine medial articular afferents at rest and during passive movements of inflamed knee joints. Brain Res 272:185–188.

Croze S, Duclaux R, Kenshalo DR (1976): The thermal sensitivity of the polymodal nociceptors in the monkey. J Physiol 263:539–562.

Curtis DR, Phillis JW, Watkins JC (1959): Chemical excitation of spinal neurones. Nature 183:611–612.

Davies SN, Lodge D (1987): Evidence for involvement of N-methyl-D-aspartate receptors in "wind-up" of class 2 neurones in the dorsal horn of the rat. Brain Res 424: 402–406.

De Koninck Y, Henry JL (1989): Bombesin, neuromedin B and neuromedin C selectively depress superficial dorsal horn neurones in the cat spinal cord. Brain Res 498: 105–117.

Devor M (1996): Pain mechanisms and pain syndromes. In Campbell JN (ed): *Pain 1996—An Updated Review*. Seattle: IASP Press, pp. 103–112.

Dickenson AH (1994a): NMDA receptor antagonists as analgesics. In Fields HL, Liebeskind JC (eds): *Pharmacological Approaches to the Treatment of Chronic Pain: New Cconcepts and Critical Issues. Progress in Pain Research and Management*, Vol. 1. Seattle: IASP Press, pp. 173–187.

Dickenson AH (1994b), Where And How Do Opioids Act? In Gebhart GF, Hammond DL, Jenson TS (eds): *Proceedings of the 7th World Congress on Pain. Progress in Pain Research and Management*, Vol. 2. Seattle: IASP Press, pp. 525–552.

Dickenson AH (1997): Mechanisms of central hypersensitivity: excitatory amino-acids mechanisms and their control. In Dickenson AH, Besson JM (eds): *The Pharmacology of Pain*, Vol. 130 of *Handbook of Experimental Pharmacology*, Springer-Verlag, Berlin, pp. 167–210.

Dickenson AH, Sullivan AF (1986): Electrophysiological studies on the effects of intrathecal morphine on nociceptive neurones in the rat dorsal horn. Pain 24:211–222.

Dickenson AH, Sullivan AF (1987): Evidence for a role of the NMDA receptor in the frequency dependent potentiation of deep rat dorsal horn nociceptive neurones following C fibre stimulation. Neuropharmacol 26:1235–1238.

Dray A (1997): Peripheral mediators of pain. In Dickenson AH, Besson JM (eds): *The Pharmacology of Pain*, Vol 130 of *Handbook of Experimental Pharmacology*, Springer-Verlag, Berlin, pp. 21–42.

Duggan AW, North RA (1984): Electrophysiology of opiods. Pharmacol Rev 35:219–281.

Duggan AW, Griersmith BT, Johnson SM (1981): Supraspinal inhibition of the excitation of dorsal horn neurones by impulses in unmyelinated primary afferents: lack of effects by strychnine and bicuculline. Brain Res 210:231–241.

Duggan AW, Morton CR, Zhao ZQ, Hendry IA (1987): Noxious heating of the skin releases immunoreactive substance P in the substantia gelatinosa of the cat: a study with antibody microprobes. Brain Res 403:345–349.

Duggan AW, Hope PJ, Jarrott B, Schaible H-G, Fleetwood-Walker SM (1990): Release, spread and persistence of immunoreactive Neurokinin A in the dorsal horn of the cat following noxious cutaneous stimulation. Studies with antibody microprobes. Neuroscience 35:195–202.

Fitzgerald M, Lynn B (1977): The sensitization of high threshold mechanoreceptors with myelinated axons by repeated heating. J Physiol 365:549–563.

Fitzgerald M, Wall PD (1980): The laminar organization of dorsal horn cells responding to peripheral C fibre stimulation. Exp Brain Res 41:36–44.

Fleetwood-Walker SM, Mitchell R, Hope PJ, El-Yassir N, Molony V, Blandon CM (1990): The involvement of neurokinin receptor subtypes in somatosensory processing in the superficial dorsal horn of the cat. Brain Res 519:169–182.

Flower RJ, Vane JR (1974): Inhibition of prostaglandin biosynthesis. Biochem Pharmacol 23:1439–1450.

Game CJA, Lodge D (1975): The pharmacology of the inhibition of dorsal horn neurones by impulses in myelinated cutaneous afferents in the cat. Exp Brain Res 23:75–84.

Gebhart GF (1995) Somatovisceral Sensation. In Conn PM (ed): *Neuroscience in Medicine*. Philadelphia: J B Lippincott Company, pp. 433–450.

Georgopoulos AP (1976): Functional properties of primary afferent units probably related to pain mechanisms in primate glabrous skin. J Neurophys 39:71–83.

Gibson SJ, Polak JM, Bloom SR, Sabate IM, Mulderry PM, Ghatei MA, McGregor GP, Morrison JFB, Kelly JS, Evans RM, Rosenfeld MG (1984): Calcitonin gene-related peptide immunoreactivity in the spinal cord of man and of eight other species. J Neurosci 4:3101–3111.

Go VLW, Yaksh TL (1987): Release of substance P from the cat spinal cord. J Physiol 391:141–167.

Haley JE, Sullivan AF, Dickenson AH (1990): Evidence for spinal N-methyl-D-aspartate receptor involvement in prolonged chemical nociception in the rat. Brain Res 518:218–226.

Hall JM (1992): Bradykinin receptors: pharmacological properties and biological roles. Pharmacol Ther 56:131–190.

Handwerker HO, Anton F, Reeh PW (1987): Discharge patterns of afferent cutaneous nerve fibers from the rat's tail during prolonged noxious mechanical stimulation. Exp Brain Res 65:493–504.

Hokfelt T (1991): Neuropeptides in perspective: the last ten years. Neuron 7:867–879.

Hokfelt T, Zhang X, Wiesenfeld-Hallin Z (1994): Messenger plasticity in primary sensory neurones following axotomy and its functional implications. Trends Neurosci 17:22–30.

Hongo T, Jankowska E, Lundberg A (1968): Post-synaptic excitation and inhibition from primary afferents in neurones of the spinocervical tract. J Physiol 199:569–592.

Jessell TM, Yoshioka K, Jahr CE (1986): Amino acid receptor-mediated transmission at primary afferent synapses in rat spinal cord. J Exp Biol 124:239–258.

Kangrga I, Randic M (1991): Outflow of endogenous aspartate and glutamate from the rat spinal dorsal horn in vitro by activation of low- and high-threshold primary afferent fibres. Modulation by μ-opioids. Brain Res 553:347–352.

Krishtal OA, Marchenko SM, Pidoplichko VI (1983): Receptors for ATP in the membrane of mammalian sensory neurones. Neurosci Lett 35:41–45.

Krishtal OA, Pidoplichko VI (1980): A receptor for protons in the nerve cell membrane. Neuroscience 5:2325–2327.

Kruger L, Perl ER, Sedivec MJ. (1981): Fine structure of myelinated mechanical nociceptor endings in cat hairy skin. J Comparative Neurology 198:137–154.

Kuraishi Y, Hirota N, Sato Y, Hino Y, Satoh M, Takagi H (1985): Evidence that substance P and somatostatin transmit separate information related to pain in the spinal dorsal horn. Brain Res 325:294–298.

LaMotte C, Pert CB, Snyder SH (1976): Opiate receptor binding in primate spinal cord: distribution and changes after dorsal root section. Brain Res 112:407–412.

Lang E, Novak PW, Reeh PW, Handwerker HO (1990): Chemosensitivity of fine afferents from rat skin in vitro. J Neurophys 63:887–901.

Light AR, Metz CB (1978): The morphology of the spinal cord efferent and afferent neurons contributing to the ventral roots of the cat. J Comp Neurol 179:501–516.

Light AR, Perl ER (1979): Spinal termination of functionally identified primary afferent neurons with slowly conducting myelinated fibres. J Comp Neurol 186:133–150.

Lundberg JM, Hokfelt T (1986): Multiple co-existence of peptides and classical transmitters in peripheral autonomic and sensory neurons—functional and pharmacological implications. Prog Brain Res 68:241–287.

Lynn B, Carpenter SE (1992): Primary afferent units from the hairy skin of the rat hind limb. Brain Res 238:29–43.

Lynn B, Shakhanbeh J (1988): Properties of Aδ high threshold mechanoreceptors in the rat hairy and glabrous skin and their response to heat. Neurosci Lett 85:71–76.

MacDonald JF, Nowak LM (1990): Mechanisms of blockade of excitatory amino acid receptor channels. Trends Pharmacol Sci 11:167–172.

Mayer ML, Westbrook GL, Guthrie PB (1984): Voltage-dependent block by Mg^{2+} of NMDA responses in spinal cord neurones. Nature 309:261–263.

Meller ST, Gebhart GF (1992): A critical review of the afferent pathways and the potential chemical mediators involved in cardiac pain. Neuroscience 48:501–524.

Melzack R, Wall PD (1965): Pain mechanism, a new theory. Science 150:971–979.

Mendell LM (1966): Physiological properties of unmyelinated fiber projection to the spinal cord. Exp Neurol 16:316–332.

Menetrey D, Giesler GJ Jr, Besson JM (1977): An analysis of response properties of spinal cord dorsal horn neurones to nonnoxious and noxious stimuli in the spinal rat. Exp Brain Res 27:15–33.

Meyer RA, Campbell JN, Raja SN (1994): Peripheral neural mechanisms of nociception. In Wall PD, Melzack R (eds): *Textbook of Pain*. Edinburgh: Churchill Livingstone, pp. 13–44.

Molander C, Xu Q, Grant G (1984): The cytoarchitectonic organization of the spinal cord in the rat. I. The lower thoracic and lumbosacral cord. J Comp Neurol 230: 133–141.

Moskowitz M (1994): Drug mechanisms in acute migraine. In Gebhart GF, Hammond DL, Jenson TS (eds): *Proceedings of the 7th World Congress on Pain. Progress in Pain Research and Management*, Vol. 2. Seattle: IASP Press, pp. 755–764.

Murase K, Ryu PD, Randic M (1989): Tachykinins modulate multiple ionic conductances in voltage-clamped rat spinal dorsal horn neurons. J Neurophys 61:854–865.

Neumann S, Doubell TP, Leslie T, Woolf CJ (1996): Inflammatory pain hypersensitivity mediated by phenotypic switch in myelinated primary sensory neurons. Nature 384: 360–364.

Noguchi K, Morita Y, Kiyama H, Ono K, Tohyama M (1988): A noxious stimulus induces the preprotachykinin-a gene expression in the dorsal root ganglion: a quantitative study using in situ hybridization histochemistry. Mol Brain Res 4:31–35.

Nowak LM, MacDonald RL (1982): Substance P: Ionic basis for depolarizing responses of mouse spinal cord neurons in cell culture. J Neurosci 2:1119–1128.

Ogawa T, Kanazawa I, Kimura S (1985): Regional distribution of substance P, neurokinin A and neurokinin B in rat spinal cord, nerve roots and dorsal root ganglia, and the effects of dorsal root section or spinal transection. Brain Res 359:152–157.

Perkins MN, Campbell E, Dray A (1993): Antinociceptive activity of the bradykinin B1 and B2 receptor antagonists, desArg^9, [Leu8]-BK and HOE 140, in two models of persistent hyperalgesia in the rat. Pain 53:191–197.

Randic M, Hecimovic H, Ryu PD (1990): Substance P modulates glutamate-induced currents in acutely isolated rat spinal dorsal horn neurones. Neurosci Lett 117:74–80.

Randic M, Miletic V (1977): Effect of substance P in cat dorsal horn neurones activated by noxious stimuli. Brain Res 128:164–169.

Rang HP, Bevan S, Dray A (1991): Chemical activation of nociceptive peripheral neurones. In Wells JCD, Woolf CJ (eds): *British Medical Bulletin*, Vol. 47. Edinburgh: Churchill Livingstone, pp. 534–548.

Reeh PW, Bayer J, Kocher L, Handwerker HO (1987): Sensitization of nociceptive cutaneous nerve fibers from the rat's tail by noxious mechanical stimulation. Exp Brain Res 65:505–512.

Ren K, Hylden JLK, Williams GM, Ruda MA, Dubner R (1992): The effects of a noncompetitive NMDA receptor antagonist, MK-801, on behavioral hyperalgesia and dorsal horn neuronal activity in rats with unilateral inflammation. Pain 50:331–344.

Rexed B (1952): The cytoarchitectonic organization of the spinal cord in the cat. J Comp Neurol 96:415–466.

Roberts LA, Beyer C, Komisaruk BR (1986): Nociceptive responses to altered GABAergic activity at the spinal cord. Life Sci 39:1667–1674.

Ryu PD, Gerber G, Murase K, Randic M (1988): Actions of calcitonin gene-related peptide on rat spinal dorsal horn neurons. Brain Res 441:357–361.

Sawynok J, Zarrindast M-R, Reid, AR, Doak GJ (1997) Adenosine A_3 receptor activation produces nociceptive behaviour and edema by release of histamine and 5-hydroxytryptamine. Eur J Pharm 333:1–7.

Schaible H-G, Schmidt RF (1983): Activation of groups III and IV sensory units in medial articular nerve by local mechanical stimulation of knee joint. J Neurophysiol 49:35–44.

Schouenborg J, Sjolund BH (1983): Activity evoked by A- and C-afferent fibres in rat dorsal horn neurones and its relation to a flexion reflex. J Neurophysiol 50: 1108–1121.

Sherman SE, Loomis CW (1994): Morphine insensitive allodynia is produced by intrathecal strychnine in the lightly anesthetized rat. Pain 56:17–29.

Simone DA, Alreja M, LaMotte RH (1991): Psychophysical studies of the itch sensation and itchy skin ("Allokinesis") produced by intracutaneous injection of histamine. Somato Motor Res 8:271–279.

Sivilotti L, Woolf CJ (1994): The contribution of $GABA_A$ and glycine receptors to central sensitization: disinhibition and touch-evoked allodynia in the spinal cord. J Neurophysiol 72:169–179.

Skilling SR, Smullin DH, Beitz AJ, Larson AA (1988): Extracellular amino acid concentrations in the dorsal spinal cord of freely moving rats following veratridine and nociceptive stimulation. J Neurochem 51:127–132.

Smith GD, Harmar AJ, McQueen DS, Seckl JR (1992): Increase in substance P and CGRP, but not somatostatin content of innervating dorsal root ganglia in adjuvant monoarthritis in the rat. Neurosci Lett 137:257–260.

Steen KH, Reeh PW, Anton F, Handwerker HO (1992): Protons selectively induce lasting excitation and sensitization to mechanical stimulation of nociceptors in rat skin, in vitro. J Neurosci 12:86–95.

Stein C (1993): Peripheral mechanisms of opioid analgesia. In Herz A (ed): *Opioids II. Handbook Exp Pharmacol*, Vol. 104. Springer-Verlag, Berlin, pp. 91–103.

Steranka LR, Manning DC, DeHaas CJ, Ferkany JW, Borosky SA, Connor JR, Vavrek RJ, Stewart JM, Snyder SH (1988): Bradykinin as a pain mediator: Receptors are localized to sensory neurons, and antagonists have analgesic actions. Proc Natl Acad Sci USA 85:3245–3249.

Sugimoto T, Bennett GJ, Kajander KC (1990): Transsynaptic degeneration in the superficial dorsal horn after sciatic nerve injury: effects of chronic constriction injury, transection, and strychnine. Pain 42:205–213.

Todd AJ, Watt C, Spike RC, Sieghart W (1996): Colocalization of GABA, glycine, and their receptors at synapses in the rat spinal cord. J Neurosci 16:974–982.

Torebjork HE, Hallin RG (1974): Identification of afferent C units in intact human skin nerves. Brain Res 67:387–403.

Urban L, Randic M (1984): Slow excitatory transmission in rat dorsal horn: possible mediation by peptides. Brain Res 290:336–341.

Van Hees J, Gybels JM (1972): Pain related to single afferent C fibres from human skin. Brain Res 48:397–400.

Wall PD (1967): The laminar organization of dorsal horn and effects of descending impulses. J Physiol 188:403–423.

Watkins JC, Evans RH (1981): Excitatory amino acid transmitters. Ann Rev Pharmacol Tox 21:165–204.

Wiesenfeld-Hallin Z, Hokfelt T, Lundberg JM, Forssmann WG, Reinecke M, Tschopp FA, Fischer JA (1984): Immunoreactive calcitonin gene-related peptide and substance P coexist in sensory neurons to the spinal cord and interact in spinal behavioral responses of the rat. Neurosci Lett 52:199–204.

Willis WD, Coggeshall RE (1991): *Sensory Mechanisms of the Spinal Cord*. New York: Plenum Press, pp. 79–151.

Woolf CJ (1991): Generation of acute pain: central mechanisms. In Wells JCD, Woolf C (eds): *British Medical Bulletin*, Vol. 47. Churchill Livingstone, pp. 523–533.

Woolf CJ, Fitzgerald M (1981): Lamina-specific alteration of C-fibre evoked activity by morphine in the dorsal horn of the rat spinal cord. Neurosci Lett 25:37–41.

Yaksh TL (1989): Behavioral and autonomic correlates of the tactile evoked allodynia produced by spinal glycine inhibition: effects of modulatory receptor systems and excitatory amino acid antagonists. Pain 37:111–123.

Yaksh TL (1993): The spinal actions of opioids. In Herz A (ed): *Opioids II. Handbook Exp Pharmacol*, Vol. 104. Springer-Verlag, pp. 53–90.

Yamamoto T, Yaksh TL (1991): Stereospecific effects of a nonpeptidic NK1 selective antagonist, CP-96, 345: Antinociception in the absence of motor dysfunction. Life Sci 49:1955–1963.

Yamamoto T, Yaksh TL (1992): Comparison of the antinociceptive effects of pre- and post treatment with intrathecal morphine and MK801, an NMDA antagonist, on the formalin test in the rat. Anesthesiol 77:757–763.

CHAPTER 2

ANIMAL MODELS OF PAIN

ALAN COWAN
Temple University School of Medicine
Philadelphia, Pennsylvania

What type of test is most commonly used in preclinical pharmacological research? Procedures involving the measurement of nociception and its suppression are likely contenders, given the regular appearance of pain-related reports in the scientific literature. Overtly simple tests from the 1940s (e.g., hot plate, tail flick) that established the antinociceptive potencies of early opioids are still in use today. The chemical nature of new analgesics has certainly changed over the years, yet the hot plate test links the assessment of meperidine by Woolfe and Macdonald in 1944 with the evaluation of, say, the delta agonist [D-Pen^2, D-Pen^5]enkephalin by Sora and colleagues in 1997. Another example: the tail flick procedure is the enduring constant, linking definitive assays of morphine and codeine in white mice (Wirth, 1952) with current comparisons of morphine and methadone in CXBK counterparts that are naturally insensitive to systemic morphine (Chang et al., 1998). Indeed, both methods (along with the phenylquinone writhing assay) continue to provide initial antinociceptive data on the assorted compounds submitted to the College on Problems of Drug Dependence for evaluation as potentially "nonaddicting" analgesics (e.g., Aceto et al., 1998).

It might be expected that after five decades of experience with these well-established tests, few practical problems would remain. This is not the case. Debate over what aspect of animal behavior represents the most appropriate nocifensive response and how the response should be quantified bedevils the whole field of analgesiometry. For example, rats can respond in a number of ways to the heat stimulus provided by the hot plate. Licking of either the forepaws or hindpaws, lifting paws off the hot surface, jumping, and squeaking represent possible end points. Some researchers record latency to the first appearance of *any* of these signs (e.g., Plone et al., 1996). Others question the equivalence of the behaviors and recommend the more exacting end points of latency to hindpaw lick or vertical jump (Hammond, 1989; Carter, 1991).

Novel Aspects of Pain Management: Opioids and Beyond, Edited by Jana Sawynok and Alan Cowan
ISBN 0-471-180173 Copyright © 1999 by Wiley-Liss, Inc.

Another ongoing debate is concerned with the relevance of drug-induced changes in tail skin temperature in interpreting data from tail flick tests (Hole and Tjølsen, 1993; Lichtman et al., 1993; Roane et al., 1998). Even an issue as basic as selecting the arbitrary cutoff time in thermal assays, first suggested by Harris and Pierson in 1964 and adopted by countless researchers since then, has been recently questioned by Carmody (1995). Thus the common practice of calculating the "maximum possible effect" (MPE) according to the following formula for each dose of test agent varies with the particular cutoff time chosen and is therefore deemed (correctly) to be "a deeply flawed concept":

$$\%\text{MPE} = \frac{(\text{Test latency} - \text{Control latency})}{(\text{Cutoff latency} - \text{Control latency})} \times 100$$

NATURE OF THE NOCICEPTIVE STIMULUS

The intensity and modality of the noxious stimulus are two experimental variables that have been investigated extensively by analgesic researchers. It is noteworthy that Woolfe and Macdonald (1944), in their pioneering study with the hot plate, examined the activity of test compounds in mice with the zinc plate set at four different temperatures (55°–70°C). More recently, findings from the following groups are of particular importance in the search for alternative analgesics to morphine, for example, agonists at kappa opioid receptors (Rajagopalan et al., 1992).

Shaw and colleagues (Delaney et al., 1986; Shaw et al., 1988) documented the subcutaneous potencies of standard opioids in several pain models and concluded that the mouse abdominal constriction test (0.4% acetic acid) was most sensitive to the opioids, and the mouse (55°C) hot plate test was least sensitive; rat tail flick and rat paw pressure tests were comparable and of intermediate rank. One conclusion to emerge from this work is well-recognized and can be restated here: the stimulus associated with the traditional mouse hot plate test is too high for satisfactory evaluation of many moderate-efficacy kappa agonists (e.g., enadoline, Hunter et al., 1990).

Parsons and Headley (1989) conducted electrophysiological studies with opioids in spinalized, anesthetized rats and demonstrated the importance of intensity of the noxious stimulus, rather than the particular modality used. These workers monitored mu- and kappa-induced suppression of firing by spinal motoneurons elicited by *matched* intensity thermal or pressure stimuli. Under these special circumstances, intravenous kappa agonists had similar effects to fentanyl (a standard mu agonist) against heat and pressure. The key concept of matching the intensity of noxious stimuli in analgesic testing was developed by Millan (1989), who examined mu and kappa agonists in rat tail flick and tail pressure procedures. Subcutaneously administered kappa agonists were equipotent with morphine and fentanyl against moderate, matched-intensity heat and pressure stimuli. Stimuli termed "moderate" were matched in the sense that a particular rat responded to both heat and pressure within 3.5–4.4 sec. Interestingly, the kappa agonists (U-50488 and tifluadom) differed from morphine and fentanyl by failing to suppress rat squeaking when electrical stimulation (a stimulus of high intensity) was applied to the animal's tail. Note, however, that subcutaneous administration of U-50488 and tifluadom *are* antinociceptive against this particular noxious stimulus under different experimental conditions, for example, when the rat's tooth pulp is stimulated electrically and the jaw opening response is monitored (Steinfels and Cook, 1986).

It is now clearly established that lowering the intensity of the noxious stimulus can uncover antinociceptive activity for a variety of compounds in, for example, hot plate (Ankier, 1974; O'Callaghan and Holtzman, 1975; Zimet et al., 1986) and tail flick/dip tests (Gray et al., 1970; Granat and Saelens, 1973; Luttinger, 1985; but see Seguin et al., 1995). The experimental strategy of lowering the temperature of the nociceptive stimulus has been taken to the extreme by Pizziketti et al. (1985), who described a cold water adaptation of the rat tail dip test. A 1:1 solution of ethylene glycol and water cooled to $-10°C$ (in a cold water circulating bath) served as the noxious stimulus. [D-Pen^2, D-Pen^5]enkephalin (DPDPE), when given intracerebroventricularly to rats, was active in this procedure but gave an unimpressive dose–response curve in the (50°C) hot water version of the test (Adams et al., 1993). This differential finding may represent a notable characteristic of delta agonists and should be studied further with additional compounds of this class. This comment also applies to dynorphin A, an endogenous kappa agonist that displays the same contrasting effect as DPDPE in the two tests (Tiseo et al., 1988).

The above introduction provides a general background to the field of nociception and antinociceptive agents. In the remainder of the chapter, recent information is summarized on those animal tests that are currently used to evaluate new analgesics.

ACUTE PAIN

Tests involving acute nociceptive noxious stimulation have been reviewed extensively in the preclinical pharmacological literature. The four key references on acute tests, listed in Table 2.1, can be strongly recommended to both seasoned investigators and newcomers to the field of algesiometry. Thus Taber (1974) presents the strengths and limitations of standard methods involving chemical, thermal, mechanical, and electrical stimuli. Such fundamental aspects of analgesic testing as stimulus intensity (discussed above), route of administration, and choice of data analysis are discussed with reference to the drugs of the time, including morphine, pentazocine, and aspirin. These issues are developed at both practical and scholarly levels by Franklin and Abbott (1989), Hammond (1989), and Dubner (1994), and it is clear that, however "old fashioned" the acute tests may seem nowadays, their appropriate use has been

TABLE 2.1 Preclinical Pain Tests Used in Screening for New Analgesics

Pain Model	Test	Key References
Acute	Hot plate, tail flick, paw pressure, tooth pulp, writhing	Taber (1974), Franklin and Abbott (1989), Hammond (1989), Dubner (1994)
Persistent	Formalin	Tjølsen et al. (1992), Porro and Cavazzuti (1993), Aloisi and Carli (1996)
Chronic	Adjuvant-induced arthritis	Colpaert (1987), Besson and Guilbaud (1988)
Incisional	Paw incision test	Brennan et al. (1996)
Visceral	Colorectal distension	Ness and Gebhart (1988), Gebhart and Sengupta (1995)
Neuropathic	Chronic constriction injury Partial nerve ligation Spinal nerve ligation Streptozotocin diabetes	Bennett and Xie (1988) Seltzer et al. (1990) Kim and Chung (1992) Courteix et al. (1993)

responsible for the initial selection and subsequent therapeutic exploitation of today's analgesics (Table 2.2). Of course, the pessimistic view would be that these procedures (although still helpful in the study of pain processes per se) have served their purpose in providing clinically useful drugs, but new approaches are now necessary to discover novel analgesics with different mechanisms of action. As indicated below, the unveiling of new animal models of, for example, neuropathic pain (not mentioned in reviews of the 1980s), along with the discovery of compounds that are active in such models, have maintained the brisk pace of research into analgesics throughout the 1990s.

Methodological Updates

The rhesus monkey warm water (50–55°C) tail withdrawal test was originally introduced by Dykstra and Woods (1986) to allow direct comparison of analgesic-induced effects on nociception, respiration, urine flow, self-administration, drug discrimination, and physical dependence in the same species. Good antinociceptive efficacy has been demonstrated recently for mu (alfentanil) and kappa (enadoline) agonists when the water was maintained at 55°C (France et al., 1994); dynorphin A-(1-13) (Butelman et al., 1995a), butorphanol (Butelman et al., 1995b), and SNC 80, the nonpeptidic delta agonist (Negus et al., 1998), were much less efficacious.

TABLE 2.2 Antinociceptive Tests Reported in Primary Papers on (Representative) Marketed Analgesics

Analgesic	Class	Test/Activity	Reference
Butorphanol	Opioid agonist–antagonist	Hot plate (+) Skin twitch (−) Tail flick (±) Writhing (+)	Pircio et al. (1976)
Buprenorphine	Mu opioid partial agonist	Tail flick (±) Tail pressure (+) Writhing (+)	Cowan et al. (1977)
Nalbuphine	Opioid agonist–antagonist	Hot plate (−) Writhing (+)	Errick and Heel (1983) Schmidt et al. (1985)
Bromfenac[a]	NSAID	Antibradykinin (+) Tail clip (−) Writhing (+)	Sancilio et al. (1987)
Tramadol	Atypical opioid	Hot plate (+) Tail flick (+) Writhing (+)	Raffa et al. (1992)
Meloxicam	COX-2 preferring NSAID	Hot plate (−) Inflamed paw pressure (+) Tail clip (−)	Engelhardt et al. (1995)

[a] Withdrawn in June 1998 because of drug-induced liver toxicity.

Dilute solutions of acetic acid and phenylquinone are injected intraperitoneally in mice to precipitate writhing/stretching in the popular abdominal constriction test. Observing the mice can be tedious and time consuming. Adachi (1994) has described a mechanoelectro transducer that automatically and objectively counts each writhe after the acetic acid. There was a good correlation between results from human observation and from the detecting unit when standard agents were assayed.

Dilute solutions of acetic acid have also been used by Stevens and colleagues to demonstrate the antinociceptive potencies of opioids, given systemically, spinally, or supraspinally to northern grass frogs (Stevens et al., 1994; Stevens, 1996; Stevens and Rothe, 1997). The test involves placing a single drop from one of 10 dilutions of acetic acid on the frog's hindlimb and observing the frog for 5 secs for a wiping response. In the absence of a response (e.g., after morphine administration), the acid is flushed away with water and the next dilution is tested, and so on until a wiping response occurs. On the basis of studies such as these, Stevens is advancing a case (on both ethical and economic grounds) for replacing rodents with frogs when new opioid agents are to be screened.

The intraperitoneal injection of endothelin-1 (ET-1) into mice causes the animals to writhe as if given acetic acid or phenylquinone. Raffa and colleagues (1996) believe, however, that the underlying mechanisms differ. Their evidence is based, partly, on differential antinociceptive ED_{50} values for 36 standard compounds tested against equieffective doses of the three noxious agents. Of particular note was the good activity of diazepam and several other benzodiazepines against (specifically) ET-1-elicited writhing. The procedure holds promise as a model for ischemic pain of visceral organs and for the discovery of compounds that otherwise are inactive in conventional writhing assays.

PERSISTENT PAIN

Formalin Test

Dubuisson and Dennis (1977) are usually given credit for bringing the rat formalin test to the attention of pain researchers. They emphasized the continuous (rather than transient) nature of the noxious stimulus and the opportunity for the animals to behave spontaneously. The injection of a dilute solution of formalin into the hindpaw of a rat elicits at least two nocifensive behaviors: flinching/shaking of the paw and/or hindquarters and licking/biting of the injected paw (Wheeler-Aceto et al., 1990). The behavioral response to formalin is biphasic. An acute/early phase lasting about 10 min is caused by activation of peripheral nociceptors. This is followed, after a short quiescent period, by a tonic/late phase persisting from 20 to 90 min after injection and linked to ongoing activity in primary afferents and increased sensitivity of dorsal horn neurons. The tonic/late phase is initiated, at least in part, by activation of *N*-methyl-D-aspartate (NMDA) receptors in the spinal cord (Dickenson and Sullivan, 1987; Haley et al., 1990).

Formalin-induced hyperalgesia represents a behavioral model of tonic chemogenic pain. The procedure has involved the use of mice (e.g., Murray et al., 1988; Shibata et al., 1989; Mogil et al., 1998), rats (Wheeler-Aceto and Cowan, 1991; Chaplan et al., 1997; Hammond et al., 1998), gerbils (Smith et al., 1994; Rupniak et al., 1996; Chapter 7 of this volume), cats (Dubuisson and Dennis, 1977), and rhesus monkeys (Alreja et al., 1984), and practical issues relevant to the model have been reviewed succinctly by Tjølsen and colleagues (1992). A simple modification, involving the injection of formalin into the vibrissal pad of rats and monitoring the duration of lip rubbing, has facilitated the study of orofacial pain and its suppression by drugs (Clavelou et al., 1989, 1995; Eisenberg et al., 1996).

The formalin test has grown enormously in popularity over the last decade and it is arguably the most commonly used model of postoperative pain in current analgesic research. An indication of this acceptance is displayed in Figure 2.1, where the papers that have appeared in the journal *Pain* and in

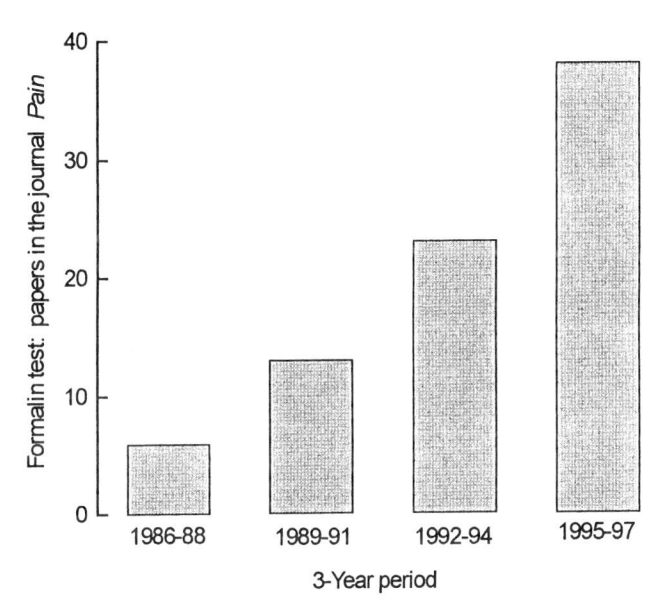

Figure 2.1 The number of papers describing the formalin test that were published in the journal *Pain* in 3-year periods between 1986 and 1997.

which the formalin test is featured are shown in 3-year histograms since 1986. The steady rise in use across time is apparent.

Methodological Update

The numerous variables associated with evaluation of antinociceptive activity in traditional (acute) procedures (Hammond, 1989) are also of concern in the formalin model. Thus such well-recognized factors as strain, age, and stress level of test animal, site/route of injection, and choice of data analysis can all influence the shape and position of a compound's dose–response curve against the formalin noxious stimulus. A perennial criticism of phasic pain studies can also be directed at accumulating data from the formalin test: how meaningful is an antinociceptive-50 value that depends entirely on a top dose of "analgesic" inducing behavioral depression and/or motor dysfunction in the animals? Or again, is the noxious stimulus (formalin) standardized such that findings may be compared across laboratories? This latter issue is considered in the following section.

Formalin Concentration and Nocifensive Behaviors. Commercially available formaldehyde solution (Merck and Co.) contains 36–38% formaldehyde along with 10–15% methanol (which acts as a stabilizer). A 1% formalin solution is made with 0.1 ml of formaldehyde in 9.9 ml of water (or, more usually, saline) so that the formaldehyde concentration is roughly 0.37% (Teng and Abbott, 1998).

Use of formalin concentrations between 1 and 5% has been recommended when studying drug-induced antagonism of tonic/late phase licking/biting in mice (Hunskaar et al., 1985; Murray et al., 1988; Rosland et al., 1990). On the basis of several recent reports, 20 µl of 2.5 or 5% formalin injected subcutaneously into either the dorsal or plantar surface of a mouse hindpaw is becoming the standard noxious stimulus in this test (e.g., Millan and Seguin, 1994; Noble et al., 1995; Wettstein and Grouhel, 1996; Bittencourt and Takahashi, 1997; Rupniak et al., 1997).

With rats, the choice of formalin concentration is no trivial matter and can influence the outcome of an assay, particularly if non-morphinelike agents are being screened (Poon and Sawynok, 1995). For example, in the more commonly monitored late phase, nociceptive responses to 50 µl of 5% formalin, but not to 50 µl of 1% formalin, were suppressed in a dose-related manner by intraperitoneal administration of the anti-inflammatory drugs ibuprofen (40–250 mg/kg) and dexamethasone (1–6.25 mg/kg) (Yashpal and Coderre, 1998). The stimulus intensity–drug response relationship can also work in the opposite direction; thus the potency of intraperitoneal caffeine against late phase flinching is increased by a factor of 8 when 20 µl of 5% formalin is replaced with 20 µl of 2% formalin (Sawynok and Reid, 1996). It is therefore prudent to study new compounds against at least two concentrations of formalin before reaching a conclusion on antihyperalgesic activity in the test. Concentrations of formalin within the 1–5% range would seem to be reasonable choices if either the incidence of late phase flinching (Ossipov et al., 1996; Dirig et al., 1997a) or a weighted-scores measure (Dubuisson and Dennis, 1977; Matthies and Franklin, 1992) is used to quantify nociceptive behavior. This is because both flinching and weighted-scores increase in a linear fashion up to the submaximal concentration of 5% formalin (Coderre et al., 1993; Wheeler-Aceto and Cowan, 1993; Jett and Michelson, 1996; but see Abbott et al., 1995 and Watson et al., 1997).

Two automated systems have been reported recently to provide an objective measure of formalin-induced nociceptive behavior in rats. Jett and Michelson (1996) described a computer-driven, dynamic-force detector that specifically quantifies nociceptive "agitation" behaviors (flinching and licking/biting) of rats placed in small polycarbonate observation tubes (Figure 2.2). A good correlation was found between the agitation response and two manual assessments: incidence of flinching and the weighted-scores measure of Coderre et al. (1993). Jourdan and colleagues (1997) described an automated system (Videotrack) based on computerized image processing that also measured pain-related behaviors (licking, biting, grooming), as well as motor activity, of rats allowed to explore a large plastic chamber. The authors validated their procedure against the weighted-scores measure of Dubuisson and Dennis (1977). It remains to be seen to what extent these automated devices will be used in pain research and drug discovery.

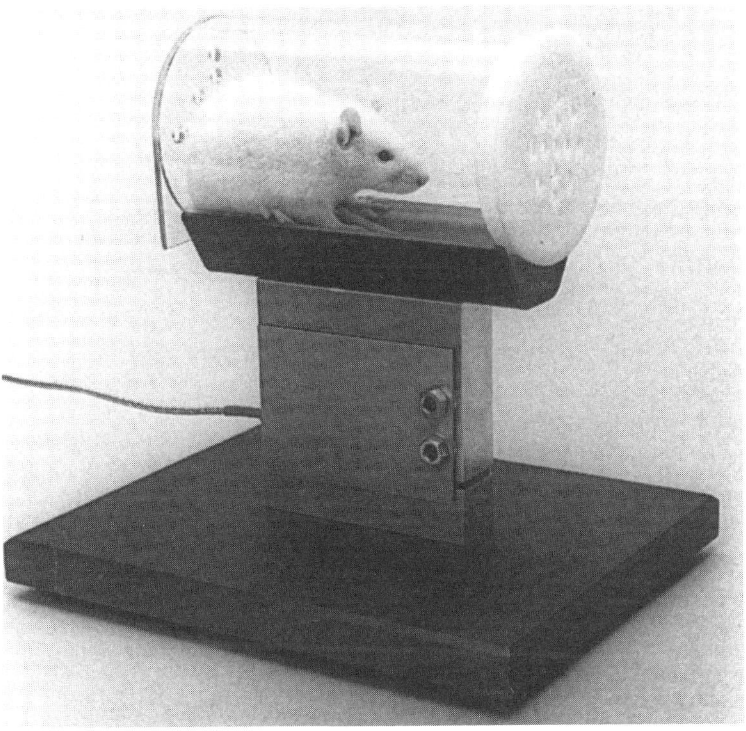

Figure 2.2 A rat (125–170 g) in an observation tube (16 cm long; 8 cm wide) positioned in the cradle of a load cell of the automated behavioral measuring system. Reproduced from Jett and Michelson (1996), with permission of the publisher. A commercial version that monitors up to 24 animals at a time is available from AccuScan Instruments (Columbus, Ohio).

Pharmacological Update

Antihyperalgesic activity has been claimed for a formidable array of compounds in the mouse/rat formalin test, particularly in the late phase. For example, in addition to positive findings with mu, kappa, and delta opioids (Pelissier et al., 1990; Murray and Cowan, 1991; Hammond et al., 1998) and several currently marketed analgesics (Table 2.3), recent results indicate activity for bradykinin antagonists (Corrêa and Calixto, 1993; Corrêa et al., 1996; Sufka and Roach, 1996), capsaicin analogues (Dray and Dickenson, 1991; Hua et al., 1997), adenosine analogues (Poon and Sawynok, 1995; Reeve and Dickenson, 1995), γ-aminobutyric acid agonists (Dirig and Yaksh, 1995; Kaneko and Hammond, 1997), nonsteroidal anti-inflammatory agents (NSAIDs) (Carrive and Meyer-Carrive, 1997; Euchenhofer et al., 1998; but see Dirig et al., 1997a), antidepressants (Acton et al., 1992; Jett et al., 1997) and antiepileptics (Field et al., 1997b; Shimoyama et al., 1997; Carlton and Zhou, 1998; and quoted in Nakamura-Craig and Follenfant, 1995).

TABLE 2.3   Potencies of Analgesics against Severe (Cancer) Pain in Humans and against Formalin-Induced Flinching in Rats

Analgesic	Equianalgesic Dose (mg, i.m.)[a]	A_{50} (mg/kg, s.c.)[b]
Buprenorphine	0.4	0.03 (0.02–0.04)
Butorphanol	2	0.14 (0.02–0.39)
Morphine	10	0.58 (0.47–0.71)
Nalbuphine	10	Curvilinear DRC; maximum antihyperalgesic effect = 57%
Pentazocine	60	0.92 (0.66–1.2)
Ketorolac	10–30[c]	Curvilinear DRC; maximum antihyperalgesic effect = 47%
Tramadol	[d]	2.1 (1.3–3.0) p.o.
Codeine	200 p.o.	25.8 (16.5–41.6) p.o.

[a]Foley (1985).
[b]Cowan et al. (1990) and Wheeler-Aceto and Cowan (unpublished results). A_{50} values and 95% confidence limits were determined by linear regression analysis from the percentage antagonism of formalin-induced (late phase) flinching.
[c]Staquet (1989); Eisenberg et al. (1994).
[d]Under study (Budd, 1995).
DRC = dose–response curve.

Two classes of pharmacological agent have been studied extensively in the formalin test, antagonists at neurokinin (NK) receptors (Seguin et al., 1995; Iyengar et al., 1997; Sakurada et al., 1997) and NMDA receptor antagonists (Kristensen et al., 1994; Elliott et al., 1995). It has been quite difficult to demonstrate *specific* antinociceptive activity for NK_1 receptor antagonists against the formalin noxious stimulus (Rupniak et al., 1995). This was a portent, perhaps, of the disappointing results obtained with these compounds in clinical trials involving migraine and dental pain (Chapter 7 of this volume). Several competitive and noncompetitive NMDA receptor antagonists are unimpressive in acute nociceptive procedures yet are active in the late phase of the formalin test (Chaplan et al., 1997; Chapter 8 of this volume). Unfortunately, the association of motor dysfunction in the animals with some of the higher intrathecal doses under test has been a confounding factor when attempting to establish dose–response relationships (Coderre and Van Empel, 1994). Nonetheless, despite concern over a narrow therapeutic window, two well-known NMDA receptor antagonists—dextromethorphan (the antitussive) and memantine (the antiparkinsonian agent)—have progressed through clinical trials. Dextromethorphan will be used primarily for treating cancer pain (when given in combination with morphine) and possibly arthritic pain (when given in combination with an NSAID) (Price et al., 1996). The indication for memantine is neuropathic pain. For present purposes, note the key role that the formalin test is playing in the primary evaluation of tomorrow's analgesics from the compound activity profiles listed in Table 2.4.

INCISIONAL PAIN

Paw Incision Test

A new model of postoperative pain involving rats has been introduced recently by Brennan et al. (1996) and validated pharmacologically by Zahn et al. (1997). The rat is anesthetized, a 1 cm longitudinal surgical incision is made through skin, fascia, and muscle in the plantar area of the animal's hindpaw and the wound is then closed. Tactile allodynia (i.e., pain due to a stimulus that does not normally provoke pain), revealed through the paw withdrawal response to calibrated von Frey filaments as well as nonpunctate and pinprick responses, ensues and this hypersensitive state lasts for several days after the incision. It is perhaps surprising that an animal model endowed with such obvious face validity (though not in itself an absolute criterion) has taken so long to appear in the analgesic literature. At any rate, morphine, given either subcutaneously or intrathecally to the rats, was active in the model (Zahn et al., 1997), as were intrathecal 6,7-dinitroquinoxaline-2,3-dione (DNQX) and 1,2,3,4-tetrahydro-6-nitro-2,3-dioxo-benzo[f]quinoxaline-7-sulfonamide disodium (NBQX), two standard non-NMDA excitatory amino acid receptor antagonists (Zahn et al., 1998). Importantly, from a predictive point of view, neither a competitive (dizocilpine) nor a noncompetitive (2-amino-5-phosphonovaleric acid) NMDA receptor antagonist was active against incisional pain at behaviorally acceptable intrathecal doses (Zahn and Brennan, 1998). The authors conclude that NMDA receptor antagonists, per se, are unlikely to be useful for pain relief after surgery.

Additional compounds are currently being evaluated in the procedure. Thus gabapentin (Field et al., 1997a), the antiepileptic agent known to be active against formalin (Singh et al., 1996) and in models of neuropathic pain (see below) (Xiao and Bennett, 1996; Hwang and Yaksh, 1997), as well as ziconotide (Table 2.4) (Wang et al., 1998) gave positive results against incisional pain. PD 154075, the selective NK_1 receptor antagonist (Gonzalez et al., 1998), was given subcutaneously to rats either pre- or postoperatively. This compound was active in the test only when given *before* the surgery.

VISCERAL PAIN

Colorectal Distension Test

Instilling irritants such as resiniferatoxin (Craft et al., 1995) and turpentine (McMahon and Abel, 1987) into the urinary bladder and distending the hollow viscera (Borgbjerg et al., 1996), are two increasingly common ways of evoking visceral nociception in animals. The testing of analgesics in unanesthetized rats using minimally invasive distension of the descending colon and rectum has become a well-recognized standard approach (Ness and Gebhart, 1988; Burton and Gebhart, 1998). Colorectal distension is effected by means of an intra-

TABLE 2.4 Representative Analgesics in Clinical Development and Pain Models in Which They Show Activity

Compound	Pharmacological Class	Formalin Test[a] (1)	CCI[b] Model (Rat) (2)	SNL[c] Model (Rat) (3)	Clinical Status
ABT-594[d] (Abbott)	Nicotinic acetylcholine receptor agonist	Flinching, licking, biting (i.p.) (4)	Tactile allodynia (i.p.) (4)	n/a	Phase I
Asimadoline (E. Merck)	Peripherally selective kappa agonist	Licking (s.c., p.o.) (5)	n/a	n/a	Rheumatic pain/osteoarthritis—Phase II
Clonidine (Roxane)	α-Adrenergic agonist	Flinching (i.th.) (6)	Heat hyperalgesia (i.th.) (7)	Tactile allodynia (i.th.) (8)	Marketed as Duraclon™ for epidural use in combination with opiates against cancer pain
Dextromethorphan (Algos)	Noncompetitive NMDA antagonist	Flinching, licking (s.c.) (9)	Heat hyperalgesia (with i.th. dextrorphan, the metabolite) (10)	Tactile allodynia (i.th.) (11)	In combination with morphine (as MorphiDex™) for cancer pain—new drug application filed

Memantine (Merz and Co.)	Noncompetitive NMDA antagonist	Flinching (i.th.) (11)	Heat hyperalgesia (i.p.) (12)	Tactile allodynia (i.p.) (13)	Neuropathic pain— Phase II
TRK-820[c] (Toray)	Kappa agonist	Flinching (s.c., intra-paw) (14)	n/a	n/a	Cancer pain—Phase II
Ziconotide (Neurex)	N-type neuronal voltage-sensitive calcium channel blocker	Flinching (i.th.) (15)	Heat hyperalgesia, tactile allodynia (bolus administration onto the site of nerve injury) (16)	Tactile allodynia (i.th.) (17)	Neuropathic/cancer pain —Phase III

[a] Mouse or rat formalin test (late phase).
[b] CCI = chronic constriction injury to rat sciatic nerve.
[c] SNL = spinal nerve ligation of L5/L6 nerves.
[d] (R)-5-(2-azetidinylmethoxy)-2-chloropyridine.
[e] 17-Cyclopropylmethyl-3,14β-dihydroxy-4,5α-epoxy-6β-[N-methyl-trans-3-(3-furyl)acrylamido]morphinan HCl.
n/a = information not available.

(1) Dubuisson and Dennis (1977); (2) Bennett and Xie (1988); (3) Kim and Chung (1992); (4) Bannon et al. (1998); (5) Barber et al. (1994); (6) Przesmycki et al. (1997); (7) Yamamoto and Nozaki-Taguchi (1996); (8) Yaksh et al. (1995); (9) Elliott et al. (1995); (10) Mao et al. (1993); (11) Chaplan et al. (1997); (12) Eisenberg et al. (1995); (13) Carlton and Hargett (1995); (14) DeHaven et al. (1998); (15) Malmberg and Yaksh (1995); (16) Xiao and Bennett (1995); (17) Bowersox et al. (1996).

anally inserted latex balloon connected to a pressure control assembly. This brief mechanical stimulus elicits tachycardia and a rise in mean arterial blood pressure. Additionally, a reproducible visceromotor response occurs—contraction of the peritoneal musculature—which can be monitored via electromyographic electrodes.

The following compounds attenuated the visceromotor and/or cardiovascular responses to colorectal distension in rats: intrathecal clonidine (Danzebrink and Gebhart, 1990), intravenous tramadol (Traub et al., 1995), and intrathecal morphine and [D-Pen^2, D-Pen^5]enkephalin (Danzebrink et al., 1995). It was notable that U-50488, the selective agonist at kappa opioid receptors, was active after intravenous injection but poorly active after intrathecal administration (Danzebrink et al., 1995). This relative inactivity of U-50488 by the intrathecal route was in agreement with similar reports by Diop et al. (1994) and Harada et al. (1995) but is at odds with the activity reported for another kappa agonist— enadoline—after intrathecal administration in the same preparation (Castex et al., 1998).

Recent results from Gebhart's laboratory, involving the recording of mechanosensitive pelvic nerve afferent fibers, suggest that U-50488 (but not mu or delta agonists) can modulate visceral nociception at a peripheral site of action, possibly on primary afferent fibers innervating the colon (Sengupta et al., 1996; Su et al., 1997). This finding hints at a possible new clinical use for peripherally selective kappa analgesics, for example, asimadoline (Table 2.4). An advance such as this shows the necessity of having a reliable model of visceral pain in place (however belatedly).

NEUROPATHIC PAIN

With painful peripheral neuropathies (e.g., postherpetic neuralgia), a spontaneous ectopic discharge from compromised primary afferents is believed to promote the central state of hyperexcitability that fosters two key symptoms: allodynia (pain due to a stimulus that does not normally provoke pain) and hyperalgesia (an increased response to a stimulus that is normally painful). Compounds of potential therapeutic value for neuropathic states have been tested primarily in one or more of the following rat behavioral models. In the chronic constriction injury model (Bennett and Xie, 1988; Attal et al., 1990), the nerve damage (strangulation) is caused by tying four ligatures loosely around the rat's sciatic nerve. Seltzer et al. (1990) describe an injury that is caused by a partial unilateral transection of the rat's sciatic nerve. The model developed by Kim and Chung (1992) involves tight ligation of the L5 and L6 spinal nerves close to their respective ganglia. Thermal hyperalgesia and mechanical allodynia in the affected hindlimb represent behavioral evidence of neuropathic pain that is common to all three approaches. Mechanical allodynia (revealed by Von Frey filaments) was most prominent with the Kim and Chung model and least obvious after the chronic constriction injury (Kim et al., 1997).

Additionally, in a model of diabetic neuropathy, a single intraperitoneal injection of streptozotocin (75 mg/kg) in rats induced hyperglycemia and glycosuria and subsequently a decrease in reaction thresholds to paw pressure and to tail immersion in water maintained at 10, 38, or 46°C (Courteix et al., 1993).

Methodological Update

The latency of paw withdrawal to noxious radiant heat is commonly measured in neuropathic rats using an apparatus originally described by Hargreaves and colleagues (1988). An updated device (Galbraith et al., 1993) consists of a glass surface (maintained at 30°C) upon which the rats are placed individually in Plexiglas containers. The thermal nociceptive stimulus originates from a movable high-intensity light source, positioned below the glass, and focused on the plantar surface of one hindpaw. An electronic timer is activated simultaneously with the light source, and both are automatically stopped when the paw is abruptly withdrawn. The sequence can be repeated, this time focusing on the other paw (see Yeomans and Proudfit, 1994). A commercial version of the instrument is displayed in Figure 2.3.

Dirig and colleagues (1997b) have analyzed the experimental variables in a modified version of the apparatus. They monitored stimulus (thermal) intensity, glass surface temperature, paw tissue temperature, and withdrawal latency and showed what other investigators may have merely assumed: increased stimulus intensity is, indeed, linked to a monotonic decrease in mean withdrawal latency.

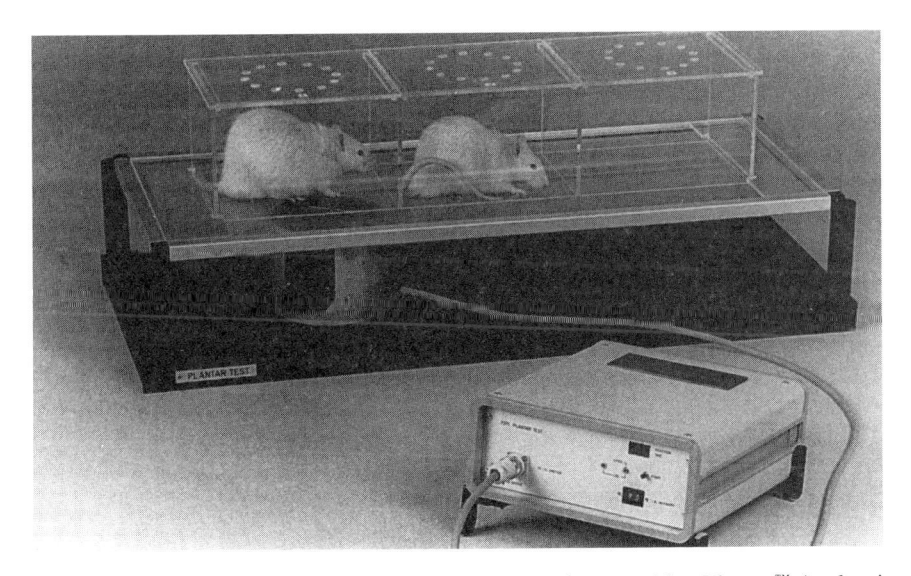

Figure 2.3 Measurement of paw withdrawal latency in rats with a Plantar™ Analgesia Instrument. The apparatus, based on the original description by Hargreaves et al. (1988), is available from Stoelting (Wood Dale, Illinois).

Additionally, they emphasized the necessity of maintaining the glass surface at 30°C to reduce variability.

Have there been recent methodological advances in the use of *cold* stimuli to test sensory processing in neuropathic rats? In this context, Jasmin and colleagues (1998) raise the following question: why is there no one accepted and standard method for checking responses to cold stimuli in rats with nerve injuries? These workers have remedied the situation by publishing a detailed account of the 5°C cold plate procedure. Rats with chronic constriction injury (CCI) of the sciatic nerve were given three 5-min test exposures to the cold plate and responded with rapid lifts of the treated hindpaw. The number of these paw lifts was reduced in a dose-related manner when the animals received subcutaneous morphine or clonidine or intravenous lidocaine. The positive result for morphine confirms the finding of Gogas et al. (1997), who tested CCI rats in what they termed a "cold bath assay." The rats were placed, individually, into a chamber containing cold water (0–4°C) to a depth of 2.5 cm above an aluminum plate. Using the latency to raise the ligated paw out of the water, Gogas et al. (1997) found subcutaneous morphine, mexiletine (sodium channel blocker), and desipramine (tricyclic antidepressant) to suppress the lifting response.

In the broader context, morphine may or may not be active against an experimental peripheral neuropathy, depending on the actual model, the stimulus used and behavior measured, and the route of administration (Lee et al., 1994, 1995; Chung and Na, 1996; Koch et al., 1996). At the clinical level, an ongoing debate continues as to the effectiveness of morphine against the various neuropathic pain syndromes.

Pharmacological Update

Studies with CCI rats and rats with spinal nerve ligation (SNL) of L5 and L6 nerves have been critical in identifying NMDA antagonists (dextromethorphan, memantine) as antihyperalgesic agents and clinical candidates (Table 2.4). Activity in CCI and/or SNL models has triggered interest in gabapentin, the antiepileptic agent (Xiao and Bennett, 1996; Hunter et al., 1997; Hwang and Yaksh, 1997), and has been key to the subsequent clinical trials of completely new types of analgesic (Table 2.4), for example, a nicotinic acetylcholine receptor agonist (ABT-594) and an N-type neuronal voltage-sensitive calcium channel blocker (ziconotide).

CONCLUSIONS

Practical aspects of antinociceptive testing have been addressed in this chapter. Until the past decade, evaluating potential drugs for various persistent, visceral, and neuropathic pain states was hampered by the lack of reliable animal models. This situation has improved to the extent that the appropriate models were in place in time to hasten NMDA receptor antagonists toward definitive clinical testing. Additionally, a comprehensive and authoritative review on antinociceptive testing by Yaksh (1997) is in place for tomorrow's analgesics.

There is no one ideal animal model of pain because not all pains are the same. In this area of vibrant research, new tests for analgesics continue to appear, for example, the mouse "grid-shock test" (Swedberg, 1994), the rat "intraplantar zymosan test" (Meller and Gebhart, 1997), and a mouse model of neuropathy (Malmberg and Basbaum, 1998). Each method will demonstrate strengths and limitations, and each, in its own way, will likely advance the field.

REFERENCES

Abbott FV, Franklin KBJ, Westbrook RF (1995): The formalin test—scoring properties of the first and second phases of the pain response in rats. Pain 60:91–102.

Aceto MD, Bowman ER, Harris LS, May EL (1998): Dependence studies on new compounds in the rhesus monkey, rat and mouse. NIDA Res Monogr 178:363–407.

Acton J, McKenna JE, Melzack R (1992): Amitriptyline produces analgesia in the formalin pain test. Exp Neurol 117:94–96.

Adachi K-I (1994): A device for automatic measurement of writhing and its application to the assessment of analgesic agents. J Pharmacol Toxicol Meth 32:79–84.

Adams JU, Tallarida RJ, Geller EB, Adler MW (1993): Isobolographic superadditivity between delta and mu opioid agonists in the rat depends on the ratio of compounds, the mu agonist and the analgesic assay used. J Pharmacol Exp Ther 266:1261–1267.

Aloisi AM, Carli G (1996): Nociceptive, environmental and neuroendocrine factors determining pain behavior in animals. In Carli G, Zimmermann M (eds): *Towards the Neurobiology of Chronic Pain*. Amsterdam: Elsevier, pp. 33–46.

Alreja M, Mutalik P, Nayar U, Manchanda SK (1984): The formalin test—a tonic pain model in the primate. Pain 20:97–105.

Ankier SI (1974): New hot plate tests to quantify antinociceptive and narcotic antagonist activity. Eur J Pharmacol 27:1–4.

Attal N, Jazat F, Kayser V, Guilbaud G (1990): Further evidence for "pain-related" behaviours in a model of unilateral peripheral mononeuropathy. Pain 41:235–251.

Bannon AW, Decker MW, Holladay MW, Curzon P, Donnelly-Roberts D, Puttfarcken PS, Bitner RS, Diaz A, Dickenson AH, Porsolt RD, Williams M, Arneric SP (1998): Broad-spectrum, non-opioid analgesic activity by selective modulation of neuronal nicotinic acetylcholine receptors. Science 279:77–81.

Barber A, Bartoszyk GD, Bender HM, Gottschlich R, Greiner HE, Harting J, Mauler F, Minck K-O, Murray RD, Simon M, Seyfried CA (1994): A pharmacological profile of the novel, peripherally selective kappa-opioid receptor agonist, EMD 61753. Br J Pharmacol 113:1317–1327.

Bennett GJ, Xie Y-K (1988): A peripheral mononeuropathy in rat that produces disorders of pain sensation like those seen in man. Pain 33:87–107.

Besson J-M, Guilbaud G (1988): *The Arthritic Rat as a Model of Clinical Pain?* Amsterdam: Excerpta Medica.

Bittencourt AL, Takahashi RN (1997): Mazindol and lidocaine are antinociceptives in the mouse formalin model: involvement of dopamine receptor. Eur J Pharmacol 330: 109–113.

Borgbjerg FM, Frigast C, Madsen JB, Mikkelsen LF (1996): The effect of intrathecal opioid-receptor agonists on visceral noxious stimulation in rabbits. Gastroenterology 110:139–146.

Bowersox SS, Gadbois T, Singh T, Pettus M, Wang Y-X, Luther RR (1996): Selective N-type neuronal voltage-sensitive calcium channel blocker, SNX-111, produces spinal antinociception in rat models of acute, persistent and neuropathic pain. J Pharmacol Exp Ther 279:1243–1249.

Brennan TJ, Vandermeulen EP, Gebhart GF (1996): Characterization of a rat model of incisional pain. Pain 64:493–501.

Budd K (1995): Tramadol—a step towards the ideal analgesic? Eur J Palliative Care 2:56–60.

Burton MB, Gebhart GF (1998): Effects of kappa-opioid receptor agonists on responses to colorectal distension in rats with and without acute colonic inflammation. J Pharmacol Exp Ther 285:707–715.

Butelman ER, France CP, Woods JH (1995a): Agonist and antagonist effects of dynorphin A-(1-13) in a thermal antinociception assay in rhesus monkeys. J Pharmacol Exp Ther 275:374–380.

Butelman ER, Winger G, Zernig G, Woods JH (1995b): Butorphanol—characterization of agonist and antagonist effects in rhesus monkeys. J Pharmacol Exp Ther 272: 845–853.

Carlton SM, Hargett GL (1995): Treatment with the NMDA antagonist memantine attenuates nociceptive responses to mechanical stimulation in neuropathic rats. Neurosci Lett 198:115–118.

Carlton SM, Zhou S (1998): Attenuation of formalin-induced nociceptive behaviors following local peripheral injection of gabapentin. Pain 76:201–207.

Carmody J (1995): Avoiding fallacies in nociceptive measurements. Pain 63:136.

Carrive P, Meyer-Carrive I (1997): Changes in formalin-evoked spinal fos expression and nociceptive behaviour after oral administration of Bufferin A (aspirin) and L-5409709 (ibuprofen + caffeine + paracetamol). Pain 70:253–266.

Carter RB (1991): Differentiating analgesic and non-analgesic drug activities on rat hot plate: effect of behavioral endpoint. Pain 47:211–220.

Castex N, Levine B, Vanderah T, Junien JL, Porreca F, Riviere PJM (1998): Spinal and peripheral kappa and mu opioid receptor agonists inhibit the response to noxious colorectal distension (CRD). Gastroenterology 114:G4639.

Chang A, Emmel DW, Rossi GC, Pasternak GW (1998): Methadone analgesia in morphine-insensitive CXBK mice. Eur J Pharmacol 351:189–191.

Chaplan SR, Malmberg AB, Yaksh TL (1997): Efficacy of spinal NMDA receptor antagonism in formalin hyperalgesia and nerve injury evoked allodynia in the rat. J Pharmacol Exp Ther 280:829–838.

Chung JM, Na HS (1996): Effects of systemic morphine on neuropathic pain behaviors in an experimental rat model. Analgesia 2:151–155.

Clavelou P, Pajot J, Dallel R, Raboisson P (1989): Application of the formalin test to the study of orofacial pain in the rat. Neurosci Lett 103:349–353.

Clavelou P, Dallel R, Orliaguet T, Woda A, Raboisson P (1995): The orofacial formalin test in rats—effects of different formalin concentrations. Pain 62:295–301.

Coderre TJ, Van Empel I (1994): The utility of excitatory amino acid (EAA) antagonists as analgesic agents. I. comparison of the antinociceptive activity of various classes of EAA antagonists in mechanical, thermal and chemical nociceptive tests. Pain 59: 345–352.

Coderre TJ, Fundytus ME, McKenna JE, Dalal S, Melzack R (1993): The formalin test—a validation of the weighted-scores method of behavioral pain rating. Pain 54: 43–50.

Colpaert FC (1987): Evidence that adjuvant arthritis in the rat is associated with chronic pain. Pain 28:201–222.

Corrêa CR, Calixto JB (1993): Evidence for participation of B_1 and B_2 kinin receptors in formalin-induced nociceptive response in the mouse. Br J Pharmacol 110:193–198.

Corrêa CR, Kyle DJ, Chakraverty S, Calixto JB (1996): Antinociceptive profile of the pseudopeptide B_2 bradykinin receptor antagonist NPC 18688 in mice. Br J Pharmacol 117:552–558.

Courteix C, Eschalier A, Lavarenne J (1993): Streptozocin-induced diabetic rats: behavioral evidence for a model of chronic pain. Pain 53:81–88.

Cowan A, Lewis JW, Macfarlane IR (1977): Agonist and antagonist properties of buprenorphine, a new antinociceptive agent. Br J Pharmacol 60:537–545.

Cowan A, Porreca F, Wheeler H (1990): Use of the formalin test in evaluating analgesics. NIDA Res Monogr 95:116–122.

Craft RM, Henley SR, Haaseth RC, Hruby VJ, Porreca F (1995): Opioid antinociception in a rat model of visceral pain: systemic versus local drug administration. J Pharmacol Exp Ther 275:1535–1542.

Danzebrink RM, Gebhart GF (1990): Antinociceptive effects of intrathecal adrenoceptor agonists in a rat model of visceral nociception. J Pharmacol Exp Ther 253:698–705.

Danzebrink RM, Green SA, Gebhart GF (1995): Spinal mu and delta, but not kappa, opioid-receptor agonists attenuate responses to noxious colorectal distension in the rat. Pain 63:39–47.

DeHaven RN, Chang AC, Daubert JD, Cassel JA, Gottshall SL, DeHaven-Hudkins DL, Mansson E, Yu G (1998): TRK-820 exhibits both kappa agonist and mu antagonist properties. Soc Neurosci Abstr 24:889.

Delaney KM, Rourke JD, Shaw JS (1986): Sensitivity of antinociceptive tests to opioid agonists and partial agonists. NIDA Res Monogr 75:438–441.

Dickenson AH, Sullivan AF (1987): Subcutaneous formalin-induced activity of dorsal horn neurones in the rat: differential response to an intrathecal opiate administered pre or post formalin. Pain 30:349–360.

Diop L, Rivière PJM, Pascaud X, Dassaud M, Junien J-L (1994): Role of vagal afferents in the antinociception produced by morphine and U-50,488H in the colonic pain reflex in rats. Eur J Pharmacol 257:181–187.

Dirig DM, Yaksh TL (1995): Intrathecal baclofen and muscimol, but not midazolam, are antinociceptive using the rat-formalin model. J Pharmacol Exp Ther 275:219–227.

Dirig DM, Konin GP, Isakson PC, Yaksh TL (1997a): Effect of spinal cyclooxygenase inhibitors in rat using the formalin test and in vitro prostaglandin E-2 release. Eur J Pharmacol 331:155–160.

Dirig DM, Salami A, Rathbun ML, Ozaki GT, Yaksh TL (1997b): Characterization of variables defining hindpaw withdrawal latency evoked by radiant thermal stimuli. J Neurosci Meth 76:183–191.

Dray A, Dickenson A (1991): Systemic capsaicin and olvanil reduce the acute algogenic and the late inflammatory phase following formalin injection into rodent paw. Pain 47:79–83.

Dubner R (1994): Methods of assessing pain in animals. In Wall PD, Melzack R (eds): *Textbook of Pain*, 3rd ed. Edinburgh: Churchill Livingstone, pp. 293–302.

Dubuisson D, Dennis SG (1977): The formalin test: a quantitative study of the analgesic effects of morphine, meperidine, and brain stem stimulation in rats and cats. Pain 4:161–174.

Dykstra LA, Woods JH (1986): A tail withdrawal procedure for assessing analgesic activity in rhesus monkeys. J Pharmacol Meth 15:263–269.

Eisenberg E, Berkey C, Carr DB, Chalmers TC, Mosteller F (1994): NSAIDs for cancer pain: meta-analysis of efficacy. In Gebhart GF, Hammond DL, Jensen TS (eds): *Proceedings of the 7th World Congress on Pain*. Seattle: IASP Press, pp. 697–707.

Eisenberg E, LaCross S, Strassman AM (1995): The clinically tested N-methyl-D-aspartate receptor antagonist memantine blocks and reverses thermal hyperalgesia in a rat model of painful mononeuropathy. Neurosci Lett 187:17–20.

Eisenberg E, Vos BP, Strassman AM (1996): The peripheral antinociceptive effect of morphine in a rat model of facial pain. Neuroscience 72:519–525.

Elliott KJ, Brodsky M, Hynansky AD, Foley KM, Inturrisi CE (1995): Dextromethorphan suppresses both formalin-induced nociceptive behavior and the formalin-induced increase in spinal cord c-fos mRNA. Pain 61:401–409.

Engelhardt G, Homma D, Schlegel K, Utzmann R, Schnitzler C (1995): Anti-inflammatory, analgesic, antipyretic and related properties of meloxicam, a new non-steroidal anti-inflammatory agent with favourable gastrointestinal tolerance. Inflamm Res 44:423–433.

Errick JK, Heel RC (1983): Nalbuphine—a preliminary review of its pharmacological properties and therapeutic efficacy. Drugs 26:191–211.

Euchenhofer C, Maihofner C, Brune K, Tegeder I, Geisslinger G (1998): Differential effect of selective cyclooxygenase-2 (COX-2) inhibitor NS 398 and diclofenac on formalin-induced nociception in the rat. Neurosci Lett 248:25–28.

Field MJ, Holloman EF, McCleary S, Hughes J, Singh L (1997a): Evaluation of gabapentin and S-(+)-3-isobutylgaba in a rat model of postoperative pain. J Pharmacol Exp Ther 282:1242–1246.

Field MJ, Oles RJ, Lewis AS, McCleary S, Hughes J, Singh L (1997b): Gabapentin (neurontin) and S-(+)-3-isobutylgaba represent a novel class of selective antihyperalgesic agents. Br J Pharmacol 121:1513–1522.

Foley KM (1985): The treatment of cancer pain. New Engl J Med 313:84–95.

France CP, Medzihradsky F, Woods JH (1994): Comparison of kappa opioids in rhesus monkeys: behavioral effects and receptor binding affinities. J Pharmacol Exp Ther 268:47–58.

Franklin KBJ, Abbott FV (1989): Techniques for assessing the effects of drugs on nociceptive responses. In Boulton AA, Baker GB, Greenshaw AJ (eds): *Neuromethods—Psychopharmacology.* Clifton, NJ: Humana Press, pp. 145–216.

Galbraith JA, Mrosko BJ, Myers RR (1993): A system to measure thermal nociception. J Neurosci Meth 49:63–68.

Gebhart GF, Sengupta JN (1995): Evaluation of visceral pain. In Gaginella TS (ed): *Handbook of Methods in Gastrointestinal Pharmacology.* Boca Raton, FL: CRC Press, pp. 359–373.

Gogas KR, Jacobson LO, Waligora D, Martin B, Hunter JC (1997): The cold bath assay: a simple and reliable method to assess cold allodynia in neuropathic rats. Analgesia 3:111–118.

Gonzalez MI, Field MJ, Holloman EF, Hughes J, Oles RJ, Singh L (1998): Evaluation of PD 154075, a tachykinin NK_1 receptor antagonist, in a rat model of postoperative pain. Eur J Pharmacol 344:115–120.

Granat FR, Saelens JK (1973): Effect of stimulus intensity on the potency of some analgetic agents. Arch Int Pharmacodyn Ther 205:52–60.

Gray WD, Osterberg AC, Scuto TJ (1970): Measurement of the analgesic efficacy and potency of pentazocine by the D'Amour and Smith method. J Pharmacol Exp Ther 172:154–162.

Haley JE, Sullivan AF, Dickenson AH (1990): Evidence for spinal N-methyl-D-aspartate receptor involvement in prolonged chemical nociception in the rat. Brain Res 518: 218–226.

Hammond DL (1989): Inference of pain and its modulation from simple behaviors. In Chapman CR, Loeser JD (eds): *Pain Measurement.* New York: Raven Press, pp. 69–91.

Hammond DL, Wang H, Nakashima N, Basbaum AI (1998): Differential effects of intrathecally administered delta and mu opioid receptor agonists on formalin-evoked nociception and on the expression of fos-like immunoreactivity in the spinal cord of the rat. J Pharmacol Exp Ther 284:378–387.

Harada Y, Nishioka K, Kitahata LM, Nakatani K, Collins JG (1995): Contrasting actions of intrathecal U50,488H, morphine, or [D-Pen^2, D-Pen^5]enkephalin or intravenous U50,488H on the visceromotor response to colorectal distension in the rat. Anesthesiology 83:336–343.

Hargreaves K, Dubner R, Brown F, Flores C, Joris J (1988): A new and sensitive method for measuring thermal nociception in cutaneous hyperalgesia. Pain 32:77–88.

Harris LS, Pierson AK (1964): Some narcotic antagonists in the benzomorphan series. J Pharmacol Exp Ther 143:141–148.

Hole K, Tjølsen A (1993): The tail-flick and formalin test in rodents: changes in skin temperature as a confounding factor. Pain 53:247–254.

Hua X-Y, Chen P, Hwang J, Yaksh TL (1997): Antinociception induced by civamide, an orally active capsaicin analogue. Pain 71:313–322.

Hunskaar S, Fasmer OB, Hole K (1985): Formalin test in mice, a useful technique for evaluating mild analgesics. J Neurosci Meth 14:69–76.

Hunter JC, Leighton GE, Meecham KG, Boyle SJ, Horwell DC, Rees DC, Hughes J (1990): CI-977, a novel and selective agonist for the κ-opioid receptor. Br J Pharmacol 101:183–189.

Hunter JC, Gogas KR, Hedley LR, Jacobson LO, Kassotakis L, Thompson J, Fontana DJ (1997): The effect of novel anti-epileptic drugs in rat experimental models of acute and chronic pain. Eur J Pharmacol 324:153–160.

Hwang JH, Yaksh TL (1997): Effect of subarachnoid gabapentin on tactile-evoked allodynia in a surgically induced neuropathic pain model in the rat. Reg Anesth 22: 249–256.

Iyengar S, Hipskind PA, Gehlert DR, Schober D, Lobb KL, Nixon JA, Helton DR, Kallman MJ, Boucher S, Couture R, Li DL, Simmons RMA (1997): LY303870, a centrally active neurokinin-1 antagonist with a long duration of action. J Pharmacol Exp Ther 280:774–785.

Jasmin L, Kohan L, Franssen M, Janni G, Goff JR (1998): The cold plate as a test of nociceptive behaviors: description and application to the study of chronic neuropathic and inflammtory pain models. Pain 75:367–382.

Jett MF, Michelson S (1996): The formalin test in rat—validation of an automated system. Pain 64:19–25.

Jett MF, McGuirk J, Waligora D, Hunter JC (1997): The effects of mexiletine, desipramine and fluoxetine in rat models involving central sensitization. Pain 69:161–169.

Jourdan D, Ardid D, Bardin L, Bardin M, Neuzeret D, Lanphouthacoul L, Eschalier A (1997): A new automated method of pain scoring in the formalin test in rats. Pain 71:265–270.

Kaneko M, Hammond DL (1997): Role of spinal γ-aminobutyric acid-A receptors in formalin-induced nociception in the rat. J Pharmacol Exp Ther 282:928–938.

Kim SH, Chung JM (1992): An experimental model for peripheral neuropathy produced by segmental spinal nerve ligation in the rat. Pain 50:355–363.

Kim KJ, Yoon YW, Chung JM (1997): Comparison of three rodent neuropathic pain models. Exp Brain Res 113:200–206.

Koch BD, Faurot GF, McGuirk JR, Clarke DE, Hunter JC (1996): Modulation of mechano-hyperalgesia by clinically effective analgesics in rats with a peripheral mononeuropathy. Analgesia 2:157–164.

Kristensen JD, Karlsten R, Gordh T, Berge O-G (1994): The NMDA antagonist 3-(2-carboxypiperazin-4-yl)propyl-1-phosphonic acid (CPP) has antinociceptive effect after intrathecal injection in the rat. Pain 56:59–67.

Lee SH, Kayser V, Desmeules J, Guilbaud G (1994): Differential action of morphine and various opioid agonists on thermal allodynia and hyperalgesia in mononeuropathic rats. Pain 57:233–240.

Lee Y-W, Chaplan SR, Yaksh TL (1995): Systemic and supraspinal, but not spinal, opiates suppress allodynia in a rat neuropathic pain model. Neurosci Lett 186:111–114.

Lichtman AH, Smith FL, Martin BR (1993): Evidence that the antinociceptive tail-flick response is produced independently from changes in either tail-skin temperature or core temperature. Pain 55:283–295.

Luttinger D (1985): Determination of antinociceptive efficacy of drugs in mice using different water temperatures in a tail-immersion test. J Pharmacol Meth 13:351–357.

Malmberg AB, Basbaum AI (1998): Partial sciatic nerve injury in the mouse as a model of neuropathic pain: behavioral and neuroanatomical correlates. Pain 76:215–222.

Malmberg AB, Yaksh TL (1995): Effect of continuous intrathecal infusion of ω-conopeptides, N-type calcium-channel blockers, on behavior and antinociception in the formalin and hot-plate tests in rats. Pain 60:83–90.

Mao J, Price DD, Hayes RL, Lu J, Mayer DJ, Frenk H (1993): Intrathecal treatment with dextrorphan or ketamine potently reduces pain-related behaviors in a rat model of peripheral mononeuropathy. Brain Res 605:164–168.

Matthies BK, Franklin KBJ (1992): Formalin pain is expressed in decerebrate rats but not attenuated by morphine. Pain 51:199–206.

McMahon SB, Abel C (1987): A model for the study of visceral pain states: chronic inflammation of the chronic decerebrate rat urinary bladder by irritant chemicals. Pain 28:109–127.

Meller ST, Gebhart GF (1997): Intraplantar zymosan as a reliable, quantifiable model of thermal and mechanical hyperalgesia in the rat. Eur J Pain 1:43–52.

Millan MJ (1989): Kappa-opioid receptor-mediated antinociception in the rat. I. Comparative actions of mu- and kappa-opioids against noxious, thermal, pressure and electrical stimuli. J Pharmacol Exp Ther 251:334–341.

Millan MJ, Seguin L (1994): Chemically diverse ligands at the glycine B site coupled to N-methyl-D-aspartate (NMDA) receptors selectively block the late phase of formalin-induced pain in mice. Neurosci Lett 178:139–143.

Mogil JS, Lichtensteiger CA, Wilson SG (1998): The effect of genotype on sensitivity to inflammatory nociception: characterization of resistant (A/J) and sensitive (C57BL/6J) inbred mouse strains. Pain 76:115–125.

Murray CW, Cowan A (1991): Tonic pain perception in the mouse: differential modulation by three receptor-selective opioid agonists. J Pharmacol Exp Ther 257:335–341.

Murray CW, Porreca F, Cowan A (1988): Methodological refinements to the mouse paw formalin test—an animal model of tonic pain. J Pharmacol Methods 20:175–186.

Nakamura-Craig M, Follenfant RL (1995): Effect of lamotrigine in the acute and chronic hyperalgesia induced by PGE_2 and in the chronic hyperalgesia in rats with streptozotocin-induced diabetes. Pain 63:33–37.

Negus SS, Gatch MB, Mello NK, Zhang X, Rice K (1998): Behavioral effects of the delta-selective opioid agonist SNC 80 and related compounds in rhesus monkeys. J Pharmacol Exp Ther 286:362–375.

Ness TJ, Gebhart GF (1988): Colorectal distension as a noxious visceral stimulus: physiologic and pharmacologic characterization of pseudaffective reflexes in the rat. Brain Res 450:153–169.

Noble F, Blommaert A, Fournie-Zaluski M-C, Roques BP (1995): A selective CCK-B receptor antagonist potentiates mu- but not delta-opioid receptor-mediated antinociception in the formalin test. Eur J Pharmacol 273:145–151.

O'Callaghan JP, Holtzman SG (1975): Quantification of the analgesic activity of narcotic antagonists by a modified hot-plate procedure. J Pharmacol Exp Ther 192:497–505.

Ossipov MH, Kovelowski CJ, Wheeler-Aceto H, Cowan A, Hunter JC, Lai J, Malan TP, Porreca F (1996): Opioid antagonists and antisera to endogenous opioids increase the nociceptive response to formalin: demonstration of an opioid kappa and delta inhibitory tone. J Pharmacol Exp Ther 277:784–788.

Parsons CG, Headley PM (1989): Spinal antinociceptive actions of μ- and κ-opioids: the importance of stimulus intensity in determining 'selectivity' between reflexes to different modalities of noxious stimulus. Br J Pharmacol 98:523–532.

Pelissier T, Paeile C, Soto-Moyano R, Saavedra H, Hernandez A (1990): Analgesia produced by intrathecal administration of the kappa opioid agonist, U-50488H, on formalin-evoked cutaneous pain in the rat. Eur J Pharmacol 190:287–293.

Pircio AW, Gylys JA, Cavanagh RL, Buyniski JP, Bierwagen ME (1976): The pharmacology of butorphanol, a 3,14-dihydroxymorphinan narcotic antagonist analgesic. Arch Int Pharmacodyn Ther 220:231–257.

Pizziketti RJ, Pressman NS, Geller EB, Cowan A, Adler MW (1985): Rat cold water tail-flick: a novel analgesic test that distinguishes opioid agonists from mixed agonist-antagonists. Eur J Pharmacol 119:23–29.

Plone MA, Emerich DF, Lindner MD (1996): Individual differences in the hotplate test and effects of habituation on sensitivity to morphine. Pain 66:265–270.

Poon A, Sawynok J (1995): Antinociception by adenosine analogs and an adenosine kinase inhibitor: dependence on formalin concentration. Eur J Pharmacol 286:177–184.

Porro CA, Cavazzuti M (1993): Spatial and temporal aspects of spinal cord and brainstem activation in the formalin pain model. Prog Neurobiol 41:565–607.

Price DD, Mao J, Lu J, Caruso FS, Frenk H, Mayer DJ (1996): Effects of the combined oral administration of NSAIDs and dextromethorphan on behavioral symptoms indicative of arthritic pain in rats. Pain 68:119–127.

Przesmycki K, Dzieciuch JA, Czuczwar SJ, Kleinrok Z (1997): Isobolographic analysis of interaction between intrathecal morphine and clonidine in the formalin test in rats. Eur J Pharmacol 337:11–17.

Raffa RB, Friderichs E, Reimann W, Shank RP, Codd EE, Vaught JL (1992): Opioid and nonopioid components independently contribute to the mechanism of action of tramadol, an 'atypical' opioid analgesic. J Pharmacol Exp Ther 260:275–285.

Raffa RB, Schupsky JJ, Lee DKH, Jacoby HI (1996): Characterization of endothelin-induced nociception in mice: Evidence for a mechanistically distinct analgesic model. J Pharmacol Exp Ther 278:1–7.

Rajagopalan P, Scribner RM, Pennev P, Schmidt WK, Tam SW, Steinfels GF, Cook L (1992): DUP 747—a new, potent, kappa opioid analgesic. Synthesis and pharmacology. Bioorg Med Chem Lett 2:715–720.

Reeve AJ, Dickenson AH (1995): The roles of spinal adenosine receptors in the control of acute and more persistent nociceptive responses of dorsal horn neurones in the anaesthetized rat. Br J Pharmacol 116:2221–2228.

Roane DS, Bounds JK, Ang C-Y, Adloo AA (1998): Quinpirole-induced alterations of tail temperature appear as hyperalgesia in the radiant heat tail-flick test. Pharmacol Biochem Behav 59:77–82.

Rosland JH, Tjølsen A, Maehle B, Hole K (1990): The formalin test in mice—effect of formalin concentration. Pain 42:235–242.

Rupniak NMJ, Webb JK, Williams AR, Carlson E, Boyce S, Hill RG (1995): Antinociceptive activity of the tachykinin NK_1 receptor antagonist, CP-99,994, in conscious gerbils. Br J Pharmacol 116:1937–1943.

REFERENCES

Rupniak NMJ, Carlson EJ, Boyce S, Webb JK, Hill RG (1996): Enantioselective inhibition of the formalin paw late phase by the NK-1 receptor antagonist L-733,060 in gerbils. Pain 67:189–195.

Rupniak NMJ, Boyce S, Webb JK, Williams AR, Carlson EJ, Hill RG, Borkowski JA, Hess JF (1997): Effects of the bradykinin B-1 receptor antagonist des-Arg^9 [Leu^8]bradykinin and genetic disruption of the B-2 receptor on nociception in rats and mice. Pain 71:89–97.

Sakurada T, Sakurada C, Tan-No K, Kisara K (1997): Neurokinin receptor antagonists—therapeutic potential in the treatment of pain syndromes. CNS Drugs 8:436–447.

Sancilio LF, Nolan JC, Wagner LE, Ward JW (1987): The analgesic and antiinflammatory activity and pharmacologic properties of bromfenac. Arzneimittelforschung 37:513–519.

Sawynok J, Reid A (1996): Caffeine antinociception: role of formalin concentration and adenosine A_1 and A_2 receptors. Eur J Pharmacol 298:105–111.

Schmidt WK, Tam SW, Shotzberger GS, Smith DH, Clark R, Vernier VG (1985): Nalbuphine. Drug Alc Dependence 14:339–362.

Seguin L, Le Marouille-Girardon S, Millan MJ (1995): Antinociceptive profiles of nonpeptidergic neurokinin-1 and neurokinin-2 receptor antagonists: a comparison to other classes of antinociceptive agent. Pain 61:325–343.

Seltzer Z, Dubner R, Shir Y (1990): A novel behavioral model of neuropathic pain disorders produced in rats by partial sciatic nerve injury. Pain 43:215–218.

Sengupta JN, Su X, Gebhart GF (1996): Kappa, but not mu or delta, opioids attenuate responses to distention of afferent fibers innervating the rat colon. Gastroenterology 111:968–980.

Shaw JS, Rourke JD, Burns KM (1988): Differential sensitivity of antinociceptive tests to opioid agonists and partial agonists. Br J Pharmacol 95:578–584.

Shibata M, Ohkubo T, Takahashi H, Inoki R (1989): Modified formalin test: characteristic biphasic pain response. Pain 38:347–352.

Shimoyama N, Shimoyama M, Davis AM, Inturrisi CE, Elliott KJ (1997): Spinal gabapentin is antinociceptive in the rat formalin test. Neurosci Lett 222:65–67.

Singh L, Field MJ, Ferris P, Hunter JC, Oles RJ, Williams RG, Woodruff GN (1996): The antiepileptic agent gabapentin (Neurontin) possesses anxiolytic-like and antinociceptive actions that are reversed by D-serine. Psychopharmacology 127:1–9.

Smith G, Harrison S, Bowers J, Wiseman J, Birch P (1994): Non-specific effects of the tachykinin NK$_1$ receptor antagonist, CP-99,994, in antinociceptive tests in rat, mouse and gerbil. Eur J Pharmacol 271:481–487.

Sora I, Funada M, Uhl GR (1997): The μ-opioid receptor is necessary for [D-Pen^2, D-Pen^5]enkephalin-induced analgesia. Eur J Pharmacol 324:R1–R2.

Staquet MJ (1989): A double-blind study with placebo control of intramuscular ketorolac tromethamine in the treatment of cancer pain. J Clin Pharmacol 29:1031–1036.

Steinfels GF, Cook L (1986): Antinociceptive profiles of mu and kappa opioid agonists in a rat tooth pulp stimulation procedure. J Pharmacol Exp Ther 236:111–117.

Stevens CW (1996): Relative analgesic potency of mu, delta and kappa opioids after spinal administration in amphibians. J Pharmacol Exp Ther 276:440–448.

Stevens CW, Rothe KS (1997): Supraspinal administration of opioids with selectivity for mu, delta and kappa opioid receptors produces analgesia in amphibians. Eur J Pharmacol 331:15–21.

Stevens CW, Klopp AJ, Facello JA (1994): Analgesic potency of mu and kappa opioids after systemic administration in amphibians. J Pharmacol Exp Ther 269:1086–1093.

Su X, Sengupta JN, Gebhart GF (1997): Effects of kappa opioid receptor-selective agonists on responses of pelvic nerve afferents to noxious colorectal distension. J Neurophysiol 78:1003–1012.

Sufka KJ, Roach JT (1996): Stimulus properties and antinociceptive effects of selective bradykinin B_1 and B_2 receptor antagonists in rats. Pain 66:99–103.

Swedberg MDB (1994): The mouse grid-shock analgesia test: pharmacological characterization of latency to vocalization threshold as an index of antinociception. J Pharmacol Exp Ther 269:1021–1028.

Taber RI (1974): Predictive value of analgesic assays in mice and rats. In Braude MC, Harris LS, May EL, Smith JP, Villarreal JE (eds): *Narcotic Antagonists*. New York: Raven Press, pp. 191–211.

Teng CJ, Abbott FV (1998): The formalin test: a dose-response analysis at three developmental stages. Pain 76:337–347.

Tiseo PJ, Geller EB, Adler MW (1988): Antinociceptive action of intracerebroventricularly administered dynorphin and other opioid peptides in the rat. J Pharmacol Exp Ther 246:449–453.

Tjølsen A, Berge O-G, Hunskaar S, Rosland JH, Hole K (1992): The formalin test—an evaluation of the method. Pain 51:5–17.

Traub RJ, Stitt S, Gebhart GF (1995): Attenuation of c-Fos expression in the rat lumbosacral spinal cord by morphine or tramadol following noxious colorectal distention. Brain Res 701:175–182.

Wang Y-X, Pettus M, Philips C, Gao D, Bowersox SS, Luther RR (1998): Antinociceptive properties of a selective, neuronal N-type calcium channel blocker, ziconotide (SNX-111), in a rat model of post-operative pain. Soc Neurosci Abstr 24:1626.

Watson GS, Sufka KJ, Coderre TJ (1997): Optimal scoring strategies and weights for the formalin test in rats. Pain 70:53–58.

Wettstein JG, Grouhel A (1996): Opioid antagonist profile of subcutaneous norbinaltorphimine in the formalin paw assay. Pharmacol Biochem Behav 53:411–416.

Wheeler-Aceto H, Cowan A (1991): Standardization of the rat paw formalin test for the evaluation of analgesics. Psychopharmacology 104:35–44.

Wheeler-Aceto H, Cowan A (1993): Naloxone causes apparent antinociception and pronociception simultaneously in the rat paw formalin test. Eur J Pharmacol 236:193–199.

Wheeler-Aceto H, Porreca F, Cowan A (1990): The rat paw formalin test—comparison of noxious agents. Pain 40:229–238.

Wirth W (1952): Methoden der Analgesieprufung am Tier. Arch Exp Path Pharmakol 216:77–83.

Woolfe G, Macdonald AD (1944): The evaluation of the analgesic action of pethidine hydrochloride (Demerol). J Pharmacol Exp Ther 80:300–307.

Xiao W-H, Bennett GJ (1995): Synthetic ω-conopeptides applied to the site of nerve injury suppress neuropathic pains in rats. J Pharmacol Exp Ther 274:666–672.

Xiao W-H, Bennett GJ (1996): Gabapentin has an antinociceptive effect mediated via a spinal site of action in a rat model of painful peripheral neuropathy. Analgesia 2: 267–273.

Yaksh TL (1997): Preclinical models of nociception. In Yaksh TL, Lynch C, Zapol WM, Maze M, Biebuyck JF, Saidman LJ (eds): *Anesthesia: Biologic Foundations*. Philadelphia: Lippincott-Raven, pp. 685–718.

Yaksh TL, Pogrel JW, Lee YW, Chaplan SR (1995): Reversal of nerve ligation-induced allodynia by spinal alpha-2 adrenoceptor agonists. J Pharmacol Exp Ther 272:207–214.

Yamamoto T, Nozaki-Taguchi N (1996): Clonidine, but not morphine, delays the development of thermal hyperesthesia induced by sciatic nerve constriction injury in the rat. Anesthesiology 85:835–845.

Yashpal K, Coderre TJ (1998): Influence of formalin concentration on the antinociceptive effects of anti-inflammatory drugs in the formalin test in rats: separate mechanisms underlying the nociceptive effects of low- and high-concentration formalin. Eur J Pain 2:63–68.

Yeomans DC, Proudfit HK (1994): Characterization of the foot withdrawal response to noxious radiant heat in the rat. Pain 59:85–94.

Zahn PK, Brennan TJ (1998): Lack of effect of intrathecally administered N-methyl-D-aspartate receptor antagonists in a rat model for postoperative pain. Anesthesiology 88:143–156.

Zahn PK, Gysbers D, Brennan TJ (1997): Effect of systemic and intrathecal morphine in a rat model of postoperative pain. Anesthesiology 86:1066–1077.

Zahn PK, Umali E, Brennan TJ (1998): Intrathecal non-NMDA excitatory animo acid receptor antagonists inhibit pain behaviors in a rat model of postoperative pain. Pain 74:213–223.

Zimet PO, Wynn RL, Ford RD, Rudo FG (1986): Effect of hot plate temperature on the antinociceptive activity of mixed opioid agonist-antagonist compounds. Drug Develop Res 7:277–280.

CHAPTER 3

RECENT ADVANCES IN THE PHARMACOLOGY OF OPIOIDS

MICHAEL H. OSSIPOV, JOSEPHINE LAI, T. PHILIP MALAN, JR., and FRANK PORRECA
University of Arizona Health Sciences Center
Tucson, Arizona

The efficacy of opioids as analgesics in conditions of acute pain is well established. Opioids are routinely used in postoperative pain and in the treatment of many painful conditions of short-term duration. Morphine, the prototypical opioid analgesic, is the reference standard against which the activity of pain treatments is measured, and morphine serves as the reference for antinociceptive activity in analgesiometric assays for acute nociception. Not all pain states respond identically to opioids, however. Pain of inflammatory origin is well treated by opioids, and evidence suggests that opioids may have enhanced activity in these conditions. In contrast, pain of neuropathic origin is generally believed, though not established, to be resistant to treatment with opioids. The changes in observed opioid activity in chronic pain situations may be related to various neurochemical and neuroanatomical changes that occur in the central nervous system and in the periphery. Such changes may include alterations in spinal dynorphin or cholecystokinin (CCK) levels, increased release of neuropeptide transmitters and excitatory amino acids leading to states of "central sensitization," sprouting of axons to enlarge the receptive fields, and phenotypic changes of primary afferent neurons. This chapter focuses on opioid activity identified in more recent studies, and on the activity of opioids in chronic pain states, with a particular emphasis on pain of neuropathic origin.

ACTIVITY OF OPIOIDS IN PAIN STATES

Pain States and Opioid Activity

In general, acute pain can be easily differentiated from chronic pain states such as those arising from inflammatory processes and nerve injury. Acute pain is

---

Novel Aspects of Pain Management: Opioids and Beyond, Edited by Jana Sawynok and Alan Cowan
ISBN 0-471-180173 Copyright © 1999 by Wiley-Liss, Inc.

defined by the International Association for the Study of Pain (IASP) as "an unpleasant sensory and emotional experience associated with actual or potential tissue damage" (for discussion, see Chaplan and Sorkin, 1997). Thus acute nociception generally elicits a protective or defensive response to a noxious stimulus. Inflammatory pain is associated with tissue damage and a resultant inflammatory response. It may be regarded as a mechanism to avoid contact with the area to allow healing to occur; thus there may be an advantage to its presence. It is no longer present once the inflammation has subsided. Neuropathic pain, on the other hand, may occur in the absence of any obvious tissue injury, and it may continue long after an original causative injury has resolved. The chronic pain states, whether of inflammatory or neuropathic origin, are often characterized by hyperalgesia and allodynia. Hyperalgesia refers to an increased response to a stimulus that is normally painful, whereas allodynia refers to pain or a nociceptive response to a stimulus that is normally not painful. In keeping with these definitions, a manipulation is considered to be *antinociceptive* when a raised threshold to a noxious stimulus occurs. A manipulation is considered to be *antihyperalgesic* when enhanced responses to nociception are returned to, but not above, baseline levels. An *antiallodynic* effect is indicated when apparently noxious responses to normally non-noxious stimuli are abolished. It is important to note that antihyperalgesic and antiallodynic manipulations are not always interchangeable, and that neither manipulation might be antinociceptive (see Chaplan and Sorkin, 1997; Willis, 1997 for discussions on pain terminology).

Acute pain is exemplified by postsurgical or postincisional pain, and opioid analgesics are well tolerated and efficacious (Arner and Meyerson, 1988). Opioids may demonstrate increased activity in inflammatory pain situations. Studies in animals with inflammatory conditions have clearly shown that morphine and other opioid agonists are more efficacious as antinociceptive agents than in normal animals (Kayser and Guilbaud, 1983; Neil et al., 1986). Stanfa and Dickenson (1993) demonstrated that the potency of morphine to inhibit evoked C-fiber activity was increased 30-fold in the carrageenan-inflamed rat. Increases in sensitivity to the antinociceptive effect of morphine following inflammation have also been shown using behavioral assays (Stanfa et al., 1994). More recently, Ossipov et al. (1995a) demonstrated enhanced efficacy of systemic or intrathecal morphine in rats with carrageenan-induced inflammation, and showed that this enhancement was sensitive to naltrindole (NTI), suggesting complex interactions among neurotransmitters in the spinal cord (see below). In other studies, rat hindpaws inflamed with Freund's complete adjuvant demonstrated greater sensitivity to systemically injected morphine or U50,488H than did the contralateral, noninflamed paw (Stein et al., 1988b). The enhanced antinociceptive effect of morphine, but not the inflammation itself, was abolished in this preparation by capsaicin, pointing to an involvement of primary afferent nociceptive C-fibers in the development of the enhanced response to morphine.

Although it is generally considered that clinical neuropathic pain is resistant to amelioration by opioids, the utility of opioid analgesics in the clinical treatment of neuropathic pain is a matter of considerable controversy. In contrast to pain arising from tissue injury, neuropathic pain was found to be resistant to treatment by intravenous infusion of morphine (Arner and Meyerson, 1988). Similar observations have been reported by a number of investigators (Twycross, 1982; Tasker et al., 1983). Max and colleagues (1988) reported in a controlled clinical study that oral codeine was ineffective against postherpetic neuralgia (PHN), another form of neuropathic pain, but failure in that study was attributed to an insufficient dose of codeine (Rowbotham et al., 1991). In a later double-blind, placebo-controlled study, it was found that intravenous morphine or lidocaine were both effective against PHN (Rowbotham et al., 1991). Many reported clinical studies of opioid efficacy against neuropathic pain have employed morphine or opioids of lesser efficacy (see Arner and Meyerson, 1988), and the use of compounds with greater analgesic efficacy must be considered. For example, fentanyl given spinally to patients with post-amputation stump pain provided immediate, long-lasting (8 hr), and complete pain relief that was considered to be superior to that of spinal lidocaine (Jacobson et al., 1990). Significantly, both in clinical situations or animal models, the ability of opioids to treat signs of neuropathic pain effectively appears to be influenced by many factors, including the etiology of the nerve injury, the type of pain involved (e.g., hyperalgesia, tactile allodynia, cold allodynia), the efficacy of the opioids given, and the route of administration employed. Neuropathic pain presents the greatest challenge in pain management, and calls for greater understanding of underlying mechanisms in order to maximize opioid therapies.

Sites of Action of Opioids

Supraspinal Sites of Opioid Activity. Opioids exert their antinociceptive actions from supraspinal, spinal, and peripheral sites, providing a multitude of areas that may be targeted in the treatment of pain with opioids. The activation of opioid receptors at supraspinal sites activate descending inhibitory systems and inhibit descending facilitatory systems. Evidence exists to establish that opioid induced antinociception is mediated in part by descending pathways arising chiefly from the ventrolateral periaqueductal gray (PAG), mesencephalic reticular formation, rostroventral medulla (RVM), nucleus gigantocellularis (NGC), and the raphe nuclei, particularly the nucleus raphe magnus (NRM) (Yaksh and Rudy, 1978). Because the prototypic opioid used in the majority of studies involving supraspinal loci of antinociceptive activity was morphine, a predominantly μ-opioid agonist, a great deal of information regarding the participation of this opioid receptor type in modulation of nociception has been gathered. For example, early studies had shown that opioids microinjected into the PAG produced antinociception (Yaksh et al., 1976; Lewis and Gebhart, 1977; Yaksh and Rudy, 1978). Morphine microinjection into the PAG has also attenuated activity of projection neurons in response to peripheral nociceptive stimuli (Bennett and Mayer, 1979). Jensen and Yaksh (1986a,b) showed that administration of morphine in the medullary reticular formation (MRF) produced antinociception in rats. More recent studies demonstrated that intracerebroventricular (i.c.v.) microinjection of [D-Ala^2,NMPhe^4,Gly-ol]enkephalin (DAMGO) (Gogas et al., 1991) or of morphine (Gogas et al., 1996) exhibited dose-dependent, naloxone-reversible attenuation of both phases of formalin-induced flinching. The antinociceptive effects correlated well with inhibition of FOS-like immunoreactivity (FLI) in the superficial laminae of the dorsal horn of the spinal cord, which is generally accepted as a marker for neuronal activity in response to nociception, although nociception may occur in the absence of increased spinal FLI and, conversely, increased spinal FLI may occur in the absence of nociception. These studies support the hypothesis that supraspinal μ-opioid activity results in an increase in descending inhibitory control (Gogas et al., 1996).

A number of recent experiments have focused on the role of δ-opioid receptors with regard to supraspinal modulation of nociception. The i.c.v. administration of selective δ-opioid agonists has produced dose-dependent antinociception in rats (Miaskowski et al., 1991) and in normal mice (Porreca et al., 1987; Heyman et al., 1989; Jiang et al., 1990), as well as in the μ-opioid receptor deficient CXBK mouse (Vaught et al., 1988). These early data with the CXBK mouse are consistent with more recent findings using μ-opioid receptor knock-out animals. In these μ-knock-out mice, i.c.v. administration of [D-Ala^2, Glu^4]deltorphin produced the same degree of antinociception in the 55°C tail-flick test as in wild-type controls (Hosohata et al., 1999). On the other hand, the potency of i.c.v. [D-Pen^{2,5}]-enkephalin (DPDPE) was decreased by approximately 30-fold in the μ-knock-out mice when compared with the wild type (Hosohata et al., 1999). Sora and colleagues (1997) suggested that i.c.v. DPDPE is inactive in animals with a genetic deletion of μ-opioid receptors, but such findings may represent differences in the observed potency of a compound with a μ-opioid receptor component of action. Similar findings were seen with intrathecal administration of [D-Ala^2, Glu^4]deltorphin, which retains full antinociceptive potency in μ-knock-out and wild-type mice, and DPDPE, which shows significantly lower potency in the μ-knock-out animals (Hosohata et al., 1999). Systemic administration of SNC 80, a selective nonpeptidic δ-opioid agonist, also showed full antinociceptive activity in μ-knock-out and wild-type control mice. These studies suggest that activation of δ-opioid receptors consistently elicits antinociception that is independent of other receptor types, including μ-opioid receptors. Animals bred to be genetically deficient in μ-opioid receptors offer significant opportunities to explore specific roles of δ-opioid receptors in modulation of nociception, and also offer insight into ultimate degrees of selectivity of experimental opioid agonists. In this regard, the antinociceptive actions of δ-opioid receptor agonists have been somewhat inconsistent in different animal models and endpoints. Some studies failed to detect antinociception produced by i.c.v. deltorphins (Negri et al., 1991) or found inconsistent results with i.c.v. DPDPE (Adams et al., 1993) using the hot water or cold water rat tail flick test, respectively. Recent data suggest that [D-Ala^2, Glu^4]deltorphin and DPDPE, administered into the rat MRF, elicit limited antinociception in a tail flick end point, but are fully active in the hot plate test, suggesting the possibility of a supraspinally integrated influence on nociceptive processes (Ossipov et al., 1994).

The serotonergic NRM has been shown to communicate with the PAG and to have serotonergic projections to the spinal cord, and thus may function as a relay for descending antinociceptive information arising from the midbrain site (Conrad et al., 1976; Basbaum and Fields, 1979). Microinjection of morphine into the NRM produces naloxone-sensitive antinociception (Oliveras et al., 1977; Dickenson et al., 1979). More recently, stimulation of the PAG produced antinociception that was attenuated by lidocaine administered into both the NRM and adjacent reticular formation, suggesting an activation of descending inhibition originating from the PAG (Sandkuhler and Gebhart, 1984). Application of morphine into the NRM or the NGC has also produced antinociception in rats by activating spinopetal (possibly serotonergic and GABAergic) mechanisms (Kiefel et al., 1993; McGowan and Hammond, 1993; Rossi et al., 1993).

Recent studies indicated that DPDPE or [D-Ala^2, Glu^4]deltorphin microinjected into the NRM and NGC produced dose-dependent antinociception in the rat tail flick, but not the 55°C hot plate, test (Thorat and Hammond, 1997). The antagonism of the antinociceptive effect of DPDPE by 7-benzylidinenaltrexone (BNTX) and of [D-Ala^2, Glu^4]deltorphin by naltriben (NTB) without cross-antagonism provided further evidence that both the δ_1- and δ_2-opioid receptors of the ventromedial medulla (VMM) contribute to descending modulation of nociception. The observation that neither antagonist alone in the VMM produced heightened nociceptive responses argued against a tonic inhibitory enkephalinergic input to the VMM (Thorat and Hammond, 1997). More recently, the microinjection of [D-Ala^2, Glu^4]deltorphin into the MRF was shown to produce dose-dependent inhibition of the first and second phases of formalin-induced flinching of the rat hindpaw, indicating antinociceptive activity of supraspinal δ_2-opioid receptors against acute nociception and against tonic nociception arising from central and/or peripheral sensitization of nociceptors (Kovelowski et al.,1998). The antinociceptive activity was accompanied by decreased FLI in the superficial laminae of the dorsal horn of the lumbar cord, supporting the behavioral observations. That activation of supraspinal δ_2-opioid receptors may modulate nociception at the spinal level was clearly demonstrated when bilateral lesions of the dorsolateral funiculus (DLF) completely abolished both the antinociceptive and spinal FLI suppressive activity of [D-Ala^2, Glu^4]deltorphin given into the MRF (Kovelowski et al., 1999). It was recently suggested that differing descending pathways, arising from several medullary nuclei and releasing different neurotransmitters in the spinal cord, may modulate different types of nociception and/or serve differing regions of the body (Proudfit and Fang, 1995). Additionally, microinjection of DAMGO into the PAG or the RVM produced antinociception against thermal noxious stimuli in the rat, and this effect was potentiated by the microinjection of [D-Ala^2, Glu^4]deltorphin into the region not receiving DAMGO, whereas co-administration of DAMGO and [D-Ala^2, Glu^4]deltorphin into the same site produced an additive effect, indicating a synergistic interaction dependent upon pathways rather than cellular interactions (Rossi et al., 1994).

The action of supraspinal κ-opioid receptor agonists with regard to modulation of nociception remains unclear. The microinjection of U50488H into the PAG or NRM was reportedly inactive against thermal noxious stimuli applied to the tail of the rat (Rossi et al., 1994). In contrast, the i.c.v. injection of the κ-opioid agonist CI-977 produced dose-dependent inhibition of both phases of formalin-induced flinching, and this effect was blocked by naloxone or nor-binaltorphimine (nor-BNI) (Gogas et al., 1996). Lesions of the DLF did not alter the antinociceptive action of i.c.v. CI-977, indicating an exclusively supraspinal modulation of nociception (Gogas et al., 1996). It is generally observed that κ-opioid agonists given supraspinally modulate nociception to noxious pressure or formalin injection, but are inactive against thermal noxious stimuli (Gogas et al., 1996). Interestingly, κ-opioid agonists have been shown to antagonize the antinociceptive action of morphine (Bhargava, 1994), an observation that was recently confirmed by in vitro electrophysiological evidence (Pan et al., 1997). Whole-cell patch clamp recordings demonstrated that U69593 or dynorphin produces a hyperpolarization of a subpopulation of NRM cells by increasing K$^+$ conductance (Pan et al., 1997). Activation of μ-opioid receptors produces a hyperpolarization of a different population of NRM neurons, which leads to a disinhibition of "primary" NRM neurons and so produces opioid-mediated antinociception through projections to the spinal cord. Hyperpolarization of these neurons, through the κ-opioid receptor, counteracts μ-opioid-mediated disinhibition (Pan et al., 1997). Parallel studies with DAMGO microinjected into the PAG and U69593 into the NRM confirmed a κ-opioid receptor-mediated antagonism of μ-opioid-mediated antinociception in the rat-tail flick (Pan et al., 1997).

Spinal Sites of Opioid Activity. A large body of evidence exists indicating that opioids also exert their antinociceptive action through the spinal cord. Opioid receptors located on the presynaptic terminals of unmyelinated nociceptor C fibers induce hyperpolarization, preventing the release of substance P (Aimone and Yaksh, 1989). Additionally, opioid receptors located postsynaptically on cell bodies of projection neurons also inhibit the ascending transmission of nociceptive input to supraspinal centers. Besse et al. (1990) found that dorsal rhizotomy produces an approximate 70% loss of δ-opioid and 60% loss of spinal μ-opioid receptors, suggesting that opioid receptor populations may exist both on primary afferent nerve terminals and on cell bodies of neurons in the dorsal horn of the spinal cord, though predominantly on the former. In situ hybridization techniques have revealed the existence of mRNA for μ- and κ-opioid receptors in soma of the dorsal root ganglia, which have axonal projections both to the spinal cord and to the periphery (Maekawa et al., 1994). Mansour and colleagues (1994, 1995) have described a possible differential distribution of mRNA for opioid receptors in cells of the dorsal root ganglion (DRG). Expression of mRNA for the μ-opioid receptor was found in medium- and large-diameter DRG cells, whereas that for the δ-opioid receptor was thought to be predominantly in large-diameter neurons, and that for the κ-opioid receptor in smaller-diameter neurons. Opioid receptor binding distributions are predominant in the DRG and the superficial layers of the dorsal horn (Mansour et al., 1995), corresponding with terminals of C fibers rather than the terminal region of larger-diameter fibers (e.g., laminae 3 and 4). Finally, Taddese and colleagues (1995), using patch-clamp techniques on isolated nociceptors, found that activation of μ-opioid receptors predictably inhibited Ca^{2+} channels of small-diameter nociceptors and not of large-diameter cells, suggesting that μ-opioid receptor activation selectively inhibits the activity of C fibers. Other evidence supports the view that the δ-opioid receptors of the spinal dorsal horn are located presynaptically on the terminals of primary afferents (C fibers) or on descending modulatory fibers (Dado et al., 1993; Arvidsson et al., 1995). Further support for this interpretation was provided by a recent study in which FLI was correlated to antinociceptive activity of spinally injected DAMGO, DPDPE, or [D-Ala^2, Glu^4]deltorphin (Hammond et al., 1998). All three opioid peptides produced dose-dependent inhibition of both phases of formalin-induced flinching. Receptor specificity was confirmed by antagonism of DAMGO by CTOP, and of DPDPE by BNTX and of [D-Ala^2, Glu^4]deltorphin by NTB without cross-antagonism. The antinociceptive effect of intrathecal DAMGO was accompanied by decreased spinal FLI, but that of either DPDPE or [D-Ala^2, Glu^4]deltorphin was not. It was concluded that unlike the μ-opioid receptors, spinal δ$_1$- and δ$_2$-opioid receptors do not modulate the activation of the immediate-early gene, *c-fos* (Hammond et al., 1998). Additionally, these data further suggest that spinal δ-opioid receptors act chiefly by presynaptic inhibition of neurotransmitter release from primary afferent fibers rather than hyperpolarizing dorsal horn neurons (Hammond et al., 1998). These findings are in contrast to recent data showing that intrathecal administration of [D-Ala^2, Glu^4]deltorphin or DPDPE can produce both a decrease in formalin flinching and FLI (Kovelowski et al., 1998). Differences in methodology appear responsible for the divergent results, with the latter study employing a lower concentration and volume of formalin (Kovelowski et al., 1998).

Peripheral Sites of Opioid Activity. In addition to central effects, opioids also exert an antinociceptive effect at peripheral sites. Local, peripheral antinociceptive actions of opioids have been demonstrated both in a large number of animal experiments and in clinical studies, and peripheral opioids appear to be more effective in the presence of inflammation (Stein and Yassouridis, 1997). The fact that peripheral opioids demonstrate dose-dependent activity and are antagonized by the selective antagonist naloxone in a stereospecific manner (Stein et al., 1988a; 1989) indicates receptor-specific effects. Functional opioid receptors of all three subtypes, μ, δ, and κ, have been identified in peripheral tissue (Barber and Gottschlich, 1992; Stein, 1993). Additionally, the endogenous opioid peptides enkephalin, dynorphin, and endorphin have also been found in immune cells in inflamed peripheral tissue (Stein et al., 1990b; Stein, 1995). Further support for a peripheral antinociceptive action of opioids is suggested by the observations that (a) locally applied morphine may be antinociceptive at less than systemic doses, (b) quaternary opioid agonists, which presumably do not cross the blood–brain barrier, have an antinociceptive effect, and (c) the antinociceptive effect of locally applied opioids may be blocked by locally applied quaternary naltrexone (see Stein et al., 1990b; Stein, 1993; Stein and Yassouridis, 1997 for reviews). Such studies serve to indicate an important function of peripheral opioid activity with regard to antinociceptive and antiinflammatory activity.

Immunocytochemical studies using an immunogold silver staining technique have identified the presence of opioid receptors on peripheral nerve terminals of small diameter primary afferent nerves (Stein et al., 1990b). The receptors were visualized with a mouse monoclonal antiidiotypic antibody raised against μ- and δ-opioid receptors. Specificity was demonstrated by an absence of staining in sections that were pre-incubated with antibody (Stein et al., 1990b). Competition studies using DAMGO, DPDPE, and U50488H to compete for human [^{125}I]β-endorphin further demonstrated the presence of opioid receptors in peripheral nerve terminals of unmyelinated and thinly myelinated primary afferent fibers of rats (Hassan et al., 1993; Stein, 1995). Similar studies have likewise visualized opioid receptors in peripheral terminals of small-diameter nerve fibers in human tissue (Stein et al., 1996). In situ hybridization studies with antisense probes to μ- and κ-opioid receptors have demonstrated the presence of mRNA for these receptors in the cell bodies in dorsal root ganglia of rats (Maekawa et al., 1994). These neurons possess axonal projections to the spinal cord and to the periphery, and transport of opioid receptors from the cell body to the peripheral terminals has been demonstrated (Hassan et al., 1993). The presence of mRNA to μ-opioid receptors in the DRG has also been shown by a ribonuclease protection assay (Schafer et al., 1995). More recently, it was demonstrated that the intrathecal injection of antisense, but not mismatch, oligodeoxynucleotide to the δ-opioid receptor blocked the antinociceptive action against formalin-induced flinching of the $δ_2$-opioid agonist [D-Ala^2, Glu^4]deltorphin, but not of the μ-opioid agonist morphine or the κ-opioid agonist CI-977, when these substances were injected directly into the paw (Bilsky et al., 1996). Similar conclusions were reached when μ-opioid receptors were targeted with intrathecal administration of antisense oligodeoxynucleotides (Khasar et al., 1996). These results indicate that, like the μ- and κ-opioid receptors, δ-opioid receptors may also be synthesized in the DRG and transported to the peripheral and central terminals of the primary afferent neurons.

The endogenous ligands for the opioid receptors in the periphery are apparently not present in normal (noninflamed) tissue. Immunocytochemistry and radioimmunoassay studies for β-endorphin, [Met^5]enkephalin, and dynorphin in rat paws revealed an absence of these substances in normal tissue (Stein et al., 1990b). However, when inflammation was induced by Freund's complete adjuvant, strong staining for β-endorphin and for [Met^5]enkephalin, but not for dynorphin, was observed and appeared to be localized in immunocytes infiltrating the site of inflammation (Stein et al., 1990b). In this and other studies, cold water swim stress antinociception in rats with inflamed paws was blocked by intraplantar injections of the immunosuppressant, cyclosporine, or by antibodies to β-endorphin, but not to [Met^5]enkephalin or to dynorphin. It was suggested that immune cells may mediate antinociception locally by the release of endogenous stores of β-endorphin, which activates opioid receptors on peripheral nerve terminals (Stein et al., 1990a,b). This observation was further strengthened by the findings that, through in situ hybridization, mRNA for proopiomelanocortin and for proenkephalin, but not for prodynorphin, was detected in inflamed but not in normal tissue obtained from rat hindpaw (Przewlocki et al., 1992). In agreement with this finding, β-endorphin and [Met^5]enkephalin, but not dynorphin, were detected in inflamed tissue and appeared to be localized in T- and B-lymphocytes, monocytes, and macrophages (Przewlocki et al., 1992). In a more recent study, Cabot and colleagues (1997) found that in rats without inflammation, β-endorphin and mRNA for proopiomelanocortin are predominant in T-lymphocytes residing in lymph nodes. In the presence of inflammation, the β-endorphin containing memory-type T lymphocytes migrates to the site of inflammation to release β-endorphin. Based on these studies, it appears that the peripheral opioid receptors act to modulate inflammatory nociception through an endogenous peripheral pain control system (Stein and Yassouridis, 1997).

It is generally believed that the peripheral antinociceptive action of morphine is mediated through actions on peripheral terminals of C fibers. In an early study, electrical stimulation of the inferior alveolar nerve was shown to induce a significant release of substance P in dental pulp of cats, which contains exclusively nociceptive sensory neurons (Brodin et al., 1983). The intravenous infusion of morphine blocked substance P release without affecting sensory nerve conduction. In later studies, it was shown that the antidromic stimulation of the sciatic nerve with stimulation parameters consistent with activation of rapidly and slowly conducting fibers (i.e., Aβ, Aδ, C fibers), or by the addition of capsaicin to the perfusate, resulted in release of substance P-like immunoreactivity (SP-LI) in the synovial perfusate of the knee joint (Yaksh, 1988). In contrast, the antidromic stimulation of rapidly conducting fibers only (i.e., Aβ fibers) did not indicate any substance P release. The addition of the μ-opioid agonists sufentanil or DAMGO or of the δ-opioid agonist DPDPE to the synovial perfusate attenuated the stimulation produced increase in SP-LI in a naloxone-reversible manner, whereas the κ-opioid agonist U50488H was without effect (Yaksh, 1988). These data were interpreted to indicate that peripheral release of SP-LI may be mediated by μ- or δ-opioid receptors on the peripheral terminals of small-diameter primary afferent neurons. Inhibition of peripheral release of substance P may also underlie an anti-inflammatory effect of peripheral opioid activity, because substance P is a mediator of peripheral sensitization and contributes to immune response of immunocytes (Stein, 1993; Stein and Yassouridis, 1997). For example, neurogenic plasma extravasation, which may be elicited by substance P release at an inflamed site, is inhibited by DAMGO or U50488H (Barber, 1993).

Electrophysiological studies also support opioid-mediated suppression of peripheral C-fiber nociceptor activity. In studies where hyperalgesia was induced by ultraviolet irradiation of the hindpaw of rats, normally quiescent polymodal nociceptors were spontaneously active in the receptive field of the inflamed skin, and this activity was enhanced by capsaicin (Andreev et al., 1994). The local injection of morphine, DAMGO, or U69593, but not of DPDPE, to the receptive field produced a suppression of spontaneous activity of the polymodal nociceptors in a dose-dependent, naloxone-reversible manner. These experiments indicate a receptor-mediated sensitivity of peripheral nociceptors to excitation by μ- and κ-opioid agonists (Andreev et al., 1994). It was also demonstrated that the intra-arterial injection of morphine or U50488H close to the inflamed knee joint of anesthetized cats produced dose-dependent, naloxone-reversible suppression of the spontaneous activity of small-diameter afferent units (Russell et al., 1987). This study provides additional electrophysiological evidence for activity of opioid receptors located at peripheral sites of primary afferent fibers.

The peripheral action of opioids is especially pronounced in the inflammatory state, both in animal models and in clinical practice. In one early study, the intraplantar injection of fentanyl blocked responses to noxious paw pressure in the hindpaws of rats with inflammation, but was without effect in normal rats (Stein et al., 1988a). This effect of fentanyl was dose-dependent and reversed by (−)- but not (+)-naloxone given locally. Intraplantar (−)-naloxone also reversed the enhanced antinociceptive effect of systemic morphine and U50488H in rats with inflammation caused by Freund's complete adjuvant (Stein et al., 1988a). Dose-dependent antinociceptive effects were also demonstrated in inflamed, but not normal, paws by intraplantar injections of DAMGO, DPDPE, and U50488H, indicating a functional role for peripheral μ-, κ- and δ-opioid receptors (Stein et al., 1989).

The enhanced antinociceptive action of peripheral opioids is believed to be due in part to increased axonal transport of opioid receptors. Ligation of the sciatic nerve in normal animals indicated a gathering of opioid binding sites proximal and distal to the ligation, as identified by in vitro autoradiography with human [^{125}I]β-endorphin as the radioligand (Hassan et al., 1993), indicating a bidirectional axonal transport of the opioid receptors. In the presence of inflammation of the rat hindpaw induced by Freund's adjuvant, there was a large increase in opioid receptors on both sides of the ligature and a corresponding increase in density in the inflamed tissue, indicating that inflammation stimulates axonal transport of opioid receptors (Hassan et al., 1993). Disruption of the perineureal barrier at the site of inflammation may also lead to increased access of peripherally administered opioids to the nerve. Antonijevic and co-workers (1995) found complementary time courses for the development of Freund's adjuvant-induced inflammation, perineureal leakage, and antinociception to intraplantar injections of U50488H, DAMGO, and DPDPE at doses inactive in the normal paw. Similarly, disruption of the perineureal barrier by hyperosmotic saline or mannitol also allowed these opioid agonists to exhibit antinociceptive activity. These findings indicate that disruption of the perineural barrier during inflammation allows endogenous opioid peptides released from immunocytes to have unrestricted transperineural passage (Antonijevic et al., 1995).

Clinical experience with peripherally applied opioids has produced mixed results. A recent meta-analysis of clinical studies over the past 30 years (1966 to 1996) in which opioids were given peripherally and excluding those studies in which intra-articular injections were made, suggested that there was insufficient evidence to support a clinically relevant peripheral analgesic activity (Picard et al., 1997). A similar type of analysis was performed regarding the analgesic benefit of intra-articular morphine after knee surgery (Kalso et al., 1997). In this review of clinical studies, a clearer clinical benefit against postoperative pain was detected, but the conclusion remained that additional and better controlled studies are needed in order to produce a firm conclusion. However, these reviews are less than definitive partly because clinical studies in which opioids or local anesthetics were given peri-operatively or when trial sample sizes were less than 10 have been excluded (Stein and Yassouridis, 1997). In several cases studied, statistically significant analgesia was detected but determined to be of insufficient magnitude to be clinically significant (Picard et al., 1997). A more comprehensive review would produce convincing evidence of a significant clinical analgesic benefit of peripherally administered opioids (Stein and Yassouridis, 1997). In one double-blind, randomized trial morphine given intra-articularly during arthroscopy produced significant lowering of pain scores postoperatively and also significantly reduced postoperative opioid consumption (Stein et al., 1991). A more recent randomized, double-blind, crossover clinical study clearly demonstrated that intra-articular morphine produced long-lasting pain relief in patients with osteoarthritis of the knee joints (Likar et al., 1997). Clinical studies have also shown that inflamed knee joints may be associated with significant synovial cellular infiltration (Stein et al., 1996). Patients with cellular infiltration showed marked increases in opioid receptor and opioid peptide levels in tissue specimens removed during arthroscopy when compared to inflamed tissue without cellular infiltration; levels were below limits of detection in normal tissue. Interestingly, the same dose of intra-articular morphine provided the same degree of analgesia, regardless of the concentration of endogenous opioid peptides or of cellular infiltration; additionally, no receptor down-regulation was observed in the presence of elevated levels of endogenous opioids. These data were taken to indicate that inflamed tissue does not produce tolerance to the analgesic effect of morphine given peripherally (Stein et al., 1996). A lack of tolerance development, along with an absence of central effects, provides a clear benefit pertaining to the development and use of peripherally acting opioids for pain relief.

NEUROCHEMICAL CHANGES IN CHRONIC PAIN STATES

Inflammatory Pain

Unilateral paw inflammation induced by a subcutaneous injection of carrageenan (Kocher et al., 1987) elicits changes in the transcription of opioid and other peptides in the spinal cord. Increases in preprodynorphin mRNA and preproenkephalin mRNA have been observed during inflammation (Dubner and Ruda, 1992). Moreover, it has clearly been shown that morphine and other opioid agonists are more efficacious as antinociceptive agents in animals with inflammatory conditions than in normal animals (Kayser and Guilbaud, 1983; Neil et al., 1986), and that the basis for the increase in morphine potency may be due, in part, to decreases in levels of spinal CCK (Stanfa et al., 1994), a peptide that has been demonstrated to act as an endogenous anti-opioid. The ability of a CCK_B antagonist to potentiate the activity of spinal morphine against C-fiber-evoked excitation of dorsal horn neurons, present in normal rats, was lost in animals with carrageenan-induced inflammation of the hindpaw. The enhanced potency of morphine in rats with carrageenan-induced inflammation was sensitive to blockade by δ-opioid receptor selective doses of naltrindole (Ossipov et al., 1995a). These data further indicate that the increased activity of spinal morphine in inflammatory states may be due to a reduction in the activity of spinal CCK (Stanfa and Dickenson, 1993).

Neuropathic Pain

Spinal CCK Is Elevated in Conditions of Neuropathy. In contrast to inflammation, neuropathy may result in increased spinal CCK levels (Stanfa et al., 1994). In situ hybridization studies have demonstrated increased preprocholecystokinin mRNA levels in the rat dorsal root ganglia or monkey dorsal horn after nerve transection (Verge et al., 1993), further suggesting a role for CCK in augmenting sensory input subsequent to nerve damage. Sciatic nerve section was found to produce autotomy (self-mutilation of the ipsilateral limb and paw) along with an upregulation of CCK mRNA in primary sensory neurons of the rat dorsal root ganglia (Xu et al., 1993). It was also demonstrated, by the same group, that incomplete ischemic injury of the spinal cord in rats produced signs of tactile allodynia, suggestive of chronic central pain in clinical cases of spinal cord injury (Xu et al., 1994a). The allodynia induced in this model was relieved by systemic injections of the selective CCK_B antagonist CI-988, and this effect was in turn blocked by naloxone. It was suggested that disruption of a normal tonic opioidergic control of nociceptive impulses following spinal cord injury may be the result of an upregulation of an endogenous spinal CCK system that allows the development of abnormal pain sensation (Xu et al., 1994a,b). Hyperalgesia might be partly mediated by descending facilitatory pathways arising from the rostral ventromedial medulla and releasing CCK in the spinal cord (Urban et al., 1996).

Elevated Opioid Peptides in Neuropathic Pain. Peripheral nerve injury has been shown to elevate spinal quantities of the endogenous opioid peptides, including enkephalins and dynorphin (Dubner and Ruda, 1992). In spite of the fact that dynorphin was originally isolated and subsequently demonstrated to have potent opioid activity, mediated primarily via κ receptors, it is clear that this peptide possesses a significant nonopioid pharmacology that may have great significance in the nerve injury state. A pathological role for endogenous spinal dynorphin may be suggested by observations that levels of endogenous dynorphin are elevated after traumatic injury of the spinal cord (Cox et al., 1985), and that behavioral sequelae of spinal cord trauma may be diminished by the intrathecal administration of antiserum to dynorphin (Faden, 1990; Shukla and Lemaire, 1994). Likewise, spinal dynorphin levels are increased after spinal nerve injury, and dynorphin antiserum given intrathecally reduces neurological impairment after such injuries (Cox et al., 1985; Faden, 1990).

NONPATHOLOGICAL INTERACTIONS OF DYNORPHIN AND OPIOIDS

In addition to the view that endogenous peptides, such as dynorphin, may be important mediators of pathological states, it is clear that physiologically relevant roles for such substances can be demonstrated under conditions of normal pain. Such a physiological role is suggested by recent studies indicating a tonic inhibitory control of afferent nociceptive input (Ossipov et al., 1996). In these studies, the formalin-induced flinch response in rats is markedly increased after naloxone, strongly suggesting that endogenous opioids released in response to peripheral nociceptive input may exert an inhibition of tonic nociception (Wheeler-Aceto and Cowan, 1993; Ossipov et al., 1996). It was also found that receptor subtype selective doses of intrathecal NTI or nor-BNI (κ-opioid antagonist), but not β-funaltrexamine (β-FNA) (μ-opioid antagonist), increased the number of flinches, suggesting an involvement of κ- and δ-opioid but not μ-opioid selective endogenous substances. Furthermore, intrathecal antisera to [Leu^5]enkephalin and dynorphin A$_{1-17}$ but not to [Met^5]enkephalin also increased flinching responses, suggesting the likelihood that endogenous [Leu^5]enkephalin and dynorphin, or like substances, may be released during tonic nociception and act to limit the nociceptive input (Ossipov et al., 1996). These studies, and those of Wheeler-Aceto and Cowan (1993), represent a clear demonstration of endogenous opioid tone. Endogenous spinal dynorphin may act as an "analgesic brake" (Iadarola et al., 1988; Hunter et al., 1996), revealing the possibility of a dual physiological and pathological role for the same endogenous peptide (dynorphin) under different conditions of pain.

Altered Analgesic Responsiveness after Peripheral Nerve Injury

It is generally believed that neuropathic pain is resistant to treatment by opioids (see above). However, the reported failure of morphine and other opioid analgesics to relieve neuropathic pain may be due to underdosing of the patient; opioid dosing should be titrated until adequate analgesia is achieved or side effects are intolerable and untreatable (Portenoy et al., 1990). Thus some clinical investigators have found evidence for efficacy of opioids in controlling pain of neuropathic origin. Infusions of intravenous hydromorphone have achieved adequate analgesia in neuropathic pain patients (Portenoy et al., 1990), but the dose–response curve was shifted to the right, possibly beyond what is normally considered to be "usual" doses for the treatment of pain of non-neuropathic origins. Portenoy and Foley (1986) and Jadad and colleagues (1992) have also reported that opioids may alleviate neuropathic pain, but at "higher than normal doses." In a double-blind, placebo-controlled study, intravenous morphine infusions successfully treated both spontaneous pain and allodynia caused by postherpetic neuralgia (Rowbotham et al., 1991). Clearly, additional investigations into the clinical utility of opioids, taking into consideration the pain modality, route of administration, dosage, and opioid compound, must be performed to evaluate opioid treatment protocols for neuropathic pain fully.

The interpretation of data collected with various animal models of neuropathic pain with regard to the efficacy of opioids is likewise unclear. Xu and co-workers (1993) showed insensitivity to morphine in a neuropathic pain model because intrathecal morphine (10 µg) did not reduce the incidence of autotomy in rats following sciatic nerve section. In contrast, the same group (Wiesenfeld-Hallin, 1984) had earlier reported that doses of intrathecal morphine, able to produce acute antinociception, also prevented autotomy after section of the sciatic nerve. Although intrathecal morphine failed to attenuate tactile allodynia in the rat after ligation injury of the L_5 and L_6 nerve roots, the high-efficacy, selective µ-opioid agonist DAMGO demonstrated a clear dose-dependent antiallodynic effect after intrathecal injection (Nichols et al., 1995), as did morphine given either systemically or i.c.v. (Bian et al., 1995; Yaksh et al., 1995). Critically, an antihyperalgesic and antinociceptive effect of intrathecal morphine, evaluated as paw withdrawal in response to thermal stimuli applied ipsilateral to the nerve injury, was demonstrated after either chronic constriction injury of the sciatic nerve (Mao et al., 1995a,b) or ligation of the L_5/L_6 spinal nerves (Wegert et al., 1997), supporting the view that mechanisms underlying allodynia and hyperalgesia are different. Interestingly, in both of these studies, the potency of intrathecal morphine to block the foot flick response in nerve-injured animals was significantly diminished (five- to sixfold) when compared to control animals regardless of whether the hyperalgesic baseline was "normalized" (with MK-801) prior to administration of morphine. Likewise, a loss of antinociceptive efficacy and potency against the tail flick reflex of intrathecal morphine has also been demonstrated (Ossipov et al., 1995c).

There is evidence of significant sprouting of large-diameter, low-threshold fibers into lamina II of the dorsal horn of the spinal cord after axotomy or crushing of the sciatic nerve or L_5/L_6 spinal nerve ligation (Woolf et al., 1992; Lekan et al., 1996). These sprouting low-threshold neurons form novel, abnormal synapses with the nociceptive transmission neurons of lamina II. The result is that the low-threshold mechanoreceptors encode nociceptive information in the neuropathic state, thus producing tactile allodynia. Because these large-diameter fibers are not likely to possess opioid receptors on the nerve terminals (Taddese et al., 1995), morphine is expected to have decreased efficacy in these circumstances owing to an action limited to the postsynaptic site. In contrast, opioids with high efficacy, and therefore large receptor reserve, still should be active, and in fact, intrathecal DAMGO produced dose-dependent antiallodynic activity in rats with L_5/L_6 spinal nerve ligation (Nichols et al., 1995).

An important consideration is that two manifestations of neuropathic pain, tactile allodynia and thermal hyperalgesia, depend on different sets of neuronal pathways. A recent study showed that spinal transection at T_8 completely abolished tactile allodynia in L_5/L_6 nerve ligated rats (Bian et al., 1998). Thermal nocifensive responses were still present after spinal transection in ligated and sham-operated rats, but thermal hyperalgesia of the hindpaws was not evident in spinal transected, L_5/L_6 nerve ligated rats. Tail withdrawal responses to tactile probing were very robust after spinal transection in both groups, demonstrating the expected loss of descending inhibition. These observations suggest that thermal hyperalgesia of the paw, seen after nerve injury, involves both spinal and supraspinal circuits, whereas tactile allodynia depends on a supraspinal loop. This difference may reflect afferent inputs associated with different fiber types. The concept that different fiber types mediate tactile allodynia and thermal hyperalgesia is further supported by the recent observation that long-term desensitization of C fibers by resiniferatoxin blocked responses to thermal nociception but did not block tactile allodynia in L_5/L_6 nerve-injured rats (Ossipov et al., 1999).

Common Substrates May Underlie Morphine Tolerance and Neuropathic Pain States. Neuropathic pain states and tolerance to morphine share common neural substrates, indicating a complex interrelationship between opioid tolerance and neuropathic pain (Mao et al., 1995a,b; Mayer et al., 1995a). Morphine-tolerant animals and rats with chronic constriction injury (CCI) (Mao et al., 1995a) or L_5/L_6 nerve ligation injury (Wegert et al., 1997) all demonstrate thermal hyperalgesia that is reversed by intrathecal injection of the NMDA antagonist MK-801. Furthermore, in all of these situations, the dose–response curve for intrathecal morphine is displaced to the right, and is not normalized by intrathecal MK-801, which "normalized" the baseline responses. Activation of NMDA receptors, which occurs during central sensitization and afferent drive related to nerve injury, results in Ca^{2+} influx and subsequent translocation of protein kinase C (PKC) from cytosol to the membrane (Mayer et al., 1995a). Increases in membrane-bound PKC have been reported in spinal cord after CCI and correlates with development of neuropathic pain behaviors (Mayer et al., 1995a). Inhibition of PKC translocation by GM1 ganglioside reduced both neuropathic pain behaviors and membrane-bound PKC in rats with CCI (Mao et al., 1995a; Mayer et al., 1995a,b). Likewise, tolerance development to morphine was associated with elevated membrane-bound PKC levels in the superficial laminae of the spinal cord, and inhibition of PKC translocation by GM1 ganglioside co-administered with intrathecal morphine attenuated the development of tolerance (Mayer et al., 1995b). These studies provide convincing evidence of a strong common mechanism underlying the development of morphine tolerance and of neuropathic pain behavior.

Blockade of NMDA Receptors Restores the Antinociceptive and Antiallodynic Action of Intrathecal Morphine. Although spinally injected morphine is inactive against tactile allodynia, it does produce dose-dependent antiallodynic effects in the presence of intrathecal MK-801 (Nichols et al., 1997). Similarly, attenuation of the presumed constant afferent barrage elicited by L_5/L_6 nerve ligation by intrathecal MK-801 restored the antiallodynic and antinociceptive efficacy of intrathecal morphine (Ossipov et al., 1995b). A similar result was observed after the application of bupivacaine at the site of nerve injury, again supporting the importance of afferent drive in limiting the activity of potential pain-relieving drugs in pathological states (Ossipov et al., 1995b). Surprisingly, however, although MK-801 reversed thermal hyperalgesia of the paw after CCI (Mao et al., 1995a) or L_5/L_6 spinal nerve ligation (Wegert et al., 1997), the antinociceptive potency of morphine was not altered, also suggesting differential mechanisms in these models of hyperalgesia.

SUMMARY AND CONCLUSIONS

The use of opioids to treat acute pain is a very well established and common practice. The use of opioids in chronic pain states is not as well established, partly because of vastly differing efficacies of opioids, depending on the etiology of the pain state. Pain of inflammatory origin is readily amenable to opioid treatment, whereas chronic pain due to nerve injury is particularly resistant to opioid treatment. Understanding the underlying mechanisms of neuropathic pain will allow us to exploit these mechanisms in order to establish effective therapeutic regimens. The combination of CCK antagonists and opioids is proposed to be significantly more efficacious than either alone, partly by blocking the anti-analgesic action of the increased endogenous release of

CCK. Likewise, abolishing afferent drive, by blockade of NMDA receptors or local anesthetics or selective Na$^+$ channel blockers, given at the site of injury and/or systemically, also should provide a means to enhance the activity of opioids against neuropathic pain states. The role of dynorphin in neuropathic pain is also of great interest, especially because of its apparently dual and opposing nature as a physiological endogenous opioid and endogenous proneuropathic agent. Increasing our knowledge of the underlying mechanisms of actions of opioids and of the physiopathic processes involved in the generation of pain states will lead to more effective therapies for all types of pain.

REFERENCES

Adams JU, Tallarida RJ, Geller EB, Adler MW (1993): Isobolographic superadditivity between delta and mu opioid agonists in the rat depends on the ratio of compounds, the mu agonist and the analgesic assay used. J Pharmacol Exp Ther 266:1261–1267.

Aimone LD, Yaksh TL (1989): Opioid modulation of capsaicin-evoked release of substance P from rat spinal cord in vivo. Peptides 10:1127–1131.

Andreev N, Urban L, Dray A (1994): Opioids suppress spontaneous activity of polymodal nociceptors in rat paw skin induced by ultraviolet irradiation. Neuroscience 58:793–798.

Antonijevic I, Mousa SA, Schafer M, Stein C (1995): Perineurial defect and peripheral opioid analgesia in inflammation. J Neurosci 15:165–172.

Arner S, Meyerson BA (1988): Lack of analgesic effect on neuropathic and idiopathic forms of pain. Pain 33:11–23.

Arvidsson U, Dado RJ, Riedl M, Lee J-H, Law PJ, Loh HH, Elde R, Wessendorf MW (1995): δ-opioid receptor immunoreactivity: distribution in brainstem and spinal cord, and relationship to biogenic amines and enkephalin. J Neurosci 15:1215–1235.

Barber A (1993): Mu- and kappa-opioid receptor agonists produce peripheral inhibition of neurogenic plasma extravasation in rat skin. Eur J Pharmacol 236:113–120.

Barber A, Gottschlich R (1992): Opioid agonists and antagonists: an evaluation of their peripheral actions in inflammation. Med Res Rev 12:525–562.

Basbaum AI, Fields HL (1979): The origin of descending pathways in the dorsolateral funiculus of the spinal cord of the cat and rat: further studies on the anatomy of pain modulation. J Comp Neurol 187:513–531.

Bennett G, Mayer DJ (1979): Inhibition of spinal cord interneurons by narcotic microinjection and focal electrical stimulation in the periaqueductal gray matter. Brain Res 172:243–257.

Besse D, Lombard MC, Zajac JM, Roques BP, Besson JM (1990): Pre- and postsynaptic distribution of μ, δ and κ opioid receptors in the superficial layers of the cervical dorsal horn of the rat spinal cord. Brain Res 521:15–22.

Bhargava HN (1994): Diversity of agents that modify opioid tolerance, physical dependence, abstinence syndrome, and self-administrative behavior. Pharmacol Rev 46:293–324.

Bian D, Nichols ML, Ossipov MH, Lai J, Porreca F (1995): Characterization of the antiallodynic efficacy of morphine in a model of neuropathic pain in rats. NeuroReport 6:1981–1984.

Bian D, Ossipov MH, Zhong CM, Malan TP, Porreca F (1998): Tactile allodynia, but not thermal hyperalgesia, of the hindlimbs is blocked by spinal transection in rats with nerve injury. Neurosci Lett 241:79–82.

Bilsky EJ, Wang T, Lai J, Porreca F (1996): Selective blockade of peripheral delta opioid agonist induced antinociception by intrathecal administration of delta receptor antisense oligodeoxynucleotide. Neurosci Lett 220:155–158.

Brodin E, Gazelius B, Panopoulos P, Olgart L (1983): Morphine inhibits substance P release from peripheral sensory nerve endings. Acta Physiol Scand 117:567–570.

Cabot PJ, Carter L, Gaiddon C, Zhang Q, Schafer M, Loeffler JP, Stein C (1997): Immune cell-derived beta-endorphin: Production, release, and control of inflammatory pain in rats. J Clin Invest 100:142–148.

Chaplan SR, Sorkin LS (1997): Agonizing over pain terminology. Pain Forum 6:81–87.

Conrad LCA, Leonard CM, Pfaff DW (1976): Connections of the median and dorsal raphe nuclei in the rat: An autoradiographic and degeneration study. J Comp Neurol 156:179–206.

Cox BM, Molineaux CJ, Jacobs TP, Rossenberger JG, Faden AI (1985): Effects of traumatic injury on dynorphin immunoreactivity in spinal cord. Neuropeptides 5:571–574.

Dado RJ, Law PY, Loh HH, Elde R (1993): Immunofluorescent identification of a delta (δ)-opioid receptor on primary afferent nerve terminals. NeuroReport 5:341–344.

Dickenson AH, Oliveras JL, Besson JM (1979): Role of the nucleus raphe magnus in opiate analgesia as studied by the microinjection technique in the rat. Brain Res 170:95–111.

Dubner R, Ruda MA (1992): Activity-dependent neuronal plasticity following tissue injury and inflammation. Trends Neurosci 15:96–103.

Faden AI (1990): Opioid and nonopioid mechanisms may contribute to dynorphin's pathophysiological actions in spinal cord injury. Ann Neurol 27:67–74.

Gogas KR, Presley RW, Levine JD, Basbaum AI (1991): The antinociceptive action of supraspinal opioids results from an increase in descending inhibitory control: correlation of nociceptive behavior and c-fos expression. Neuroscience 42:617–628.

Gogas KR, Levine JD, Basbaum AI (1996): Differential contribution of descending controls to the antinociceptive actions of kappa and mu opioids: an analysis of formalin-evoked C-fos expression. J Pharmacol Exp Ther 276:801–809.

Hammond DL, Wang H, Nakashima N, Basbaum AI (1998): Differential effects of intrathecally administered delta and mu opioid receptor agonists on formalin-evoked nociception and on the expression of fos-like immunoreactivity in the spinal cord of the rat. J Pharmacol Exp Ther 284:378–387.

Hassan AH, Ableitner A, Stein C, Herz A (1993): Inflammation of the rat paw enhances axonal transport of opioid receptors in the sciatic nerve and increases their density in the inflamed tissue. Neuroscience 55:185–195.

Heyman JS, Jiang Q, Rothman RB, Mosberg HI, Porreca F (1989): Modulation of mu-mediated antinociception by delta agonists: characterization with antagonists. Eur J Pharmacol 169:43–52.

Hosohata Y, Vanderah TW, Burkey TH, Ossipov MH, Kovelowski CJ, Bian D, Sora I, Uhl GR, Zhang X, Rice KC, Roeske WR, Hruby VJ, Yamamura HI, Porreca F (1999): Opioid delta receptor agonist activity in mu-opioid receptor "knock-out" mice. Submitted.

Hunter JC, Woodburn VL, Durieux C, Pettersson EKE, Poat JA, Hughes J (1996): C-fos antisense oligodeoxynucleotide increases formalin-induced nociception and regulates preprodynorphin expression. Neuroscience 65:485–492.

Iadarola MJ, Brady LS, Draisci G, Dubner R (1988): Enhancement of dynorphin gene expression in spinal cord following experimental inflammation: stimulus specificity, behavioral parameters and opioid receptor binding. Pain 35:313–326.

Jacobson L, Chabal C, Brody MC, Mariano AJ, Chaney EF (1990): A comparison of the effects of intrathecal fentanyl and lidocaine on established postamputation stump pain. Pain 40:137–141.

Jadad AR, Carroll D, Glynn CJ, Moore RA, McQuay HJ (1992): Morphine responsiveness of chronic pain: doubleblind randomized cross-over study with patient-controlled analgesia. Lancet 339:1367–1371.

Jensen TS, Yaksh TL (1986a): I. Comparison of antinociceptive action of morphine in the periaqueductal gray, medial and paramedial medulla in rat. Brain Res 363:99–113.

Jensen TS, Yaksh TL (1986b): III. Comparison of the antinociceptive action of mu and delta opioid ligands in the periaqueductal gray matter, medial and paramedial ventral medulla in the rat as studied by microinjection techniques. Brain Res 372:301–312.

Jiang Q, Mosberg HI, Porreca F (1990): Modulation of the potency and efficacy of mu-mediated antinociception by delta agonists in the mouse. J Pharmacol Exp Ther 254:683–689.

Kalso E, Tramer MR, Carroll D, McQuay HJ, Moore RA (1997): Pain relief from intra-articular morphine after knee surgery: a qualitative systematic review. Pain 71:127–134.

Kayser V, Guilbaud G (1983): The analgesic effects of morphine but not those of the enkephalinase inhibitor thiorphan are enhanced in the arthritic rat. Brain Res 267:131–138.

Khasar SG, Gold MS, Dastmalchi S, Levine JD (1996): Selective attenuation of mu-opioid receptor-mediated effects in rat sensory neurons by intrathecal administration of antisense oligodeoxynucleotides. Neurosci Lett 218:17–20.

Kiefel JM, Rossi GC, Bodnar RJ (1993): Medullary mu and delta opioid receptors modulate mesencephalic morphine analgesia in rats. Brain Res 624:151–161.

Kocher L, Anton F, Reeh PW, Handwerker HO (1987): The effect of carrageenan-induced inflammation on the sensitivity of unmyelinated skin nociceptors in the rat. Pain 29:363–373.

Kovelowski CJ, Ossipov MH, Porreca F (1999): Lesion of the dorsolateral funiculus (DLF) blocks antinociception and suppression of spinal fos-like immunoreactivity (FLI) elicited by medullary micro-injection of [D-Ala^2,Glu^4]deltorphin (DELT). Pain, in press.

Lekan HA, Carlton SM, Coggeshall RE (1996): Sprouting of A beta fibers into lamina II of the rat dorsal horn in peripheral neuropathy. Neurosci Lett 208:147–150.

Lewis VA, Gebhart GF (1977): Evaluation of the periaqueductal central gray (PAG) as a morphine-specific locus of action and examination of morphine-induced and stimulation-produced analgesia at coincident PAG loci. Brain Res 124:283–303.

Likar R, Schafer M, Paulak F, Sittl R, Pipam W, Schalk H, Geissler D, Bernatzky G (1997): Intraarticular morphine analgesia in chronic pain patients with osteoarthritis. Anesth Analg 84:1313–1317.

Maekawa K, Minami M, Masuda T, Satoh M (1994): Expression of µ- and κ-, but not δ-, opioid receptor mRNAs is enhanced in the spinal dorsal horn of the arthritic rats. Pain 64:365–371.

Mansour A, Fox CA, Thompson RC, Akil H, Watson SJ (1994): µ-Opioid receptor mRNA expression in the rat CNS: comparison to µ-receptor binding. Brain Res 643:245–265.

Mansour A, Fox CA, Akil H, Watson SJ (1995): Opioid-receptor mRNA expression in the rat CNS: anatomical and functional implications. Trends Neurosci 18:22–29.

Mao J, Price DD, Mayer DJ (1995a): Experimental mononeuropathy reduces the antinociceptive effects of morphine: implications for common intracellular mechanisms involved in morphine tolerance and neuropathic pain. Pain 61:353–364.

Mao J, Price DD, Mayer DJ (1995b): Mechanisms of hyperalgesia and morphine tolerance: A current view of their possible interactions. Pain 62:259–274.

Max MB, Schafer SC, Culnane M, Dubner R, Gracely RH (1988): Association of pain relief with drug side effects in postherpetic neuralgia: a single dose study of clonidine, codeine, ibuprofen, and placebo. Clin Pharmacol Ther 43:363–371.

Mayer DJ, Mao J, Price DD (1995a): The association of neuropathic pain, morphine tolerance and dependence, and the translocation of protein kinase C. NIDA Res Monograph 147:269–298.

Mayer DJ, Mao J, Price DD (1995b): The development of morphine tolerance and dependence is associated with translocation of protein kinase C. Pain 61:365–374.

McGowan MK, Hammond DL (1993): Antinociception produced by microinjection of L-glutamate into the ventromedial medulla of the rat: mediation by spinal GABA$_A$ receptors. Brain Res 620:86–96.

Miaskowski C, Taiwo YO, Levine JD (1991): Contribution of supraspinal µ- and δ-opioid receptors to antinociception in the rat. Eur J Pharmacol 205:247–252.

Negri L, Noviello V, Angelucci F (1991): Behavioural effects of deltorphins in rats. Eur J Pharmacol 209:163–168.

Neil A, Kayser V, Gacel G, Besson JM, Guilbaud G (1986): Opioid receptor types and antinociceptive activity in chronic inflammation: both κ- and µ-opiate agonistic effects are enhanced in arthritic rats. Eur J Pharmacol 130:203–208.

Nichols ML, Bian D, Ossipov MH, Lai J, Porreca F (1995): Regulation of opioid antiallodynic efficacy by cholecystokinin in a model of neuropathic pain in rats. J Pharmacol Exp Ther 275:1339–1345.

Nichols ML, Lopez Y, Ossipov MH, Bian D, Porreca F (1997): Enhancement of the antiallodynic and antinociceptive efficacy of spinal morphine by antisera to dynorphin A(1-13) or MK-801 in a nerve-ligation model of peripheral neuropathy. Pain 69:317–322.

Oliveras JL, Hosobuchi Y, Redjemi F, Guilbaud G, Besson JM (1977): Opiate antagonist, naloxone, strongly reduces analgesia induced by stimulation of a raphe nucleus (centralis inferior). Brain Res 120:221–229.

Ossipov MH, Kovelowski CJ, Nichols ML, Hruby VJ, Porreca F (1994): Characterization of supraspinal antinociceptive actions of opioid delta agonists in the rat. Pain 62:287–293.

Ossipov MH, Kovelowski CJ, Porreca F (1995a): The increase in morphine antinociceptive potency produced by carrageenan-induced hindpaw inflammation is blocked by NTI, a selective δ-opioid antagonist. Neurosci Lett 184:173–176.

Ossipov MH, Lopez Y, Nichols ML, Bian D, Porreca F (1995b): The loss of antinociceptive efficacy of spinal morphine in rats with nerve ligation injury is prevented by reducing spinal afferent drive. Neurosci Lett 199:87–90.

Ossipov MH, Nichols ML, Bian D, Porreca F (1995c): Inhibition by spinal morphine of the tail-flick response is attenuated in rats with nerve ligation injury. Neurosci Lett 199:83–86.

Ossipov MH, Kovelowski CJ, Wheeler-Aceto H, Cowan A, Hunter JC, Lai J, Porreca F (1996): Opioid antagonists and antisera to endogenous opioids increase the nociceptive response to formalin: Demonstration of an opioid κ and δ inhibitory tone. J Pharmacol Exp Ther 277:784–788.

Ossipov MH, Bian D, Porreca F (1999): Lack of involvement of capsaicin-sensitive primary afferents in nerve-ligation injury induced tactile allodynia in rats. Pain 79:127–133.

Pan ZZ, Tershner SA, Fields HL (1997): Cellular mechanism for anti-analgesic action of agonists of the kappa-opioid receptor. Nature 389:382–385.

Picard PR, Tramer MR, McQuay HJ, Moore RA (1997): Analgesic efficacy of peripheral opioids (all except intra-articular): a qualitative systematic review of randomised controlled trials. Pain 72:309–318.

Porreca F, Heyman JS, Mosberg HI, Omnaas JR, Vaught JL (1987): Role of mu and delta receptors in the supraspinal and spinal analgesic effects of [D-Pen2, D-Pen5]enkephalin in the mouse. J Pharmacol Exp Ther 241:393–400.

Portenoy RK, Foley KM (1986): Chronic use of opioid analgesics in non-malignant pain: report of 38 cases. Pain 25:171–186.

Portenoy RK, Foley KM, Inturrisi CE (1990): The nature of opioid responsiveness and its implications for neuropathic pain: new hypotheses derived from studies of opioid infusions. Pain 43:273–286.

Proudfit HK, Fang F (1995): The neuronal pathways that mediate the antinociception produced by microinjection of morphine in the rat periaqueductal gray. Soc Neurosci Abstr 21:1168.

Przewlocki R, Hassan AH, Lason W, Epplen C, Herz A, Stein C (1992): Gene expression and localization of opioid peptides in immune cells of inflamed tissue: functional role in antinociception. Neuroscience 48:491–500.

Rossi GC, Pasternak GW, Bodnar RJ (1993): Synergistic brainstem interactions for morphine analgesia. Brain Res 624:171–180.

Rossi GC, Pasternak GW, Bodnar RJ (1994): Mu and delta opioid synergy between the periaqueductal gray and the rostro-ventral medulla. Brain Res 665:85–93.

Rowbotham MC, Reisner-Keller LA, Fields HL (1991): Both intravenous lidocaine and morphine reduce the pain of postherpetic neuralgia. Neurology 41:1024–1028.

Russell NJ, Schaible HG, Schmidt RF (1987): Opiates inhibit the discharges of fine afferent units from inflamed knee joint of the cat. Neurosci Lett 76:107–112.

Sandkuhler J, Gebhart GF (1984): Relative contributions of the nucleus raphe magnus and adjacent medullary reticular formation to the inhibition by stimulation in the periaqueductal gray of a spinal nociceptive reflex in the pentobarbital-anesthetized rat. Brain Res 305:77–87.

Schafer M, Imai Y, Uhl GR, Stein C (1995): Inflammation enhances peripheral mu-opioid receptor-mediated analgesia, but not mu-opioid receptor transcription in dorsal root ganglia. Eur J Pharmacol 279:165–169.

Shukla VK, Lemaire S (1994): Non-opioid effects of dynorphins: possible role of the NMDA receptor. Trends Pharmacol Sci 15:420–424.

Sora I, Funada M, Uhl GR (1997): The mu-opioid receptor is necessary for [D-Pen^2,D-Pen^5]enkephalin-induced analgesia. Eur J Pharmacol 324:R1–R2.

Stanfa LC, Dickenson AH (1993): Cholecystokinin as a factor in the enhanced potency of spinal morphine following carrageenan inflammation. Br J Pharmacol 108:967–973.

Stanfa L, Dickenson A, Xu X-J, Weisenfeld-Hallin Z (1994): Cholecystokinin and morphine analgesia: variations on a theme. Trends Pharmacol Sci 15:65–66.

Stein C (1993): Peripheral mechanisms of opioid analgesia. Anesth Analg 76:182–191.

Stein C (1995): The control of pain in peripheral tissue by opioids. New Engl J Med 332:1685–1690.

Stein C, Yassouridis A (1997): Peripheral morphine analgesia. Pain 71:119–121.

Stein C, Millan MJ, Shippenberg TS, Herz A (1988a): Peripheral effect of fentanyl upon nociception in inflamed tissue of the rat. Neurosci Lett 84:225–228.

Stein C, Millan MJ, Yassouridis A, Herz A (1988b): Antinociceptive effects of μ- and κ-agonists in inflammation are enhanced by a peripheral opioid receptor-specific mechanism. Eur J Pharmacol 155:255–264.

Stein C, Millan MJ, Shippenberg TS, Peter K, Herz A (1989): Peripheral opioid receptors mediating antinociception in inflammation. Evidence for involvement of mu, delta and kappa receptors. J Pharmacol Exp Ther 248:1269–1275.

Stein C, Gramsch C, Herz A (1990a): Intrinsic mechanisms of antinociception in inflammation: local opioid receptors and beta-endorphin. J Neurosci 10:1292–1298.

Stein C, Hassan AH, Przewlocki R, Gramsch C, Peter K, Herz A (1990b): Opioids from immunocytes interact with receptors on sensory nerves to inhibit nociception in inflammation. Proc Natl Acad Sci USA 87:5935–5939.

Stein C, Comisel K, Haimerl E, Yassouridis A, Lehrberger K, Herz A, Peter K (1991): Analgesic effect of intraarticular morphine after arthroscopic knee surgery. New Engl J Med 325: 1123–1126.

Stein C, Pfluger M, Yassouridis A, Hoelzl J, Lehrberger K, Welte C, Hassan AH (1996): No tolerance to peripheral morphine analgesia in presence of opioid expression in inflamed synovia. J Clin Invest 98:793–799.

Taddese A, Nah S-Y, McCleskey EW (1995): Selective opioid inhibition of small nociceptive neurons. Science 270:1366–1369.

Tasker RR, Buda T, Hawrylyshyn P (1983): Clinical neurophysiological investigation of deafferentation pain. In Bonica JJ, Lindblom U, Iggo I (eds): *Advances in Pain Research and Therapy*, Vol. 5. New York: Raven Press, pp. 713–738.

Thorat SN, Hammond DL (1997): Modulation of nociception by microinjection of delta-1 and delta-2 opioid receptor ligands in the ventromedial medulla of the rat. J Pharmacol Exp Ther 283:1185–1192.

Twycross RG (1982): Morphine and diamorphine in the terminally ill patient. Acta Anesthesiol Scand 74(Suppl.):128–134.

Urban M, Jiang MC, Gebhart GF (1996): Participation of central descending nociceptive facilitatory systems in secondary hyperalgesia produced by mustard oil. Brain Res 737:83–91.

Vaught JL, Mathiasen JR, Raffa RB (1988): Examination of the involvement of supraspinal and spinal mu and delta opioid receptors in analgesia using the mu receptor deficient CXBK mouse. J Pharmacol Exp Ther 245:13–16.

Verge VMK, Wiesenfeld-Hallin Z, Hokfelt T (1993): Cholecystokinin in mammalian primary sensory neurons and spinal cord: in situ hybridization studies in rat and monkey. Eur J Neurosci 5:240–250.

Wegert S, Ossipov MH, Nichols ML, Bian D, Vanderah T, Malan TP, Porreca F (1997): Differential activities of intrathecal MK-801 or morphine to alter responses to thermal and mechanical stimuli in normal or nerve-injured rats. Pain 71:57–64.

Wheeler-Aceto H, Cowan A (1993): Naloxone causes apparent antinociception and pronociception simultaneously in the rat paw formalin test. Eur J Pharmacol 236:193–199.

Wiesenfeld-Hallin Z (1984): The effects of intrathecal morphine and naltrexone on autotomy in sciatic nerve sectioned rats. Pain 18:267–278.

Willis WD (1997): Pain terminology as it applies to animal experiments. Pain Forum 6:88–91.

Woolf CJ, Shortland P, Coggeshall RE (1992): Peripheral nerve injury triggers central sprouting of myelinated afferents. Nature 355:75–78.

Xu X-J, Puke MJC, Verge VMK, Wiesenfeld-Hallin ZW, Hughes J, Hokfelt T (1993): Up-regulation of cholecystokinin in primary sensory neurons is associated with morphine insensitivity in experimental neuropathic pain in the rat. Neurosci Lett 152:129–132.

Xu X-J, Hao J-X, Seiger A, Hughes J, Hokfelt T, Wiesenfeld-Hallin ZW (1994a): Chronic pain-related behaviors in spinally injured rats: evidence for functional alterations of the endogenous cholecystokinin and opioid systems. Pain 56:271–277.

Xu X-J, Hokfelt T, Hughes J, Wiesenfeld-Hallin ZW (1994b): The CCK-B antagonist CI988 enhances the reflex-depressive effect of morphine in axotomized rats. NeuroReport 5:718–720.

Yaksh TL (1988): Substance P release from knee joint afferent terminals: modulation by opioids. Brain Res 458:319–324.

Yaksh TL, Rudy TA (1978): Narcotic analgesics: CNS sites and mechanisms of action as revealed by intracerebral injection techniques. Pain 4:299–359.

Yaksh TL, Yeung JC, Rudy TA (1976): Systemic examination in the rat of brain sites sensitive to the direct application of morphine: Observation of differential effects within the periaqueductal gray. Brain Res 114:83–103.

Yaksh TL, Pogrel JW, Lee YW, Chaplan SR (1995): Reversal of nerve ligation-induced allodynia by spinal alpha-2 adrenoceptor agonists. J Pharmacol Exp Ther 272:207–214.

CHAPTER 4

SOME NEW INSIGHTS INTO THE PHARMACOLOGY OF NONSTEROIDAL ANTI-INFLAMMATORY DRUGS

KEITH McCORMACK
McCormack Limited
Leighton Buzzard, Bedfordshire, United Kingdom

This chapter reviews recent findings that provide new insights into the use of currently available NSAIDs, as well as a recently launched NSAID (lornoxicam). In addition, I allude to the possibilities for the design of novel compounds. The chapter is restricted to a review and subsequent discussion of NSAID pharmacology that may provide a basis for their improved use and possibly greater efficacy in managing the symptomatology of chronic inflammatory disorders. Generally, this chapter is also restricted to pharmacological differences that relate to derived effects and not adverse effects. The issue of cyclooxygenase (COX) selectivity is not discussed in detail. Finally, I have chosen to review the pharmacology of NSAIDs in the management of chronic inflammatory disorders for two reasons. First, the use of NSAIDs in the treatment of chronic disorders, such as the arthritides, arguably represents their most important clinical application. Second, translation of in vitro/in vivo effects will almost certainly be greater following repeat multiple dosing at high doses by comparison, for example, with occasional use for short periods at lower doses in the management of acute disorders such as dental pain or headaches.

REVISITING NSAIDs AND CHRONIC INFLAMMATORY DISORDERS

Combination Therapy

Arthritic pain is a common and frequently debilitating chronic pain condition characteristic of a variety of arthritic diseases such as osteoarthritis (OA), ju-

---

Novel Aspects of Pain Management: Opioids and Beyond, Edited by Jana Sawynok and Alan Cowan
ISBN 0-471-180173   Copyright © 1999 by Wiley-Liss, Inc.

venile arthritis, rheumatoid arthritis (RA), gout, psoriatic arthritis, and ankylosing spondylitis. Many people suffer from arthritic pain, which is a common cause of the loss of working ability. Currently, NSAIDs supplemented with glucocorticosteroids represent an important therapeutic regime. Putatively, this treatment approach targets peripheral factors causing arthritic pain (Buritova et al., 1996). Thus, in addition to the inhibitory effect of an NSAID upon COX activity, it is assumed that further benefit will accrue from the added effects of a glucocorticosteroid upon eicosanoid metabolism through attenuation of phospholipase A_2 activity (Schalkwijk et al., 1991; O'Banion et al., 1992; Glaser et al., 1993), and inhibition of activity of the transcription factors, nuclear factor κB (NF-κB) and activator protein-1 (Cato and Wade, 1996; Blackwell and Christman, 1997; Chen et al., 1997; Heck et al., 1997; van der Burg et al., 1997) (see section on Salicylate for further discussion of NF-κB). Indeed, in the freely moving rat, co-administration of diclofenac and dexamethasone, using doses that had negligible effects when administered separately, significantly reduced both the total number of carrageenan-evoked spinal c-Fos protein like neuronal immunoreactivity and the peripheral edema (Buritova et al., 1996). On this basis, Buritova et al. (1996) propose that in the treatment of chronic inflammatory disorders, apparent interactions between the mechanisms of action of NSAIDs and glucocorticosteroids suggest that in clinical practice, cotherapy may produce beneficial anti-inflammatory and analgesic effects in the absence of excessive side effects.

Whereas the use of NSAIDs, in combination with glucocorticosteroid, targets the involvement of eicosanoids in the pathogenesis of arthritic pain, recent insights also indicate a critical involvement of central nervous system excitatory amino acid (EAA) receptors (Dougherty et al., 1992; Sluka et al., 1992; Sorkin et al., 1992; Westlund et al., 1992; Neugebauer et al., 1993). The results of these studies suggest that in humans, the development of arthritic pain is associated with the release of EAAs within the spinal cord (Sluka et al., 1992; Sorkin et al., 1992; Sluka and Westlund, 1993a,b). Activation of spinal cord N-methyl-D-aspartate (NMDA) receptors facilitates (Dougherty et al., 1992), whereas blockade of these receptors inhibits (Neugebauer et al., 1993) spinal cord nociceptive transmission associated with a presumed arthritic pain condition in experimental animals. Given these observations, Price et al. (1996) reasoned that an NSAID in combination with an NMDA receptor antagonist may represent a potentially useful treatment strategy for managing arthritic pain. If NSAIDs downregulate the output from sensitized nociceptors, then enhanced analgesia may be derived from the additional effects of an NMDA receptor antagonist upon central sensitization that follows central EAA receptor-mediated mechanisms. Unfortunately, the use of NMDA receptor antagonists in humans may be associated with distressing side effects such as hallucinations and mood changes. However, the capacity of the morphinan dextromethorphan to antagonize NMDA receptor activity appears not to be associated with such adverse outcomes. Indeed, dextromethorphan is an established antitussive drug that is approved for peroral administration.

Using a rat model of adjuvant-induced arthritis, Price et al. (1996) evaluated the effects of combining single oral doses of dextromethorphan with oral doses of either ibuprofen, naproxen, piroxicam, etodolac, diclofenac, or ketorolac upon paw withdrawal thresholds using the Randall–Sellito test (Butler et al., 1992; Perrot et al., 1993). Their finding that dextromethorphan, at doses that are ineffective by themselves, potently facilitates the analgesic effects of NSAIDs in a rat model of arthritic pain provides further support for the earlier suggestion (Ren, 1994) that NMDA receptor antagonists may be optimally useful when used in combination with other classes of analgesics. Price et al. (1996) conclude that the combination of dextromethorphan and an NSAID may represent a novel analgesic approach to the improved management of arthritic pain.

Despite the apparent clinical utility of an NSAID in combination with either a glucocorticosteroid or an NMDA receptor antagonist, it remains to be determined whether differences exist between the effects of different NSAIDs when used in the management of chronic inflammatory disorders, such as arthritis. Notwithstanding differences between pharmacokinetic profiles, any differences in effects upon the symptomatology and perhaps progression of the various arthritides, for example, may reflect the capacity of a particular NSAID to modulate nociceptive processing by a mechanism(s) that operates in addition to an inhibition of prostaglandin (PG) synthesis. Indeed, the likelihood that some NSAIDs may have greater clinical utility is both seductive and provocative, and continues to represent a topic that attracts much debate (see McCormack 1994a;1994b for review). In the following section, recent findings are reported that fuel the notion that some NSAIDs, at least when used to manage arthritis, may exert clinically relevant "novel" effects. However, whether these effects translate into any real therapeutic advantages has yet to be determined.

Novel NSAIDs/Novel Effects

Salicylate. In spite of its origins in antiquity, recent data (Kopp and Ghosh, 1994; Weber et al., 1995; Grilli et al., 1996; Osnes et al., 1996; Sakurada et al., 1996; Bitko et al., 1997; Chen et al., 1997; Mitchell et al., 1997; Schmedtje et al., 1997) suggest that sodium salicylate and aspirin may possibly be distinguished through inhibitory effects upon nuclear translocation and activity of the transcription factor NF-κB, which is critical for the inducible expression of multiple cellular genes involved in immune and inflammatory responses. The products of these genes include cytokines such as the interleukins (ILs) IL-1, IL-6, and IL-8, interferon β (IFN-β), tumor necrosis factor alpha (TNF-α), PGH (PG endoperoxide)-synthase 2, and the cell adhesion molecules endothelial leukocyte adhesion molecule-1 (ELAM-1), intercellular adhesion molecule-1 (ICAM-1), vascular cell adhesion molecule-1 (VCAM-1), and granulocyte macrophage colony stimulating factor. NF-κB is an inducible eukaryotic transcription factor of the *rel* family (Grilli et al., 1993) which exists in an inactive form in the cytoplasm of most cells where it is bound to an inhibitory protein, IκB. NF-κB is activated in response to a number of stimulants including bacterial lipopolysaccharide, double-stranded RNA, phorbol esters, IL-1, TNF-α (Grilli et al., 1993), and nerve growth factor (Carter et al., 1996), and likely has a pivotal role in the pathogenesis of RA (Sakurada et al., 1996). Stimulation triggers the release of NF-κB from IκB, resulting in the translocation of NF-κB from the cytoplasm to the nucleus, where NF-κB binds to DNA and regulates transcription of specific genes. Interestingly, both sodium salicylate and aspirin inhibited NF-κB activity in the human Jurkat T cell line at concentrations that likely could be achieved within chronically inflamed sites following repeated administration of high therapeutic doses (Kopp and Ghosh, 1994; McCormack, 1994a;1994b; Mitchell et al., 1997). In another study (Grilli et al., 1996), at concentrations compatible with those during chronic anti-inflammatory therapy, both aspirin and sodium salicylate were found to protect against neurotoxicity elicited by the EAA glutamate in primary neuronal cultures and hippocampal slices. The site of action of both drugs appeared to be downstream from glutamate receptors, and to involve specific inhibition of glutamate-mediated induction of NF-κB. These results implicate a role for aspirin and sodium salicylate in preventing neurodegeneration and consequently may influence long-term outcomes in the management of chronic inflammatory disorders (Grilli and Memo, 1997).

Although the effects of other NSAIDs upon NF-κB activity have yet to be investigated, in the study by Kopp and Ghosh (1994) it is noteworthy that neither acetaminophen (a weak inhibitor of COX activity) nor indomethacin (a potent inhibitor of COX activity) had any significant effect upon NF-κB activity, even at concentrations significantly higher than those administered clinically.

Although it is tempting to speculate on the implications of inhibiting the activity of a key factor such as NF-κB in the cytokine network, it must be emphasised that the available data (Kopp and Ghosh, 1994; Mitchell et al., 1997) suggest that a salicylate-mediated inhibition of NF-κB activity would be evident only at high doses. Moreover, given the emerging enthusiasm for the potential clinical utility of NSAIDs with preferential inhibitory effects upon COX 2 activity over COX 1 activity in the treatment of arthritis, it is difficult to envisage renewed focus on the salicylates, notably aspirin, which are perceived as having a greater potential for adverse events with chronic dosing at the top of the therapeutic range (Rainsford, 1989; Levy, 1990; Brune and McCormack, 1994).

Finally, in spite of the perceived role of aspirin in the management of the arthritides, the salicylates continue to generate surprising observations. It has been reported that a number of viruses, including the human immunodeficiency virus (HIV)-1, exploit NF-κB for their replication (Nabel and Baltimore, 1987; Grilli et al., 1993). Because the HIV-1 long terminal repeat (LTR) contains two inducible NF-κB sites (Nabel and Baltimore, 1987; Griffin et al., 1989), treatment of chronically infected cells with agents that produce the activation of NF-κB also lead to an increase in the level of viral replication (Pomerantz et al., 1989; Demarchi et al., 1996). Indeed, it has been demonstrated that, at high doses, both sodium salicylate and aspirin can inhibit NF-κB-dependent transcription from the HIV-1 LTR in the Jurkat human T cell line (Kopp and Ghosh, 1994). This transcriptional inhibition by salicylate may perhaps underlie preliminary reports that aspirin may have a role in treating HIV infection (MacIlwain, 1993). Additionally, it was also recently suggested that as inhibitors of NF-κB activation, sodium salicylate and aspirin may be of use in managing viral pathogenesis during respiratory syncytial viral infection (Bitko et al., 1997).

Lornoxicam. Rheumatoid arthritis is a chronic inflammatory disease characterized by the progressive destruction of joints. Histomorphological studies have indicated that articular cartilage destruction in RA occurs predominantly in areas contiguous with transformed-appearing synovial lining cells (Fassbender, 1983), which are generally described as fibroblast-like (Shiozawa and Tokuhisa, 1992). Such synovial fibroblast-like cells (synoviocytes) are regarded as the final mediator of joint destruction in RA; they secrete collagenase, stromelysin, and other proteolytic enzymes that are prominent in the degradation of cartilage (Dayer et al., 1976; Chin et al., 1985; He et al., 1989).

Kumkumian et al. (1989) have investigated the effects of platelet-derived growth factor (PDGF) and IL-1 upon the regulation of synoviocytes from patients with RA. They observed that IL-1 inhibited PDGF-stimulated synoviocyte proliferation, and that exogenous PGE$_2$, a PG known to be produced in response to IL-1, dramatically inhibited synoviocyte proliferation induced by PDGF. Importantly, when these same cells were treated with PDGF and IL-1 in the presence of indomethacin, PDGF and IL-1 operated synergistically to stimulate synoviocyte proliferation whereas the DNA synthetic response to IL-1 was unaffected. More recently, these results were confirmed by Lin et al. (1989) and Hamilton et al. (1994). Using NIH-3T3 fibroblasts, it was observed that aspirin pretreatment increased both the rate and amplitude of PDGF-stimulated PGH synthase mRNA induction. Taken together, these results suggest that PGs negatively modulate PDGF-mediated effects upon fibroblast/fibroblast-like synthetic activity (Hamilton et al., 1994). Moreover, PGs, notably PGD$_2$, PGE$_1$, and PGI$_2$ also inhibit the release of PDGF from platelets (Stürzebecher et al., 1986, 1989; Takacs and Jellinek, 1987; Willis et al., 1987). Thus, given that both the platelet (Yaron and Djaldetti, 1978; Endresen, 1981, 1984, 1989; Farr et al., 1981, 1984; de Gaetano et al., 1989; Endresen and Førre, 1992; Uhlin-Hansen et al., 1992, Ertenli et al., 1996; Lin et al., 1996; Mannaioni et al., 1997) and PDGF (Kumkumian et al., 1989; Guerne and Vischer, 1991; Remmers et al., 1991a,b; Reuterdahl et al., 1991; Ridderstadt et al., 1991; Smith et al., 1991; Thornton et al., 1991; Goddard et al., 1992; Harvey et al., 1993; Monier et al., 1994; Ohba et al., 1996; Lemaire et al., 1997) occupy a crucial role in the hyperplastic response of synovial connective tissue cells in RA, intervention by NSAIDs apparently represents a paradox. Thus, whereas inhibition of PG synthesis likely diminishes pain through an attenuation of peripheral sensitization (Schaible and Grubb, 1993), this may result paradoxically in disinhibition of both PDGF release and PDGF-mediated synoviocyte proliferation as well as PGH synthase mRNA induction.

Faced with this possible therapeutic dilemma, it is interesting to review the new NSAID, lornoxicam (launched in 1997) (Fig. 4.1), which, in addition to inhibiting COX activity potently (Pruss et al., 1990), also has been demonstrated to inhibit dramatically the release of PDGF from human platelets in vitro (Pruss et al., 1990; Nycomed Pharma, 1990, unpublished observations). Importantly, this dose-related effect takes place at levels of lornoxicam that are entirely consistent with levels of free drug in the synovial fluid of chronically inflamed joints of patients with either RA or OA, following single or repeat dosing (Nycomed Pharma, 1990, unpublished observations).

Whether this new NSAID has any special attributes in the management of RA is an issue that will become apparent only with accumulating clinical experience. Indeed, the results of preclinical studies (discussed below) prompted the earlier proposal (Hitzenberger et al., 1990) that lornoxicam may possess disease-modifying effects. Comparative studies to test this intriguing notion have not yet been undertaken (Nycomed Pharma, 1997, personal communication). Also, it would be interesting to determine whether lornoxicam can inhibit PDGF from lining layer cells and sublining macrophage-like cells within the rheumatoid synovium (Remmers et al., 1991b). In light of the above observations of a possible dual action of lornoxicam, the effects of this NSAID upon bone and cartilage destruction in the adjuvant arthritic rat-injected paw (Pruss et al., 1990) (Fig. 4.2) are worthy of comment. In addition to published results (Pruss et al., 1990), unpublished observations (kindly supplied by Nycomed Pharma, 1997) demonstrate that the lowest daily dose of lornoxicam (0.03 mg/kg perorally) tested in this model significantly prevented the degenerative bone changes that follow the subplantar injection of mycobacterium butyricum. These results are impressive because they occur at a dose that, when directly extrapolated to the human, represents an amount that is actually considerably below the recommended dose for managing RA (Berry and Ollier, 1990). On a comparative basis, it should be noted that the effects of other NSAIDs upon degenerative bone changes in this model are often limited (Blackham et al., 1977; Engelhardt et al., 1995; Aota et al., 1996; Yamamoto et al., 1996) or require high doses (Awouters et al., 1975; Rainsford, 1989; Engelhardt et al.,

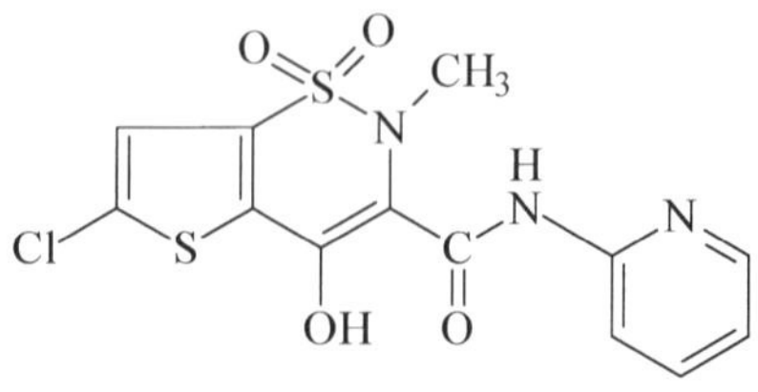

Figure 4.1 Lornoxicam.

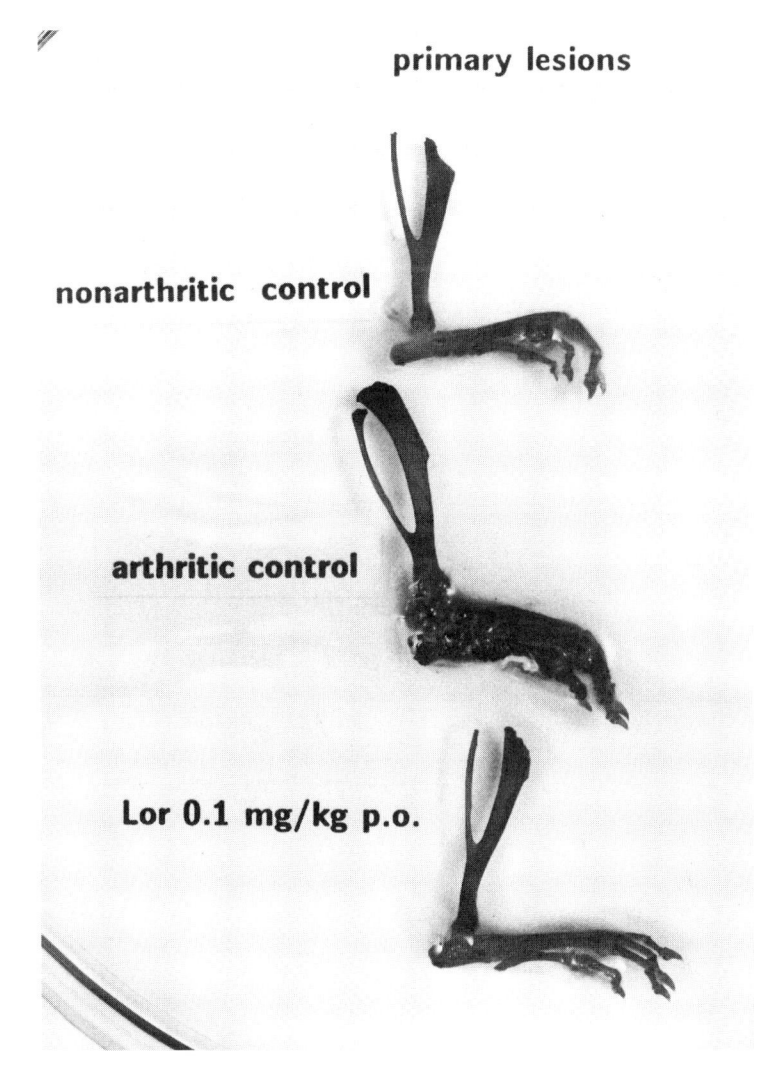

Figure 4.2 Preventive effect of lornoxicam on the primary bone changes in the adjuvant arthritic rat-injected paw. Photograph reproduced from Pruss et al. (1990) with kind permission

1995). Interestingly, attenuation of the progress of degenerative changes by an NSAID does not appear to be simply related to an inhibition of PG synthesis (Aota et al., 1996; Yamamoto et al., 1996). Inhibition of ossification, for example, can occur using an NSAID at a dose that produces no obvious antiinflammatory activity (Lussier and de Medicis, 1983). However, it is important to mention that when attempting to compare the effects of different NSAIDs in this model, possible differences in pharmacokinetics, such as protein binding

(Ferdinandi et al., 1982) and clearance (Rainsford, 1989), may complicate the extrapolation of doses from the rat to the human. Also, reported differences between NSAIDs may possibly reflect differences between methods used to assess joint destruction. Finally, although adjuvant arthritis in the rat is an established model of chronic polyarthritis, which has been used successfully to develop compounds exhibiting therapeutic benefit in humans, the relationship of this model to human RA is limited. Indeed, there are conflicting reports on the effectiveness of disease modifying antirheumatic drugs (gold, D-penicillamine, chloroquine, hydroxychloroquine) in adjuvant arthritis (Graeme et al., 1966; Liyanage and Currey, 1972; Lewis et al., 1980; Carlson et al., 1985; Garrett et al., 1985).

Pravadoline. Pravadoline was originally synthesised as a putative COX inhibitor in which the inclusion of a basic amine was designed to limit gastric irritancy relative to that of typical acidic NSAIDs. Indeed, pravadoline proved to be a COX-inhibiting antinociceptive agent, apparently devoid of gastrointestinal toxicity. However, although the clinical attractiveness suggested by its comparative superior preclinical profile prompted further intensive investigations of this compound, pravadoline was not developed further when evidence of nephrotoxicity was observed following multiple administration in humans (Ward, 1994). Pravadoline, however, merits attention because unexpectedly this compound was found to possess several additional, and potentially useful, properties, uncharacteristic of typical acidic NSAIDs. Remarkably, when tested in a range of nociceptive assays, but particularly in the adjuvant arthritis rat model, pravadoline clearly has greater antinociceptive efficacy than the classical acidic NSAIDs. This profile is marked in the adjuvant arthritic rat model, where, in contrast with zomepirac, and in a manner more similar to morphine, pravadoline produces steep dose–response curves and a high maximal effect.

Pravadoline, in addition to an inhibition of COX activity, also possesses agonist activity at cannabinoid receptors (Ward et al., 1990a,b; Burstein et al., 1992; Howlett, 1995; Xie et al., 1995). The mechanism by which pravadoline displays greater efficacy than classical acidic NSAIDs when tested in the adjuvant arthritic rat is likely a consequence of its dual actions (Burstein et al., 1992; Ward, 1994). Elucidation of the mechanism by which pravadoline and structurally related COX inhibitors apparently lack the gastrointestinal liabilities of many NSAIDs could lead to important new therapeutic agents (Ward, 1994).

Ibuprofen. Whether the current regulatory climate would have precluded general clinical application of pravadoline is a matter of speculation, for it was claimed "frank THC (i.e., Δ^9-tetrahydrocannabinol)-like highs" were not evident in clinical use (Ward, 1994). Clearly this is an interesting area for further research. However, although THC-type 7-oic acids have been proposed as candidates for a new class of NSAID (Burstein et al., 1992), with in vivo effects that may result in disease-modifying activity in the management of RA, for example (Burstein et al., 1992), current legislation may restrict further research. Given this likely barrier, it is interesting to report the recent findings of Fowler et al. (1997) that ibuprofen inhibits the metabolism of the endogenous cannabimimetic agent, anandamide.

It is now well established that many of the pharmacological actions of cannabinoids are mediated by cannabinoid receptors (Pertwee, 1993), and in recent years endogenous cannabimimetic agents have been identified (Hanus et al., 1993). The first of these to be isolated, anandamide [N-(2-hydroxyethyl)-5,8,11,14-eicosatetraenamide] (Devane et al., 1992), has been shown both in vivo and in vitro to produce many of the pharmacological and biochemical effects of cannabinoids secondary to interaction with cannabinoid receptors (Mackie et al., 1993; Vogel et al., 1993; Smith et al., 1994). Anandamide is rapidly metabolized by a membrane-bound amidase to produce arachidonic acid (Hillard et al., 1995; Ueda et al., 1995a–c). On reviewing the reports that the greater antinociceptive efficacy of pravadoline may derive from agonist activity at cannabinoid receptors (see above), Fowler et al. (1997) reasoned that a concomitant inhibition of anandamide amidase together with inhibition of COX activity might also result in enhanced antinociceptive activity. Accordingly, they undertook an evaluation of the effects of selected NSAIDs upon the activity of anandamide amidase.

Preliminary studies using a rat cerebellar membrane preparation revealed that in the absence of anandamide, ibuprofen, aspirin, sulindac, and acetaminophen did not affect the specific binding of the high-affinity cannabinoid agonist ligand [^{3}H] WIN55212-2. This result is consistent with the report that these compounds, unlike pravadoline, do not inhibit neuronally stimulated contractions of mouse vas deferens preparations (Haubrich et al., 1990). On the other hand, nabumetone was found to inhibit the binding of [^{3}H] WIN55212-2. Because nabumetone acts as a prodrug in vivo (Blower, 1992), the clinical relevance of this finding remains unknown. However, this observation demonstrates that nonacidic NSAIDs other than pravadoline and its analogues (D'Ambra et al., 1992) may affect cannabinoid receptor function.

Incubation of the membranes with anandamide produced inhibition of [^{3}H] WIN 55212-2 binding. The duration of this inhibitory effect was prolonged by ibuprofen but not by aspirin, sulindac, acetaminophen, ketoprofen, and naproxen. Using a direct assay of anandamide amidase with [^{14}C]anandamide as ligand, Omeir et al. (1995) confirmed the inhibitory effect of ibuprofen upon anandamide metabolism, and gave an IC$_{50}$ value of ~400 μM at a [^{14}C]anandamide concentration of 27.7 μM. For comparison, IC$_{50}$ values for inhibition by ibuprofen of COX 1 and COX 2 activities in broken cells are approximately 15 and 800 μM, respectively (Mitchell et al., 1993). On this basis, and following a brief review of the literature, Fowler et al. (1997) conclude that, particularly in the case of individuals taking higher doses of ibuprofen for the management of RA, therapeutic concentrations of ibuprofen may affect the metabolism of anandamide. Of course, whether such an effect contributes to the clinical profile of this drug, or distinguishes ibuprofen in the management of RA, is a matter that awaits elucidation.

Finally, it has been demonstrated recently that both $R(-)$-ibuprofen (IC$_{50}$: 121.8 μM) and S(+)-ibuprofen (IC$_{50}$:61.7 μM) inhibit the activation of NF-κB n response to T-cell stimulation (Brune, 1997, personal communication; Scheuren et al., 1997) (see also section on salicylate, above). The effect of ibuprofen was specific because, at concentrations up to 10 mM, ibuprofen did not affect the heat shock transcription factor and the activation of NF-κB by PGE$_2$. Very high concentrations of ibuprofen (20 mM) did not prevent NF-κB binding to DNA in vitro. Immunofluorescence and nuclear import experiments indicate that the site of ibuprofen action appears to be upstream of the dissociation of the NF-κB-IκB complex. Clearly, given the pivotal role of NF-κB in RA (Handel et al., 1995; Sakurada et al., 1996), the effects of NSAIDs upon the activity of NF-κB merit further investigation. Moreover, such studies may provide exciting opportunities for the development of novel therapies in the management of chronic inflammatory disorders. Indeed, it now seems possible that PGH synthase-1 peroxidase, putatively an NSAID-insensitive activity of PGH synthase-1, through its effects in mediating NF-κB activity, may provide a new and important target for anti-inflammatory therapy (Munroe et al., 1995).

Acetaminophen. Often classified as an NSAID, the biochemical properties of acetaminophen, which include weak inhibitory activity on COX activity (Mitchell et al., 1993; Vane and Botting, 1995), together with its ability to cross the blood–brain barrier, suggest a central activity, which has been reported in several studies both in animals (Carlsson et al., 1988) and in humans (Chen and Chapman, 1980). The classical view that, unlike aspirin, acetaminophen has little or no anti-inflammatory effect has been challenged by Lökken et al. (1995) following the recent observations that acetaminophen reduces the development of polyarthritis and inflammatory signs together with Fos-like immunoreactivity, in models of both adjuvant-arthritis and carrageenan-induced inflammation, respectively (Abbadie and Besson, 1994; Honoré et al., 1995).

Reviewing the published literature, Lökken et al. (1995) support the earlier view expressed by Honoré et al. (1995), that the traditional dogma that acetaminophen lacks anti-inflammatory activity, needs reappraisal. Indeed, the recent results of Abbadie and Besson (1994) and those of Honoré et al. (1995) confirm those of previous studies showing an anti-inflammatory effect of acetaminophen in a variety of acute and chronic inflammatory tests in rodents (Vinegar et al., 1976; Glenn et al., 1977; Wong and Gardocki, 1983; Higuchi et al., 1984; Mburu et al., 1988; McQueen et al., 1991; Abbadie and Besson, 1994) and following oral surgery in humans (Skjelbred and Lökken, 1979; Skjelbred et al., 1984; Olstad and Skjelbred, 1986a,b). Taken together, the results of these studies indicate that under some conditions, acetaminophen may exert greater anti-inflammatory activity than aspirin (Lökken et al., 1995). Given the reduced risk of gastrointestinal bleeding with acetaminophen with therapeutic dosing (Brune and McCormack, 1994), the origination of studies designed to clarify the anti-inflammatory use of acetaminophen appears warranted. Additional insights into an analgesic effect, which might be secondary to an anti-inflammatory effect, would also follow.

FUTURE NSAIDs AND STRATEGIES

Whether NSAID-mediated analgesia, and indeed other effects, involve an interaction with the heterotrimeric GTP-binding proteins (G proteins) is an area that has attracted scant attention despite the publication of several very tantalizing reports (Abramson et al., 1985, 1990, 1991a,b, 1994; Bomalaski et al., 1986; Longheu et al., 1988; Weissman, 1991; Tissot et al., 1992; for review see McCormack, 1994a;1994b). More recently, Shackelford et al. (1997) provide the first report that the stabilization of the NF-κB inhibitory protein, IκB, by aspirin at therapeutic doses is pertussis toxin (PTX) sensitive (which indicates the involvement of a PTX-sensitive G protein). Further studies here are important, and will likely also provide additional insights into the not infrequent reports that in both animals (Björkman et al., 1990) and humans (Vescovi et al., 1987), NSAID-mediated analgesia involves a naloxone-sensitive component, which in some situations may involve a direct interaction at the opioid receptor (Pini et al., 1997).

Further scope for developing novel NSAIDs may derive from our greater understanding of the adenosine cyclic-3′,5′-monophosphate (cAMP) signaling pathway, notably the regulation and function of the adenylyl cyclase (AC) enzyme superfamily. PGs, on activating the PG receptor subtypes EP_1, EP_2, or EP_3 (Coleman et al., 1990), can activate either stimulatory (Gs) or inhibitory (Gi/o) alpha subunits of G proteins (Kumazawa et al., 1994). Classically, it is generally accepted that the pain-enhancing effects of PGs result through Gsα-mediated increases in cAMP (Ferreira, 1981), with this system becoming down-regulated through the inhibitory effects of an NSAID upon COX activity. Today, nine mammalian isoforms of the AC enzyme (which converts ATP to cAMP) have been discovered within nervous tissue (Sunahara et al., 1996; Hanoune et al., 1997). Importantly, however, it is now evident that some of these isoforms can be regulated by the G protein βγ dimer (Gβγ) (AC I, II, and IV), the calcium-binding protein, calmodulin (AC I, III, VIII), and calcium (AC V and VI) (for review see Sunahara et al., 1996; Hanoune et al., 1997). Until such discoveries, it was generally believed that activity of AC was regulated solely by the G protein alpha subunits (Gsα—stimulation of AC, Giα/Goα—inhibition of AC). Of particular relevance is the further discovery that several of these AC isoforms (listed above) can be regulated by coincident, but not necessarily simultaneous, inputs and that the subsequent effect upon AC activity is nonlinear. Clearly, this greater understanding of the AC enzyme superfamily provides the opportunity to target individual AC isoforms by NSAIDs which have, for example, the additional capacity to modulate Gβγ levels through effects at receptors that couple to Gi (an abundant supply of

Gβγ). Moreover, this new knowledge may provide further insights into the synergism demonstrated to occur in pain models when NSAIDs are used in combination with ligands which activate Gi/o (Malmberg and Yaksh, 1993).

CONCLUSION

It is a sobering thought that many of our effective medicines in use today did not originate from intellectualism, but were culled from the hedgerows and derived from ancient folklore remedies. The NSAIDs, which today command the worldwide attention of industrialists, economists, stock market analysts, researchers, and physicians alike, represent a category of drugs with origins that are truly lost in antiquity and myth. In accepting the ubiquitous nature of these compounds to inhibit COX activity, we should not overlook the rich structural and pharmacological diversity which, likewise, is a hallmark of this category. With our greater understanding of both peripheral and central processing of nociceptive input, the opportunities exist to explore the clinical significance of such diversity. Interest in undertaking such new studies, however, will ultimately be driven by the need to provide greater benefit to the patient. If such goals are not in sight, then understandably research funding incentives will become limited for compounds that may be viewed as less exciting than the newest basic science hypotheses. Progress in science, however, is generally not a reasonable process with quantum leaps in discovery; rather, it is one of struggle and development through the repeated acquisition of small gains. Consequently, we should not understate either the contribution of NSAID pharmacology to our current understanding or the potential of this group for yielding novel entities.

ACKNOWLEDGMENT

The author gratefully acknowledges the expertise and advice of Helen Millins on methods of literature searching and retrieval.

REFERENCES

Abbadie C, Besson J-M (1994): Chronic treatments with aspirin or acetaminophen reduce both the development of polyarthritis and Fos-like immunoreactivity in rat lumbar spinal cord. Pain 57:45–54.

Abramson S, Korchak H, Ludewig R, Edelson H, Haines K, Levin RI, Herman R, Rider L, Kimmel S, Weissman G (1985): Modes of action of aspirin-like drugs. Proc Natl Acad Sci USA 82:7227–7231.

Abramson SB, Cherksey B, Gude D, Leszczynska-Piziak J, Philips MR, Blau L, Weissman G (1990): Nonsteroidal antiinflammatory drugs exert differential effects on neutrophil function and plasma membrane viscosity: Studies in human neutrophils and liposomes. Inflammation 14:11–30.

Abramson SB, Leszczynska-Piziak J, Haines K, Reibman J (1991a): Non-steroidal anti-inflammatory drugs: Effects on a GTP binding protein within the neutrophil plasma membrane. Biochem Pharmacol 41:1567–1573.

Abramson SB, Leszczynska-Piziak J, Weissman G (1991b): Arachidonic acid as a second messenger. Interactions with a GTP-binding protein of human neutrophils. J Immunol 147:231–236.

Abramson SB, Leszczynska-Piziak J, Clancy RM, Philips M, Weissmann G (1994): Inhibition of neutrophic function by aspirin-like drugs (NSAIDs): Requirement for assembly of heterotrimeric G proteins in bilayer phospholipid. Biochem Pharmacol 47:563–572.

Aota S, Nakamura T, Suzuki K, Tanaka Y, Okazaki Y, Segawa Y, Miura M, Kikuchi S (1996): Effects of indomethacin administration on bone turnover and bone mass in adjuvant-induced arthritis in rats. Calcif Tissue Int 59:385–391.

Awouters F, Niemeggers CJE, Lenaerts FM, Janssen PAJ (1975): The effects of suprofen in rats with mycobacterium butyricum-induced arthritis. Arzneim-Forsch (Drug Res) 25:1526–1537.

Berry H, Ollier S (1990): Lornoxicam in clinical practice. Postgrad Med J 66:S41–S45.

Bitko V, Velazquez A, Yang L, Yang YC, Barik S (1997): Transcriptional induction of multiple cytokines by human respiratory syncytial virus requires activation of NF-κB and is inhibited by sodium salicylate and aspirin. Virology 232:369–378.

Björkman R, Hedner J, Hedner T, Henning M (1990): Central naloxone-reversible antinociception by diclofenac in the rat. Naunyn Schmiedebergs Arch Pharmacol 342:171–176.

Blackham A, Burns JW, Farmer JB, Radziwonik H, Westwick J (1977): An X-ray analysis of adjuvant arthritis in the rat. The effect of prednisolone and indomethacin. Agents Actions 7:145–151.

Blackwell TS, Christman JW (1997): The role of nuclear factor-κB in cytokine gene regulation. Am J Respir Cell Mol Biol 17:3–9.

Blower PR (1992): The unique pharmacologic profile of nabumetone. J Rheumatol 19:13–19.

Bomalaski JS, Hirata F, Clark MA (1986): Aspirin inhibits phospholipase C. Biochem Biophys Res Commun 139:115–121.

Brune K, McCormack K (1994): The over-the-counter use of nonsteroidal anti-inflammatory drugs and other antipyretic analgesics. In Lewis AJ, Furst DE (eds): *Nonsteroidal Anti-inflammatory Drugs. Mechanisms and Clinical Uses*, 2nd ed. New York: Marcel Dekker, pp. 97–126.

Buritova J, Honoré P, Chapman V, Besson J-M (1996): Enhanced effects of co-administered dexamethasone and diclofenac on inflammatory pain processing and associated spinal c-Fos expression in the rat. Pain 64:559–568.

Burstein SH, Audetie CA, Breuer A, Devane WA, Colodner S, Doyle SA, Mechoulam R (1992): Synthetic nonpsychotropic cannabinoids with potent antiinflammatory, analgesic, and leukocyte adhesion activities. J Med Chem 35:3135–3141.

Butler SH, Godefroy F, Besson JM, Weil-Fugazzo J (1992): A limited arthritic model for chronic pain studies in the rat. Pain 48:73–81.

Carlson RP, Datko LJ, O'Neill-Davis L, Blazek EM, DeLustro F, Beideman R, Lewis AJ (1985): Comparison of inflammatory changes in established type II collagen- and adjuvant-induced arthritis using outbred Wistar rats. Int J Immunopharmacol 7: 811–826.

Carlsson KH, Monzel W, Jurna I (1988): Depression by morphine and the non-opioid analgesic agents, metamizol (dipyrone), lysine acetylsalicylate and paracetamol of activity in rat thalamus neurons evoked by electrical stimulation of nociceptive afferents. Pain 32:313–326.

Carter BD, Kaltschmidt C, Kaltschmidt B, Offenhuser N, Bohm-Matthaei R, Baeuerle PA, Barde YA (1996): Selective activation of NF-κB by nerve growth factor through the neurotrophin receptor p75. Science 272:542–545.

Cato AC, Wade E (1996): Molecular mechanisms of anti-inflammatory action of glucocorticoids. Bioessays 18:371–378.

Chen AC, Chapman CR (1980): Aspirin analgesia evaluated by event-related potentials in man: possible central action in brain. Exp Brain Res 39:359–364.

Chen F, Sun S, Kuhn DC, Gaydos LJ, Shi X, Lu Y, Demers LM (1997): Involvement of NF-κB in silica-induced cyclooxygenase II gene expression in rat alveolar macrophages. Am J Physiol 272:L779–L786.

Chin JR, Murphy G, Werb Z (1985): Stromelysin, a connective tissue-degrading metalloendopeptidase secreted by stimulated rabbit synovial fibroblasts in parallel with collagenase. Biosynthesis, isolation, characterization, and substrates. J Biol Chem 260:12367–12376.

Coleman RA, Kennedy I, Humphrey PPA, Bunce K, Lumley P (1990): Prostanoids and their receptors. In Emmet J (ed): *Membranes and Receptors. Comprehensive Medical Chemistry*, Vol. 3, Oxford: Pergamon Press, pp. 643–714.

D'Ambra TE, Estep KG, Bell MR, Eissenstat MA, Josef KA, Ward SJ, Haycock DA, Baizman ER, Casiano FM, Beglin NC (1992): Conformationally restrained analogues of pravadoline: nanomolar potent, enantioselective, (aminoalkly)indole agonists of the cannabinoid receptor. J Med Chem 35:124–135.

Dayer JM, Krane SM, Russell RG, Robinson DR (1976): Production of collagenase and prostaglandins by isolated adherent rheumatoid synovial cells. Proc Natl Acad Sci USA 73:945–949.

de Gaetano G, Cerletti C, Nanni-Costa MP, Poggi I (1989): The blood platelet as an inflammatory cell. Eur Respir J 2:441s–445s.

Demarchi F, d'Adda di Fagagna F, Falaschi A, Giacca M (1996): Activation of transcription factor NF-κB by the Tat protein of human immunodeficiency virus type 1. J Virol 70:4427–4437.

Devane WA, Hanus L, Breuer A, Pertwee RG, Stevenson LA, Griffin G, Gibson D, Mandelbaum A, Etinger A, Mechoulam R (1992): Isolation and structure of a brain constituent that binds to the cannabinoid receptor. Science 258:1946–1949.

Dougherty PM, Sluka KM, Sorkin LS, Westlund KN, Willis WD (1992): Neural changes in acute arthritis in monkeys. I. Parallel enhancement of responses of spinothalamic tract neurons to mechanical stimulation and excitatory amino acids. Brain Res Rev 17:1–13.

Endresen GK (1981): Investigation of blood platelets in synovial fluid from patients with rheumatoid arthritis. Scand J Rheumatol 10:204–208.

Endresen GK (1984): Demonstration of fibronectin associated with platelets in synovial fluid from patients with rheumatoid arthritis. Scand J Rheumatol 13:351–356.

Endresen GKM (1989): Evidence for activation of platelets in the synovial fluid from patients with rheumatoid arthritis. Rheumatol Int 9:9–24.

Endresen GKM, Førre Ø (1992): Human platelets in synovial fluid. A focus on the effects of growth factors on the inflammatory responses in rheumatoid arthritis. Clin Exp Rheumatol 10:181–187.

Engelhardt G, Homma D, Schnitzler C (1995): Meloxicam: A potent inhibitor of adjuvant arthritis in the Lewis rat. Inflamm Res 44:548–555.

Ertenli I, Haznedaroglu IC, Kiraz S, Celik I, Calguneri M, Kirazhi S (1996): Cytokines affecting megakaryocytopoiesis in rheumatoid arthritis with thrombocytosis. Rheumatol Int 16:5–8.

Farr M, Scott DL, Constable T, Hawker R, Hawkins CF (1981): Platelets and rheumatoid arthritis. Ann Rheum Dis 40:617–618.

Farr M, Wainwright A, Salmon M, Hollywell CA, Bacon PA (1984): Platelets in the synovial fluid of patients with rheumatoid arthritis. Rheumatol Int 4:13–17.

Fassbender HG (1983): The significance of inflammatory processes in osteoarthrosis. Z Rheumatol 42:145–152.

Ferdinandi ES, Cayen MN, Pace-Asciak C (1982): Disposition of etodolac, other antiinflammatory pyranoindole-1-acetic acids and furobufen in normal and adjuvant arthritic rats. J Pharmacol Exp Ther 220:417–426.

Ferreira SH (1981): Local control of inflammatory pain. Agents Actions 11:636–638.

Fowler CJ, Stenström A, Tiger G (1997): Ibuprofen inhibits the metabolism of the endogenous cannabimimetic agent anandamide. Pharmacol Toxicol 80:103–107.

Garrett IR, Whitehouse MW, Vernon Roberts B, Brooks PM (1985): Ambivalent properties of gold drugs in adjuvant induced polyarthritis in rats. J Rheumatol 12: 1079–1082.

Glaser KB, Sung A, Bauer J, Weichman BM (1993): Regulation of eicosanoid biosynthesis in the macrophage. Involvement of protein tyrosine phosphorylation and modulation by selective protein tyrosine kinase inhibitors. Biochem Pharmacol 45:711–721.

Glenn EM, Bowman BJ, Rohloff NA (1977): Anti-inflammatory and PG inhibitory effects of phenacetin and acetaminophen. Agents Actions 7:513–516.

Goddard DH, Grossman SL, Newton R, Clark MA, Bomalaski JS (1992): Regulation of synovial cell growth: basic fibroblast growth factor synergizes with interleukin 1 beta stimulating phospholipase A2 enzyme activity, phospholipase A2 activity protein production and release of prostaglandin E2 by rheumatoid arthritis synovial cells in culture. Cytokine 4:377–384.

Graeme ML, Fabry E, Sigg EB (1966): Mycobacterial adjuvant periarthritis in rodents and its modification by antiinflammatory agents. J Pharmacol 153:373–380.

Griffin GE, Leung K, Folks TM, Kunkel S, Nabel GJ (1989): Activation of HIV gene expression during monocyte differentiation by induction of NF-kappa-B. Nature 339: 70–73.

Grilli M, Memo M (1997): Transcriptional pharmacology of neurodegenerative disorders: novel venue towards neuroprotection against excitotoxicity. Mol Psychiatry 2: 192–194.

Grilli M, Chiu JJ-S, Lenardo M (1993): NF-κB and Rel: participants in a multiform transcriptional regulatory system. Int Rev Cytol 143:1–62.

Grilli M, Pizzi M, Memo M, Spano P (1996): Neuroprotection by aspirin and sodium salicylate through blockade of NF-κB activation. Science 274:1383–1385.

Guerne PA, Vischer TL (1991): L'interleukine-6, parmi les autres cytokines, dans les rheumatismes. Méd Hyg 49:869–873.

Hamilton JA, Butler DM, Stanton H (1994): Cytokine interactions promoting DNA synthesis in human synovial fibroblasts. J Rheumatol 21:797–803.

Handel ML, McMorrow LB, Gravallese EM (1995): Nuclear factor-kappa B in rheumatoid synovium. Localization of p50 and p65. Arthritis Rheum 38:1762–1770.

Hanoune J, Pouille Y, Tzavara E, Shen T, Lipskaya L, Miyamoto N, Suzuki Y, Defer N (1997): Adenylyl cyclases: structure, regulation and function in an enzyme superfamily. Mol Cell Endocrinol 128:179–194.

Hanus L, Gopher A, Almog S, Mechoulam R (1993): Two new unsaturated fatty acid ethanolamides in brain that bind to the cannabinoid receptor. J Med Chem 36:3032–3034.

Harvey AK, Stack ST, Chandrasekhar S (1993): Differential modulation of degradative and repair responses of interleukin-1-treated chondrocytes by platelet-derived growth factor. Biochem J 292:129–136.

Haubrich DR, Ward SJ, Baizman E, Bell MR, Bradford J, Ferrari R, Miller M, Perrone M, Pierson AK, Saelens JK (1990): Pharmacology of pravadoline: a new analgesic agent. J Pharmacol Exp Ther 255:511–522.

He CS, Wilhelm SM, Pentland AP, Marmer BL, Grant GA, Eisen AZ, Goldberg GI (1989): Tissue cooperation in a proteolytic cascade activating human interstitial collagenase. Proc Natl Acad Sci USA 86:2632–2636.

Heck S, Bender K, Kullmann M, Gottlicher M, Herrlich P, Cato ACB (1997): IκBα-independent downregulation of NF-κB activity by glucocorticoid receptor. EMBO J 16:4698–4707.

Higuchi S, Osada Y, Shioiri Y, Tanaka N, Otomo S (1984): Effect of anti-inflammatory drugs on the lame walking reaction in adjuvant-induced edematous rats. Nippon Yakurigaku Zasshi 84:243–249.

Hillard CJ, Wilkinson DM, Edgemond WS, Campbell WB (1995): Characterization of the kinetics and distribution of N-arachidonylethanolamine (anandamide) hydrolysis by rat brain. Biochim Biophys Acta 1257:249–256.

Hitzenberger G, Radhofer-Welte S, Takacs F, Rosenow D (1990): Pharmacokinetics of lornoxicam in man. Postgrad Med J 66:S22–S26.

Honoré P, Buritova J, Besson J-M (1995): Aspirin and acetaminophen reduced both Fos expression in rat lumbar spinal cord and inflammatory signs produced by carrageenin inflammation. Pain 63:365–375.

Howlett AC (1995): Pharmacology of cannabinoid receptors. Ann Rev Pharmacol Toxicol 35:607–634.

Kopp E, Ghosh S (1994): Inhibition of NF-κB by sodium salicylate and aspirin. Science 265:956–959.

Kumazawa T, Mizumura K, Koda H (1994): Different mechanisms (receptor subtypes and second messenger actions) implicated in PGE$_2$-induced sensitization of the responses to bradykinin and to heat of polymodal receptors. In Gebhart GF, Hammond DL, Jensen TS (eds): *Proceedings of the 7th World Congress on Pain. Progress in Research and Management.* Seattle: IASP Press, pp. 265–276.

Kumkumian GK, Lafyatis R, Remmers EF, Case JP, Kim SJ, Wilder RL (1989): Platelet-derived growth factor and IL-1 interactions in rheumatoid arthritis. Regulation of synoviocyte proliferation, prostaglandin production, and collagenase transcription. J Immunol 143:833–837.

Lemaire R, Huet G, Zerimech F, Grard G, Fontaine C, Duquesnoy B, Flipo RM (1997): Selective induction of the secretion of cathepsins B and L by cytokines in synovial fibroblast-like cells. Br J Rheumatol 36:735–743.

Levy M (1990): Unwanted drug effects of antipyretic analgesics: epidemiological data. In Brune K (ed): *New Pharmacological and Epidemiological Data in Analgesic Research.* Basel: Birkhäuser Verlag, pp. 39–47.

Lewis AJ, Cottney J, White DD, Fox PK, McNeillie A, Dunlop J, Smith WE, Brown DH (1980): Action of gold salts in some inflammatory and immunological models. Agents Actions 10:63–77.

Lin AH, Bienkowski MJ, Gorman RR (1989): Regulation of prostaglandin H synthase mRNA levels and prostaglandin biosynthesis by platelet-derived growth factor. J Biol Chem 264:17379–17383.

Lin MK, Farewell V, Vadas P, Bookman AA, Keystone EC, Pruzanski W (1996): Secretory phospholipase A$_2$ as an index of disease activity in rheumatoid arthritis. Prospective double blind study of 212 patients. J Rheumatol 23:1162–1166.

Liyanage SP, Currey HL (1972): Failure of oral D-penicillamine to modify adjuvant arthritis or immune response in the rat. Ann Rheum Dis 31:521–523.

Lökken P, Skoglund LA, Skjelbred P (1995): Anti-inflammatory efficacy of treatments with aspirin and acetaminophen. Pain 60:231–232.

Longheu M, Roccesalva N, Parenti M, Groppetti A (1988): Effect of pertussis toxin on aspirin-mediated analgesia. Pharmacol Res Commun 20:133.

Lussier A, de Medicis R (1983): Correlation between ossification and inflammation using a rat experimental model. J Rheumatol (Suppl. 11)10:114–117.

MacIlwain C (1993): Aspirin on trial as HIV treatment. Nature 364:369.

Mackie K, Devane WA, Hille B (1993): Anandamide, an endogenous cannabinoid, inhibits calcium currents as a partial agonist in N18 neuroblastoma cells. Mol Pharmacol 44:498–503.

Malmberg AB, Yaksh TL (1993): Pharmacology of the spinal action of ketorolac, morphine, ST-91, U50488H, and L-PIA on the formalin test and an isobolographic analysis of the NSAID interaction. Anesthesiology 79:270–281.

Mannaioni PF, Di Bello G, Masini E (1997): Platelets and inflammation: Role of platelet-derived growth factor, adhesion molecules and histamine. Inflamm Res 46:4–18.

Mburu DN, Mbugua SW, Skoglund LA, Lokken P (1988): Effects of paracetamol and acetylsalicylic acid on the post-operative course after experimental orthopaedic surgery in dogs. J Vet Pharmacol Ther 11:163–170.

McCormack K (1994a): Non-steroidal anti-inflammatory drugs and spinal nociceptive processing. Pain 59:9–43.

McCormack K (1994b): The spinal actions of NSAIDs and the dissociation between antiinflammatory and analgesic effects. Drugs 47:28–45.

McQueen DS, Iggo A, Birrell GJ, Grubb BD (1991): Effects of paracetamol and aspirin on neural activity of joint mechanonociceptors in adjuvant arthritis. Br J Pharmacol 104:178–182.

Mitchell JA, Akarasereenont P, Thiemermann C, Flower RJ, Vane JR (1993): Selectivity of nonsteroidal antiinflammatory drugs as inhibitors of constitutive and inducible cyclooxygenase. Proc Natl Acad Sci USA 90:11693–11697.

Mitchell JA, Saunders M, Barnes PJ, Newton R, Belvisi MG (1997): Sodium salicylate inhibits cyclo-oxygenase-2 activity independently of transcription factor (nuclear factor κB) activation: role of arachidonic acid. Mol Pharmacol 51:907–912.

Monier S, Rème T, Cognot C, Gao Q-L, Travaglio-Encinoza A, Cuchacovich M, Gaillard J-P, Jorgensen C, Sany J, Dupuy D'angeac A, Jullien P (1994): Growth factor activity of IL-6 in the synovial fluid of patients with rheumatoid arthritis. Clin Exp Rheumatol 12:595–602.

Munroe DG, Wang EY, MacIntyre JP, Tam SS, Lee DH, Taylor GR, Zhou L, Plante RK, Kazmi SM, Bauerle PA (1995): Novel intracellular signaling function of prostaglandin H synthase-1 by NF-κB activation. J Inflamm 45:260–268.

Nabel G, Baltimore D (1987): An inducible transcription factor activates expression of human immunodeficiency virus in T cells. Nature 326:711–713.

Neugebauer V, Kornhuber J, Lucke T, Schaible HG (1993): The clinically available NMDA receptor antagonist memantine is antinociceptive on rat spinal cord neurons. NeuroReport 4:1259–1262.

O'Banion MK, Winn VD, Young DA (1992): cDNA cloning and functional activity of a glucocorticoid-regulated inflammatory cyclooxygenase. Proc Natl Acad Sci USA 89:4888–4892.

Ohba T, Takase W, Ohhara M, Kasukawa R (1996): Thrombin in the synovial fluid of patients with rheumatoid arthritis mediates proliferation of synovial fibroblast-like cells by induction of platelet derived growth factor. J Rheumatol 23:1505–1511.

Olstad OA, Skjelbred P (1986a): Comparison of the analgesic effect of a corticosteroid and paracetamol in patients with pain after oral surgery. Br J Clin Pharmacol 22:437–442.

Olstad OA, Skjelbred P (1986b): The effects of indoprofen vs paracetamol on swelling, pain and other events after surgery. Int J Clin Pharmacol Ther Toxicol 24:34–38.

Omeir RL, Chin S, Hong Y, Ahern DG, Deutsch DG (1995): Arachidonoyl ethanolamide-(1,2-14C) as a substrate for anandamide amidase. Life Sci 56:1999–2005.

Osnes LT, Foss KB, Joo GB, Okkenhaug C, Westvik AB, Ovstebo R, Kierulf P (1996): Acetylsalicylic acid and sodium salicylate inhibit LPS-induced NF-κB/c-Rel nuclear translocation, and synthesis of tissue factor (TF) and tumor necrosis factor alfa (TNF-alpha) in human monocytes. Thromb Haemost 76:970–976.

Perrot S, Attal N, Ardid D, Guilbaud G (1993): Are mechanical and cold allodynia in mononeuropathic and arthritic rats relieved by systemic treatment with calcitonin or guanethidine. Pain 52:41–47.

Pertwee R (1993): The evidence for the existence of cannabinoid receptors. Gen Pharmacol 24:811–824.

Pini LA, Vitale G, Ottani A, Sandrini M (1997): Naloxone-reversible antinociception by paracetamol in the rat. J Pharmacol Exp Ther 280:934–940.

Pomerantz JL, Mauxion F, Yoshida M, Greene WC, Sen R (1989): A second sequence element located 3 to the NF-kappa-b binding site regulates IL-2 receptor-alpha gene induction. J Immunol 143:4275–4281.

Price DD, Mao J, Lu J, Caruso S, Frenk H, Mayer DJ (1996): Effects of the combined oral administration of NSAIDs and dextromethorphan on behavioural symptoms indicative of arthritic pain in rats. Pain 68:119–127.

Pruss TP, Stroißnig H, Radhofer-Welte S, Wendtlandt W, Mehdi N, Takacs F, Fellier H (1990): Overview of the pharmacological properties, pharmacokinetics and animal safety assessment of lornoxicam. Postgrad Med J 66:S18–S21.

Rainsford KD (1989): The mode of action of azapropazone in relation to its therapeutic actions in rheumatic conditions and its major side-effects. In Rainsford KD (ed): *Azapropazone, 20 Years of Clinical Use.* Lancaster, UK: Kluwer Academic Publishers, pp. 31–52.

Remmers EF, Sano H, Lafyatis R, Case JP, Kumkumian GK, Hla T, Maciag T, Wilder RL (1991a): Production of platelet derived growth factor B chain (PDGF-B/*c-sis*) mRNA and immunoreactive PDGF B-like polypeptide by rheumatoid synovium: Coexpression with heparin binding acidic fibroblast growth factor-1. J Rheumatol 18:7–13.

Remmers EF, Sano H, Wilder RL (1991b): Platelet-derived growth factors and heparin-binding (fibroblast) growth factors in the synovial tissue pathology of rheumatoid arthritis. Semin Arthritis Rheum 21:191–199.

Ren K (1994): Wind-up and the NMDA receptor: from animal studies to humans. Pain 59:157–158.

Reuterdahl C, Tingstrom A, Terracio L, Funa K, Heldin CH, Rubin K (1991): Characterization of platelet-derived growth factor beta-receptor expressing cells in the vasculature of human rheumatoid synovium. Lab Invest 64:321–329.

Ridderstadt A, Abedi-Valugerdi M, Möller E (1991): Cytokines in rheumatoid arthritis. Ann Med 23:219–223.

Sakurada S, Kato T, Okamoto T (1996): Induction of cytokines and ICAM-1 by proinflammatory cytokines in primary rheumatoid synovial fibroblasts and inhibition by N-acetyl-L-cysteine and aspirin. Int Immunol 8:1483–1493.

Schaible HG, Grubb BD (1993): Afferent and spinal mechanisms of joint pain. Pain 55:5–54.

Schalkwijk C, Vervoordeldonk M, Pfeilschifter J, Marki F, van den Bosch H (1991): Cytokine- and forskolin-induced synthesis of group II phospholipase A_2 and prostaglandin E_2 in rat mesangial cells is prevented by dexamethasone. Biochem Biophys Res Commun 180:46–52.

Scheuren N, Bang H, Münster T, Brune K, Pahl A (1997): Modulation of transcription factor NF-κB by enantiomers of the nonsteroidal drug ibuprofen. Br J Pharmacol 123:645–652.

Schmedtje JR Jr, Ji Y-S, Liu W-L, DuBois RN, Runge MS (1997): Hypoxia induces cyclooxygenase-2 via the NF-κB p65 transcription factor in human vascular endothelial cells. J Biol Chem 262:601–608.

Shackelford RE, Alford PB, Xue Y, Thai SF, Adams DO, Pizzo S (1997): Aspirin inhibits tumor necrosis factor alpha gene expression in murine tissue macrophages. Mol Pharmacol 52:421–429.

Shiozawa S, Tokuhisa L (1992): Contribution of synovial mesenchymal cells to the pathogenesis of rheumatoid arthritis. Semin Arthritis Rheum 21:267–273.

Skjelbred P, Lökken P (1979): Paracetamol versus placebo: effects on post-operative course. Eur J Clin Pharmacol 15:27–33.

Skjelbred P, Skoglund LA, Lökken P (1984): The anti-inflammatory effects of acetylsalicylic acid and paracetamol. Tandlaegebladet 88:816–818.

Sluka KA, Westlund KN (1993a): An experimental arthritis model in rats: the effects of NMDA and non-NMDA antagonists on aspartate and glutamate release in the dorsal horn. Neurosci Lett 149:99–102.

Sluka KA, Westlund KN (1993b): Spinal cord amino acid release and content in an arthritis model: the effects of pretreatment with non-NMDA, NMDA and NK1 receptor antagonists. Brain Res 627:89–103.

Sluka KA, Dougherty PM, Sorkin LS, Willis WD, Westlund KN (1992): Neural changes in acute arthritis in monkeys. III. Changes in substance P, calcitonin, gene-related peptide and glutamate in the dorsal horn of the spinal cord. Brain Res Rev 17:29–38.

Smith PB, Compton DR, Welch SP, Razdan RK, Mechoulam R, Martin BR (1994): The pharmacological activity of anandamide, a putative endogenous cannabinoid, in mice. J Pharmacol Exp Ther 270:219–227.

Smith RJ, Justen JM, Sam LM, Rohloff NA, Ruppell PL, Brunden MN, Chin JE (1991): Platelet-derived growth factor potentiates cellular responses of articular chondrocytes to interleukin-1. Arthritis Rheum 34:697–706.

Sorkin LS, Westlund KN, Sluka KA, Dougherty PM, Willis WD (1992): Neural changes in acute arthritis in monkeys. IV. Time-course of amino acid release in the lumbar dorsal horn. Brain Res Rev 17:39–50.

Stürzebecher S, Haberey M, Müller B, Schillinger E, Schröder G, Skubella W, Stock G, Vorbrüggen H, Witt W (1986): Pharmacological profile of a novel carbacyclin derivative with high metabolic stability and oral activity in the rat. Prostaglandins 31:95–109.

Stürzebecher S, Nieuweboer B, Matthes S, Schillinger E (1989): Effects of PGD_2, PGE_1, and PGI_2-analogues on PDGF-release and aggregation of human gelfiltered platelets. In Schrör K, Singzinger H (eds): *Prostaglandins in Clinical Research: Cardiovascular System*. New York: Alan R Liss, pp. 365–369.

Sunahara RK, Dessauer CW, Gilman AG (1996): Complexity and diversity of mammalian adenylyl cyclases. Ann Rev Pharmacol Toxicol 36:461–480.

Takacs E, Jellinek H (1987): Early morphological changes of vessels in an experimental model system. Inter Angio 6:7–19.

Thornton SC, Por SB, Penny R, Richter M, Shelley L, Breit SN (1991): Identification of the major fibroblast growth factors released spontaneously in inflammatory arthritis as platelet derived growth factor and tumour necrosis factor-alpha. Clin Exp Immunol 86:79–86.

Tissot M, Roch-Arveiller M, Fontagne J, Giroud JP (1992): Effects of niflumic acid on polyphosphoinositide and oxidative metabolism in polymorphonuclear leukocytes from healthy and thermally injured rats. Inflammation 16:645–657.

Ueda N, Kurahashi Y, Yamamoto S, Tokunaga T (1995a): Partial purification and characterization of the porcine brain enzyme hydrolyzing and synthesizing anandamide. J Biol Chem 270:23823–23827.

Ueda N, Yamamoto K, Kurahashi Y, Yamamoto S, Ogawa M, Matsuki N, Kudo I, Shinkai H, Shirakawa E, Tokunaga T (1995b): Oxygenation of arachidonylethanolamide (anandamide) by lipoxygenases. Adv Prostaglandin Thromboxane Leukot Res 23:163–165.

Ueda N, Yamamoto K, Yamamoto S, Tokunaga T, Shirakawa E, Shinkai H, Ogawa M, Sato T, Kudo I, Inoue K (1995c): Lipoxygenase-catalyzed oxygenation of arachidonylethanolamide, a cannabinoid receptor agonist. Biochim Biophys Acta 1254:127–134.

Uhlin-Hansen L, Langvoll D, Wik T, Kalset SO (1992): Blood platelets stimulate the expression of chondroitin sulfate proteoglycon in human monocytes. Blood 80:1058–1065.

van der Burg B, Liden J, Okret S, Delaunay F, Wissink S, Van der Saag PT, Gustafsson JA (1997): Nuclear factor-κB repression in antiinflammation and immunosuppression by glucocorticoids. Trends Endocrinol Metab 8:152–157.

Vane JR, Botting RM (1995): New insights into the mode of action of anti-inflammatory drugs. Inflamm Res 44:1–10.

Vescovi PP, Gerra G, Ippolito L (1987): Nicotinic acid effectiveness in the treatment of benzodiazepine withdrawal. Curr Ther Res Clin Exp 41:1017–1021.

Vinegar R, Truax JF, Selph JL (1976): Quantitative comparison of the analgesic and anti-inflammatory activities of aspirin, phenacetin and acetaminophen in rodents. Eur J Pharmacol 37:23–30.

Vogel Z, Barg J, Levy R, Saya D, Heldman E, Mechoulam R (1993): Anandamide, a brain endogenous compound, interacts specifically with cannabinoid receptors and inhibits adenylate cyclase. J Neurochem 61:352–355.

Ward SJ (1994): Pravadoline. A dual-mechanism aminoalkylindole analgesic. In Lewis AJ, Furst DE (eds): *Nonsteroidal Anti-inflammatory Drugs. Mechanisms and Clinical Uses*, 2nd ed. New York: Marcel Dekker, pp. 297–316.

Ward SJ, Baizman ER, Bell M, Childers S, D'Ambra T, Eissenstat M, Estep K, Haycock D, Howlett A, Luttinger D, Miller M, Pacheco M (1990a): Aminoalkylindoles (AAIs): a new route to the cannabinoid receptor? Natl Inst Drug Abuse Monogr 105:304–305.

Ward SJ, Mastriani D, Casiano F, Arnold R (1990b): Pravadoline: profile in isolated tissue preparations. J Pharmacol Exp Ther 255:1230–1239.

Weber C, Erl W, Pietsch A, Weber PC (1995): Aspirin inhibits nuclear factor-κB mobilization and monocyte adhesion in stimulated human endothelial cells. Circulation 91:1914–1917.

Weissman G (1991): Aspirin. Sci Am 264:58–64.

Westlund KN, Sun YC, Sluka KA, Dougherty PM, Sorkin LS, Willis WD (1992): Neural changes in acute arthritis in monkeys. II. Increased glutamate immunoreactivity in the medial articular nerve. Brain Res Rev 17:15–27.

Willis AL, Smith DL, Vigo C, Kluge A, O'Yang C, Kertesz D, Wu H (1987): Orally active prostacyclin-mimetic RS-93427: Therapeutic potential in vascular occlusive disease associated with atherosclerosis. In Samuelson B, Paoletti R, Ramwell W (eds): *Advances in Prostaglandin, Thromboxane, and Leukotriene Research.* New York: Raven Press, pp. 254–265.

Wong S, Gardocki JF (1983): Anti-inflammatory and antiarthritic evaluation of acetaminophen and its potentiation of tolmetin. J Pharmacol Exp Ther 226:625–632.

Xie XQ, Eissenstat M, Makriyannis A (1995): Common cannabimimetic pharmacophoric requirements between aminoalkyl indoles and classical cannabinoids. Life Sci 56:23–24.

Yamamoto N, Sakai F, Yamazaki H, Kawai Y, Nakahara K, Okuhara M (1996): Effect of FR133605, a novel cytokine suppressive agent, on bone and cartilage destruction in adjuvant arthritic rats. J Rheumatol 23:1778–1783.

Yaron M, Djaldetti M (1978): Platelets in synovial fluid (letter). Arthritis Rheum 21: 607–608.

CHAPTER 5

PERIPHERALLY ACTING ANALGESIC AGENTS

HUMPHREY P. RANG, STUART J. BEVAN, and MARTIN N. PERKINS
Novartis Institute for Medical Sciences
London, United Kingdom

This chapter is concerned with analgesic agents that act in the periphery, directly or indirectly, to reduce the activity of sensory neurons. In pathological pain states, as distinct from acute "physiological" pain, which is associated with nociceptor discharge in response to an intense stimulus, there are changes in (*a*) the properties of peripheral sensory nerve terminals, and (*b*) the central processing of the afferent input. These changes mean that nociceptive afferent fibers may be activated by stimuli of low intensity (hyperalgesia) and also that activation of low-threshold afferent fibers, particularly mechanoreceptors, can elicit pain rather than a touch sensation (allodynia).

In most cases, these two changes—peripheral and central sensitization—are driven by pathological events in the periphery, usually inflammation or nerve damage, or a combination of the two. Tissue inflammation alters the chemical environment of sensory nerve terminals, mainly as a result of the release of different inflammatory mediators to which the nerves respond, either directly or indirectly. Nerve damage results in a distinct pattern of functional changes within the sensory nerves and their central connections associated with neuropathic pain states, which are discussed in Chapters 1 and 2.

In this chapter we focus on pharmacological strategies for blocking the response of sensory neurons to inflammatory mediators, because it is in this area that new therapies are expected to be developed in the foreseeable future. The main mediators, targets, and effects are indicated in Figure 5.1 and Table 5.1.

Other chapters in this book deal with other potential targets for peripherally acting analgesic drugs, namely, peripheral opiate receptors (Chapter 3) and capsaicin receptors (Chapter 6).

Novel Aspects of Pain Management: Opioids and Beyond, Edited by Jana Sawynok and Alan Cowan
ISBN 0-471-180173 Copyright © 1999 by Wiley-Liss, Inc.

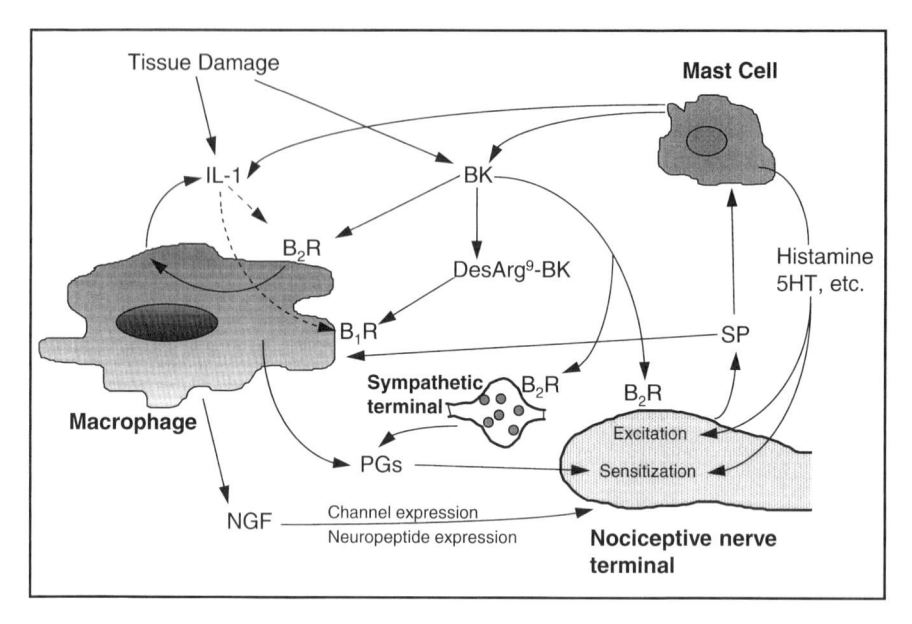

Figure 5.1 Postulated interactions between different peripheral cell types and mediators in the pathogenesis of inflammatory pain. BK = bradykinin; SP = substance P; PGs = prostanoids; NGF = nerve growth factor; B_1R, B_2R = bradykinin B_1 and B_2 receptors; 5HT = 5-hydroxytryptamine; IL-1 = interleukin-1. Dotted arrows represent receptor upregulation by IL-1.

PROSTANOID ANTAGONISTS—POTENTIAL AS PERIPHERALLY ACTING ANALGESIC DRUGS

A role for prostanoids in the genesis of inflammatory hyperalgesia is well established, the evidence coming partly from the proven therapeutic efficacy of nonsteroidal anti-inflammatory drugs (NSAIDs) as analgesics (see Chapter 4) and partly from the evidence showing that administration of prostanoids in the periphery causes hyperalgesia associated with sensitization of nociceptive afferent neurons. Many of the basic observations have been known for a long time, but there has been little progress so far in the search for specific prostanoid antagonists with potential for use as analgesic drugs.

Following on from the success in the purification and cloning of the TP (thromboxane) receptor, all of the members of the prostanoid receptor family have now been cloned (designated DP, EP, FP, and IP; see reviews by Coleman et al., 1994; Negishi et al., 1995; Pierce et al., 1995; Ushikubi et al., 1995). All of them are G-protein-coupled receptors, and their main characteristics are summarized in Table 5.2.

Several studies have addressed the underlying mechanisms, as well as the receptor types involved in the production of hyperalgesia by prostanoids (see

TABLE 5.1 Inflammatory Mediators Known to Affect Nociceptive Nerve Terminals

Mediator	Molecular Target	Cellular Location	Effects
Bradykinin	B_2 receptor	Nociceptive nerve terminals	Excitation Sensitization
	B_2 receptor	Inflammatory cells	Cytokine release Prostanoid release
[DesArg⁹]bradykinin	B_1 receptor	Inflammatory cells	Cytokine release Prostanoid release
Prostanoids	EP, IP receptors	Nociceptive nerve terminals	Excitation Sensitization
Histamine	H_1 receptor	Nociceptive nerve terminals (? "itch" subset)	Excitation (itch)
Serotonin	$5HT_3$ receptors	Nociceptive nerve terminals	Excitation
Nerve growth factor	TrkA receptor	Nociceptive nerves	Increased peptide and ion channel expression Sprouting
		Mast cells	Histamine release
Tachykinins	NK_1/NK_2 receptor	Mast cell	Histamine release
Protons	? receptor	Nociceptive nerve terminals	Excitation

TABLE 5.2 Prostanoid Receptor Subtypes[a]

Receptor	Eicosanoid Potency	Selective Agonists[b]	Selective Antagonists[b]	Transduction Pathway
TP	$T > D_2 > F_2 > E_2$	Yes	Yes	↑ PI turnover
IP	$I > E_1 > D_2 > T > F_2$	Yes	No	↑ cAMP
DP	$D_2 \gg T > E_2, I_2, F_2$	Yes	Yes	↑ cAMP
FP	$F_2 > F_1 > D_2 > T > E_2$	Yes	No	↑ PI turnover
EP_1	$E_2 > E_1 > F_2 > D_2$	Yes	Yes	↑ PI turnover
EP_2	$E_2 = E_1 \gg D_2 = F_2$	Yes	No	↑ cAMP
EP_3	$E_2 = E_1 \gg D_2 > F_2$	Yes	No	↓ cAMP

[a]Compiled from Coleman et al., 1994; Narumiya, 1995.
[b]For details, see Coleman et al., 1994.

Khasar et al., 1995, and reviews by Kress and Reeh, 1996; Mizumura and Kumazawa, 1996). By measuring behavioral responses in intact animals, or by recording single-unit discharges in intact or isolated preparations, prostanoid-induced sensitization of nociceptors has been demonstrated by many groups (see reviews by Rang et al., 1991; Dray, 1995). Most studies show that prostanoids do not cause direct activation of nociceptors—except articular afferents (Schaible and Schmidt, 1988; Birrell et al., 1991)—but rather sensitize them to the excitatory effects of other stimuli, including chemical, mechanical, and thermal stimuli. Two questions are particularly relevant to the feasibility of developing prostanoid antagonists as potential analgesic agents: (1) Which prostanoids and which receptors are involved? (2) Do the effects of prostanoids discriminate between different types of excitatory stimulus?

Receptor Specificity

Comparison of the effects of various endogenous and synthetic prostanoids on nociceptors points to the involvement of certain receptor types, but the limited availability of selective agonists is a drawback. Studies by Kumazawa and his colleagues (see Kumazawa et al., 1996) on testicular nociceptor responses in the dog implicate mainly the EP_2 and EP_3 receptor, linked respectively to stimulation and inhibition of adenylate cyclase. On the other hand, McQueen et al. (1991) and Birrell et al. (1993) showed that cicaprost, a selective agonist at the IP receptor, enhanced the mechanosensitivity of articular afferents in inflamed rat knee joint. DP, FP, and TP receptors are probably not involved, for various studies have reported agonists at these receptors to be inactive. Using the Randall–Sellito paw pressure test in the rat, Khasar et al. (1995) found evidence for the involvement of multiple prostanoid receptors, including EP_1, in the mechanical hyperalgesia produced by different prostanoids injected into the paw. In situ hybridization studies have shown a high level of expression of EP_3 and IP receptors in sensory neurons (Sugimoto et al., 1994; Oida et al., 1995). Though expression of receptor mRNAs was limited to subpopulations of cells, there was no obvious correlation with other markers of the nociceptor phenotype, such as cell size or peptide expression. Comparable studies have not yet been reported for other receptor subtypes.

Overall, the identification of specific receptor subtypes responsible for prostanoid-induced hyperalgesia remains confusing. Studies on intact tissues generally implicate several receptor types and show discrepancies between different studies, which may be partly species-related. So far, specific antagonists for EP_1, but not for other EP or IP receptors, are known.

Stimulus Specificity

There is evidence that the sensitizing action of prostaglandins shows specificity between the three main types of stimulus that have been studied, namely, thermal, mechanical, and chemical (especially bradykinin). Sensitization of bradykinin-induced excitation is observed consistently, and generally requires lower concentrations of prostanoids than are needed for sensitization to other stimuli.

Kumazawa et al. (1993) concluded that sensitization of dog testicular nociceptors to bradykinin was mediated by the EP_3 receptor, which is coupled to inhibition of adenylate cyclase. They also showed that manipulations that raise intracellular cyclic AMP (cAMP) tend to inhibit bradykinin-evoked responses, consistent with a negative effect of cAMP on responsiveness to bradykinin. However, others (Birrell and McQueen, 1993; Rueff and Dray, 1993) have found that cicaprost causes sensitization of nociceptors to bradykinin. This receptor is coupled to activation of adenylate cyclase, and Dray et al. (1992) showed that dibutyryl cAMP sensitizes cutaneous afferent fibers in the rat to bradykinin, an effect opposite to that observed by Kumazawa et al. (1993). Furthermore, studies on sensory neurons in culture by Cui and Nicol (1995) also showed that cAMP enhances sensitivity to bradykinin in cultured neurons. It is possible that species differences, or the use of neonatal tissues by Dray et al. (1992) and by Cui and Nicol (1995), may account for these discrepancies. The special synergy between prostanoids and bradykinin that has been described for nociceptors in situ suggests that prostanoids may influence, in a specific way, the signal transduction pathway through which bradykinin causes excitation of nociceptors. This mechanism is thought to involve activation of protein kinase C, leading to an inward cation current (Burgess et al., 1989). Through a similar mechanism, bradykinin has also been reported to enhance the inward current activated by temperatures in the noxious range (Cesare and McNaughton, 1996). Nicol and Cui (1994) showed that the bradykinin-evoked depolarization in cultured sensory neurons was not affected by prostaglandin E_2 (PGE_2), so there is currently no explanation at the cellular level of the specific synergism reported in other functional studies.

The facilitation by prostanoids of nociceptive responses to thermal stimuli is well established, and probably reflects a nonspecific increase in the excitability of nociceptive nerve terminals. The effect has been reported for E-series prostaglandins, as well as prostacyclins and cicaprost, so it is believed that both EP and IP receptors play a role, and there is evidence that this type of sensitization is associated with an increased intracellular cAMP concentration (Mizumura et al., 1993; Kumazawa et al., 1996). Sensitization of mechanoceptors by prostaglandins is less clear-cut, having been demonstrated electrophysiologically only for cat articular nociceptors (Schaible and Schmidt, 1988), but not in rat or dog tissues (Mizumura et al., 1987; Lang et al., 1990; Grubb et al., 1991), even though numerous reports have shown mechanical hyperalgesia in behavioral tests (e.g., Khasar et al., 1995).

Two possible ionic mechanisms by which prostanoids may increase membrane excitability have been described. Weinreich and his colleagues (Fowler et al., 1985; Weinreich and Wonderlin, 1987) have shown that prostanoids, acting through increased cAMP formation, suppress a slow spike afterhyperpolarization seen in nodose ganglion neurons. This hyperpolarization results from the opening of calcium-activated K$^+$ channels, and has the effect of inhibiting repetitive firing in response to a maintained depolarizing current. The effect of prostanoids is thus to facilitate repetitive firing. Some dorsal root ganglion neurons show a similar after-hyperpolarization, which is inhibited by PGE$_2$ (Gold et al., 1996b). In nodose ganglion cells, prostaglandin I$_2$ (PGI$_2$) as well as other prostaglandins (PGs) elicits this response; it is also seen with bradykinin, and a recent study (Weinreich et al., 1995) suggests that bradykinin acts on B$_2$ receptors to stimulate PGI$_2$ production by the neurons.

A second ionic mechanism by which prostanoids, acting through increased cAMP formation, increase excitability is by an effect on the gating of tetrodotoxin-resistant (TTX-R) sodium channels (England et al., 1996; Gold et al., 1996a), which are expressed in nociceptive neurons. The opening of these channels in response to depolarization is facilitated, mainly due to a hyperpolarizing shift in their activation curve. The nature of the prostanoid receptor causing this effect has not yet been elucidated, but the fact that it is associated with stimulation of adenylate cyclase suggests that EP$_2$ and/or IP receptors may be involved.

In summary there is evidence that prostanoids, though not directly excitatory to sensory neurons, can facilitate their excitation either specifically, in response to bradykinin, or nonspecifically to all stimuli. In the most fully studied system, the dog testicular nociceptors, the receptor type, and transduction mechanism responsible for sensitization to bradykinin (EP$_3$-receptor causing inhibition of adenylate cyclase) appear to be different from those mediating heat sensitization (EP$_2$-receptor causing activation of adenylate cyclase), but this distinction is less clear for other test systems. Because dorsal root ganglion neurons express both EP$_3$ and IP receptors, which exert opposite effects on adenylate cyclase, the end result of prostanoid action may well depend on relative concentrations of different prostanoids produced at different times and in different tissues. Following the cloning of all the main prostanoid receptor subtypes, it should now be possible to perform gene knock-out experiments to determine the importance of peripheral prostanoids in sustaining inflammatory hyperalgesia. New therapies coming from this approach will probably have to await the discovery of antagonists at EP and IP receptors.

KININS AND KININ RECEPTORS IN HYPERALGESIA

Kinins are small peptides of which bradykinin (Arg-Pro-Pro-Gly-Phe-Ser-Pro-Phe-Arg) and kallidin (Lys-bradykinin), together with their truncated analogues, des-Arg^{9}bradykinin and des-Arg^{10}kallidin, are the best known examples. They are formed from precursor molecules in response to tissue injury, trauma, or inflammation. Bradykinin is produced in plasma from high molecular weight kininogen and kallidin is formed in tissue from low molecular weight kininogen (see Bhoola et al., 1992).

There are two kinin receptors, the B_1 and B_2 receptors (Hall, 1992), and the recent cloning of their genes show them to be typical G-protein-coupled receptors (McEachern et al., 1991; Hess et al., 1992), although there is little sequence homology between them (Menke et al., 1994).

The preferential agonists for the B_2 receptor are bradykinin and kallidin, and this receptor is thought to mediate the majority of the acute pharmacological effects of these kinins. The ligands for the B_1 receptor are the only active metabolites of bradykinin and kallidin, des-Arg^{9}bradykinin and des-Arg^{10}kallidin, respectively, which are formed by specific kininases.

Although kinins have many effects, it is their action on nociceptive neurons that is most relevant to their potential use as peripherally acting analgesics, and there is evidence that both B_1 and B_2 receptors may play a role.

B_2 receptors are expressed on nociceptive neurons, and their activation causes both excitation and sensitization. Bradykinin causes depolarization of the sensory neuron, owing to an increase in sodium ion conductance, and this involves activation of phospholipase C with subsequent stimulation of protein kinase C (Burgess et al., 1989; Dray et al., 1992). It causes neuronal discharges in C-fibers in vitro and in vivo (Mizumura et al., 1990; Dray et al., 1992; Sengupta and Gebhart, 1994); it induces nocifensor responses indicative of pain in animals (Ferreira et al., 1993; Khasar et al., 1993; Davis et al., 1994) and overt pain in humans (Whalley et al., 1987; Kindgen-Milles and Klement, 1992). Bradykinin also sensitizes nociceptors to noxious stimuli (Khan et al., 1991; Birrell et al., 1993; Rueff and Dray, 1993), an effect that may underlie the persistent tenderness associated with inflammation in humans.

Although B_1 receptors are not expressed on sensory neurons (Davis et al., 1996), there is evidence that they play a role in the development of inflammatory hyperalgesia. B_1 kinin receptor antagonists are antinociceptive in vivo in models of persistent inflammatory hyperalgesia (Correa and Calixto, 1993; Dray and Perkins, 1993; Perkins et al., 1993; Perkins and Kelly, 1993). It is likely that induced expression of B_1 receptors by non-neuronal cells is caused by cytokines, particularly interleukin-1β, which are produced during inflammation (Regoli et al., 1990; Dray and Perkins, 1993; Galizzi et al., 1994). B_1 receptor activation in turn causes the release of other inflammatory and sensitizing agents (e.g., prostaglandins and cytokines) from non-neuronal cell types such as macrophages and other inflammatory cells.

Kinin Antagonists as Analgesic Agents

The evidence for an involvement of kinins in inflammatory hyperalgesia supports the possibility that kinin antagonists might be useful as analgesic drugs. Considerable effort has been expended in recent years in developing selective B_2 receptor antagonists. The first such compounds were peptide analogues of bradykinin, one of which, HOE 140 (Hock et al., 1991), has been widely studied. HOE 140 and related peptide antagonists have been shown to be antinociceptive in several models of inflammatory hyperalgesia in vivo (Steranka et al., 1988; Heapy et al., 1993; Perkins et al., 1993). They are not, however, orally active, and therefore have not been developed for clinical use as analgesic drugs. Figure 5.2 shows that mechanical hyperalgesia induced in the rat paw by inflammation in response to injection of Freund's adjuvant, interleukin-1, or capsaicin can be fully reversed by local injection of either a B_1- or a B_2-receptor antagonist. This result suggests that both receptors play a role, and that both must be activated to produce hyperalgesia. The details of this interplay between B_1 and B_2 receptors are not yet clear, and the relative merits of selective versus nonselective bradykinin antagonists for therapeutic use as analgesics are likely to be decided only when such compounds enter clinical trials. Orally active nonpeptide antagonists at the B_2 receptor have recently been described, the most potent and selective of these being FR173657 (Asano et al., 1997; Griesbacher and Legat, 1997). Such compounds have not yet been tested in

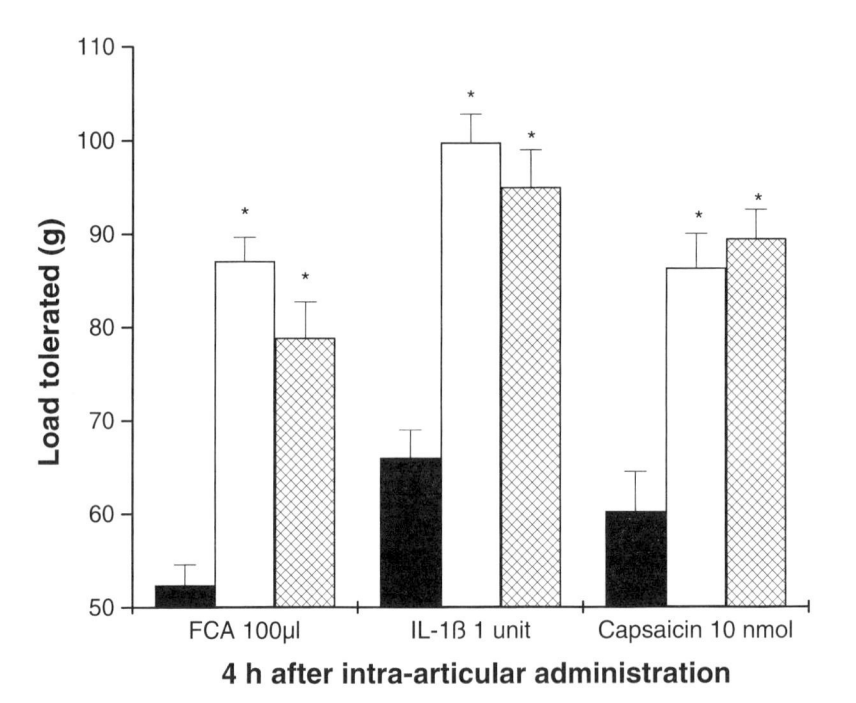

Figure 5.2 Inhibition of hyperalgesia by bradykinin B_1- and B_2-receptor antagonists in the rat. Rat knee joints were injected with Freund's complete adjuvant (FCA), IL-1β, or capsaicin, as shown, and the load tolerated was measured 4 hr later (black bars). Hyperalgesia is indicated by the reduction in the tolerated load compared with that of vehicle-injected joints (about 110 g, not shown). Intravenous injection of [DesArg⁹Leu⁸]BK, 10 nmol/kg (open bars) or HOE 140 0.1 nmol/kg (cross-hatched bars), 30 min before testing, reversed the hyperalgesia in all cases, compared with saline-injected controls (black bars). ANOVA/Tukey's test: * = $p < 0.05$. Data from Davis and Perkins (1994).

humans, but appear to have considerable potential for clinical use in the treatment of pain and a variety of inflammatory conditions.

In summary, the use of kinin antagonists as analgesic agents is not yet proven clinically but there are several compounds about to enter clinical trials, and there is good reason to expect that this new class of compound will find a place in the treatment of inflammatory pain.

CYTOKINES AND PERIPHERAL HYPERALGESIA

There is strong evidence suggesting that cytokines have a major role in modulating nociception in the periphery, though the details are not yet well understood. The majority of the evidence relates to interleukin-1β (IL-1β), which is extremely potent in inducing hyperalgesia following local or systemic administration in animals (Ferreira et al., 1988; Follenfant et al., 1989; Davis and Perkins, 1994; Perkins and Kelly, 1994; Watkins et al., 1994; 1995). Whether this hyperalgesic action of IL-1β is due to a direct excitatory action on nociceptive neurons, or results from changes in the release of secondary mediators, is not clear. IL-1β elicits activity in both somatic and visceral sensory nerves (Fukuoka et al., 1994; Watkins et al., 1995; Kelly et al., 1996) and, like kinins, it also increases neuronal responses to noxious thermal and mechanical stimulation (Fukuoka et al., 1994). Recently, it has been demonstrated in vitro that IL-1β excites joint mechanonociceptors (Kelly et al., 1996), consistent with either a direct or indirect action. Evidence that IL-1β acts directly on nociceptive neurons is provided by a study demonstrating that IL-1β induced an increase in intracellular Ca^{2+} in acutely dissociated dorsal root ganglion cells (Kawatani and Birder, 1992). IL-1β is unique among cytokines in having an endogenous competitive antagonist, IL-1ra, acting at the IL-1β receptor. This, together with other mechanisms, tightly regulates the production and action of IL-1β in the body (Arend, 1993; Colotta et al., 1993; Dayer and Burger, 1994; Re et al., 1994).

There is less evidence for a role for other excitatory cytokines in nociception but several of them have been shown to be hyperalgesic in vivo, namely, tumor necrosis factor-α (TNF-α) and interleukin-2, -6, and -8 (Follenfant et al., 1989; Cunha et al., 1991; Davis and Perkins, 1994). In some cases this action seems to depend on the subsequent production of IL-1β (Numerof et al., 1988; Tilg et al., 1993; 1994). IL-2 has been shown to activate cutaneous nociceptors in the rat, although this could be indirect (Martin and Murphy, 1995). An involvement of the sympathetic nervous system has also been suggested for the cytokine IL-8 (Cunha et al., 1991; 1992).

Experimental evidence suggests that antagonism of cytokines may be a useful therapeutic approach to controlling pain. Antibodies directed against cytokines are available, and one of these, an engineered antibody (CDP571) to TNF-α, produced symptomatic improvement, including pain relief, in patients with rheumatoid arthritis (Rankin et al., 1995).

The most direct approach to targeting these excitatory cytokines would be the development of receptor antagonists. This has proved difficult to achieve, but recently a relatively low molecular weight peptide antagonist, AF12198, at the human IL-1β receptor has been synthesized (Akeson et al., 1996). AF12198 blocks IL-1β-induced IL-8 production in vitro and IL-1β induction of IL-6 in vivo. It will be interesting to see whether this peptide is also effective in hyperalgesia models in vivo. Another approach is to inhibit the synthesis of cytokines. Inhibition of IL-1β converting enzyme (ICE) by an orally active synthetic inhibitor, SDZ 224-015, has been shown to reduce lipopolysaccharide-induced inflammation and pyrexia (Elford et al., 1995), but its analgesic activity has not yet been assessed. Other approaches, not yet tested clinically, are to inhibit various points on the kinase cascade through which cytokines produce their cellular effects (see McKinnon et al., 1996).

Inhibitory Cytokines

The role of so-called "inhibitory" cytokines has recently been uncovered. These cytokines, the best characterized of which are IL-4, IL-10, and IL-13, have been shown to be anti-inflammatory, but there is only one study to date assessing the antinociceptive actions of an inhibitory cytokine (Poole et al., 1995). In this study, IL-10 was shown to inhibit the hyperalgesia produced by bradykinin, IL-1β, TNF-α, or IL-6 in the rat. There are several possible mechanisms for such an inhibitory action of these cytokines, including inhibition of prostanoid formation (Dechanet et al., 1995) by the suppression of the inducible isoform of cyclooxygenase (Niiro et al., 1995). Alternatively, these cytokines have been shown to reduce production of IL-1β (Chomarat et al., 1995), probably by suppressing IL-1 gene transcription (Donnelly et al., 1991), and to inhibit nuclear localization of NF-κB, a transcription factor involved in the expression of inflammatory cytokine genes (Wang et al., 1995). There is, however, little direct experimental evidence for a role for these cytokines in modulating hyperalgesia, although monoclonal antibodies to IL-10 have been shown to potentiate carrageenin-induced hyperalgesia (Poole et al., 1995).

This area of research is a new one, and so far, few compounds are known that interfere with cytokine signaling pathways. Progress in defining the role of cytokines in the production of pain has been modest.

NERVE GROWTH FACTOR

The Role of Nerve Growth Factor in Hyperalgesia

There is now a considerable body of experimental evidence that one of the neurotrophins, nerve growth factor (NGF), plays a critical role in the regulation of sensory neuron properties, and that it plays a role in inflammatory pain (see reviews by McMahon et al., 1995 and Woolf et al., 1996). NGF is a protein of about 13 kDa, which is synthesized and secreted by cells in the target tissues, such as keratinocytes and fibroblasts. At physiological concentrations, NGF exists as a homodimer and exerts its biological effects largely through an interaction with a tyrosine kinase receptor (trkA) which is expressed by a subset of neural crest-derived sensory neurons. During early development, NGF acts to support the survival and differentiation of these neurons, and exposure of developing animals to blocking antibodies leads to the absence of small sensory neurons expressing the neuropeptides, substance P, and calcitonin gene-related peptide (CGRP) (see Lewin and Mendell, 1993 for review). In addition, transgenic animals with null mutations of the genes encoding either NGF (Crowley et al., 1994) or the trkA receptor (Smeyne et al., 1994) have at birth only about 30% of the normal number of dorsal root ganglion (DRG) neurons and show a profound loss of small-diameter neurons and a corresponding impairment of responsiveness to noxious thermal and mechanical stimuli (Crowley et al., 1994).

Lack of NGF in the postnatal period does not cause loss of sensory neurons (Lewin et al., 1992). Throughout life, however, trkA-expressing neurons remain responsive to NGF, which regulates a range of neuronal properties and acts as an important mediator of inflammatory hyperalgesia. In particular, NGF is required for the expression of a range of important proteins such as the precursors of substance P and CGRP (Lindsay and Harmar, 1989; Lindsay et al., 1989) and the capsaicin- and proton-activated ion channels (Winter et al., 1988; Bevan and Winter, 1995). Injection of NGF into the target tissues raises the levels of the two neuropeptides in the sciatic nerve (Donnerer et al., 1992; Woolf et al., 1994) and increases the numbers of DRG neurons that express preprotachykinin and CGRP mRNA (Leslie et al., 1995).

Nerve growth factor production is increased in experimental inflammation (Donnerer et al., 1992; Woolf et al., 1994) and in chronic inflammatory disorders such as rhematoid arthritis (Aloe et al., 1992). A link between NGF production and inflammatory hyperalgesia is suggested by several pieces of evidence. First, experimental administration of NGF leads to hyperalgesia and allodynia in both rats (Lewin et al., 1993; Della Seta et al., 1994; Woolf et al., 1994) and humans (Petty et al., 1994; Dyck et al., 1997). Second, transgenic mice that overexpress NGF in the skin show marked hyperalgesia, whereas mice expressing antisense DNA to inhibit NGF production show hypoalgesia (Davis et al., 1993). Third, inhibiting the action of NGF with either antibodies to NGF (Lewin et al., 1994; Woolf et al., 1994; Fig. 5.3) or with a fusion protein consisting of the extracellular, NGF-binding domain of the trkA receptor linked to an F_c fragment of immunoglobulin (McMahon et al., 1995; Dmitrieva et al., 1997) substantially reduces inflammatory hyperalgesia.

The mechanisms underlying NGF-induced hyperalgesia may, in part, involve the observed increase in substance P levels in the sensory nerves innervating inflamed tissues (see e.g. Smith et al., 1992; Woolf et al., 1994). The mechanical allodynia seen after a single systemic dose of NGF in rats is associated with substance P receptor activation in the neonatal rat spinal cord (Thompson

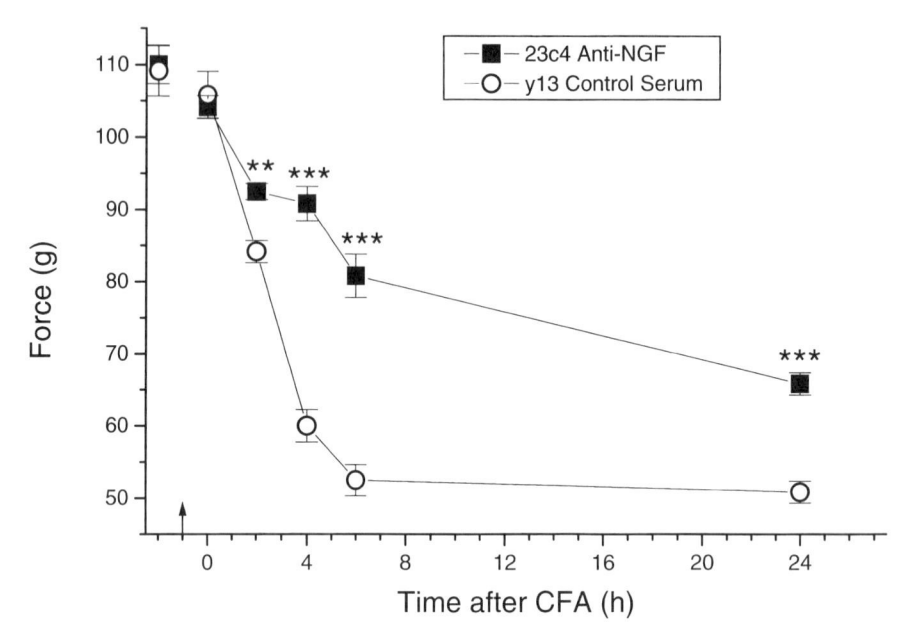

Figure 5.3 Effect of a neutralizing antibody to NGF on the development of inflammatory hyperalgesia in the rat paw. The foot withdrawal threshold was measured before, and at intervals after, intraplantar injection of Freund's complete adjuvant (CFA) at time zero. One hour before CFA injection, animals were injected intraperitoneally with either control serum (open symbols, or anti-NGF (closed symbols). The hyperalgesia, measured as a reduction in the normal paw withdrawal threshold, was inhibited in the anti-NGF group. (JM Winter, unpublished). ANOVA/Tukey's HSD: *** = $p < 0.001$; ** = $p < 0.01$.

et al., 1995). Both A- and C-fiber-mediated responses were blocked by a neurokinin-1 (NK_1) receptor antagonist, suggesting that NGF induces some myelinated neurons to synthesize substance P, even though they lack the trkA receptor (see Leslie et al., 1995). It has been postulated that NGF stimulation of trkA-bearing sensory neurons evokes the paracrine release of mediators, such as brain-derived neurotrophic factor (BDNF), which acts on adjacent neurons. Nerve growth factor has also been shown to influence the pattern of afferent connectivity in the adult spinal cord (Lewin et al., 1992), which may be directly related to changes in neuropeptide content. Evidence for a neuropeptide involvement in adult rats is lacking, however, and Rueff et al. (1996) failed to show any receptor-mediated effect of a NK_1 receptor antagonist on NGF-induced mechanical or thermal hyperalgesia.

Besides sensory neurons, other trkA-bearing cells in the periphery include postganglionic sympathetic neurons and inflammatory cells. Nerve growth factor can stimulate inflammatory cells (Bischoff and Dahinden, 1992) and degranulates mast cells to liberate histamine and 5-hydroxytryptamine (Horigome et al., 1993; Tal and Liberman, 1997), both of which stimulate or sensitize nociceptive afferents. Similarly, it has been proposed that NGF stimulation of sympathetic neurons can release arachidonic acid derivatives that can induce hyperalgesia (see Heller et al., 1994). The finding that thermal hyperalgesia was inhibited by a 5-lipoxygenase inhibitor (Amann et al., 1996) also suggests that some indirect effects of NGF result from the action of lipid mediators. These indirect effects of NGF on nociception predominate during the early phase of the hyperalgesia, which is inhibited by sympathectomy (Andreev et al., 1995; Woolf et al., 1996) and by pretreatment with a mast cell degranulating agent (Lewin et al., 1994). Furthermore, a transient increase in thermal, but not mechanical, sensitivity induced by NGF in a skin-nerve preparation in vitro is inhibited when the preparation is taken from mast cell-depleted animals (Rueff and Mendell, 1996).

Nerve growth factor may be an important factor in the hyperalgesia induced by cytokines such as TNF-α and IL-1β (see above). TNF-α production usually precedes the elevation of IL-1β in the cytokine cascade (Vassalli, 1992) and TNF-α stimulates the synthesis and release of NGF from non-neuronal cells (Hattori et al., 1993). TNF-α-induced hyperalgesia is significantly attenuated by prior administration of anti-NGF (Woolf et al., 1997). Furthermore, the rise in NGF levels and the inflammatory hyperalgesia seen after injection of complete Freund's adjuvant is inhibited by IL-1ra (Safieh-Garabedian et al., 1995).

NGF Inhibitors as Analgesic Agents

From the above discussions, it is clear that drugs that inhibit the hyperalgesic actions of NGF may prove useful for the treatment of chronic inflammatory pain. Large proteins such as antibodies or fusion proteins are unlikely to be of general use as analgesic agents. A major requirement will be for drugs that do not show appreciable blood–brain barrier penetration, for NGF regulates the properties of some CNS neurons, notably cholinergic basal forebrain neurons (Hartikka and Hefti, 1988; Vantini et al., 1989; Crowley et al., 1994). Unwanted peripheral effects of NGF inhibitors may still pose a problem because, unlike primary afferent neurons, postganglionic sympathetic neurons remain dependent on NGF in adult animals. This fact reduces the attractiveness of receptor antagonists as potential analgesic agents. Given the complexity of the signaling pathways for NGF and the evidence that, in PC12 cells at least, different pathways are responsible for survival and transcription (see, e.g., Tolkovsky, 1997), it may be possible to find agents that selectively inhibit the intracellular pathways that mediate the NGF-mediated changes responsible for hyperalgesia.

CONCLUSIONS

In this chapter, we have reviewed the possible role of various peripheral mediators—prostaglandins, kinins, cytokines, and NGF—in the genesis of inflammatory pain. Identifying the role of such mediators furnishes possible new points of attack for analgesic drugs, on which rational drug discovery programs can be based. Of the mediators discussed, there is a good chance that selective prostaglandin and kinin antagonists will be developed within the next few years; NGF is a more difficult target, and the development of small-molecule inhibitors is more remote.

REFERENCES

Akeson AL, Woods CW, Hsieh LC, Bohnke RA, Ackermann L, Chan KY, Robinson JL, Yanofsky D, Jacobs JW, Barrett RW, Bowlin TL (1996): AF12198, a novel low molecular weight antagonist, selectively binds the human type I interleukin (IL)-1 receptor and blocks in vivo responses to IL-1. J Biol Chem 271:30517–30523.

Aloe L, Tuveri MA, Carcassi U, Levi-Montalcini R (1992): Nerve growth factor in the synovial fluid of patients with chronic arthritis. Arthritis Rheum 35:351–355.

Amann R, Schuligoi R, Lanz I, Peskar BA (1996): Effect of a 5-lipoxygenase inhibitor on nerve growth factor-induced thermal hyperalgesia in the rat. Eur J Pharmacol 306:89–91.

Andreev NY, Dimitrieva N, Koltzenburg M, McMahon SB (1995): Peripheral administration of nerve growth factor in the adult rat produces a thermal hyperalgesia that requires the presence of sympathetic post-ganglionic neurones. Pain 63:109–115.

Arend WP (1993): Interleukin-1 receptor antagonist. Adv Immunol 54:167–227.

Asano M, Inamura N, Hatori C, Sawai H, Fujiwara T, Katayama A, Kayakiri H, Satoh S, Abe Y, Inoue T, Sawada Y, Nakahara K, Oku T, Okuhara M (1997): The identification of an orally active, nonpeptide bradykinin B_2 receptor antagonist, FR173657. Br J Pharmacol 120:617–624.

Bevan S, Winter J (1995): Nerve growth factor (NGF) differentially regulates the chemosensitivity of adult rat cultured sensory neurons. J Neurosci 15:4918–4926.

Bhoola KD, Figueroa CD, Worthy K (1992): Bioregulation of kinins: kallikreins, kininogens and kininases. Pharmacol Rev 44:1–80.

Birrell GJ, McQueen DS (1993): The effects of capsaicin, bradykinin, PGE_2 and cicaprost on the discharge of articular sensory receptors in vitro. Brain Res 611:103–107.

Birrell GJ, McQueen DS, Iggo A, Coleman RA, Grubb BD (1991): PGI_2-induced activation and sensitization of articular mechanonociceptors. Neurosci Lett 124:5–8.

Birrell GJ, McQueen DS, Iggo A, Grubb BD (1993): Prostanoid-induced potentiation of the excitatory and sensitizing effects of bradykinin on articular mechanonociceptors in the rat ankle joint. Neuroscience 54:537–544.

Bischoff SC, Dahinden CA (1992): Effect of nerve growth factor on the release of inflammatory mediators by mature human basophils. Blood 79:2662–2669.

Burgess GM, Mullaney I, McNeill M, Dunn PM, Rang HP (1989): Second messengers involved in the mechanism of action of bradykinin in sensory neurons in culture. J Neurosci 9:3314–3325.

Cesare P, McNaughton P (1996): A novel heat-activated current in nociceptive neurons and its sensitization by bradykinin. Proc Natl Acad Sci USA 93:15435–15439.

Chomarat P, Vannier E, Dechanet J, Rissoan MC, Banchereau J, Dinarello CA, Miossec P (1995): Balance of IL-1 receptor antagonist/IL-1 beta in rheumatoid synovium and its regulation by IL-4 and IL-10. J Immunol 154:1432–1439.

Coleman RA, Smith WL, Navumiya S (1994): International Union of Pharmacology classification of prostanoid receptors: properties, distribution and structure of the receptors and their subtypes. Pharm Rev 46:205–229.

Colotta F, Re F, Muzio M, Bertini R, Polentarutti N, Sironi M, Giri JG, Dower SK, Sims JE, Mantovani A (1993): Interleukin-1 type II receptor: a decoy target for IL-1 that is regulated by IL-4. Science 261:472–475.

Correa CR, Calixto JB (1993): Evidence for participation of B_1 and B_2 kinin receptors in formalin-induced nociceptive response in the mouse. Br J Pharmacol 110:193–198.

Crowley C, Spencer SD, Nishimura MC, Chen KS, Pitts-Meek S, Armanini MP, Ling LH, McMahon SB, Shelton DL, Levinson AD (1994): Mice lacking nerve growth factor display perinatal loss of sensory and sympathetic neurons yet develop basal forebrain cholinergic neurons. Cell 76:1001–1011.

Cui M, Nicol GD (1995): Cyclic AMP mediates the prostaglandin E2-induced potentiation of bradykinin excitation in rat sensory neurons. Neuroscience 66:459–466.

Cunha FQ, Lorenzetti BB, Poole S, Ferreira SH (1991): Interleukin-8 as a mediator of sympathetic pain. Br J Pharmacol 104:765–767.

Cunha FQ, Poole S, Lorenzetti BB, Ferreira SH (1992): The pivotal role of tumour necrosis factor alpha in the development of inflammatory hyperalgesia. Br J Pharmacol 107:660–664.

Davis AJ, Perkins MN (1994): The involvement of bradykinin B_1 and B_2 receptor mechanisms in cytokine-induced mechanical hyperalgesia in the rat. Br J Pharmacol 113:63–68.

Davis BM, Lewin GR, Mendell LM, Jones ME, Albers KM (1993): Altered expression of nerve growth factor in the skin of transgenic mice leads to changes in response to mechanical stimuli. Neuroscience 56:789–792.

Davis AJ, Kelly D, Perkins MN (1994): The induction of des-Arg^9-bradykinin-mediated hyperalgesia in the rat by inflammatory stimuli. Braz J Med Biol Res 27:1793–1802.

Davis CL, Naeem S, Phagoo SB, Campbell EA, Urban L, Burgess GM (1996): B_1 receptors and sensory neurones. Br J Pharmacol 118:1469–1476.

Dayer JM, Burger D (1994): Interleukin-1, tumor necrosis factor and their specific inhibitors. Eur Cytokine News 5:563–571.

Dechanet J, Rissoan MC, Banchereau J, Miossec P (1995): Interleukin 4, but not interleukin 10, regulates the production of inflammation mediators by rheumatoid synoviocytes. Cytokine 7:176–183.

Della Seta D, de Acetis L, Aloe L, Alleva E (1994): NGF effects on hot plate behaviours in mice. Pharmacol Biochem Behav 49:701–705.

Dmitrieva N, Shelton D, Rive ASC, McMahon SB (1997): The role of nerve growth factor in a model of visceral inflammation. Neuroscience 78:449–459.

Donnelly RP, Fenton MJ, Kaufman JD, Gerrard TL (1991): IL-1 expression in human monocytes is transcriptionally and posttranscriptionally regulated by IL-4. J Immunol 146:3431–3436.

Donnerer J, Schuligoi R, Stein C (1992): Increased content and transport of substance P and calcitonin gene-related peptide in sensory nerves innervating inflamed tissue: evidence for a regulatory function of nerve growth factor in vivo. Neuroscience 49: 693–698.

Dray A (1995): Inflammatory mediators of pain. Br J Anaesth 75:125–131.

Dray A, Perkins MN (1993): Bradykinin and inflammatory pain. Trends Neurosci 16: 99–104.

Dray A, Patel IA, Perkins MN, Rueff A (1992): Bradykinin-induced activation of nociceptors: receptor and mechanistic studies on the neonatal rat spinal cord-tail preparation in vitro. Br J Pharmacol 107:1129–1134.

Dyck PJ, Peroutka S, Rask C, Burton E, Baker MK, Lehman KA, Gillen DA, Hokanson JL, O'Brien PC (1997): Intradermal recombinant human nerve growth factor induces pressure allodynia and lowered heat-pain threshold in humans. Neurology 48:501–505.

Elford PR, Heng R, Revesz L, MacKenzie AR (1995): Reduction of inflammation and pyrexia in the rat by oral administration of SDZ 224-015, an inhibitor of the interleukin-1beta converting enzyme. Br J Pharmacol 115:601–606.

England S, Bevan S, Docherty RJ (1996): PGE_2 modulates the tetrodotoxin-resistant sodium current in neonatal rat dorsal root ganglion neurones via the cyclic AMP-protein kinase A cascade. J Physiol 495:429–440.

Ferreira SH, Lorenzetti BB, Bristow AF, Poole S (1988): Interleukin-1beta as a potent hyperalgesic agent antagonized by a tripeptide analogue. Nature 334:698–700.

Ferreira SH, Lorenzetti BB, Cunha FQ, Poole S (1993): Bradykinin release of TNF-alpha plays a key role in the development of inflammatory hyperalgesia. Agents Actions 38:7–9.

Follenfant RL, Nakamura-Craig M, Henderson B, Higgs GA (1989): Inhibition by neuropeptides of interleukin-1 beta-induced, prostaglandin-independent hyperalgesia. Br J Pharmacol 98:41–43.

Fowler JC, Wonderlin WF, Weinreich D (1985): Prostaglandins block a Ca^{2+}-dependent slow spike afterhyperpolarisation independent of effects on Ca^{2+} influx in visceral afferent neurons. Brain Res 345:345–349.

Fukuoka H, Kawatani M, Hisamitsu T, Takeshige C (1994): Cutaneous hyperalgesia induced by peripheral injection of interleukin-1 beta in the rat. Brain Res 657: 133–140.

Galizzi JP, Bodinier MC, Chapelain B, Ly SM, Coussy L, Giraud S, Neliat G, Jean G (1994): Upregulation of $[^3H]$-des-Arg^{10}-kallidin binding to bradykinin B_1 receptor by interleukin-1β in isolated smooth muscle cells: correlation with B_1 agonist-induced PGI_2 production. Br J Pharmacol 113:389–394.

Gold MS, Reichling DB, Shuster MJ, Levine JD (1996a): Hyperalgesic agents increase a tetrodotoxin-resistant Na+ current in nociceptors. Proc Natl Acad Sci USA 93: 1108–1112.

Gold MS, Shuster MJ, Levine JD (1996b): Role of a Ca(2+)-dependent slow afterhyperpolarization in prostaglandin E2-induced sensitization of cultured rat sensory neurons. Neurosci Lett 205:161–164.

Griesbacher T, Legat FJ (1997): Effects of FR173657, a non-peptide B_2 antagonist, on kinin-induced hypotension, visceral and peripheral oedema formation and bronchoconstriction. Br J Pharmacol 120:933–939.

Grubb BD, Birrell GJ, McQueen DS, Iggo A (1991): The role of PGE$_2$ in the sensitization of mechanoreceptors in normal and inflamed ankle joints of the rat. Exp Brain Res 84:383–392.

Hall JM (1992): Bradykinin receptors: pharmacological properties and biological roles. Pharmacol Ther 56:131–190.

Hartikka J, Hefti F (1988): Development of septal cholinergic neurons in culture: plating density and glial cells modulate effects of NGF on survival, fiber growth, and expression of transmitter-specific enzymes. J Neurosci 8:2967–2985.

Hattori A, Tanaka E, Murase K, Ishida N, Chatani Y, Tsujimoto M, Hayashi K, Kohno M (1993): Tumor necrosis factor stimulates the synthesis and secretion of biologically active nerve growth factor in non-neuronal cells. J Biol Chem 268:2577–2582.

Heapy CG, Shaw JS, Farmer SC (1993): Differential sensitivity of antinociceptive assays to the bradykinin antagonist Hoe 140. Br J Pharmacol 108:209–213 (Abstract).

Heller PH, Green PG, Tanner KD, Miao FJ-P, Levine JD (1994): Peripheral contributions to inflammation. In Fields HL, Liebeskind JC (eds): *Pharmacological Approaches to The Treatment of Chronic Pain: New Concepts and Critical Issues*. Seattle: IASP Press, pp. 31–42.

Hess JF, Borkowski JA, Young GS, Strader CD, Ransom RW (1992): Cloning and pharmacological characterisation of a human bradykinin (BK-2) receptor. Biochem Biophys Res Commun 184:260–268.

Hock FJ, Wirth K, Albus U, Linz W, Gerhards HJ, Wiemer G, Henke S, Breipohl G, Konig W, Knolle J, Scholkens BA (1991): Hoe 140 a new potent and long acting bradykinin-antagonist: In vitro studies. Br J Pharmacol 102:769–773.

Horigome K, Pryor JC, Bullock ED, Johnson EM Jr (1993): Mediator release from mast cells by nerve growth factor. Neurotrophin specificity and receptor mediation. J Biol Chem 268:14881–14887.

Kawatani M, Birder L (1992): Interleukin facilitates Ca^{2+} release in acutely dissociated dorsal root ganglion (DRG) cells of rat. Neuroscience 18:691 (Abstract).

Kelly DC, Ashgar AUR, McQueen DS (1996): Effects of bradykinin and desArg-bradykinin on afferent neural discharge in interleukin-1β-treated knee joints. Br J Pharmacol 117(Suppl.):90(P).

Khan AA, Raja SN, Manning DC, Campbell JN, Meyer RA (1991): The effects of bradykinin and sequence-related analogs on the response properties of cutaneous nociceptors in monkeys. Somatosens Mot Res 9:97–106.

Khasar SG, Green PG, Levine JD (1993): Comparison of intradermal and subcutaneous hyperalgesic effects of inflammatory mediators in the rat. Neurosci Lett 153:215–218.

Khasar SG, Ouseph AK, Chou B, Ho T, Green PG, Levine JD (1995): Is there more than one prostaglandin E receptor subtype mediating hyperalgesia in the rat hindpaw? Neuroscience 64:1161–1165.

Kindgen-Milles D, Klement W (1992): Pain and inflammation evoked in the human skin by bradykinin receptor antagonists. Eur J Pharmacol 218:183–185.

Kress M, Reeh PW (1996): Chemical excitation and sensitization in nociceptors. In Belmonte C, Cervero F (eds): *Neurobiology of Nociceptors*. Oxford: Oxford University Press, pp. 258–297.

Kumazawa T, Mizumura K, Koda H (1993): Involvement of EP_3 subtype of prostaglandin E receptors in PGE_2-induced enhancement of the bradykinin response of nociceptors. Brain Res 632:321–324.

Kumazawa T, Mizumura K, Koda H, Fukusako H (1996): EP receptor subtypes implicated in the PGE_2-induced sensitization of polymodal receptors in response to bradykinin and heat. J Neurophysiol 75:2361–2368.

Lang E, Novak A, Reeh PW, Handwerker HO (1990): Chemosensitivity of fine afferents from rat skin in vitro. J Neurophysiol 63:887–901.

Leslie TA, Emson PC, Dowd PM, Woolf CJ (1995): Nerve growth factor contributes to the up-regulation of growth-associated protein 43 and preprotachykinin A messenger RNAs in primary sensory neurons following peripheral inflammation. Neuroscience 67:753–761.

Lewin GR, Mendell LM (1993): Nerve growth factor and nociception. Trends Neurosci 16:353–359.

Lewin GR, Winter J, McMahon SB (1992): Regulation of afferent connectivity in the adult spinal cord by nerve growth factor. Eur J Neurosci 4:700–707.

Lewin GR, Ritter AM, Mendell LM (1993): Nerve growth factor-induced hyperalgesia in the neonatal and adult rat. J Neurosci 13:2136–2148.

Lewin GR, Rueff A, Mendell LM (1994): Peripheral and central mechanisms of NGF-induced hyperalgesia. Eur J Neurosci 6:1903–1912.

Lindsay RM, Harmar AJ (1989): Nerve growth factor regulates expression of neuropeptide genes in adult sensory neurons. Nature 337:362–364.

Lindsay RM, Lockett C, Sternberg J, Winter J (1989): Neuropeptide expression in cultures of adult sensory neurons: modulation of substance P and calcitonin gene-related peptide levels by nerve growth factor. Neuroscience 33:53–65.

Martin HA, Murphy PR (1995): Interleukin-2 activates a sub-population of cutaneous c-fibre polymodal nociceptors in the rat hairy skin. Arch Physiol Biochem 103: 136–148.

McEachern AE, Shelton ER, Bhakta S, Obernolte R, Bach C, Zuppan P, Fujisaka J, Aldrich RW, Jarnagin K (1991): Expression cloning of a rat B_2 bradykinin receptor. Proc Natl Acad Sci USA 88:7724–7728.

McKinnon M, Proudfoot AEI, Wells TNC, Solari R (1996): Strategies for the discovery of cytokine receptor antagonists. Drug News Perspect 9:389–398.

McMahon SB, Bennett DL, Priestley JV, Shelton DL (1995): The biological effects of endogenous nerve growth factor on adult sensory neurons revealed by a trkA-IgG fusion molecule. Nat Med 1:740–741.

McQueen DS, Iggo A, Birrell GJ, Grubb BD (1991): Effects of paracetamol and aspirin on neural activity of joint mechanonociceptors in adjuvant arthritis. Br J Pharmacol 104:178–182.

Menke JG, Borkowski JA, Bierilo KK, MacNeil T, Derrick AW, Schneck KA, Ransom RW, Strader CD, Linemeyer DL, Hess JF (1994): Expression cloning of a human B_1 Bradykinin receptor. J Biol Chem 269:21583–21586.

Mizumura K, Kumazawa T (1996): Modification of nociceptor responses by inflammatory mediators and second messengers implicated in their action—a study in canine testicular polymodal nociceptors. Prog Brain Res 113:115–141.

Mizumura K, Sato J, Kumazawa T (1987): Effects of prostaglandins and other putative chemical intermediaries on the activity of canine testicular polymodal receptors studied in vitro. Pflugers Arch 408:565–572.

Mizumura K, Minagawa M, Tsujii Y, Kumasawa T (1990): The effects of bradykinin agonists and antagonists on visceral polymodal receptor activities. Pain 40:221–227.

Mizumura K, Koda H, Kumazawa T (1993): Augmenting effects of cyclic AMP on the heat response of canine testicular polymodal receptors. Neurosci Lett 162:75–77.

Narumiya S (1995): Structures, properties and distributions of prostanoid receptors. Adv Prostaglandin Thromboxane Leukot Res 23:17–22.

Negishi M, Sugimoto Y, Ichikawa A (1995): Molecular mechanisms of diverse actions of prostanoid receptors. Biochem Biophys Acta 1259:109–119.

Nicol GD, Cui M (1994): Enhancement by prostaglandin E2 of bradykinin activation of embryonic rat sensory neurones. J Physiol 480:485–492.

Niiro H, Otsuka T, Tanabe T, Hara S, Kuga S, Nemoto Y, Tanaka Y, Nakashima H, Kitajima S, Abe M, Niho Y (1995): Inhibition by interleukin-10 of inducible cyclooxygenase expression in lipopolysaccharide-stimulated monocytes: its underlying mechanism in comparison with interleukin-4. Blood 85:3736–3745.

Numerof RP, Aronson FR, Mier JW (1988): IL-2 stimulates the production of IL-1 alpha and IL-1 beta by human peripheral blood mononuclear cells. J Immunol 141:4250–4257.

Oida H, Namba T, Sugimoto Y, Ushikubi F, Ohishi H, Ichikawa A, Narumiya S (1995): In situ hybridization studies of prostacyclin receptor mRNA expression in various mouse organs. Br J Pharmacol 116:2828–2837.

Perkins MN, Kelly D (1993): Induction of bradykinin B_1 receptors in vivo in a model of ultra-violet irradiation-induced thermal hyperalgesia in the rat. Br J Pharmacol 110:1441–1444.

Perkins MN, Kelly D (1994): Interleukin-1β induced-desArg⁹bradykinin-mediated thermal hyperalgesia in the rat. Neuropharmacology 33:657–660.

Perkins MN, Campbell E, Dray A (1993): Antinociceptive activity of the bradykinin B_1 and B_2 receptor antagonists, desArg⁹(Leu⁸)-Bk and HOE 140, in two models of persistent hyperalgesia in the rat. Pain 53:191–197.

Petty BG, Cornblath DR, Adornato BT, Chaudhry V, Flexner C, Wachsman M, Sinicropi D, Burton LE, Peroutka SJ (1994): The effect of systematically administered recombinant human growth factor in healthy human subjects. Ann Neurol 36:244–246.

Pierce KL, Gil DW, Woodward DF, Regan JW (1995): Cloning of human prostanoid receptors. Trends Pharmacol Sci 16:253–256.

Poole S, Cunha FQ, Selkirk S, Lorenzetti BB, Ferreira SH (1995): Cytokine-mediated inflammatory hyperalgesia limited by interleukin-10. Br J Pharmacol 115:684–688.

Rang HP, Bevan SJ, Dray A (1991): Chemical activation of nociceptive peripheral neurones. In Wells JCD, Woolf CJ (eds): *Pain Mechanisms and Management*. London: The British Council, pp. 534–548.

Rankin EC, Choy EH, Kassimos D, Kingsley GH, Sopwith AM, Isenberg DA, Panayi GS (1995): The therapeutic effects of an engineered human anti-tumour necrosis factor alpha antibody (CDP571) in rheumatoid arthritis. Br J Rheumatol 34:334–342.

Re F, Muzio M, De Rossi M, Polentarutti N, Giri JG, Mantovani A, Colotta F (1994): The type II "receptor" as a decoy target for interleukin-1 in polymorphonuclear leukocytes: Characterization of induction by dexamethasone and ligand binding properties of the released decoy receptor. J Exp Med 179:739–743.

Regoli D, Rhaleb NE, Drapeau G, Dion S (1990): Kinin receptor subtypes. J Cardiovasc Pharmacol 15(Suppl. 6):S30–S38.

Rueff A, Dray A (1993): Sensitization of peripheral afferent fibres in the in vitro neonatal rat spinal cord-tail by bradykinin and prostaglandins. Neuroscience 54:527–535.

Rueff A, Mendell M (1996): Nerve growth factor and NT-5 induce increased thermal sensitivity of cutaneous nociceptors in vitro. J Neurophysiol 76:3593–3596.

Rueff A, Dawson AJ, Mendell LM (1996): Characteristics of nerve growth factor induced hyperalgesia in adult rats: dependence on enhanced bradykinin-1 receptor activity but not neurokinin-1 receptor activation. Pain 66:359–372.

Safieh-Garabedian B, Poole S, Allchorne A, Winter J, Woolf CJ (1995): Contribution of interleukin-1β to the inflammation-induced increase in nerve growth factor levels and inflammatory hyperalgesia. Br J Pharmacol 115:1265–1275.

Schaible HG, Schmidt RF (1988): Excitation and sensitization of fine articular afferents from cat's knee joint by prostaglandin E2. J Physiol 403:91–104.

Sengupta JN, Gebhart GF (1994): Characterization of mechanosensitive pelvic nerve afferent fibres innervating the colon of the rat. J Neurophysiol 71:2046–2060.

Smeyne RJ, Klein R, Schnapp A, Long LK, Bryant S, Lewin A, Lira SA, Baracid M (1994): Severe sensory and sympathetic neuropathies in mice carrying a disrupted Trk/NGF receptor gene. Nature 368:193.

Smith GD, Harmar AJ, McQueen DS, Seckl JR (1992): Increase in substance P and CGRP, but not somatostatin content of innervating dorsal root ganglion in adjuvant monoarthritis in the rat. Neurosci Lett 137:257–260.

Steranka LR, Manning DC, DeHaas CJ, Ferkany JW, Borosky SA, Connor JR, Vavrek RJ, Stewart JM, Snyder SH (1988): Bradykinin as a pain mediator: Receptors are localized to sensory neurons, and antagonists have analgesic actions. Proc Natl Acad Sci USA 85:3245–3249.

Sugimoto Y, Shigemoto R, Namba T, Negishi M, Mizuno N, Narumiya S, Ichikawa A (1994): Distribution of the messenger RNA for the prostaglandin E receptor subtype EP_3 in the mouse nervous system. Neuroscience 62:919–928.

Tal M, Liberman R (1997): Local injection of nerve growth factor (NGF) triggers degranulation of mast cells in rat paw. Neurosci Lett 221:129–132.

Thompson SWN, Dray A, McCarson KE, Krause JE, Urban L (1995): Nerve growth factor induces mechanical allodynia associated with novel A fiber-evoked spinal reflex activity and enhanced neurokinin-1 receptor activation in the rat. Pain 62:219–231.

Tilg H, Shapiro L, Atkins MB, Dinarello CA, Mier JW (1993): Induction of circulating and erythrocyte-bound IL-8 by IL-2 immunotherapy and suppression of its in vitro production by IL-1 receptor antagonist and soluble tumor necrosis factor receptor (p75) chimera. J Immunol 151:3299–3307.

Tilg H, Shapiro L, Vannier E, Poutsiaka DD, Trehu E, Atkins MB, Dinarello CA, Mier JW (1994): Induction of circulating antagonists to IL-1 and TNF by IL-2 administration and their effects on IL-2 induced cytokine production in vitro. J Immunol 152:3189–3198.

Tolkovsky A (1997): Neurotrophic factors in action—new dogs and new tricks. Trends Neurosci 20:1–3.

Ushikubi F, Hirata M, Narumiya S (1995): Molecular biology of prostanoid receptors; an overview. J Lipid Mediat Cell Signal 12:343–359.

Vantini G, Schiavo N, Di Martino A, Polato P, Triban C, Callegaro L, Toffano G, Leon A (1989): Evidence for a physiological role of nerve growth factor in the central nervous system of neonatal rats. Neuron 3:267–273.

Vassalli P (1992): The pathophysiology of tumor necrosis factors. Ann Rev Immunol 10:411–452.

Wang P, Wu P, Siegel MI, Egan RW, Billah MM (1995): Interleukin (IL)-10 inhibits nuclear factor kappa β (NF kappa β) activation in human monocytes. IL-10 and IL-4 suppress cytokine synthesis by different mechanisms. J Biol Chem 270:9558–9563.

Watkins LR, Wiertelak EP, Goehler LE, Smith KP, Martin D, Maier SF (1994): Characterization of cytokine-induced hyperalgesia. Brain Res 654:15–26.

Watkins LR, Goehler LE, Relton J, Brewer MT, Maier SF (1995): Mechanisms of tumor necrosis factor-alpha (TNF-alpha) hyperalgesia. Brain Res 692:244–250.

Weinreich D, Wonderlin WF (1987): Inhibition of calcium-dependent spike after hyperpolarization increases excitability of rabbit visceral afferent neurons. J Physiol 394:415–427.

Weinreich D, Koschorke GM, Undem BJ, Taylor GE (1995): Prevention of the excitatory actions of bradykinin by inhibition of PGI_2 formation in nodose neurones of the guinea-pig. J Physiol 483:735–746.

Whalley ET, Clegg S, Stewart JM, Vavrek RJ (1987): The effect of kinin agonists and antagonists on the pain response of the human blister base. Naunyn-Schmiedeberg's Arch Pharmacol 336:652–655.

Winter J, Forbes CA, Sternberg J, Lindsay RM (1988): Nerve growth factor (NGF) regulates adult rat dorsal root ganglion neuron responses to the excitotoxin capsaicin. Neuron 1:973–981.

Woolf CJ, Safieh-Garabedian B, Ma Q-P, Crilly P, Winter J (1994): Nerve growth factor contributes to the generation of inflammatory sensory hypersensitivity. Neuroscience 62:327–331.

Woolf CJ, Ma Q-P, Allchorne A, Poole S (1996): Peripheral cell types contributing to the hyperalgesic action of nerve growth factor in inflammation. J Neurosci 16:2716–2723.

Woolf CJ, Allchorne A, Safieh-Garabedian B, Poole S (1997): Cytokines, nerve growth factor and inflammatory hyperalgesia: the contribution of tumor necrosis factor alpha. Br J Pharmacol 121:417–424.

CHAPTER 6

VANILLOIDS AS ANALGESICS

ANDY DRAY
Astra Research Centre Montreal
Montreal, Quebec, Canada

Capsaicin (obtained from hot chili peppers) is a naturally occurring vanilloid (Fig. 6.1) that selectively *activates*, and at higher doses selectively *inactivates* and ultimately damages, several types of primary afferent C and Aδ fibers. It has been one of the most important tools for investigating the function of these fibers, particularly with regard to nociception and neurogenic inflammation (Dray, 1992; Wood, 1993). Other fine peripheral fibers, such as sympathetic fibers are insensitive to capsaicin, as are afferent fibers from species other than mammals, for example, avians (Szolcsányi et al., 1986; Winter et al., 1990).

Although application of capsaicin to skin or mucus membranes produces a burning pain and hyperalgesia, repeated application leads to loss of sensitivity to capsaicin, and higher concentrations block C-fiber conduction, resulting in a long-lasting sensory deficit. These properties of capsaicin have been exploited to treat many painful conditions, such as cluster headache and neuropathic pain, that are resistant to conventional analgesics. The development of other vanilloid analogues has been vigorously pursued to make better analgesics than conventional opioids or nonsteroidal anti-inflammatory drugs. This chapter describes the effects and putative mechanism of action of vanilloids in relation to pain and antinociception and summarizes the progress made in the development of related analgesics.

VANILLOIDS IN HUMANS: EFFECTS OF CAPSAICIN AND THERAPEUTIC EFFICACY

Acute intradermal injection or repeated topical application of capsaicin to the skin produces an initial concentration-dependent burning sensation and a flare response. The immediate area of capsaicin administration usually becomes in-

---

Novel Aspects of Pain Management: Opioids and Beyond, Edited by Jana Sawynok and Alan Cowan
ISBN 0-471-180173 Copyright © 1999 by Wiley-Liss, Inc.

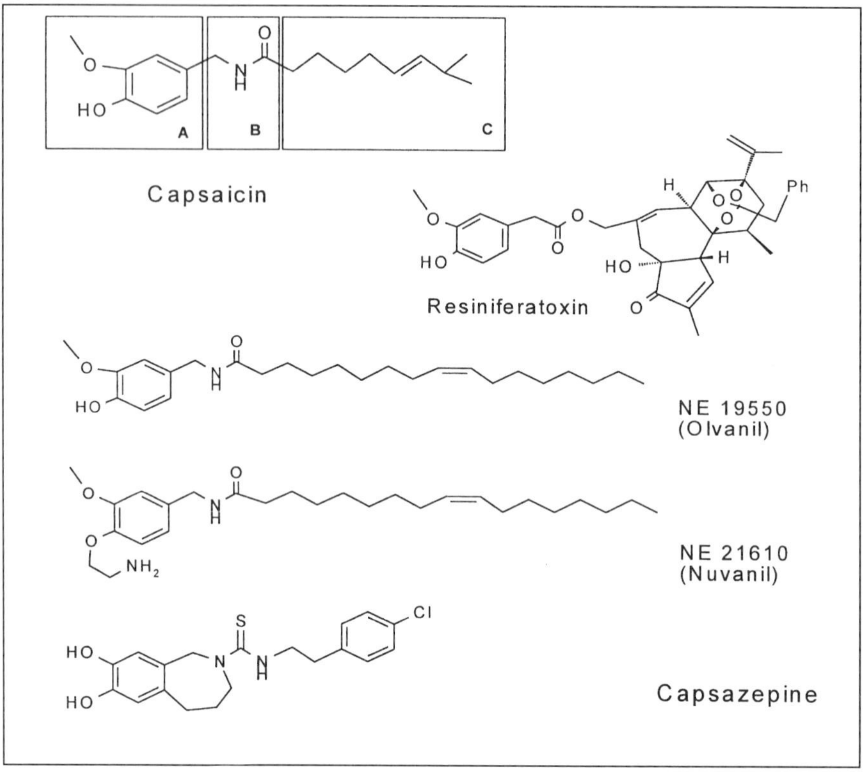

Figure 6.1 Chemical structures of the naturally occurring vanilloids capsaicin and resiniferatoxin and other synthetic vanilloid agonists (olvanil and nuvanil), as well as the vanilloid *antagonist*, capsazepine. The capsaicin molecule has been divided into three modular sites A, B, and C for systematic synthesis of analogues for structure–activity studies.

sensitive to further mechanical or thermal stimulation for several hours. Within the area of the flare, a primary hyperalgesia is produced with an increase in perceived pain to mechanical and thermal stimuli, and an area of secondary (mechanical) allodynia extends beyond the flare (Simone et al., 1989; LaMotte et al., 1991; Magnusson and Koskinen, 1996). This pattern of effects has been utilized extensively as a convenient and reversible method for studying pain mechanisms in humans, for example, the identification of "silent nociceptors" (Schmelz et al., 1994), central sensitization mechanisms (Sang et al., 1996), the involvement of peripheral sympathetic fibers in nociception (Liu et al., 1996), and the evaluation of several types of analgesic agents (Andersen et al., 1996; Kinnman et al., 1997).

In rodents, local application of capsaicin produces afferent nerve excitation and increased sensitivity to thermal and mechanical stimuli (Kenins, 1982;

McMahon et al., 1991). These effects diminish with repeated administration and can be accompanied by reduced sensitivity to noxious chemical, mechanical, and thermal stimuli. In humans, topical capsaicin also produces analgesia (Simone et al., 1989; Beydouin et al., 1996) and loss of flare responses to a variety of stimuli only after several days or weeks of treatment (Anand et al., 1983; Bjerring and Arendt-Nielsen, 1990). Overall, analgesia produced by topical capsaicin appears variable and dependent on the amount of capsaicin that penetrates the skin (Kenins, 1982; Carter and Francis, 1991; McMahon et al., 1991; Lynn et al., 1992), so that the frequency of capsaicin administration and the choice of vehicle or formulation are important considerations.

It is worth noting that topical capsaicin reduces plasma extravasation and vasodilatation (Lynn et al., 1992), but reduced skin levels of substance P or calcitonin gene-related peptide are unlikely to account for this (McMahon et al., 1991).

Administration of capsaicin or another vanilloid, resiniferatoxin (RTX), into the urinary bladder inhibits afferent nerve functions, and is used to treat bladder hyperreflexia or bladder pain after spinal cord injury or cystitis, respectively (Chandiramani et al., 1996; Lazzeri et al., 1996, 1997). Topical capsaicin can also prevent itching and has been used to treat chronic pruritus (psoriasis, posthemodialysis, notalgia paresthetica, brachioradial pruritus, aquagenic pruritus) of differing etiology (Leibsohn, 1992; Ellis et al., 1993; Knight and Hayashi, 1994; Tarng et al., 1996). The antipruritic activity is also due to selective inactivation of a specific subset of C fibers (Lynn, 1992; McMahon and Kotzenburg, 1992).

Systemic capsaicin depletes substance P from sensory fibers innervating the joint synovium, though inactivation of these fibers rather than neuropeptide depletion accounts for the reduction of joint inflammation and hyperalgesia (Colpaert et al., 1983; Perkins and Campbell, 1992). In humans, topical capsaicin is inconsistent in reducing joint pain, possibly due to variability in the concentrations of capsaicin achieved in joint afferents (Deal et al., 1991). Although no significant improvement is seen in patients with rheumatoid arthritis of the hands (McCarthy and McCarty, 1992), double-blind studies in osteoarthritis consistently show that prolonged topical treatment with capsaicin cream provides pain relief (Deal et al., 1991; McCarthy and McCarty, 1992; Altman et al., 1994).

Capsaicin pretreatment of neonatal rats, to induce C-fiber degeneration, attenuates the thermal, but not mechanical, allodynia seen after a peripherally induced neuropathy (chronic constriction injury or partial ligation of the sciatic nerve in the adult animals) (Shir and Seltzer, 1990; Meller et al., 1992), but capsaicin treatment does not affect the Aβ fiber mediated allodynia produced by spinal administration of the convulsant strychnine (Sherman and Loomis, 1996). Thus vanilloids affect only centrally induced pain states that depend on fine afferent fiber activation. In keeping with this, intrathecal administration of capsaicin or direct application around the sciatic nerve 1 week after its ligation attenuates thermal hyperalgesia (Yamamoto and Yaksh, 1992).

Prolonged (weeks to months) topical application of capsaicin is considered to be of therapeutic benefit in post-mastectomy pain (Watson et al., 1989; Dini et al., 1993), stump pain (Rayner et al., 1989), reflex sympathetic dystrophy (Sinoff and Hart, 1993), oral neuropathic pain (Epstein and Marcoe, 1994), trigeminal neuralgia (Fusco et al., 1991), and fibromyalgia (McCarty et al., 1994), although the greatest experience has been in diabetic neuropathy (Capsaicin Study Group, 1991) and postherpetic neuralgia (Bernstein et al., 1987; Bjerring et al., 1990; Watson et al., 1993). With diabetic neuropathy, significant improvement was reported in pain and other scores for up to 2 years after treatment without adverse side effects. Generally, the effects of capsaicin take several weeks to develop, but in many studies patients drop out in the earlier weeks of treatment owing to intolerance of the irritation and burning caused by capsaicin.

Prolonged nasal application of capsaicin produces significant improvement in cluster headache and in some cases the symptoms disappeared (Sicuteri et al., 1989; Fusco et al., 1991; Marks et al., 1993). These studies suggest that sensory neurones around the nasal mucosa, as well as fine trigeminal afferent fibers, may be involved in the pathogenesis of headache. Thus the likely mechanism of headache relief is the selective inactivation of these groups of fibers (Strassman et al., 1996).

VANILLOIDS AND SENSORY FIBER ACTIVATION

Capsaicin induces concentration-dependent activation of fine afferent fibers and subsets of isolated sensory neurons (large as well as small neurons) (Petersen and LaMotte, 1991; Seno and Dray, 1993; Liu and Simon, 1996). This is due to membrane depolarization and an increase in membrane permeability to cations, particularly to calcium and sodium ions (Wood and Docherty, 1997). It has been claimed that vanilloid-operated ion channels may have a higher selectivity for calcium ions (Caterina et al., 1997) or sodium ions (Oh et al., 1996), respectively. An increase in membrane cation conductance also occurs via voltage-gated ion channels (calcium, sodium), but this makes a small contribution compared with the ionic conductance occurring through capsaicin-operated ion channels.

The capsaicin-operated channel is unique in that it is insensitive to conventional calcium and sodium ion-channel blockers such as dihydropyridines, ω-conotoxin, and tetrodotoxin, respectively (Bevan and Geppetti, 1994; Wood and Docherty, 1997). However, it is selectively blocked by low concentrations of ruthenium red, which attenuates both the activation of sensory neurons and the release of sensory neuropeptides induced by capsaicin and other vanilloids, but not by other sensory nerve stimulants (Maggi et al., 1988; Amann et al., 1990; Dray et al., 1990b). As a secondary result of calcium entry into nerve cells, capsaicin-induced activation stimulates an increase in inositol trisphosphate turnover and arachidonic acid release, and increases intracellular levels of cGMP, diacyl glycerol, and nitric oxide (Wood et al., 1989; Farkas-Szállási et al., 1995).

VANILLOID RECEPTORS

Structure–activity studies with vanilloid analogues suggest the presence of a membrane receptor for vanilloids. Such studies indicate that substitutions in the "A" ring and the "B" region are critical for agonistic activity (Fig. 6.1). Agonistic potency is increased in compounds with increased chain length, and is optimal with compounds having 8–12 carbons in the lipophilic side chain "C" region. Activity decreases with longer chain length (Walpole et al., 1993a–c).

Studies to characterize a capsaicin binding protein have not been successful, owing to the poor characteristics of radio-labeled capsaicin as a binding ligand. However, another labeled vanilloid, RTX, obtained from the latex of *Euphorbia resinifera* shows specific, saturable, capsaicin-displaceable binding (Szállási and Blumberg, 1990). This potent irritant (Fig. 6.1) also activates small sensory neurons in a manner identical to that of capsaicin (Blumberg et al., 1993; Winter et al., 1990, 1993a). [^{3}H]RTX binding shows positive cooperativity indicative of two interactive binding sites that may be the same or different vanilloid receptors (Szállási, 1994). [^{3}H]RTX has also been valuable in localizing capsaicin-displaceable binding in the spinal dorsal horn and to a number of sensory nuclei in the brainstem (nucleus of the solitary tract, area postrema, trigeminal nucleus) but not sympathetic neurons (Winter et al., 1993a; Acs et al., 1994; 1996b; Szállázi, 1994; Szállázi et al., 1995). [^{3}H]RTX binding in the human spinal cord differs in affinity (K_d = 11 nM) from that seen in the rat (K_d = 25 pM) but resembles that in the guinea pig (Szállási and Goso, 1994; Szállási et al., 1994), indicating possible species differences in vanilloid receptors and possible intraspecies differences in the efficacy of vanilloid ligands. Ligation of the vagus or sciatic nerve produces an accumulation of RTX binding proximal to the ligation, suggesting that the high RTX binding in spinal dorsal horn and sensory ganglia is due to transportation of binding proteins (Szállási et al., 1995).

Some descriptions of capsaicin and RTX binding indicate large differences in affinity and agonist potency (30–40 thousandfold) (Maggi et al., 1990; Szallási et al., 1993b), whereas other studies indicate smaller differences (20-fold) (e.g., Wardle et al., 1997). Several explanations may account for this; receptor subtypes with different ligand binding affinity may exist, receptor effector coupling may differ between tissues (Acs et al., 1994; Szállási, 1994), or there may be a lack of correspondence between RTX binding and functional activity (Acs et al., 1996a; 1997; Farkas-Szállási et al., 1996).

Radiation-inactivation analysis of the [^{3}H]RTX binding protein has suggested that the binding complex has a molecular weight of 270 kDa (Szállási and Blumberg, 1991) and may exist as a multimeric complex of protein subunits. If so, this would explain the difficulty in cloning the correct configuration of subunits required to reconstitute the vanilloid receptor (James et al., 1993). Molecular cloning of an RTX-binding protein has indicated two sites, one present in sensory neurons and another in non-neural or vanilloid-insensitive neural tissues (Ninkina et al., 1994). The former site was encoded by a 235 amino acid protein with molecular weight of 26,000 (termed RBP-26, resiniferatoxin binding protein 26). Because this sensory neuron site binds RTX with high affinity (K_d = 10 nM), it appears to resemble closely the binding site described by others (see Szállási, 1994).

Further evidence for vanilloid receptors has come from using the competitive capsaicin antagonist, capsazepine (Fig. 1). This compound selectively inhibits the excitatory effects of capsaicin both in vivo and in vitro (Dickenson and Dray, 1991; Bevan et al., 1992) as well as the secondary release of neuropeptides (Franco-Cereceda and Lundberg, 1992; Wardle et al., 1997). Molecular studies with RTX and capsazepine have further indicated differences in vanilloid receptors and possible receptor heterogeneity in different tissues (spinal cord versus airways; Szállási et al., 1993a; Wardle et al., 1997). Indeed, there may be receptor heterogeneity within sensory neurons. Thus capsazepine is less effective at inhibiting [^{3}H]RTX binding in sensory neurons than inhibiting the functional responses (calcium uptake) to RTX and capsaicin (Acs et al., 1996a). In addition, capsaicin and other vanilloid analogues evoke two types of activation in the same subpopulation of sensory neurons (Petersen et al., 1995; Liu et al., 1997). Capsazepine attenuates only a proportion (early component) of the afferent fiber response to capsaicin and protects this from the desensitization that follows prolonged exposure to capsaicin (Dray et al., 1992).

Recently, a gene coding for a vanilloid receptor has been found in small sensory neurons (Caterina et al., 1997). The receptor protein (838 amino acids, molecular weight 95 kDa) is an integral part of the nerve cell membrane and, when expressed in HEK 293 cells or xenopus oocytes, exhibits similar sensitivity to capsaicin, RTX, and capsazepine as the native receptor in sensory nerves. The cooperativity of [^{3}H]RTX binding suggests that there is more than one binding site and it may be that the ion channel pore is formed by several protein subunits (at least three or four), each with six transmembrane domains. The vanilloid recognition site may be located within the membrane, for capsaicin is efficacious when administered on either side of the membrane. As with the native receptor, desensitization to the repeated administration of capsaicin requires the presence of calcium and at least two components of the response are distinguishable by the fact that only one undergoes rapid densitization. In addition, capsaicin-induced neurotoxicity is possible only when the vanilloid receptor is present in cells.

The cloned receptor protein could not be located in areas known to exhibit capsaicin sensitivity such as the nodose ganglion or preoptic hypothalamus, suggesting receptor heterogeneity. Accordingly, the cloned receptor was named VR1, indicating that it is likely to be a receptor subtype.

The vanilloid receptor complex may also be a heat transducer (Caterina et al., 1997). Thus its concomitant activation explains the burning quality of capsaicin-containing foods and capsaicin-induced pain. Other experiments argue against this identity because responses to capsaicin are sensitive to capsazepine and ruthenium red whereas those to heat stimuli are not. In addition, responsiveness to capsaicin can be selectively desensitized without affecting responses to heat stimuli (Dray et al., 1990a; Reichling and Levine, 1997).

AN ENDOGENOUS VANILLOID LIGAND?

By analogy with other systems, a natural ligand for the vanilloid binding protein should exist. Protons have been a principal candidate for this role, because protons are produced in conditions such as ischemia and inflammation, and can activate or sensitize nociceptors. Indeed, proton and capsaicin-induced activation of sensory neurons have identical ion conductance mechanisms (Bevan and Geppetti, 1994). However, there is only partial overlap between sensory fiber sensitivity to protons and to capsaicin (Steen et al., 1992; Baumann et al., 1996; Chen et al., 1997), and their exact mechanism of action differs because both increase intracellular calcium (Garcia-Hirschfeld et al., 1995), but the response to each agent is still observed after selective desensitization to the other (Dray et al., 1992; Garcia-Hirschfeld et al., 1995; Chen et al., 1997). Finally, application of protons to the cloned VR1 receptor is usually ineffective alone (Caterina et al., 1997) but the effect of capsaicin is potentiated in the presence of protons. Presently it is not clear where or how this interaction occurs.

There may be several binding domains on the vanilloid receptor, because capsazepine has little effect on proton-induced activation of sensory neurons (Dray et al., 1990a; Bevan and Geppetti, 1994; Chen et al., 1997). Conversely, proton-induced activation of trigeminal or tracheal afferent neurons (Liu and Simon, 1994; Fox et al., 1995) and the proton-induced neuropeptide release from visceral sensory neurons (heart, trachea) are inhibited by capsazepine (Franco-Cereceda and Lundberg, 1992). It may be that protons induce the release of an endogenous vanilloid (Franco-Cereceda et al., 1994).

CAPSAICIN-INDUCED DESENSITIZATION AND NERVE INACTIVATION

Prolonged or frequent administration of capsaicin leads to a progressive decline in the response to capsaicin without affecting responses to other stimuli (Dray et al., 1990a; Holzer, 1991). The molecular mechanism for desensitization has not been fully elucidated, but is likely to be a receptor-mediated event, because it can be prevented in part by "protecting" the vanilloid receptor with capsazepine (Dray et al., 1992).

Desensitization is calcium-dependent, involving a dephosphorylation mechanism via the calcium- and calmodulin-dependent cytosolic enzyme protein phosphatase 2B (calcineurin) (Wood and Docherty, 1997). Inhibition of calcineurin by complexing with cyclosporin A and its cytoplasmic binding protein, cyclophilin, prevents desensitization. Conversely, raising intracellular levels of cyclic AMP increases capsaicin responses (Pitchford and Levine, 1991), further suggesting that capsaicin sensitivity is regulated by phosphorylation of a key protein; this may be part of the vanilloid receptor ion channel complex.

Sensory fiber inactivation, with a reduction or loss of responsiveness to all stimuli, usually occurs with high concentrations of capsaicin (Dray et al., 1990a). Extracellular calcium is also required for this type of desensitization (Wood and Docherty, 1997), and it can be prevented by ruthenium red, which blocks the ion channels activated by capsaicin (Maggi et al., 1988; Amann et al., 1990). This type of functional desensitization, supplemented by inhibition of sensory neurochemical release described below, explains the short-lasting analgesic and anti-inflammatory effects of capsaicin.

Neurochemical release occurs by two distinct mechanisms of calcium entry: via the capsaicin-operated channel and via voltage-gated channels that are activated following membrane depolarization (Dray, 1992). The initial calcium entry induced by capsaicin leads to inactivation of voltage-gated calcium conductance (Docherty et al., 1991) and to a reversible inhibition of sensory neurotransmitter release in the spinal cord, as well as inhibition of neurochemical release in the periphery. Indeed, the inactivation of neurochemical release occurs *with little effect on tissue concentrations*, suggesting that compromised sensory nerve function occurs without depletion of sensory neurochemicals (Dray et al., 1989; McMahon et al., 1991). Other explanations for the prolonged antinociceptive effects have been proposed. Thus spinal substance P, released by capsaicin, may be metabolized to an *N*-terminal fragment [SP(1-7)] that inhibits further substance P release (Goettl et al., 1997).

CAPSAICIN-INDUCED NEUROTOXICITY

Initial excitation by capsaicin is followed by insensitivity to noxious stimuli. Antinociception lasts from a few hours (after 1–10 mg/kg) to several months after a single dose (50 mg/kg) or cumulative doses (total of 950 mg/kg). Capsaicin-induced neurotoxicity can be lifelong, particularly after pretreatments in neonatal animals. However, in adults, localized administration of capsaicin induces reversible injury of the peripheral receptive area of sensory fibers leaving cell bodies intact with the capability of nerve terminal regeneration (Chung et al., 1990; Winter et al., 1993a). After perineural application of capsaicin, C fibers degenerate distally, and extensive axonal sprouting can be seen from the proximal nerve. Although neurons with damaged axons attempt to regenerate, they do not necessarily reinnervate their original targets in vivo (Pini et al., 1990; Jancsó, 1992; Winter et al., 1993b) and this may produce permanent sensory deficits. Neurotoxicity is thought to be a consequence of intense excitation and increased membrane permeability to cations. The damage is partially osmotic, owing to loading sodium ions, and partially because of calcium entry causing activation of calcium-sensitive proteases (Winter et al., 1990). In vivo, the severity of these effects depends on the age of the animal at the time of treatment, the route of administration, and the dose of capsaicin used.

It is noteworthy that neural degeneration following high systemic doses of capsaicin has also been observed in a number of central sensory and nonsensory areas including the retina and brain (vagus, trigeminal tract, hypothalamus) (Ritter and Dinh, 1993). The implications of these findings are unclear and further studies are indicated.

CAPSAICIN-INDUCED ANTINOCICEPTION

Though treatment with capsaicin produces antinociception (Faulkner and Growcott, 1980; Hayes and Tyers, 1980; Hayes et al., 1981a,b), loss of responsiveness to a thermal stimulus has been less consistent, with reports of no change as well as increased thermal nociceptive thresholds (Hayes et al., 1981a,b; Cervero and McRitchie, 1983). This variability may be due to differences in dosing regimes, or possible plasticity and regeneration of sensory neurons. Because of the rapid access of capsaicin to the central nervous system, analgesia probably results from an acute, short-lasting inactivation of sensory nerve conduction and neurotransmitter release at central nerve terminals (Dickenson et al., 1990a,b). However, other mechanisms including release of inhibitory tachykinin metabolites (Goettl et al., 1997) or of opioid peptides such as β-endorphin (Back and Yaksh, 1995), have been proposed to contribute to the prolonged antinociception induced by capsaicin. Anti-inflammatory activity is likely to involve short-lasting inactivation of neurochemical release in the periphery. Neither of these reversible effects is likely to be caused by an acute central or peripheral sensory fiber neurotoxicity.

VANILLOID ANALOGUES

Vanilloids that induce analgesia without unwanted side effects, such as initial irritability, are highly desirable. Indeed, a number of studies have described vanilloids with these properties (Brand et al., 1987; 1990; Sietsema et al., 1988; Chen et al., 1992; Yang et al., 1992; Wrigglesworth et al., 1996). For example, analgesic and anti-inflammatory activity occur with NE19550 (olvanil) (Fig. 6.1) (Brand et al., 1987; Campbell et al., 1989; 1993; Dickenson et al., 1990a; Dray and Dickenson, 1991), and NE21610 (nuvanil) (Fig. 6.1) has improved solubility, increased oral efficacy, and reduced irritancy. However, NE21610 and NE19550 also caused profound hypothermia (Campbell et al., 1993), but notably in humans, NE21610 is less excitatory than capsaicin and effectively inhibits burn-induced hyperalgesia and allodynia (Davis et al., 1995). Indeed, several other nonpungent vanilloid analogues exhibit reduced activation of vagally mediated blood pressure reflexes, yet retain antinociceptive activity (Chen et al., 1992; Hua et al., 1997).

Capsazepine shows no vanilloid side effects but inhibits capsaicin-induced analgesia. In models of acute experimental pain, it does not exhibit significant analgesic or anti-inflammatory activity (Perkins and Campbell, 1992). Other studies show that capsazepine attenuates the proton-induced activation of sensory fibers and sensory neuropeptide release (Franco-Cereceda and Lundberg 1992; Fox et al., 1995). Presently it is unclear whether or not capsazepine interacts with endogenous "vanilloid" factors.

SUMMARY AND CONCLUSIONS

The analgesic and anti-inflammatory activity of capsaicin and other naturally occurring vanilloids has been of intense interest for a number of years. These compounds show unique features. Vanilloids produce pain and subsequent concentration-dependent insensitivity to sensory stimuli via a specific membrane receptor. Structure–activity studies with vanilloids, including RTX and the use of capsazepine, support the existence of vanilloid receptor subtypes whose molecular characterization has been difficult because the receptor exists in a multimeric form and is difficult to reconstitute. However, there has been an increase in the use of capsaicin itself, particularly as a topical analgesic, in a variety of pain conditions that have responded poorly to conventional analgesic therapy. A systemically effective vanilloid analgesic is desirable, and the clinical data to date encourage a more intensive effort to develop other compounds of this type. This will be considerably enhanced by the recent cloning of a vanilloid VR1 receptor that can be expressed in a suitable form for a more intensive chemical screening and drug discovery effort.

REFERENCES

Acs G, Palkovits M, Blumberg PM (1994): [^{3}H]Resiniferatoxin binding by the human vanilloid (capsaisin) receptor. Brain Res Mol Brain Res 23:185–190.

Acs G, Lee J, Marquez VE, Blumberg PM (1996a): Distinct structure activity relations for stimulation of ^{45}Ca uptake and for high affinity binding in cultured dorsal root ganglion neurons and dorsal root ganglion membranes. Brain Res Mol Brain Res 35:173–182.

Acs G, Palkovits M, Blumberg PM (1996b): Comparison of [^{3}H]resiniferatoxin binding by the vanilloid (capsaicin) receptor in dorsal root ganglia, spinal cord, dorsal vagal complex, sciatic and vagal nerve and urinary bladder of the rat. Life Sci 55:1017–1026.

Acs G, Biro T, Acs P, Modarres S, Blumberg PM (1997): Differential activation and desensitization of sensory neurons by resiniferatoxin. J Neurosci 17:5622–5628.

REFERENCES

Altman RD, Aven A, Holmburg CE, Pfeifer LM, Sack M, Young GT (1994): Capsaicin cream 0.025% as monotherapy for osteoarthritis: a double-blind study. Semin Arthritis Rheum 23:25–33.

Amann R, Donnerer J, Lembeck F (1990): Activation of primary afferent neurons by thermal stimulation: Influence of ruthenium red. Naunyn-Schmiedeberg's Arch Pharmacol 341:108–113.

Anand P, Bloom SR, McGregor GP (1983): Topical capsaicin pretreatment inhibits axon reflex vasodilatation caused by somatostatin and vasoactive intestinal peptide in human skin. Br J Pharmacol 78:665–669.

Andersen OK, Felsby S, Nocolaisen L, Bjerring P, Jensen TS, Arendt-Nielsen L (1996): The effect of ketamine on stimulation of primary and secondary hyperalgesic areas induced by capsaicin—a double-blind, placebo-controlled, human experimental study. Pain 66:51–61.

Back FW, Yaksh TL (1995): Release of beta-endorphin immunoreactivity into ventriculo-cisternal perfusate by lumbar intrathecal capsaicin in the rat. Brain Res 701:192–200.

Baumann TK, Burchiel KJ, Ingram SL, Martenson ME (1996): Responses of adult human dorsal root ganglion neurons in culture to capsaicin and low pH. Pain 65:31–38.

Bernstein JE, Bickers DR, Dahl MV, Roshal JY (1987): Treatment of chronic postherpetic neuralgia with topical capsaicin. J Am Acad Dermatol 17:93–96.

Bevan S, Geppetti P (1994): Protons: small stimulants of capsaicin-sensitive sensory nerves. Trends Neurosci 17:509–512.

Bevan SJ, Hothi S, Hughes GA, James IF, Rang HP, Shah K, Walpole CJS, Yeats JC (1992): Capsazepine: A competitive antagonist of the sensory neurone excitant, capsaicin. Br J Pharmacol 107:544–552.

Beydouin A, Dyke DB, Morrow TJ, Casey KL (1996): Topical capsaicin selectively attenuates heat pain and A delta fiber-mediated laser-evoked potentials. Pain 65:189–196.

Bjerring P, Arendt-Nielsen L (1990): Inhibition of histamine skin flare reaction following repeated topical application of capsaicin. Allergy 45:121–125.

Bjerring P, Arendt-Nielsen L, Soderberg U (1990): Argon laser induced cutaneous sensory and pain thresholds in post-herpetic neuralgia. Quantitative modulation by topical capsaicin. Acta DermVenereol 70:121–125.

Blumberg PM, Szállási A, Ács G (1993): Resiniferatoxin—an ultrapotent capsaicin analogue. In Wood J N (ed): *Capsaicin in the Study of Pain*. London: Academic Press, pp. 45–62.

Brand LM, Berman E, Schwen R, Loomans M, Janusz J, Bohne R, Maddin C, Gardner J, LaHann T, Farmer R, Jones L, Chiabrando C, Fanelli R (1987): NE-19550: a novel, orally active anti-inflammatory analgesic. Drugs Exp Clin Res 13:259–265.

Brand LM, Skare KL, Loomans ME, Reller HH, Schwen RJ, Lade DA, Bohne RL, Maddin CS, Moorehead DP, Fanelli R, Chiabrando C, Castelli MG, Tai HH (1990): Anti-inflammatory pharmacology and mechanism of the orally active capsaicin analogs, NE-19950 and NE-28345. Agents Actions 31:329–340.

Campbell EA, Dray A, Perkins MN, Shaw W (1989): Comparison of capsaicin and olvanil as antinociceptive agents in vivo and in vitro. Br J Pharmacol 98:907P.

Campbell EA, Bevan S, Dray A (1993): Clinical applications of capsaicin and its analogues. In Wood J N (ed): *Capsaicin in the Study of Pain*. London: Academic Press, pp. 255–272.

Capsaicin Study Group (1991): Treatment of painful diabetic neuropathy with topical capsaicin. A multi-centre, double-blind, vehicle-controlled study. Arch Intern Med 151:2225–2229.

Carter RB, Francis WR (1991): Capsaicin desensitization to plasma extravasation evoked by antidromic C-fiber stimulation is not associated with antinociception in the rat. Neurosci Lett 127:49–52.

Caterina MJ, Schumacher MA, Tominga M, Rosen TA, Levine JD, Julius D (1997): The capsaicin receptor: a heat-activated ion channel in the pain pathway. Nature 389:816–824.

Cervero F, McRitchie HA (1983): Effect of neonatal administration of capsaicin in several nociceptive systems of the rat. In Bonica JJ, Liebeskind JC, Albe-Fessard DG (eds): *Advances in Pain Research and Therapy*, Vol. 4, New York: Raven Press, pp. 87–94.

Chandiramani VA, Peterson T, Duthie GS, Fowler CJ (1996): Urodynamic changes during therapeutic intravesical instillations of capsaicin. Br J Urol 77:792–797.

Chen IJ, Yang JM, Yeh JL, Wu BN, Lo YC, Chen SJ (1992): Hypotensive and antinociceptive effects of ether-linked and relatively non-pungent analogues of N-nonanoyl vanillylamide. Eur J Med Chem 27:187–192.

Chen X, Belmonte C, Rang HP (1997): Capsaicin and carbon dioxide act by distinct mechanisms on sensory nerve terminal in the cat cornea. Pain 70:23–29.

Chung K, Klein CM, Coggeshall RE (1990): The receptive part of the primary afferent axon is most vulnerable to systemic capsaicin in adult rats. Brain Res 511:222–226.

Colpaert FC, Donnerer J, Lembeck F (1983): Effects of capsaicin in inflammation and on the substance P content of nervous tissue in rats with adjuvant arthritis. Life Sci 32:1827–1834.

Davis KD, Meyer RA, Turnquist JL, Fillon TG, Pappagallo M, Campbell JN (1995): Cutaneous pretreatment with the capsaicin analog NE-21610 prevents the pain to a burn and subsequent hyperalgesia. Pain 62:373–378.

Deal CL, Schnitzer TJ, Lipstein E, Seibold JR, Stevens RM, Levy MD, Albert D, Renold F (1991): Treatment of arthritis with topical capsaicin: a double-blind trial. Clin Ther 13:383–395.

Dickenson AH, Dray A (1991): Selective antagonism of capsaicin by capsazepine: evidence for a spinal receptor site in capsaicin-induced antinociception. Br J Pharmacol 104:1045–1049.

Dickenson A, Hughes C, Rueff A, Dray A (1990a): A spinal mechanism of action is involved in the antinociception produced by the capsaicin analogue olvanil. Pain 43:353–362.

Dickenson AH, Ashwood N, Sullivan AF, James I, Dray A (1990b): Antinociception produced by capsaicin: spinal or peripheral mechanism? Eur J Pharmacol 187:225–233.

Dini D, Bertelli G, Gozza A, Formo GG (1993): Treatment of the post-mastectomy pain syndrome with topical capsaicin. Pain 54:223–226.

Docherty RJ, Robertson B, Bevan S (1991): Capsaicin causes prolonged inhibition of voltage-activated calcium currents in adult rat dorsal root ganglion neurons in culture. Neuroscience 40:513–521.

Dray A (1992): Neuropharmacological mechanisms of capsaicin and related compounds. Biochem Pharmacol 44:611–615.

Dray A, Dickenson A (1991): Systemic capsaicin and olvanil reduce the acute algogenic and the late inflammatory phase following formalin injection into rodent paw. Pain 47:79–83.

Dray A, Hankins MW, Yeats JC (1989): Desensitization and capsaicin-induced release of substance P like immunoreactivity (SPLI) from the guinea pig ureter in vitro. Neuroscience 31:479–483.

Dray A, Bettany J, Forster P (1990a): Actions of capsaicin on peripheral nociceptors of the neonatal rat spinal cord-tail *in-vitro*: dependence of extracellular and independence of second messengers. Br J Pharmacol 101:727–733.

Dray A, Forbes C, Burgess GM (1990b): Ruthenium red blocks the capsaicin-induced increase in intracellular calcium and activation of membrane currents in sensory neurons, as well as the activation of peripheral nociceptors in vitro. Neurosci Lett 110:52–59.

Dray A, Patel I, Naeem S, Rueff A, Urban L (1992): Studies with capsazepine on peripheral nociceptor activation by capsaicin and low pH: evidence for a duel effect of capsaicin. Br J Pharmacol 107:236P.

Ellis CN, Berberian B, Sulica VI, Dodd WA, Jarratt MT, Katz HI, Prawer S, Krueger G, Rex IH Jr, Wolf JE (1993): A double-blind evaluation of topical capsaicin in pruritic psoriasis. Am Acad Dermatol 29:438–442.

Epstein JB, Marcoe JH (1994): Topical application of capsaicin for treatment of oral neuropathic pain and trigeminal neuralgia. Oral Surg Oral Med Oral Pathol 77: 135–140.

Farkas-Szállási T, Lundberg JM, Wiesenfeld-Hallin Z, Hökfelt T, Szállási A (1995): Increased levels of GMAP, VIP and nitric oxide synthase, and their mRNAs, in lumbar dorsal root ganglia of the rat following systemic resiniferatoxin treatment. NeuroReport 6:2230–2234.

Farkas-Szállási T, Bennett GJ, Blumberg PM, Hökfelt T, Lundberg JM, Szállási A (1996): Vanilloid receptor loss is independent of the messenger plasticity that follows systemic resiniferatoxin administration. Brain Res 719:213–218.

Faulkner DC, Growcott JW (1980): Effects of neonatal capsaicin administration on the nociceptive response of the rat to mechanical and chemical stimuli. J Pharm Pharmacol 32:657–658.

Fox AJ, Urban L, Barnes PJ, Dray A (1995): Effects of capsazepine against capsaicin- and proton-evoked excitation of single airway C-fibres and vagus nerve from the guinea pig. Neuroscience 67:741–752.

Franco-Cereceda A, Lundberg JM (1992): Capsazepine inhibits low pH- and lactic acid evoked release of calcitonin gene-related peptide from sensory nerves in guinea-pig heart. Eur J Pharmacol 221:183–184.

Franco-Cereceda A, Kallner G, Lundberg JM (1994): Cyclo-oxygenase products released by low pH have capsaicin-like actions on sensory nerves in the isolated guinea pig heart. Cardiovasc Res 28:365–369.

Fusco BM, Geppetti P, Fanciullacci M, Sicuteri F (1991): Local application of capsaicin for the treatment of cluster headache and idiopathic trigeminal neuralgia. Cephalgia 11:234–235.

García-Hirschfeld J, López-Briones LG, Belmonte C, Valdeolmillos M (1995): Intracellular free calcium responses to protons and capsaicin in cultured trigeminal neurons. Neuroscience 67:235–243.

Goettl VM, Larson DL, Portoghese PS, Larson AA (1997): Inhibition of substance P release from spinal cord tissue after pretreatment with capsaicin does not mediate the antinociceptive effect of capsaicin in adult mice. Pain 71:271–278.

Hayes AG, Tyers MB (1980): Effect of capsaicin on nociceptive heat, pressure and chemical thresholds and on substance P levels in the rat. Brain Res 189:561–564.

Hayes AG, Scadding JW, Skingle M, Tyers MB (1981a): Effects of neonatal administration of capsaicin on nociceptive thresholds in the mouse and rat. J Pharm Pharmacol 33:183–185.

Hayes AG, Skingle M, Tyers MB (1981b): Effects of single doses of capsaicin on nociceptive thresholds in the rodent. Neuropharmacology 20:505–511.

Holzer P (1991): Capsaicin: Cellular targets, mechanisms of action, and selectivity for thin sensory neurons. Pharmacol Rev 43:143–201.

Hua X-Y, Chen P, Hwang J-H, Yaksh TL (1997): Antinociception induced by civamide, an orally active capsaicin analogue. Pain 71:313–322.

James IF, Ninkina N, Wood JN (1993): The capsaicin receptor. In Wood J (ed): *Capsaicin in the Study of Pain*. London: Academic Press, pp. 83–104.

Jancsó G (1992): Pathobiological responses of C-fibre primary sensory neurons to peripheral nerve injury. Exp Physiol 77:405–431.

Kenins P (1982): Response of single nerve fibres to capsaicin applied to the skin. Neurosci Lett 29:83–88.

Kinnman E, Nygards EB, Hansson P (1997): Peripherally administered morphine attenuates capsaicin-induced mechanical hypersensitivity in humans. Anesth Analg 84:595–599.

Knight TE, Hayashi T (1994): Solar (brachioradial) pruritus—response to capsaicin cream. Int Dermatol 33:206–209.

LaMotte RH, Shian CN, Simone DA, Tsai E-Fun P (1991): Neurogenic hyperalgesia: psychophysical studies of underlying mechanisms. Neurophysiol 66:190–211.

Lazzeri M, Beneforti P, Benaim G, Maggi CA, Lecci A, Turini D (1996): Intravesical capsaicin for treatment of severe bladder pain: a randomized placebo controlled study. J Urol 156:947–952.

Lazzeri M, Beneforti P, Turini D (1997): Urodynamic effects of intravesicular resiniferatoxin in humans-preliminary results in stable and unstable detrusor. J Urol 158:2093–2096.

Leibsohn E (1992): Treatment of notalgia paresthetica with capsaicin. Cutis 49:335–336.

Liu L, Simon SA (1994): A rapid capsaicin-activated current in rat trigeminal ganglion neurons. Proc Natl Acad Sci USA 91:738–741.

Liu L, Simon SA (1996): Similarities and differences in the currents activated by capsaicin, peperine and zingerone in rat trigeminal ganglion cells. J Neurophysiol 76:1858–1869.

Liu L, Lo Y-C, Chen I-L, Simon SA (1997): The responses of rat trigeminal ganglion neurons to capsaicin and two nonpungent vanilloid receptor agonists, olvanil and glyceryl nonamide. J Neurosci 17:4101–4111.

Liu M, Max MB, Parada S, Rowan JS, Bennett GJ (1996): The sympathetic nervous system contributes to capsaicin-evoked mechanical allodynia but not pinprick hyperalgesia in humans. J Neurosci 16:7331–7335.

Lynn B (1992): Capsaicin: actions on C fibre afferents that may be involved in itch. Skin Pharmacology 5:9–13.

Lynn B, Ye W, Cotsell B (1992): The actions of capsaicin applied topically to the skin of the rat on C-fibre afferents, antidromic vasodilatation and substance P levels. Br J Pharmacol 107:400–406.

Maggi CA, Patacchini R, Santicioli P, Giuliani S, Geppetti P, Meli A (1988): Protective action of ruthenium red toward capsaicin desensitization of sensory fibers. Neurosci Lett 88:201–205.

Maggi CA, Patacchini R, Tramontana M, Amann R, Guiliani S, Santicioli P (1990): Similarities and differences in the action of resiniferatoxin and capsaicin on central and peripheral endings of primary sensory neurones. Neuroscience 37:531–539.

Magnusson BM, Koskinen LO (1996): Effects of topical application of capsaicin to human skin: a comparison of effects evaluated by visual assessment, sensation registration, skin blood flow and cutaneous impedance measurements. Acta Derm Venereol 76:129–132.

Marks DR, Rapoport A, Padla D, Weeks R, Rosum R, Sheftell F, Arrowsmith F (1993): A double-blind placebo-controlled trial of intranasal capsaicin for cluster headache. Cephalgia 13:114–116.

McCarthy GM, McCarty DJ (1992): Effects of topical capsaicin in the painful osteoarthritis of the hands. Rheumatol 19:604–607.

McCarty DJ, Csuka M, McCarthy G, Trotter D (1994): Treatment of pain due to fibromyalgia with topical capsaicin: a pilot study. Semin Arthritis Rheum 23(Suppl. 3): 41–47.

McMahon SB, Kotzenburg M (1992): Itching for an explanation. Trends Neurosci 15: 497–501.

McMahon SB, Lewin G, Bloom SR (1991): The consequences of long-term topical capsaicin application in the rat. Pain 44:301–310.

Meller ST, Gebhart GF, Mayes TJ (1992): Neonatal capsaicin treatment prevents the development of the thermal hyperalgesia produced in a model of neuropathic pain in the rat. Pain 51:317–321.

Ninkina NN, Willoughby JJ, Beech MM, Coote PR, Wood JN (1994): Molecular cloning of a resiniferatoxin-binding protein. Mol Brain Res 22:39–48.

Oh U, Hwang SW, Kim D (1996): Capsaicin activates a non selective cation channel in cultured neonatal dorsal root ganglion neurons. J Neurosci 16:1659–1667.

Perkins MN, Campbell EA (1992): Capsazepine reversal of the analgesic action of capsaicin in vivo. Br J Pharmacol 107:329–333.

Petersen M, Lamotte RH (1991): Relationship between capsaicin sensitivity of mammalian sensory neurons, cell size and type of voltage gated Ca-current. Brain Res 561:20–26.

Petersen M, LaMotte RH, Klusch A, Kniffki K-D (1995): Capsaicin elicits inward current with two components differing in time course and response to pH in adult rat sensory neurons. Soc Neurosci 21:648.

Pini A, Baranowski R, Lynn B (1990): Long-term reduction in the number of C-fibre nociceptors following capsaicin treatment of a cutaneous nerve in adult rats. Eur J Neurosci 2:89–97.

Pitchford S, Levine JD (1991): Prostaglandins sensitize nociceptors in cell culture. Neurosci Lett 132:105–108.

Rayner HC, Atkins RC, Westerman RA (1989): Relief of local stump pain by capsaicin cream. Lancet 2:1276–1277.

Reichling D, Levine JD (1997): Heat transduction in rat sensory neurons by calcium-dependent activation of a cation channel. Proc Natl Acad Sci USA 94:7006–7011.

Ritter S, Dinh TT (1993): Capsaicin-induced degeneration in the rat brain and retina. In Wood J N (ed): *Capsaicin in the Study of Pain*. London: Academic Press, pp. 105–138.

Sang CN, Gracely RH, Max MB, Bennett GJ (1996): Capsaicin-evoked mechanical allodynia and hyperalgesia cross nerve territories. Evidence for a central mechanism. Anesthesiol 85:491–496.

Schmelz M, Schmidt R, Ringkamp M, Handwerker HO, Torebjork HE (1994): Sensitization of insensitive branches of C nociceptors in human skin. J Physiol 480:389–394.

Seno N, Dray A (1993): Capsaicin induced activation of fine afferent fibres from rat skin in vitro. Neuroscience 55:563–569.

Sherman SE, Loomis CW (1996): Strychnine-sensitive modulation is selective for non-noxious somatosensory input in the spinal cord of the rat. Pain 66:321–330.

Shir Y, Seltzer Z (1990): A-fibers mediate mechanical hyperesthesia and allodynia and C-fibers mediate thermal hyperalgesia in a new model of causalgiform pain disorders in rats. Neurosci Lett 115:62–67.

Sicuteri F, Fusco BM, Marabini S, Campagnolo V, Maggi CA, Geppetti P, Fanciullacci M (1989): Beneficial effect of capsaicin application to the nasal mucosa in cluster headache. Clin Pain 5:49–53.

Sietsema WK, Berman EF, Farmer RW, Maddin CS (1988): The antinociceptive effect and pharmacokinetics of olvanil following oral and subcutaneous dosing in the mouse. Life Sci 43:1385–1391.

Simone DA, Baumann TK, LaMotte RH (1989): Dose-dependent pain and mechanical hyperalgesia in humans after intradermal injection of capsaicin. Pain 38:99–107.

Sinoff SE, Hart MB (1993): Topical capsaicin and burning pain. Clin Pain 9:70–73.

Steen KH, Reeh PW, Anton F, Handwerker HO (1992): Protons selectively induce lasting excitation and sensitization to mechanical structure of nociceptors in rat skin in vitro. J Neurosci 12:86–95.

Strassman AM, Raymond SA, Burnstein R (1996): Sensitization of meningeal sensory neurons and the origin of headaches. Nature 384:560–564.

Szállási A (1994): The vanilloid (capsaicin) receptor: receptor types and species differences. Gen Pharmacol 25:223–243.

Szállási A, Blumberg PM (1990): Specific binding of resiniferatoxin, an ultrapotent capsaicin analog, to dorsal root ganglion membranes. Brain Res 524:106–111.

Szállási A, Blumberg PM (1991): Molecular target size of the vanilloid (capsaicin) receptor in pig dorsal root ganglia. Life Sci 48:1863–1869.

Szállási A, Goso C (1994): Characterization by [^{3}H]resiniferatoxin binding of a human vanilloid (capsaicin) receptor in post-mortem spinal cord. Neurosci Lett 165:101–104.

Szállási A, Goso C, Blumberg PM, Manzini S (1993a): Competitive inhibition by capsazepine of [^{3}H]resiniferatoxin binding to central (spinal cord and dorsal root ganglia) and peripheral (urinary bladder and airways) vanilloid (capsaicin) receptors in the rat. J Pharmacol Exp Ther 267:728–733.

Szállási A, Lewin NA, Blumberg PM (1993b): Vanilloid (capsaicin) receptor in the rat: positive cooperativity of resiniferatoxin binding and its modulation by reduction and oxidation. J Pharmacol Exp Ther 266:678–683.

Szállási A, Blumberg PM, Nilsson S, Hökfelt T, Lundberg JM (1994): Visualizing [3H]resiniferatoxin autoradiography of capsaicin-sensitive neurons in the rat, pig and man. Eur J Pharmacol 264:217–221.

Szállási A, Nilsson S, Farkas-Szállási T, Blumberg P, Hökfelt T, Lundberg J (1995): Vanilloid (capsaicin) receptors in the rat: distribution in the brain, regional differences in the spinal cord, axonal transport to the periphery, and depletion by systemic vanilloid treatment. Brain Res 703:175–183.

Szolcsányi J, Sann H, Pierau F-K (1986): Nociception in pigeons is not impaired by capsaicin. Pain 27:247–260.

Tarng DC, Cho YL, Liu HN, Juang TP (1996): Hemodialysis-related pruritus: a double-blind, placebo-controlled, crossover study of capsaicin 0.025% cream. Nephron 72:617–622.

Walpole CSJ, Wrigglesworth R, Bevan S, Campbell EA, Dray A, James IF, Masdin KJ, Perkins MN, Winter J (1993a): Analogues of capsaicin with agonist activity as novel analgesic agents; structure-activity studies. 2. The amide bond "B-region." J Med Chem 36:2373–2380.

Walpole CSJ, Wrigglesworth R, Bevan S, Campbell EA, Dray A, James IF, Masdin KJ, Perkins MN, Winter J (1993b): Analogues of capsaicin with agonist activity as novel analgesic agents; structure-activity studies. 3. The hydrophobic side-chain "C-region." J Med Chem 36:2362–2372.

Walpole CSJ, Wrigglesworth R, Bevan S, Campbell EA, Dray A, James IF, Perkins MN, Reid DJ, Winter J (1993c): Analogues of capsaicin with agonist activity as novel analgesic agents; structure-activity studies. 1. The aromatic "A-region." J Med Chem 36:2362–2372.

Wardle KA, Ranson J, Sange GJ (1997): Pharmacological characterization of the vanilloid receptor in the rat dorsal spinal cord. Br J Pharmacol 121:1012–1016.

Watson CPN, Evans RJ, Watt VR (1989): The post-mastectomy pain syndrome and the effect of topical capsaicin. Pain 38:177–186.

Watson CPN, Tyler KL, Bickers DR, Millikan LE, Smith S, Coleman E (1993): A randomized vehicle-controlled trial of topical capsaicin in the treatment of postherpetic neuralgia. Clin Ther 15:510–526.

Winter J, Dray A, Wood JN, Yeats JC, Bevan S (1990): Cellular mechanism of action of resiniferatoxin: a potent sensory neuron excitotoxin. Brain Res 520:131–140.

Winter J, Walpole CSJ, Bevan S, James IF (1993a): Characterization of resiniferatoxin binding sites on sensory neurons: co-regulation of resiniferatoxin binding and capsaicin-sensitivity in adult rat dorsal root ganglia. Neuroscience 57:747–757.

Winter J, Woolf C, Lynn B (1993b): Degenerative and regenerative responses of sensory neurons to capsaicin-induced damage. In Wood J N (ed): *Capsaicin in the Study of Pain*. London: Academic Press, pp. 139–160.

Wood JN (1993): "Capsaicin in the study of pain." London: Academic Press.

Wood JN, Docherty RJ (1997): Chemical activators of sensory neurons. Ann Rev Physiol 59:457–482.

Wood JN, Coote PR, Minhas A, Mullaney I, McNeil M, Burgess GM (1989): Capsaicin-induced ion fluxes increase cyclic GMP but not cyclic AMP levels in rat sensory neurones in culture. J Neurochem 53:1203–1211.

Wrigglesworth R, Walpole CSJ, Bevan S, Campbell EA, Dray A, Hughes GA, James I, Masdin KJ, Winter J (1996): Analogues of capsaicin with agonist activity as novel analgesic agents: structure-activity studies. 4. Potent, orally active analgesics. J Med Chem 39:4942–4951.

Yamamoto T, Yaksh TL (1992): Effects of intrathecal capsaicin and NK-1 antagonist, CP,96-345, on the thermal hyperalgesia observed following unilateral constriction of the sciatic nerve in the rat. Pain 51:329–334.

Yang JM, Wu BN, Chen IJ (1992): Depressor response of sodium nonivamide acetate: a newly synthesised non-pungent analogue of capsaicin. Asia Pacific J Pharmacol 7:95–102.

CHAPTER 7

NEUROKININ ANTAGONISTS

NADIA M. J. RUPNIAK and RAYMOND G. HILL
Merck Sharp and Dohme Research Laboratories
Neuroscience Research Centre
Terlings Park, Harlow, Essex, United Kingdom

Substance P was the first tachykinin (or neurokinin) to be discovered and is the best characterized. Other tachykinins that share a common C-terminal sequence, Phe-X-Gly-Leu-Met-NH$_2$ (where X is Phe, Tyr, Val, or Ile), notable for their widespread distribution in mammalian tissues including the peripheral and central nervous system, are neurokinin A and B. The actions of these three tachykinins are respectively mediated through G-protein linked receptors designated NK$_1$, NK$_2$ and NK$_3$ (Cascieri et al., 1992). However, the receptor selectivity of these peptides is relatively poor. There is a mismatch between tachykinin-containing neurons and fibers, and their corresponding receptor in certain brain regions; this is particularly apparent in the case of neurokinin A, because NK$_2$ receptor expression appears to be in extremely low abundance in the adult mammalian nervous system (Saffroy et al., 1987). The only sure way to establish the role of particular neurokinins in nociception is by appropriate investigation of functional receptor pharmacology.

The characterization of neurokinin actions was difficult in the past because the only available antagonists were themselves peptides and were difficult to deliver in an intact and active form to the site at which they were expected to act. Some peptide antagonists have agonist properties (e.g., Salt et al., 1982) or are frankly neurotoxic (Hokfelt et al., 1981; Rodriguez et al., 1983). We focus here on the experiments conducted with the selective and potent nonpeptide antagonists for tachykinin receptors that have been recently discovered. The effects of these compounds on nociceptive processes have been studied extensively in animal assays and the findings generally support the prediction that tachykinin, especially NK$_1$ receptor, antagonists would be clinically useful as analgesics in a variety of pain conditions. However, as reports of clinical

---

Novel Aspects of Pain Management: Opioids and Beyond, Edited by Jana Sawynok and Alan Cowan
ISBN 0-471-180173   Copyright © 1999 by Wiley-Liss, Inc.

trials with these agents have begun to emerge, it has become increasingly apparent that this expectation has not been borne out in humans.

EVIDENCE FOR A ROLE OF TACHYKININS IN NOCICEPTION

Both substance P and neurokinin A, but not neurokinin B, appear to act as primary afferent neurotransmitters, because the gene precursor for these (preprotachykinin A) is in unmyelinated primary sensory afferent neurons (Weihe, 1990; Duggan and Weihe, 1991). Substance P and neurokinin A are synthesized in the cell bodies of sensory nerve fibers (located in spinal or cranial sensory ganglia) from which they are transported both centrally and peripherally, and can be released from terminals within the central nervous system (CNS) and within peripheral tissues (see Hill, 1986). Some afferent fibers contain substance P alone, whereas others contain both substance P and neurokinin A, and both may co-exist with other peptides such as calcitonin gene-related peptide (CGRP) (Weihe, 1990) and also with excitatory amino acids (Duggan and Weihe, 1991).

The first clear association between substance P and nociception came from the finding that treatment of neonatal rats with the sensorotoxin capsaicin caused depletion of the peptide from primary afferents, and this was accompanied by hypoalgesia (Gasparovic et al., 1964). It is now realized that capsaicin is not selective for neurons containing substance P, or even for tachykinins as a class, but will deplete small primary afferents of most, if not all, of their peptide content (Weihe, 1990). Noxious cutaneous stimuli can release neurokinin A into the dorsal horn of the spinal cord under most experimental circumstances, whereas the release of substance P appears to require prolonged stimuli of a higher intensity (Duggan and Weihe, 1991). Radioligand binding and immunocytochemical studies have shown that NK_1 receptors predominate within the spinal dorsal horn, consistent with the suggestion that substance P and neurokinin A are important messengers here (Bleazard et al., 1994). Yashpal et al. (1990) have described binding of [^{125}I]neurokinin A to spinal cord in the adult rat, suggesting the presence of NK_2 receptors, but the precise location of these sites is incompletely defined as yet, and it is likely that at least some of this binding is to NK_1 receptors. Studies with a highly selective NK_2 antagonist, MEN 10376, failed to find any NK_2 receptor binding within the rat CNS including the spinal cord (Humpel and Saria, 1993). Binding of [^{125}I]eledoisin (presumably to NK_3 receptors, although this ligand is somewhat unselective) was restricted to lamina I and the outer part of lamina II, although the distribution of [^{125}I]eledoisin binding changes with development, being widespread in the neonatal rat but circumscribed in the adult (Beresford et al., 1992).

Electrophysiological Studies *in vitro*

Substance P depolarizes the ventral root of an isolated rat spinal cord preparation (Konishi and Otsuka, 1974). The slow depolarization produced by sustained electrical stimulation of the dorsal root in the same segment resembled that produced by exogenous substance P in the solution bathing the preparation. It was therefore suggested that substance P might function as a neurotransmitter in pain perception. Similar findings have been obtained using single neuron intracellular recording from isolated spinal cords or slices; the late slow excitatory postsynaptic potential (EPSP) generated in dorsal horn neurons by high-intensity electrical stimulation of a dorsal rootlet again resembled the action of exogenous substance P (Urban et al., 1985). Substance P, neurokinin A, and other tachykinins have been shown to excite and/or depolarize neurons in isolated spinal cord preparations, and it is likely that most of these responses are expressed via NK_1 receptors that are well represented in this tissue, with a smaller contribution from NK_3 sites. In studies on the larger laminae IV and V neurons, the selective NK_1 agonist, $[Sar^9, Met(O_2)^{11}]$substance P, was the most potent ligand tested (Morris et al., 1992). The smaller neurons of the substantia gelatinosa are not readily excited by tachykinins (Bleazard and Morris, 1993), even though this region has an abundant innervation with fibers shown immunocytochemically to contain substance P and other tachykinins. Recent immunocytochemical studies have shown that the substantia gelatinosa has few if any NK_1 receptors (Bleazard et al., 1994). Studies on the pharmacology of neurokinin receptors in immature spinal cord or slices may give misleading results, as receptor distribution and density changes with age (Ireland et al., 1992). Bentley and Gent (1995), using iontophoretic application of peptides in an adult rat spinal cord preparation, did find excitatory and inhibitory responses to the NK_1 receptor agonist, GR 73632, on substantia gelatinosa neurons.

Electrophysiological Studies *in vivo*

Henry (1976) showed that substance P excites those dorsal horn neurons that also respond to noxious stimuli but does not excite neurons that are excited only by low-intensity cutaneous stimuli. Others have shown, however, that low- and high-threshold dorsal horn neurons and also motoneurons were excited by substance P in cats (Zieglgansberger and Tulloch, 1979). In the cat trigeminal complex, only nucleus caudalis neurons that were excited by cutaneous noxia or by electrical stimulation of tooth pulp were excited by substance P (Andersen et al., 1978; Henry et al., 1980), although in the rat, nociceptive and non-nociceptive neurons are both readily excited by substance P (Hill et al., 1980; Crozier et al., 1981; Salt et al., 1983). Weak excitation of nociceptive dorsal horn neurons by iontophoretic substance P has been observed in the anesthetized rhesus monkey (Dougherty and Willis, 1991).

Using iontophoretic application of substance P and neurokinin A, Salter and Henry (1991) demonstrated that presumed NK_1 receptor activation preferentially excited nociceptive neurons, whereas presumed NK_2 receptor activation by neurokinin A excited neurons responding to both noxious and non-noxious stimuli. Fleetwood-Walker et al. (1987) reported that the NK_1 selective agonist [Met-O-Me^{11}]substance P excited neurons in laminae IV and V of cat spinal cord, but when injected in the superficial laminae of the cord, it exhibited only inhibitory effects, and these were restricted to non-nociceptive neurons. In contrast, the NK_2 agonist neurokinin A produced a selective facilitation of the responses to noxious heat without affecting the responses to non-noxious stimuli. Characteristic flexion reflexes are evoked by noxious stimuli, and these are facilitated by the presence of tissue inflammation or by high-intensity electrical stimuli applied to peripheral nerves sufficient to excite C-nociceptor fibers (Woolf, 1983; Ferrell et al., 1988). Intrathecal administration of substance P to a decerebrate, spinalized rat was found to facilitate the hamstring flexion reflex (Wiesenfeld-Hallin and Duranti, 1987), suggesting that release of substance P in the spinal cord may mediate hyperalgesia following tissue injury.

Conscious Animal Assays

When administered by intrathecal or intracisternal/ventricular injection to mice, NK_1 and NK_2 receptor agonists produce a distinctive behavioral syndrome of caudally directed biting and scratching (see Vaught, 1988). However, the specificity of such behaviors as indicators of pain perception is highly questionable (Bossut et al., 1988; Frenk et al., 1988). More convincing evidence for a role of spinal tachykinins in nociception comes from experiments in which nociceptive thresholds to mechanical and thermal stimuli were shown to be reduced by central administration of tachykinins. Both NK_1 and NK_2 agonists are active, but their rank order of potency suggests that NK_1 receptor activation may be the common denominator; interestingly, agonists selective at NK_3 receptors do not reduce nociceptive response latency (Cridland and Henry, 1986; Laneuville et al., 1988; Picard et al., 1993).

NONPEPTIDE TACHYKININ RECEPTOR ANTAGONISTS

The first nonpeptide tachykinin antagonist was the NK_1 receptor selective antagonist CP-96,345, discovered at Pfizer (Snider et al., 1991). Following the discovery of this quinuclidine agent, a large number of structurally diverse nonpeptide antagonists at NK_1, NK_2, and NK_3 receptors have been described (reviewed by Longmore et al., 1995; Lowe and MacLean, 1995; Swain and Hargreaves, 1996). The majority are NK_1 receptor antagonists and single nonpeptide NK_2 and NK_3 receptor antagonists, SR48968 and SR142801, respectively, are available, both of which have been developed by Sanofi (Emonds-Alt et al., 1993; Croci et al., 1995). These developments have provided excellent research tools with which to elucidate the role of tachykinins in nociception, and yet these studies have proved surprisingly difficult to perform.

Marked species variants in NK_1 receptor pharmacology exist. Thus CP-96,345 was found to have high affinity for the NK_1 receptor expressed in human, gerbil, rabbit, guinea pig, cat, and monkey brain and low affinity for the murine and rat NK_1 receptor; conversely, RP 67580 bound with higher affinity to the rat than to the human NK$_1$ receptor (Beresford et al., 1991; Gitter et al., 1991; Fong et al., 1992; Beaujouan et al., 1993). The current record for difference in affinity is probably held by MEN 10930, which has subnanomolar affinity at the human receptor but is inactive up to 10 μM at the murine receptor (Astolfi et al., 1997). Because most conventional animal assays employ rats and mice, preclinical assessment of compounds selective for the human NK$_1$ receptor necessitated nociception assays in other species, notably gerbils, guinea pigs, and rabbits. Proof of concept studies performed on rats were difficult to interpret unless using compounds with high affinity for the rat NK$_1$ receptor. Few such compounds have been developed, and poor pharmacokinetics has limited the usefulness of the prototypic rat-selective antagonist RP 67580 for in vivo studies (Laird et al., 1993).

Other features of these compounds further complicated their evaluation in animal nociception assays. The first generation NK$_1$ antagonists (CP-96,345 and RP 67580) blocked sodium and calcium channels at high concentrations (Caeser et al., 1993; Rupniak et al., 1993); this action itself caused analgesia independently of any antinociceptive effects resulting from blockade of NK$_1$ receptors (Nagahisa et al., 1992; Rupniak et al., 1993). All in vivo studies should therefore be controlled by use of enantiomeric pairs of compounds, one having high affinity for the NK$_1$ receptor and the other low affinity; only antinociceptive activity that is confined to the high affinity enantiomer can be attributed to NK$_1$ receptor blockade. Unspecific ion channel pharmacology is also an unwanted property of the NK$_2$ antagonist, SR48968 (Lombet and Spedding, 1994).

The ability of NK$_1$ receptor antagonists to penetrate the CNS following systemic administration is a key determinant of their activity in nociception assays. Poorly brain-penetrant compounds include SR140333, LY 303870, RPR 100893, and CGP 49823, whereas those with exceptionally good CNS penetration include the piperidines CP-99,994 and GR203040, the piperidine ether L-733,060, and morpholines such as L-742,694 (Rupniak et al., 1996, 1997). Moreover, a long *duration* of central NK$_1$ receptor blockade is critical for unequivocal demonstration of enantioselective antinociceptive effects in certain assays (Rupniak et al., 1996; see following section).

EVIDENCE FOR ANTINOCICEPTIVE EFFECTS OF NK$_1$ AND NK$_2$ RECEPTOR ANTAGONISTS

Electrophysiological Studies

Electrophysiological studies show a selective inhibitory effect of NK$_1$ receptor antagonists on facilitated nociceptive spinal reflexes. Prolonged ventral root depolarizations evoked by stimulation of the dorsal root in isolated spinal cords of rats were found to be resistant to application of the NK$_1$ antagonist CP-96,345, although reduction in this potential was seen after application of the peptide NK_2 antagonist MEN 10376 (Thompson et al., 1993a). In spinal cords taken from animals in which thermal and mechanical hyperalgesia had been produced by ultraviolet irradiation, the amplitude of the ventral root potential was reduced by CP-96,345 (Thompson et al., 1993b). This suggests that activation of NK_1 receptors becomes relevant in the presence of peripheral inflammation.

CP-96,345 readily blocked the excitation produced by iontophoretic substance P and that produced by nociceptive inputs to dorsal horn neurons in cats (Radhakrishnan and Henry, 1991) and rhesus monkeys (Dougherty et al., 1993). Neugebauer et al. (1994, 1995) have studied the role of NK_1 receptor activation in the excitatory responses of anesthetized rat dorsal horn neurons following intense joint stimulation. The activation of dorsal horn cells required the same intensity of noxious stimulation needed to cause substance P release, and CP-96,345, applied iontophoretically, reduced the response to noxious but not to innocuous stimuli. Although CP-96,345 has poor selectivity at the rat receptor, these studies were controlled by showing that its inactive isomer, CP-96,344, was without effect. It has been shown that the sensitization of spinothalamic tract neurons, following acute inflammation of the knee in anesthetized rhesus monkeys, was reversed by intrathecal CP-99,994 (Rees et al., 1995).

Studies in which CP-96,345 was given intrathecally to rats have demonstrated that this agent blocks the flexor reflex facilitation produced either by C-fiber conditioning stimulation or by intrathecal application of substance P (Xu et al., 1992). Similar experiments with RP 67,580, a rodent NK_1-selective antagonist, confirmed that blockade of NK_1 receptors in the spinal cord of an anesthetized rat prevented facilitation of flexor reflexes but did not reduce the size of the baseline reflex or wind-up (Laird et al., 1993). Low doses of RP 67,580 (3–30 μg/kg i.v.), which are adequate to maintain plasma concentrations in the region of 3–20 nM, blocked facilitation, and this is consistent with its affinity of 4 nM at the rodent NK_1 receptor. Its less active enantiomer, RP 68,651, was without effect on facilitation of the flexor reflex. RP 67,580 also inhibited the hypersensitivity of the spinal flexor reflex during persistent inflammation in rats (Parsons et al., 1996; Ma and Woolf, 1997). In anesthetized rabbits, a species with humanlike NK_1 receptor pharmacology, CP-99,994 was found to attenuate potently the facilitation produced by electrical stimulation of the skin (ID_{50} 2.7 μg/kg i.v.), again with no effects on the baseline reflex (Boyce et al., 1993).

The involvement of NK_2 receptor activation in pain perception is more difficult to characterize given the limited amount of work published to date. A recent study investigated the processing of nociceptive inputs from the knee joint to the spinal cord in rats. The nonpeptide NK_2 antagonist SR 48,968 reduced the response to noxious and innocuous pressure applied to both normal and inflamed knee joints; these effects were not seen with the less active enantiomer, SR 48,965 (Neugebauer et al., 1996). Neurokinin A has been shown to facilitate flexor reflexes when given intrathecally (Xu and Wiesenfeld-Hallin,

1992) and this facilitation, but not that produced by substance P, was blocked by the peptide NK_2 antagonist MEN 10,207 (Xu et al., 1992).

Conscious Animal Assays

In contrast to the electrophysiological studies described above, convincing evidence for antinociceptive activity of NK_1 antagonists in conscious animal assays has proved difficult to establish. The receptor selectivity of intrathecal injection of tachykinins on nociceptive thresholds has been confirmed by use of the nonpeptide antagonists CP-96,345 and SR 48,968, confirming that potentiation of nociception can occur following activation of either NK_1 or NK_2 receptors (Picard et al., 1993). Enantioselectivity of the effects at the NK_1 receptor has been established for CP-96,345 and CP-99,994 (Malmberg and Yaksh, 1992; Yashpal et al., 1993; Rupniak et al., 1995).

Early studies demonstrated antinociceptive effects following systemic administration of nonpeptide NK_1 antagonists in certain rodent assays. However, the doses of NK_1 receptor antagonists employed in behavioral experiments were substantially higher (mg/kg range) than those required to block facilitated reflexes in electrophysiological experiments (μg/kg range). Thus the rodent NK_1 receptor selective antagonist RP 67,580 exhibited antinociceptive activity in mice, inhibiting writhing induced by phenylbenzoquinone or acetic acid and the nociceptive response to intraplantar injection of formalin, but was inactive in tests using thermal or mechanical noxious stimuli (Garret et al., 1991; Moussaoui et al., 1992; Rupniak et al., 1993). However, RP 67,580 exhibited equally potent antinociceptive effects in species with humanlike NK_1 receptor pharmacology, and evidence for significant ion channel blocking activity of this compound challenged the NK_1 receptor specificity of these observations (Rupniak et al., 1993). Other nonpeptide antagonists have been used in a number of studies. A well designed study by Yashpal et al. (1993) demonstrated that facilitation (but not the *baseline* reflex) of the tail flick response in the rat caused by immersion of the tail in hot water was attenuated enantioselectively by CP-96,345 at a dose of 5 mg/kg. CP-96,345 was also active in the rat formalin and carrageenan paw tests (Yamamoto and Yaksh, 1991; Birch et al., 1992; Nagahisa et al., 1992; Yashpal et al., 1993), mouse acetic acid-induced writhing test (Nagahisa et al., 1992), and mouse hot plate test (Lecci et al., 1991), but enantioselectivity was marginal or absent (Nagahisa et al., 1992; unpublished observations). The nonspecific antinociceptive effects of CP-96,345 appear to be attributable to ion channel blockade (Schmidt et al., 1992; Karlsson et al., 1994).

The second-generation NK_1 antagonist CP-99,994 had low affinity for the L-type calcium channel in vitro (McLean et al., 1993) and CP-99,994 thus appeared to represent an ideal compound with which to examine the involvement of NK_1 receptor activation in nociception. However, findings with this compound proved disappointing. CP-99,994 inhibited the early- and late-phase nociceptive response to intraplantar injection of formalin in rats and gerbils, but this occurred only at high doses ($\geq$ 10 mg/kg), with little or no separation between the effects of CP-99,994 and its less active enantiomer CP-100,263 (Smith et al., 1994; Rupniak et al., 1995). The inability to demonstrate clear antinociceptive effects of NK_1 antagonists in the formalin paw assay was perplexing in view of electrophysiological experiments in which the excitation of spinal dorsal horn neurons elicited by intraplantar injection of formalin was enantioselectively inhibited by intrathecal injection of RP 67,580 in rats (Chapman and Dickenson, 1993). Moreover, it has been established that injection of formalin into peripheral tissues results in increased levels of substance P in the dorsal horn (McCarson and Goldstein, 1990). Yamamoto and Yaksh (1991) had also shown that the late-phase response to formalin in rats was blocked by *intrathecal* injection of CP-96,345, but not by its less active enantiomer, CP-96,344. Several other studies also reported differential inhibition of the late- rather than the early-phase response to formalin in rats by CP-96,345 (Birch et al., 1992; Nagahisa et al., 1992; Yashpal et al., 1993). However, because CP-96,345 has relatively weak affinity for the rat NK_1 receptor, the high doses required to overcome this might explain the difficulty in showing clear separation between the effects of the low- and high-affinity enantiomers. Attempts to overcome this concern using more appropriate species, gerbils or guinea pigs, were confounded by the failure to detect a measurable late-phase response to formalin in these species (Rupniak et al., 1993; Smith et al., 1994; Rupniak et al., 1995).

These confounding factors were resolved in a recent study using a long-acting NK_1 antagonist, L-733,060, in gerbils (Rupniak et al., 1996). We reasoned that the poor enantiomeric separation achieved in the formalin paw assay when NK_1 antagonists were administered systemically might be attributable to an anesthetic-like nerve block caused by unspecific effects on ion channels in peripheral tissues (the paw itself, and/or the peripheral nerve), and that this masked the selective antinociceptive effects of blocking NK_1 receptors in the spinal cord. The use of an NK_1 receptor antagonist with a long central duration of action enabled a direct test of this hypothesis because it permitted us to maintain blockade of central NK_1 receptors at a time when peak plasma drug levels had subsided, and the nonspecific effects of these compounds in peripheral tissues could therefore be minimized. In this study, we found that CP-99,994 was extremely brain penetrant but that its ability to block central NK_1 receptors was critically dependent on maintaining high levels of this compound in the plasma. In contrast, central NK_1 receptor blockade could be maintained for several hours after administration of L-733,060, even when plasma concentrations were relatively low. The ability to pretreat gerbils with L-733,060 3 hours before they were challenged with formalin allowed an extended period of habituation to their observation cages such that it became possible to observe a distinct, late phase response to formalin. Under these conditions we demonstrated for the first time a clear separation (> 50-fold) in the potency of L-733,060 and its less active enantiomer L-733,061 to inhibit the late phase paw licking response to formalin in gerbils. The inhibition of paw licking by L-733,060 appeared to be due to central NK_1 receptor blockade, because the μg/kg potency coincided with that required to inhibit foot tapping induced by central NK_1 agonist challenge.

Attempts to establish an assay of carrageenan-induced hyperalgesia in gerbils have been less successful, but recently experiments have been described in which mechanical and thermal hyperalgesia in guinea pigs have been studied (Patel et al., 1996). In this preliminary report, orally administered CP-99,994, RPR 100,893, and SR 140,333 were all found to cause modest inhibition (approximately 25–35%) of carrageenan-induced hyperalgesia at high doses (30–100 mg/kg). The novel NK_1 antagonist SDZ NKT 343 inhibited carrageenan-induced hyperalgesia in guinea pigs by 68%, with an ID_{50} of approximately 1 mg/kg perorally (Campbell et al., 1997). Recently, we also obtained evidence for complete inhibition of carrageenan-induced mechanical hyperalgesia in guinea pigs using L-733,060, but not its less active enantiomer L-733,061, at 3 mg/kg subcutaneous (unpublished observations).

In summary, evidence for an antinociceptive profile of NK_1 antagonists in conscious animal assays has proved difficult to establish, and it is clear that this class of compounds does not display the broad spectrum of antinociceptive activity associated with morphine. Activity in acute nociception tests that involve inflammation more closely resembles that of nonsteroidal antiinflammatory drugs (Table 7.1). Both electrophysiological and behavioral studies indicate that NK_1 antagonists have little effect on protective spinal nociceptive reflexes but are able to inhibit facilitation or hyperalgesia induced by prolonged, intense noxious stimuli.

A recent study by Sluka et al. (1997) compared the NK_1 antagonist CP-99,994 with the NK_2 antagonist SR 48,968 on thermal hyperalgesia induced by intra-articular kaolin and carrageenan in rats. CP-99,994 was able to reverse, but not *prevent*, the induction of hyperalgesia when administered either spinally or systemically. In contrast, opposite findings were obtained with SR 48,968, which prevented the induction of hyperalgesia when given as a pretreatment,

TABLE 7.1 Analgesic Profile of NK_1 Receptor Antagonists in Conscious Animal Assays

Assay	Morphine	Indomethacin	NK_1 Antagonist
Tail flick/hot plate	Yes	No	No
Paw pressure	Yes	No	No
Writhing	Yes	Yes	Yes[a]
Formalin paw	Yes	Yes	Yes[a]
Carrageenan paw	Yes	Yes	Yes[a]

[a]Activity seen at high (mg/kg) doses is complicated by unspecific pharmacology (e.g., ion channel blockade).

but failed to reverse hyperalgesia after it had been established. These findings suggest a differential role of spinal tachykinin receptors in the development (NK_2) and maintenance (NK_1) of inflammatory hyperalgesia. Conclusions on the role of NK_2 receptors should be cautious, however, in view of the limited evidence for their existence in the CNS and the demonstration of multiple affinity states for the NK_1 receptor (Maggi and Schwartz, 1997).

Immunocytochemical Assays

Additional evidence for a role for substance P acting at NK_1 receptors in nociception has come from studies in which a selective antibody for the NK_1 receptor has been used to visualize these receptors within the dorsal horn of the spinal cord. These receptors are found in laminae I, III–VI, and X (Bleazard et al., 1994; Littlewood et al., 1995). Retrograde labeling of spinothalamic tract cells shows that more than 70% of projecting lamina I cells have the NK_1 receptor as do about 35% of cells projecting from deeper laminae (Marshall et al., 1996). Following either inflammation of a paw with Freund's adjuvant or sciatic nerve section in rats, an increase in NK_1 receptor immunoreactivity in superficial laminae was observed (Abbadie et al., 1996). Noxious stimuli have been found to initiate internalization of the NK_1 receptor on lamina I cells (Mantyh et al., 1995), and this can be blocked with NK_1 receptor antagonist drugs (Abbadie et al., 1997).

Immediate early gene induction can also be evoked in dorsal horn neurons by a noxious peripheral stimulus. C-fos protein expression in lumbar dorsal horn neurons following intraplantar injection of formalin in the rat was reduced in a dose-related fashion by intravenous RP 67580 (Chapman et al., 1996). A much larger reduction was seen when threshold doses of the NK_1 receptor antagonist were given together with an NMDA receptor blocking drug. In cervical dorsal horn (trigeminal nucleus caudalis), the activation of *c-fos*, by either noxious chemical stimulation of the meninges or direct electrical stimulation of the trigeminal ganglion, was seen to be reduced but not abolished following NK_1 receptor blockade (Cutrer et al., 1995; Shepheard et al., 1995).

CLINICAL POTENTIAL OF NK_1 RECEPTOR ANTAGONISTS: EXPECTATION AND OUTCOME

Recent studies on the plasticity of sensory neurotransmission have emphasized that the role of nociceptive fibers is more than simple carriage of a message from the peripheral tissues to the CNS. Maintained activation of these fibers can lead to reprogramming of central circuits and changes in responsiveness to subsequent noxious stimuli. Changes in the sensitivity of pain pathways under pathological conditions such as inflammation and sensory nerve damage are postulated by Cervero and Laird (1991). Phase 1 pain represents the normal protective reflex response to a brief noxious stimulus, whereby the stimulus is removed as soon as pain is registered. Evidence presented in the preceding section suggests that activation of tachykinin NK_1 receptors is unlikely to be an important part of this phase of pain perception. Phase 2 pain is the situation after a damaging stimulus that produces prolonged activation of nociceptor fibers and also activates a population of nociceptor fibers that are normally silent. This raises the CNS to a higher state of excitability that may persist even in the absence of further stimulation. NK_1 receptors appear to be involved in this process particularly in inflammatory hyperalgesia. Moreover, inflammation may cause a phenotypic switch in a subpopulation of myelinated Aβ fibers so that they, like C fibers, express substance P and hence acquire the ability to excite dorsal horn neurons following innocuous stimulation (Neumann et al., 1996). Phase 3 pain is the state of affairs that might occur in an abnormal pain syndrome, such as following peripheral nerve damage. Here, pain thresholds may be greatly reduced and spontaneous pain can arise. There is growing evidence that NK_1 antagonists are able to inhibit hyperalgesia in animals with experimental peripheral neuropathy (see below).

There has been a strong expectation that NK_1 antagonists will be clinically efficacious analgesics, especially in conditions associated with inflammation, and clinical trials are currently in progress.

Dental Pain

Assessment of pain following molar extraction represents a simple and rapid method to evaluate analgesic drugs in humans. Several studies have now been conducted with NK_1 antagonists, with equivocal findings (see Table 7.2). The first compared the effects of CP-99,994 with ibuprofen and suggested that NK_1 receptor blockade was indeed associated with analgesia in humans (Dionne et al., 1996). In that study, CP-99,994 was administered at a dose of 750 µg/kg as an intravenous infusion over 5 hr. Although comparable clinical efficacy to ibuprofen was observed with CP-99,994, findings with other NK_1 antagonists have been less encouraging. A second orally active, CNS penetrant NK_1 antag-

TABLE 7.2 Analgesic Activity of NK_1 Receptor Antagonists: Preliminary Findings from Clinical Trials

Clinical Condition	Compound	Outcome
Dental pain	CP-99,994 (750 µg/kg i.v.)	Analgesia equal to ibuprofen
	CP-122,721 (200 mg p.o.)	Weak analgesia
	L-754,030 (300 mg p.o.)	No analgesia
Osteoarthritis	LY 303870 (600 mg p.o. b.i.d.)	No analgesia
Neuropathic pain	CP-99,994 (100 µg/kg i.v.)	No analgesia
Migraine	RPR 100893 (20 mg p.o.)	No analgesia
	LY 303870 (240 mg p.o.)	No analgesia

onist, L-754,030 (300 mg perorally), was recently reported to be ineffective as an analgesic for postoperative dental pain (Reinhardt et al., 1998). It is noteworthy that this latter compound has been shown to be a clinically effective NK_1 antagonist against the effects of substance P on forearm blood flow in humans (Newby et al., 1997).

Arthritis

There is circumstantial evidence that substance P may play an integral role in the pathophysiology of inflammatory joint diseases, the most common of which is rheumatoid arthritis. It has been proposed that the nervous system contributes to the symmetry of joint inflammation in rheumatoid arthritis (Kidd et al., 1989); substance P may be involved in such a neurogenic process.

The only reported clinical study with an NK_1 antagonist examined the effects of LY 303870 (lanepitant) in osteoarthritis patients with moderate joint pain. LY 303870 was without effect given acutely in single doses of up to 600 mg perorally; however, no effect of the reference analgesic, naproxen, was detected in this trial. Unlike naproxen (375 mg perorally), LY 303870 was also found to be ineffective when given as a twice daily treatment at doses up to 600 mg perorally for 3 weeks (Goldstein, 1998; see Table 7.2).

Neuropathic Pain

Peripheral nerve injury may be associated with disturbing sensory abnormalities, such as persistent burning pain and tactile allodynia, accompanied by receptive field expansion in some patients (Gracely et al., 1992). Animals with ligated peripheral nerves display behavior suggestive of spontaneous pain and have enhanced reflex responses to both noxious and innocuous stimuli (Bennett and Xie, 1988). In such animals, NK_1 receptors may be upregulated following peripheral nerve injury (Aanonsen et al., 1992). We examined the effect of GR 205171, an NK_1 receptor antagonist that has similar affinities for the rat and human NK_1 receptor (pK_i 9.5 vs. 10.6, respectively; Gardner et al., 1996), on behavioral and electrophysiological correlates of experimental peripheral neuropathy in rats. Response latencies to innocuous mechanical stimulation were reduced and the receptive fields of dorsal horn neuron were enlarged 7–14 days after ligation of the sciatic nerve. GR 205171 (3 mg/kg intravenously) reversed both the facilitated reflexes and the receptive field expansion to a level indistinguishable from those of the contralateral, control limbs; this effect was shown to be enantioselective (Cumberbatch et al., 1998).

These preclinical studies suggest that NK_1 receptor blockade might be able to alleviate heightened pain sensitivity in patients with peripheral nerve damage. The findings of a single study have been presented to date, and in this CP-99,994 ($\leq$ 100 µg/kg intravenously, infused over 2 hr) had no analgesic effect in patients with painful peripheral neuropathy (Suarez et al., 1994; see Table 7.2). However, it should be noted that this dose of CP-99,994 was lower than that employed in the dental pain trial where analgesic efficacy was seen (see above).

Migraine

Migraine headache is characterized by an intense unilateral throbbing pain. Although the precise mechanisms involved in the genesis of a migraine attack are not fully understood, it is likely that the pain is vascular in origin. The vasculature of meningeal tissues such as the dura mater are densely innervated by C-fiber sensory afferents that run in the trigeminal nerve and contain substance P and other neuropeptides (Liu-Chen et al., 1983). It is considered that the release of neuropeptides from these sensory fibers during a migraine attack causes neurogenic inflammation within the meninges, resulting in the activation of nociceptive afferents projecting to the trigeminal nucleus caudalis (Uddman and Edvinsson, 1989; Shepheard et al., 1993).

The trigeminal nucleus caudalis is the primary relay station for nociceptive transmission from the meninges and cranial conduit arteries. Highly CNS-penetrant NK_1 antagonists, such as CP-99,994, can attenuate increases in *c-fos* expression (an immediate early gene marker of neuronal activation) in this region (see above and Shepheard et al., 1995). These findings suggest that NK_1 antagonists should provide an effective anti-migraine therapy. Findings from two clinical studies examining the ability of NK_1 antagonists to abort migraine headache have been presented. The first study employed RPR 100,893 at doses up to 20 mg (Diener, 1995); the second examined the effects of LY 303,870 at doses up to 240 mg (Goldstein et al., 1997). Neither agent was found to give headache relief (see Table 7.2).

CONCLUSIONS

This review reflects a substantial and growing body of preclinical evidence that blocking the actions of tachykinins, particularly substance P, can reduce the hypersensitivity of nociceptive pathways that is thought to contribute to pathological pain in humans. Despite the strength of this rationale, the outcome from available clinical trials is that NK_1 receptor blockade does not appear to result in analgesia in humans. Interpretation of these preliminary clinical findings requires caution, however, because not all studies have been performed with compounds that are brain penetrant (see Rupniak et al., 1996, 1997). It is of interest that the only positive clinical trial showing analgesic effects of an NK_1 antagonist is the dental pain study using intravenous infusion of CP-99,994; studies with other agents administered orally or using poorly brain-penetrant compounds have proved negative.

The majority of clinical trials to date have also employed only acute administration of NK_1 antagonists and results from more long-term clinical investigations, for example, to evaluate the potential prophylactic effects of NK_1

receptor antagonists in preventing migraine recurrence or in retarding the spread and progression of arthritis, are probably necessary before their clinical utility can be adequately assessed.

REFERENCES

Aanonsen LM, Kajander KC, Bennett GJ, Seybold VS (1992): Autoradiographic analysis of ^{125}I-substance P binding in rat spinal cord following chronic constriction injury of the sciatic nerve. Brain Res 596:259–268.

Abbadie C, Brown JL, Mantyh PW, Basbaum AI (1996): Spinal cord substance P receptor immunoreactivity increases in both inflammatory and nerve injury models of persistent pain. Neuroscience 70:201–209.

Abbadie C, Trafton JA, Marchand S, Wang H, Mantyh PW, Basbaum AI (1997): Pharmacological regulation of noxious stimulus evoked internalisation of the NK_1 receptor in the dorsal horn of the rat spinal cord. Soc Neurosci Abs 23:446.

Anderson RK, Lund JP, Puil E (1978): Enkephalin and substance P effects related to trigeminal pain. Can J Phys Pharm 56:216–222.

Astolfi M, Patacchini R, Maggi M, Manzinin S (1997): Improved discriminatory properties between human and murine tachykinin NK_1 receptors of MEN 10930: a new potent and competitive antagonist. Neuropeptides 31:373–379.

Beaujouan JC, Heuillet E, Petitet F, Saffroy M, Torrens Y, Glowinski J (1993): Higher potency of RP67580 in the mouse and the rat compared with other non-peptide and peptide tachykinin NK_1 antagonists. Br J Pharmacol 108:793–800.

Bennett GJ, Xie Y-K (1988): A peripheral mononeuropathy in rat that produces disorders of pain sensation like those seen in man. Pain 33:87–107.

Bentley GN, Gent PJ (1995): Neurokinin actions on substantia gelatinosa neurones in an adult rat longitudinal spinal cord preparation. Brain Res 673:101–111.

Beresford IJM, Birch PJ, Hagan RM, Ireland SJ (1991): Investigation into species variants in tachykinin NK_1 receptors by the use of the non-peptide antagonist, CP-96,345. Br J Pharmacol 104:292–293.

Beresford IJM, Ireland SJ, Stables J, Hagan RM (1992): Ontogeny and characterisation of ^{125}I-Bolton Hunter-eledoisin binding sites in rat spinal cord by quantitative autoradiography. Neuroscience 46:225–232.

Birch PJ, Harrsion MM, Hayes AG, Rogers H, Tyers MB (1992): The non-peptide NK_1 receptor antagonist, ($\pm$)-CP-96,345, produces antinociceptive and anti-oedema effects in the rat. Br J Pharmacol 105:508–510.

Bleazard L, Morris R (1993): Paradoxical lack of action of neurokinin agonists on substantia gelatinosa neurons of the rat spinal cord: An in vitro study. Proc 32nd Int Phys Congr 209:1P.

Bleazard L, Hill RG, Morris R (1994): The correlation between the distribution of the NK1 receptor and the actions of tachykinin agonists in the dorsal horn of the rat indicates that substance P does not have a functional role on substantia gelatinosa (lamina II) neurons. J Neurosci 14:7655–7664.

Bossut D, Frenk H, Mayer DJ (1988): Is substance P a primary afferent neurotransmitter for nociceptive input? II. Spinalization does not reduce and intrathecal morphine potentiates behavioral responses to substance P. Brain Res 455:232–239.

Boyce S, Laird JMA, Tattersall FD, Rupniak NMJ, Hargreaves RJ, Hill RG (1993): Antinociceptive effects of NK$_1$ receptor antagonists: comparison of behavioural and electrophysiological tests. 7th World Congress on Pain (Abstract 641):231.

Caeser M, Seabrook GR, Kemp JA (1993): Block of voltage-dependent sodium currents by the substance P receptor antagonist (±)-CP-96,345 in neurones cultured from rat cortex. Br J Pharmacol 109:918–924.

Campbell EA, Walpole CSJ, Gentry C, Patel S, Panesar M, Urban L (1997): The NK$_1$ receptor antagonist, SDZ NKT 343 inhibits inflammatory and neuropathic hyperalgesia. Abs European Neuropeptide Club, Marburg.

Cascieri MA, Huang R-RC, Fong TM, Cheung AH, Sadowski S, Ber E, Strader CD (1992): Determination of the amino acid residues in substance P conferring selectivity and specificity for the art neurokinin receptors. Mol Pharmacol 41:1096–1099.

Cervero F, Laird JMA (1991): One pain or many pains? A new look at pain mechanisms. NIPS 6:268–273.

Chapman V, Dickenson AH (1993): The effect of intrathecal administration of RP67580, a potent neurokinin$_1$ antagonist, on nociceptive transmission in the rat spinal cord. Neurosci Lett 157:149–152.

Chapman V, Buritova J, Honore P, Besson JM (1996): Physiological contributions of neurokinin 1 receptor activation and interactions with NMDA receptors, to inflammatory evoked spinal c-fos expression. J Neurophysiol 76:1817–1827.

Cridland RA, Henry JL (1986): Comparison of the effects of substance P, neurokinin A, physalaemin and eledoisin in facilitating a nociceptive reflex in the rat. Brain Res 381:93–99.

Croci T, Landi M, Emonds-Alt X, Le Fur G, Manara L (1995): Neuronal NK$_3$ receptors in guinea-pig ileum and taenia caeci—in vitro characterization by their first non-peptide antagonist, SR142801. Life Sci 57:PL361–PL366.

Crozier CS, Hill RG, Salt TE (1981): The effects of capsaicin pre-treatment on substance P levels and sensory responses of neurons in the rat trigeminal nucleus caudalis. J Physiol 324:78P.

Cumberbatch MJ, Carlson E, Wyatt A, Boyce S, Hill RG, Rupniak NMJ (1998): Reversal of behavioural and electrophysiological correlates of experimental peripheral neuropathy by the NK$_1$ receptor antagonist GR205171 in rats. Neuropharmacol 37: 1535–1543.

Cutrer FM, Moussaoui S, Garret C, Moskowitz MA (1995): The non-peptide neurokinin-1 antagonist, RPR-100893, decreases c-fos expression in trigeminal nucleus caudalis following noxious chemical meningeal stimulation. Neuroscience 64:741–750.

Diener HC for the RPR 100893-201 migraine study group (1995): Substance P antagonist RPR 100893 is not effective in human migraine attacks. Abs 6th Int Headache Res Sem, Copenhagen.

Dionne RA, Max MB, Parada S, Gordon SM, MacLean DB (1996): Evaluation of a neurokinin$_1$ antagonist, CP-99,994, in comparison to ibuprofen and placebo in the oral surgery model. Clin Pharmacol Therap 59:216.

Dougherty PM, Willis WD (1991): Enhancement of spinothalamic neuron responses to chemical and mechanical stimuli following combined micro-iontophoretic application of N-methyl-D-aspartic acid and substance P. Pain 47:85–93.

Dougherty PM, Palecek J, Paleckova V, Sorkin LS, Willis WD (1993): The role of NMDA, non-NMDA, and NK_1 receptors in the excitation of spinothalamic tract neurons in anaesthetized monkeys. J Physiol 459:209P.

Duggan AW, Weihe E (1991): Central transmission of impulses in nociceptors: events in the superficial dorsal horn. In Basbaum A, Besson JM (eds): *Towards a New Pharmacology of Pain*. Chichester: John Wiley & Sons, pp. 35–67.

Emonds-Alt X, Golliot F, Pointeau P, Le Fur G, Breliere JC (1993): Characterisation of the binding sites of [^{3}H]SR48968, a potent non-peptide radioligand antagonist of the neurokinin-2 receptor. Biochem Biophys Res Comm 191:1172–1177.

Ferrell WR, Wood L, Baxendale RH (1988): The effect of acute joint inflammation on flexion reflex excitability in the decerebrate, low spinal cat. Q J Exp Physiol 73: 95–102.

Fleetwood-Walker SM, Mitchell R, Hope PJ, El-Yassir N, Molony V (1987): The roles of tachykinin and opioid receptor types in nociceptive and non-nociceptive processing in superficial dorsal horn. In Schmidt RF, Schaible HG, Vahle-Hinz C (eds): *Fine Afferent Nerve Fibers and Pain*. Weinheim: VCH, pp. 239–247.

Fong TM, Yu H, Strader CD (1992): Molecular basis for the species selectivity of the neurokinin-1 receptor antagonists CP-96,345 and RP 67580. J Biol Chem 267: 25668–25671.

Frenk H, Bossut D, Urca G, Mayer DJ (1988): Is substance P a primary afferent neurotransmitter for nociceptive input? I. Analysis of pain-related behaviors resulting from intrathecal administration of substance P and 6 excitatory compounds. Brain Res 455:223–231.

Gardner CJ, Armour DR, Beattie DT, Gale JD, Hawcock AB, Kilpatrick GJ, Twissell DJ, Ward P (1996): GR 205171: A novel antagonist with high affinity for the tachykinin NK_1 receptor, and potent broad-spectrum anti-emetic activity. Regulat Pept 65:45–53.

Garret C, Carruette A, Fardin V, Moussaoui S, Peyronnel J-F, Blanchard J-C, Laduron PM (1991): Pharmacological properties of a potent and selective nonpeptide substance P antagonist. Proc Natl Acad Sci USA 88:10208–10212.

Gasparovic K, Hadzovik S, Stern P (1964): Contribution to the theory that substance P has a transmitter role in sensory pathways. Med Exp 10:303–306.

Gitter BD, Waters DC, Bruns RF, Mason NR, Nixon JA, Howbert JJ (1991): Species differences in affinities of non-peptide antagonists for substance P receptors. Eur J Pharmacol 197:237–238.

Goldstein D (1998): Lanipetant in osteoarthritic pain. Clin Pharmacol Therap 63:PI 24.

Goldstein D, Wang O, Saper JR, Stolz R, Silberstein SD, Mathew NT (1997): Ineffectiveness of neurokinin-1 antagonist in acute migraine: a crossover study. Cephalalgia 17:785–790.

Gracely RH, Lynch SA, Bennett GJ (1992): Painful neuropathy: altered central processing maintained dynamically by peripheral input. Pain 51:175–194.

Henry JL (1976): Effects of substance P on functionally identified units in cat spinal cord. Brain Res 114:439–451.

Henry JL, Sessle BJ, Lucier GE, Hu JW (1980): Effects of substance P on nociceptive and non-nociceptive trigeminal brain stem neurons. Pain 8:33–45.

Hill RG (1986): Current perspectives on pain. Sci Prog Oxf 70:95–107.

Hill RG, Hoddinott ML, Keen PM (1980): Action of substance P on trigeminal nucleus caudalis neurons in capsaicin-treated rats. In Ajmone-Marsan C, Traczyck WZ (eds): *Neuropeptides and Neural Transmission.* New York: Raven Press, pp. 31–41.

Hokfelt T, Vinvent S, Hellsten L, Rosell S, Folkers K, Markey K, Goldstein M, Cuello C (1981): Immunohistochemical evidence for a 'neurotoxic' action of (D-Pro^2,D-Trp^{7,9})-substance P, an analogue with substance P antagonistic activity. Acta Physiol Scand 113:571–573.

Humpel C, Saria A (1993): Characterisation of neurokinin binding sites in rat brain membranes using highly selective ligands. Neuropeptides 25:65–71.

Ireland SJ, Wright IK, Jordan CC (1992): Characterization of tachykinin-induced ventral root depolarization in the neonatal rat spinal cord. Neuroscience 46:217–223.

Karlsson U, Nasstrom J, Berge O-G (1994): (±)-CP-96,345, an NK$_1$ receptor antagonist, has local anaesthetic-like effects in a mammalian sciatic nerve preparation. Regulat Pept 52:39–46.

Kidd BL, Mapp PI, Gibson SJ, Polak JM, O'Higgins F, Buckland-Wright JC, Blake DR (1989): A neurogenic mechanism for symmetrical arthritis. Lancet ii:1128–1130.

Konishi S, Otsuka M (1974): Excitatory action of hypothalamic substance P on spinal motoneurons of newborn rats. Nature 252:734–735.

Laird JMA, Hargreaves RJ, Hill RG (1993): Effect of RP67580, a non-peptide neurokinin-1 receptor antagonist, on facilitation of a nociceptive spinal flexion reflex in the rat. Br J Pharmacol 109:713–718.

Laneuville O, Dorais J, Couture R (1988): Characterization of the effects produced by neurokinins and three antagonists selective for neurokinin receptor subtypes in a spinal nociceptive reflex of the rat. Life Sci 42:1295–1305.

Lecci A, Giuliani S, Patacchini R, Viff G, Maggi CA (1991): Role of NK$_1$ tachykinin receptors in thermonociception: effect of (±)CP-96,345, a non-peptide substance P antagonist, on the hot plate test in mice. Neurosci Lett 129:299–302.

Littlewood NK, Todd AJ, Spike RC, Watt C, Shehab SAS (1995): The types of neuron in spinal dorsal horn which possess neurokinin-1 receptors. Neuroscience 66:597–608.

Liu-Chen L-Y, Mayberg MR, Moskowitz MA (1983): Immunohistochemical evidence for a substance P-containing trigeminovascular pathway to pial arteries in cats. Brain Res 268:162–166.

Lombet A, Spedding M (1994): Differential effects of non-peptidic tachykinin receptor antagonists on Ca^{2+} channels. Eur J Pharmacol 267:113–155.

Longmore J, Swain CJ, Hill RG (1995): Neurokinin receptors. Drug News Perspect 8:5–23.

Lowe JA, McLean S (1995): Tachykinin antagonists. Curr Pharm Des 1:269–278.

Ma Q-P, Woolf CJ (1997): Tachykinin NK$_1$ receptor antagonist RP67580 attenuates progressive hypersensitivity of flexor reflex during experimental inflammation in rats. Eur J Pharmacol 322:165–171.

Maggi CA, Schwartz TW (1997): The dual nature of the tachykinin binding sites (NK$_1$, NK$_2$, NK$_3$ ligands) in the rat brain. Trends Pharmacol Sci 18:351–354.

Malmberg AB, Yaksh TL (1992): Hyperalgesia mediated by spinal glutamate or substance P receptor blocked by spinal cyclooxygenase inhibition. Science 257:1276–1278.

Mantyh PW, DeMaster E, Malhotra E, Ghilardi JR, Rogers SD, Mantyh CR, Liu H, Basbaum AI, Vigna SR, Maggio JE, Simone DA (1995): Receptor endocytosis and dendrite reshaping in spinal neurones after somatosensory stimulation. Science 268:1629–1632.

Marshall GE, Shehab SAS, Spike RC, Todd AJ (1996): Neurokinin-1 receptors on spinothalamic neurons in the rat. Neuroscience 72:255–263.

McCarson KE, Goldstein BD (1990): Timecourse of the alteration in substance P levels in the dorsal horn following formalin: blockade by naloxone. Pain 41:95–100.

McLean S, Ganong A, Seymour PA, Snider RM, Desai MC, Rosen T, Bryce DK, Longo KP, Reynolds LS, Robinson G, Schmidt AW, Siok C, Heym J (1993): Pharmacology of CP-99,994; a nonpeptide antagonist of the tachykinin NK_1 receptor. J Pharmacol Exp Ther 267:472–479.

Morris R, Bleazard L, Hill RG (1992): The responses of neurons, in the deep dorsal horn of rat spinal cord slices in vitro, to the application of neurokinin agonists are correlated with their responses to peripheral nerve stimulation. J Physiol 452:252P.

Moussaoui SM, Carruette A, Montier F, Garret C (1992): RP67580, a non-peptide substance P antagonist inhibits neurogenic inflammation and possesses antinociceptive activities in rodents. Neuropeptides 22:46.

Nagahisa A, Asai R, Kanai Y, Murase A, Tsuchiya-Nakagaki M, Nakagaki T, Shieh TC, Taniguchi K (1992): Non-specific activity of (±)-CP-96,345 in models of pain and inflammation. Br J Pharmacol 107:273–275.

Neugebauer V, Schaible H-G, Weiretter F, Freudenberger U (1994): The involvement of substance P and neurokinin-1 receptors in the responses of rat dorsal horn neurons to noxious but not to innocuous mechanical stimuli applied to the knee joint. Brain Res 666:207–215.

Neugebauer V, Weiretter F, Schaible H-G (1995): Involvement of substance P and neurokinin-1 receptors in the hyperexcitability of dorsal horn neurons during development of acute arthritis in rat's knee joint. J Neurophysiol 73:1574–1582.

Neugebauer V, Rumenapp P, Schaible HG (1996): The role of spinal neurokinin-2 receptors in the processing of nociceptive information from the joint and in the generation and maintenance of inflammation-evoked hyperexcitability of dorsal horn neurons in the rat. Eur J Neurosci 8:249–260.

Neumann S, Doubell TP, Leslie T, Woolf CJ (1996): Inflammatory pain hypersensitivity mediated by phenotypic switch in myelinated primary sensory neurons. Nature 384:360–364.

Newby DE, Sciberras DG, Ferro CJ, Mendel CM, Gertz BJ, Majumdar A, Lowry RC, Webb DJ (1999): Antagonism of substance P induced forearm vasodilatation by the neurokinin type 1 receptor antagonist, L-745,030. Br J Clin Pharmacol (in press).

Parsons AM, Honda CN, Jia Y-P, Budai D, Xu X-J, Weisenfeld-Hallin Z, Seybold VS (1996): Spinal NK_1 receptors contribute to the increased excitability of the nociceptive flexor reflex during persistent peripheral inflammation. Brain Res 739:263–275.

Patel S, Gentry CT, Campbell EA (1996): A model for the in vivo evaluation of tachykinin NK_1 receptor antagonists using carrageenan-induced hyperalgesia in the guinea-pig paw. Br J Pharmacol 117:248P.

Picard P, Boucher S, Regoli D, Gitter BD, Howbert JJ, Couture R (1993): Use of non-peptide tachykinin receptor antagonists to substantiate the involvement of NK_1 and NK_2 receptors in a spinal nociceptive reflex in the rats. Eur J Pharmacol 232:255–261.

Radhakrishnan V, Henry JL (1991): Novel substance P antagonist, CP-96,345, blocks responses of cat spinal dorsal horn neurons to noxious cutaneous stimulation and to substance P. Neurosci Lett 132:39–43.

Rees H, Sluka KA, Tsuruoka M, Chen PS, Willis WD (1995): The effects of NK1 and NK2 receptor antagonists on the sensitization of STT cells following acute inflammation in the anaesthetised primate. J Physiol 483:152P.

Reinhardt RB, Laub JB, Fricke JR, Polis AB, Gertz BJ (1998): Comparison of a neurokinin$_1$ antagonist, L-754,030, to placebo, acetaminophen and ibuprofen in the dental pain model. Clin Pharmacol Therap 63:PI–124.

Rodriguez RE, Salt TE, Cahusac PMB, Hill RG (1983): The behavioural effects of intrathecally administered [D-Pro^2,D-Trp^{7,9}]-substance P, an analogue with presumed antagonist actions, in the rat. Neuropharmacology 22:173–176.

Rupniak NMJ, Boyce S, Williams AR, Cook G, Longmore J, Seabrook GR, Caeser M, Iversen SD, Hill RG (1993): Antinociceptive activity of NK_1 receptor antagonists: non-specific effects of racemic RP67580. Br J Pharmacol 110:1607–1613.

Rupniak NMJ, Webb JK, Williams AR, Carlson E, Boyce S, Hill RG (1995): Antinociceptive activity of the tachykinin NK_1 receptor antagonist, CP-99,994, in conscious gerbils. Br J Pharmacol 116:1937–1943.

Rupniak NMJ, Carlson EJ, Boyce S, Webb JK, Hill RG (1996): Enantioselective inhibition of the formalin paw late phase by the NK_1 receptor antagonist L-733,060 in gerbils. Pain 67:189–195.

Rupniak NMJ, Tattersall FD, Williams AR, Rycroft W, Carlson EJ, Cascieri MA, Sadowski S, Ber E, Hale JJ, Mills SG, MacCoss M, Seward E, Huscroft I, Owen S, Swain CJ, Hill RG, Hargreaves RJ (1997): In vitro and in vivo predictors of the anti-emetic activity of NK_1 receptor antagonists. Eur J Pharmacol 326:201–209.

Saffroy M, Beaujouan JC, Torrens Y, Besseyre J, Bergstrom L, Glowinski J (1987): Localization of tachykinin binding sites (NK_1, NK_2, NK_3 ligands) in the rat brain. Peptides 9:227–241.

Salt TE, De Vries GJ, Cahusac PMB, Morris R, Hill RG (1982): Evaluation of [D-Pro^2,D-Trp^{7,9}]-substance P as an antagonist of substance P responses in the rat central nervous system. Neurosci Lett 30:291–295.

Salt TE, Morris R, Hill RG (1983): Distribution of substance P-responsive and nociceptive neurons in relation to substance P-immunoreactivity within caudal trigeminal nucleus of the rat. Brain Res 273:217–228.

Salter MW, Henry JL (1991): Responses of functionally identified neurons in the dorsal horn of the cat spinal cord to substance P, neurokinin A and physalaemin. Neuroscience 43:601–610.

Schmidt AW, McLean S, Heym J (1992): The substance P receptor antagonist CP-96,345 interacts with Ca^{2+} channels. Eur J Pharmacol 219:491–492.

Shepheard SL, Williamson DJ, Hill RG, Hargreaves RJ (1993): The non-peptide neurokinin$_1$ receptor antagonist RP67580, blocks neurogenic plasma extravasation in the dura mater of rats. Br J Pharmacol 108:11–12.

Shepheard SL, Williamson DJ, Williams J, Hill RG, Hargreaves RJ (1995): Comparison of the effects of sumatriptan and the NK$_1$ antagonist CP-99,994 on plasma extravasation in dura mater and c-fos mRNA expression in trigeminal nucleus caudalis of rats. Neuropharmacology 34:255–261.

Sluka KA, Milton MA, Willis WD, Westlund KN (1997): Differential roles of neurokinin 1 and neurokinin 2 receptors in the development and maintenance of heat hyperalgesia induced by acute inflammation. Br J Pharmacol 120:1263–1273.

Smith G, Harrison S, Bowers J, Wiseman J, Birch P (1994): Non-specific effects of the tachykinin NK$_1$ receptor antagonist CP-99,994 in antinociceptive tests in rat, mouse and gerbil. Eur J Pharmacol 271:481–487.

Snider RM, Constantine JW, Lowe JA, Longo KP, Lebel WS, Woody HA, Drozda SE, Desai MC, Vinick FJ, Spencer RW, Hess HJ (1991): A potent nonpeptide antagonist of the substance P (NK$_1$) receptor. Science 251:435–439.

Suarez GA, Opfer-Gehrking TL, MacLean DB, Low PA (1994): Double-blind, placebo-controlled study of the efficacy of a substance P (NK1) receptor antagonist in painful peripheral neuropathy. Neurology 44:373P.

Swain CJ, Hargreaves RJ (1996): Neurokinin receptor antagonists. Ann Rep Med Chem 31:111–120.

Thompson SWN, Dray A, Urban L (1993a): The contribution of tachykinin receptor activation to C fiber evoked responses in the neonatal rat spinal cord in vitro. J Physiol 459:464P.

Thompson SWN, Dray A, Urban L (1993b): NMDA and tachykinin receptor-mediated contributions to the C-fiber-evoked response in the neonatal rat spinal cord in vitro are enhanced following peripheral inflammation. Br J Pharmacol 108:22P.

Uddman R, Edvinsson L (1989): Neuropeptides in the cerebral circulation. Cerebrovasc Brain Metab Rev 1:230–252.

Urban L, Willets J, Randic M, Papka RE (1985): The acute and chronic effects of capsaicin on slow excitatory transmission in rat dorsal horn. Brain Res 330:390–396.

Vaught JL (1988): Substance P antagonists and analgesia: a review of the hypothesis. Life Sci 43:1419–1431.

Weihe E (1990): Neuropeptides in primary afferent neurons. In Zenker W, Neuhuber W (eds): *Primary Afferent Neurones*. New York: Plenum Press, pp. 127–159.

Wiesenfeld-Hallin Z, Duranti R (1987): D-Arg^1,D-Try^{7,9},Leu^{11}-substance P (spantide) does not antagonise substance P-induced hyperexcitability of the nociceptive flexion withdrawal reflex in the rat. Acta Physiol Scand 129:55–59.

Woolf CJ (1983): Evidence for a central component of postinjury pain hypersensitivity. Nature 306:686–688.

Xu XJ, Dalsgaard CJ, Wiesenfeld-Hallin Z (1992): Intrathecal CP-96,345 blocks reflex facilitation induced in rats by substance P and C-fiber-conditioning stimulation. Eur J Pharmacol 216:337–344.

Xu XJ, Wiesenfeld-Hallin Z (1992): Intrathecal neurokinin A facilitates the spinal nociceptive flexor reflex evoked by thermal and mechanical stimuli and synergistically interacts with substance P. Acta Physiol Scand 144:163–168.

Yamamoto T, Yaksh TL (1991): Stereospecific effects of a nonpeptidic NK$_1$ selective antagonist, CP-96,345: antinociception in the absence of motor dysfunction. Life Sci 49:1955–1963.

Yashpal K, Dam TV, Quirion R (1990): Quantitative autoradiographic distribution of multiple neurokinin binding sites in rat spinal cord. Brain Res 506:259–266.

Yashpal K, Radhakrishnan V, Coderres TJ, Henry JL (1993): CP-96,345, but not its stereoisomer, CP-96,344, blocks the nociceptive responses to intrathecally administered substance P and to noxious thermal and electrical stimuli in the rat. Neuroscience 52:1039–1047.

Zieglgansberger W, Tulloch IF (1979): Effects of substance P on neurons in the dorsal horn of the spinal cord of the cat. Brain Res 166:273–282.

CHAPTER 8

EXCITATORY AMINO ACID ANTAGONISTS: POTENTIAL ANALGESICS FOR PERSISTENT PAIN

TERENCE J. CODERRE
Clinical Research Institute of Montreal, Université de Montréal,
McGill University
Montreal, Quebec, Canada

Over the past 10 years, it has become more and more apparent that the excitatory amino acids (EAAs) glutamate and aspartate play a role in nociception. Much of the evidence indicates a critical role of the N-methyl-D-aspartate (NMDA) and the other ionotropic glutamate receptors (iGluRs), ($\pm$)-α-amino-3-hydroxy-5-methylisoxazole-4-propionic acid (AMPA) and kainic acid, in spinal cord nociceptive processing, as well as in plasticity in the spinal cord, which leads to persistent nociception (Coderre, 1993; Dickenson, 1994). There is also an emerging field of research that points to a contribution of metabotropic glutamate receptors (mGluRs) in nociception (Neugebauer et al., 1994; Young et al., 1995; Fisher and Coderre, 1996a,b). In this chapter, we examine evidence for a contribution of both iGluRs and mGluRs to persistent nociception and discuss the potential utility of EAA antagonists as analgesic agents.

HISTORICAL EVIDENCE FOR A ROLE OF GLUTAMATE IN NOCICEPTION

Evidence for a role of glutamate in nociceptive processing appeared in the late 1950s, when Watkins and colleagues (Curtis et al., 1959) demonstrated that iontophoretic application of glutamate depolarized spinal cord neurons. Further evidence was provided when glutamate was found in the central terminals of primary afferent nerves (Graham et al., 1967; Johnson, 1978), as well as within intrinsic dorsal horn neurons (Miller et al., 1988). Glutamate was also observed

---

Novel Aspects of Pain Management: Opioids and Beyond, Edited by Jana Sawynok and Alan Cowan
ISBN 0-471-180173 Copyright © 1999 by Wiley-Liss, Inc.

to be released from *in vitro* spinal cord preparations after electrical (Hopkin and Neal, 1971) or chemical (Ueda et al., 1995) stimulation, and into spinal cerebrospinal fluid (CSF) *in vivo* after noxious chemical stimulation of the hindpaw (Skilling et al., 1988; Ueda et al., 1994) or after chronic joint inflammation (Sluka and Westlund, 1992; Yang et al., 1996). The presence of glutamate receptors in spinal cord dorsal horn has been confirmed in autoradiographic studies in both rats (Greenamyre et al., 1984; Monaghan and Cotman, 1985) and humans (Jansen et al., 1990; Shaw et al., 1991).

A contribution of iGluRs to nociceptive processing was originally suggested by the ability of AMPA/kainate, and particularly NMDA, receptor antagonists to produce analgesic effects in both phasic and tonic nociceptive tests in rats (Cahusac et al., 1984; Näsström et al., 1992). In addition, AMPA antagonists have been found to produce an inhibition of miniature end-plate potentials in dorsal horn neurons (Hori et al., 1992) and dorsal root potentials evoked by single shock C-fiber stimulation (Thompson et al., 1992). NMDA antagonists also prevent the development of wind-up that occurs in spinal cord dorsal horn neurons in response to repetitive C fiber stimulation (Davies and Lodge, 1987; Dickenson and Sullivan, 1987; Woolf and Thompson, 1991). Furthermore, tetanic electrical stimulation of the primary afferent fibers *in vitro* (Randic et al., 1993) or *in vivo* (Liu and Sandkuhler, 1995) induces a long-term potentiation of the C-fiber-evoked potentials in dorsal horn neurons that is prevented by superfusion with NMDA antagonists.

Further evidence for a role of iGluRs in nociception came from studies of the behavioral effects produced by spinal administration of iGluR agonists. Thus the intrathecal administration of NMDA (Aanonsen and Wilcox, 1987; Björkman et al., 1994), AMPA (Brambilla et al., 1996; Björkman et al., 1994), and kainate (Sun and Larson, 1991) produce spontaneous nociceptive behaviors in rats or mice. It has also been demonstrated that intrathecal injection of NMDA or non-NMDA agonists produces either thermal (Meller et al., 1996; Kolhekar et al., 1994; Malmberg and Yaksh, 1993) or mechanical (Meller et al., 1993) hyperalgesia.

Ionotropic glutamate receptors have also been implicated in the sensitization of dorsal horn neurons. Iontophoretic application of AMPA, kainate, or NMDA produces enhanced dorsal horn neuronal responses to non-noxious and noxious mechanical stimulation (Aanonsen et al., 1990; Dougherty and Willis, 1991; Cumberbatch et al., 1994). In addition, dorsal horn neurons that are sensitized following peripheral tissue injury or inflammation show increased responsiveness to iontophoretic application of AMPA, kainate, and NMDA (Dougherty and Willis, 1992), and exhibit a reduction in responsiveness or sensitization following administration of AMPA/kainate or NMDA antagonists (Schaible et al., 1991; Dougherty et al., 1992; Neugebauer et al., 1993). NMDA antagonists also reduce the facilitation of flexion reflexes to both noxious (Woolf and Thompson, 1991) and non-noxious stimuli (Ma and Woolf, 1995) induced by electrical nerve (C-fiber) stimulation or cutaneous application of the chemical irritant mustard oil, as well as reducing hyperreflexia in a model of visceral pain (Rice and McMahon, 1994).

Finally, there is recent evidence that EAAs may have effects on the peripheral terminals of primary afferent nerves. First, a significant number of unmyelinated axons in the glabrous skin of the rat hindpaw are labeled after immunohistochemical staining for NMDA, AMPA, and kainate receptors (Carlton et al., 1995). Second, the administration of L-glutamate, NMDA, AMPA, or kainic acid to the rat hindpaw has been found to produce an activation of primary afferent neurons, to elicit nociceptive reflexes (Ault and Hildebrand, 1993a,b), and to produce both mechanical (Carlton et al., 1995; Zhou et al., 1996) and thermal (Jackson et al., 1995) hyperalgesia/allodynia, which is attenuated by either NMDA or non-NMDA antagonists (Zhou et al., 1996). Third, intraplantar hindpaw injections of both NMDA and non-NMDA antagonists produce a reduction in thermal hyperalgesia induced by hindpaw injection of carrageenan (Jackson et al., 1995), as well as nociceptive behaviors in the formalin test (Davidson et al., 1997).

CLINICAL UTILITY OF IONOTROPIC GLUTAMATE RECEPTOR ANTAGONISTS

Studies in Animal Models of Persistent Pain

Much attention has been placed on iGluR antagonists, and particularly NMDA receptor antagonists, as potential novel treatments for chronic pain. Systemic (Davar et al., 1991; Smith et al., 1995) or intrathecal (Mao et al., 1992a,b; Yamamoto and Yaksh, 1992b) administration of the noncompetitive NMDA antagonist dizocilpine maleate (MK-801) has been found to reduce hyperalgesia and allodynia in rat models of neuropathic pain, as well as to reduce autotomy behavior in rats and mice with peripheral nerve sections (Seltzer et al., 1991; Banos et al., 1994). Persistent hyperalgesia after chronic constriction injury of the sciatic nerve in rats was also reduced by systemic or intrathecal treatment with the noncompetitive NMDA antagonists dextrorphan (Mao et al., 1993; Tal and Bennet, 1994), dextromethorphan (Chaplan et al., 1997), 3-Amino-1-hydroxypyrrolidin-2-one (HA-966) (Mao et al., 1992a), ketamine (Mao et al., 1993; Qian et al., 1996), magnesium (Xiao and Bennett, 1994), and memantine (Carlton and Hargett, 1995; Eisenberg et al., 1995), as well as the AMPA/kainate antagonist 6-Cyano-7-nitroquinoxaline-2,3-dione (CNQX) (Mao et al., 1992a). Systemic administration of NMDA (Hao and Xu, 1996) or AMPA/kainate (Xu et al., 1993) antagonists also dose-dependently suppresses mechanical allodynia in spinal cord injured rats, or following the spinal injection of strychnine (Onaka et al., 1996; Sorkin and Puig, 1996).

NMDA antagonists, including 2-Amino-5-phosphonopentanoic acid (AP-5) (Ren and Dubner, 1993), memantine (Eisenberg et al., 1994), and MK-801 (Ren et al., 1992), as well as the AMPA/kainate antagonist 6,7-Dinitroquinoxaline-

2,3-dione (DNQX) (Coutinho et al., 1996), have also been found to reduce effectively hyperalgesia in animal models of inflammatory pain. Furthermore, NMDA receptor antagonists have been demonstrated to reduce the hyperalgesia that develops after thermal (Coderre and Melzack, 1991) and visceral (Kolhekar and Gebhart, 1994) injury. Finally, persistent nociceptive responses induced by formalin injections in the hindpaw of mice and rats have been reduced with the NMDA antagonists AP-5 (Murray et al., 1991; Coderre and Melzack, 1992; Näsström et al., 1992), 2-Amino-7-phosphonoheptanoic acid (AP-7) (Näsström et al., 1992), CGP 34879 (Millan and Sequin, 1994), CGS 19755 (Hunter and Singh, 1994; Millan and Sequin, 1994), 3-(2-Carboxypiperazin-4-yl)-propyl-1-phosphonic acid (CPP) (Kristensen et al., 1994; Näsström et al., 1992), dextromethorphan (Elliot et al., 1995), ketamine (Näsström et al., 1992; Millan and Sequin, 1994), memantine (Eisenberg et al., 1993; Millan and Sequin, 1994), and MK-801 (Coderre and Melzack, 1992; Näsström et al., 1992; Yamamoto and Yaksh, 1992a), as well as the AMPA/kainate antagonists CNQX (Näsström et al., 1992), 2,3-Dioxo-6-nitro-1,2,3,4-tetrahydrobenzo[f]quinoxaline-7-)sulphonamide (NBQX) (Hunter and Singh, 1994), and DNQX (Näsström et al., 1992).

Studies of Human Clinical or Experimental Pain

There is a growing literature in human research that points to a role of excitatory amino acids in nociceptive processing. Experimental studies have been performed using the clinically available agents ketamine and dextromethorphan. Arendtnielsen et al. (1995) showed that whereas ketamine infusion did not alter reflex responses and pain rating to a single electrical nerve stimulus or a single brief noxious mechanical or thermal stimulus, it did reduce facilitation of the withdrawal reflex to, and pain rating of, repeated electrical nerve or noxious thermal or mechanical stimuli. Ilkjaer et al. (1996) demonstrated that ketamine reduces the magnitude of both primary and secondary hyperalgesia after thermal injury, and also pain evoked by prolonged noxious heat stimulation, without altering phasic heat pain thresholds in undamaged skin. It has also been shown that ketamine significantly reduces the ongoing pain and hyperalgesia produced by intradermal capsaicin injection (Park et al. 1995; Andersen et al., 1996); however, this effect was not found using clinically relevant doses of dextromethorphan (Kauppila et al., 1995). Furthermore, although dextromethorphan was unable to reduce pain induced by experimental ischemia (Kauppila et al., 1995), it did reduce temporal summation of second pain, a human correlate of wind-up in dorsal horn neurons (Price et al., 1994). Consistent with the animal studies with EAA antagonists (Davidson et al., 1997; Jackson et al., 1995), it has also been shown that local injection of ketamine inhibits the development of primary and secondary hyperalgesia after burn injury (Warncke et al., 1997).

In human clinical trials, it has been demonstrated that back (Cherry et al., 1995), headache (Nicolodi and Sicuteri, 1995), ischemic (Maurset et al., 1989), oral facial (Mathisen et al., 1995), neuropathic (Backonja et al., 1994; Felsby et al., 1996; Oye et al., 1996), phantom limb (Stannard and Porter, 1993; Nikolajsen et al., 1996), acute postoperative (Eide et al., 1995a; Maurset et al., 1989; Mathisen et al., 1995), chronic postoperative (Eide et al., 1995a; Persson et al., 1995), post-traumatic (Max et al., 1995), and spinal cord injury (Eide et al., 1995b) pain, as well as the pain associated with cancer (Oshima et al., 1990; Mercadante et al., 1995), fibromyalgia (Oye et al., 1996; Sorensen et al., 1995), post-herpetic neuralgia (Eide et al., 1994; Hoffmann et al., 1994), and reflex sympathetic dystrophy (Kishimoto et al., 1995) are suppressed by subanesthetic doses of the noncompetitive NMDA antagonist ketamine. Furthermore, intrathecal administration of the competitive NMDA antagonist CPP abolished afterdischarges and spreading pain and hyperalgesia in a patient with neuropathic pain (Kristensen et al, 1992). Suzuki et al. (1996) also demonstrated that dextromethorphan reduced pain and allodynia associated with postherpetic neuralgia; however, it has been found to be ineffective in a study of neuropathic pain (McQuay et al., 1994). It should be noted that much of this clinical evidence is preliminary and based on small group sizes. Furthermore, many of the above clinical trials have used the noncompetitive NMDA antagonist ketamine, which, as pointed out by Meller (1996), has significant effects on other neurotransmitter systems and ion channels.

MOTOR DEFICITS AND OTHER SIDE EFFECTS OF iGluR ANTAGONISTS

In spite of the growing excitement about NMDA antagonists, studies assessing the potential usefulness of iGluR antagonists as analgesic agents have generated mixed conclusions. The initial study of Cahusac et al. (1984) indicated that intrathecal administration of the selective NMDA antagonist 2-Amino-5-phosphoponovaleric acid (APV), or the nonselective glutamate antagonist gamma-D-Glutamylaminomethylsulphonic acid, produced antinociceptive effects in tail flick, hot plate, and paw pressure tests in rats. The doses required to produce antinociception on these measures were, however, quite high and were found to produce extensor paralysis in the rat hindquarters. We have found that doses of EAA receptor antagonists that produce antinociceptive effects in both phasic and tonic nociceptive tests also produce evidence of motor dysfunction (Coderre and Van Empel, 1994a). Rats exhibited poor placing, grasping, and righting reflexes in the case of competitive NMDA antagonists, and balance loss, weaving, and falling in the case of the open-channel blocker MK-801. It is also true that competitive NMDA antagonists such as APV do not easily cross the blood–brain barrier (Meldrum, 1985), so clinical administration of these agents is limited to situations where central administration is possible. In addition, the open-channel blockers (ketamine and MK-801) produce psychotomimetic effects (Domino et al., 1965; Oye et al., 1992), and may produce neurotoxicity at the higher dose levels (Olney, 1990), limiting their effective dose range.

Despite the disappointing results of studies assessing the antinociceptive effects and motor dysfunction produced by EAA antagonists, evidence with the use of agents acting at varying sites within the NMDA receptor complex or combination therapies, presented below, suggests that EAA antagonists may prove to be useful therapeutic agents for the treatment of clinical pain after all.

NMDA RECEPTOR COMPLEX, ALLOSTERIC SITES, AND ANALGESIC COMBINATIONS

Most studies assessing the analgesic potential of NMDA receptor antagonists have used competitive antagonists that act directly at the NMDA/glutamate binding site or noncompetitive antagonists that act as open-channel blockers at the phencyclidine site in the NMDA receptor channel. There are, however, additional sites in the NMDA receptor complex that are capable of modulating NMDA receptor activity, including strychnine-insensitive glycine receptors and polyamine receptors that are allosterically coupled to the NMDA receptor and enhance its activity. Recent evidence suggests that the use of NMDA antagonists, which act at glycine-allosteric and polyamine sites in the NMDA receptor complex, may provide solutions to the problems encountered with open-channel blockers and competitive NMDA antagonists. Thus both allosteric-glycine (Willetts et al., 1990; Hargreaves et al., 1991) and polyamine (Perrault et al., 1990; Carter et al., 1990) antagonists easily cross the blood–brain barrier and produce potent NMDA receptor antagonism at doses that do not induce neurotoxic or behavioral stimulant effects. The potential for glycine-allosteric antagonists as analgesics is indicated by the finding that selective antagonists and partial agonists of the allosteric glycine site reduce the wind-up of dorsal horn neurons in response to repeated C-fiber afferent nerve stimulation (Dickenson and Aydar, 1991), as well as reducing behavioral (Hunter and Singh, 1994; Millan and Seguin, 1994; Vaccarino et al., 1993; Lutfy and Weber, 1996) and neuronal (Dickenson and Aydar, 1991; Chapman and Dickenson, 1995) responses to subcutaneous injection of formalin in the rat hindpaw.

It may also be possible to enhance the analgesic effects of competitive and noncompetitive NMDA antagonists by using combinations of agents that increase the binding of antagonists to their receptors. For example, the endogenous polyamines spermine and spermidine increase the binding of open-channel blockers (MK-801, ketamine) when they bind to a polyamine receptor site within the NMDA receptor complex (Ransom and Stec, 1988; Williams et al., 1989). Thus it is possible that significant analgesic effects could be obtained by much lower doses of open-channel blockers without producing undesired side effects. Because glycine also potentiates competitive binding at the NMDA receptor site, by binding to the allosteric-glycine site (Johnson and Ascher, 1987), it is possible that glycine may be used to enhance the effectiveness of antagonists acting at the NMDA receptor by potentiating their competitive binding at the NMDA receptor. We recently demonstrated that the antinociceptive activity of the open-channel blocker MK-801 was dramatically enhanced by combination with a nonanalgesic dose of the polyamine agonist spermine. Furthermore, we showed that the antinociceptive effect of the competitive NMDA antagonist D-AP5 was significantly enhanced by a specific action of glycine at the allosteric-glycine site in the NMDA receptor complex (Coderre and Van Empel, 1994b).

METABOTROPIC GLUTAMATE RECEPTORS AND NOCICEPTION

Recently, a family of metabotropic glutamate receptors (mGluR1 to mGluR8) that are linked through G proteins to intracellular second messenger systems have been identified and distinguished from iGluRs (see Fig. 8.1). Activation of class I mGluRs (mGluR1 or mGluR5) produces phosphatidylinositol hydrolysis (Abe et al., 1992), increases in cyclic adenosine 3′,5′-monophosphate (cAMP) (by mGluR1α) (Aramori and Nakanishi, 1992), and intracellular Ca^{2+} mobilization (Masu et al., 1991; Aramori and Nakanishi, 1992). Class II (mGluR2,3) and Class III (mGluR4,6-8) mGluRs are linked to G proteins, which inhibit cAMP, and are distinguished by a differential agonist and antagonist selectivity (Jane et al., 1994).

Recent data suggest that in addition to iGluRs, mGluRs also play a significant role in nociception. Specifically, it has been demonstrated that iontophoretic application of the mGluR antagonists L-AP3 or (R,S)-2-Chloro-5-hydroxyphenylglycine (CHPG), attenuates rat dorsal horn neuronal activity associated with repeated mustard oil application (Young et al., 1994; 1995) and knee joint inflammation (Neugebauer et al., 1994). Furthermore, low doses of the mGluR agonists trans-1-Aminocyclopentane-1,3-dicarboylic acid (ACPD) or (1S,3R)-ACPD produce a depolarization of dorsal horn neurons (Young et al., 1994; 1995) and an increase in the response of spinothalamic tract neurons to innocuous mechanical stimulation (Palecek et al., 1994). It has also been shown that application of (1S,3R)-ACPD produces a dose-dependent, reversible ventral root depolarization in neonatal rat spinal cord *in vitro*, and that the ventral root depolarization and wind-up evoked by electrical stimulation of the dorsal roots or capsaicin application is blocked by the mGluR antagonist (+)-MCPG (Boxall et al., 1996). We have found that late-phase nociceptive responses in the rat formalin test are enhanced by intrathecal pretreatment with the mGluR agonists (1S,3R)-ACPD and (R,S)-DHPG, and slightly but significantly reduced by intrathecal pretreatment with the selective mGluR 1/5 antagonists S(+)α-amino-4-carboxy-benzeneacetic acid (S)-4CPG and (S)-4-carboxy-3-hydroxyphenylglycine (S)-4C3HPG (Coderre and Melzack, 1992; Fisher and Coderre, 1996b).

A role of mGluRs in nociception is further suggested because the intrathecal administration of quisqualate, an agonist at both mGluRs and AMPA receptors, produces mechanical (Aanonsen et al., 1990) and thermal (Kolhekar et al., 1994) hyperalgesia, as well as spontaneous nociceptive behaviors (Sun and Larson, 1991) in rodents. Similar spontaneous behaviors are induced by the mGluR agonist (1S,3R)-ACPD (Meller et al., 1996; Fisher and Coderre, 1996a),

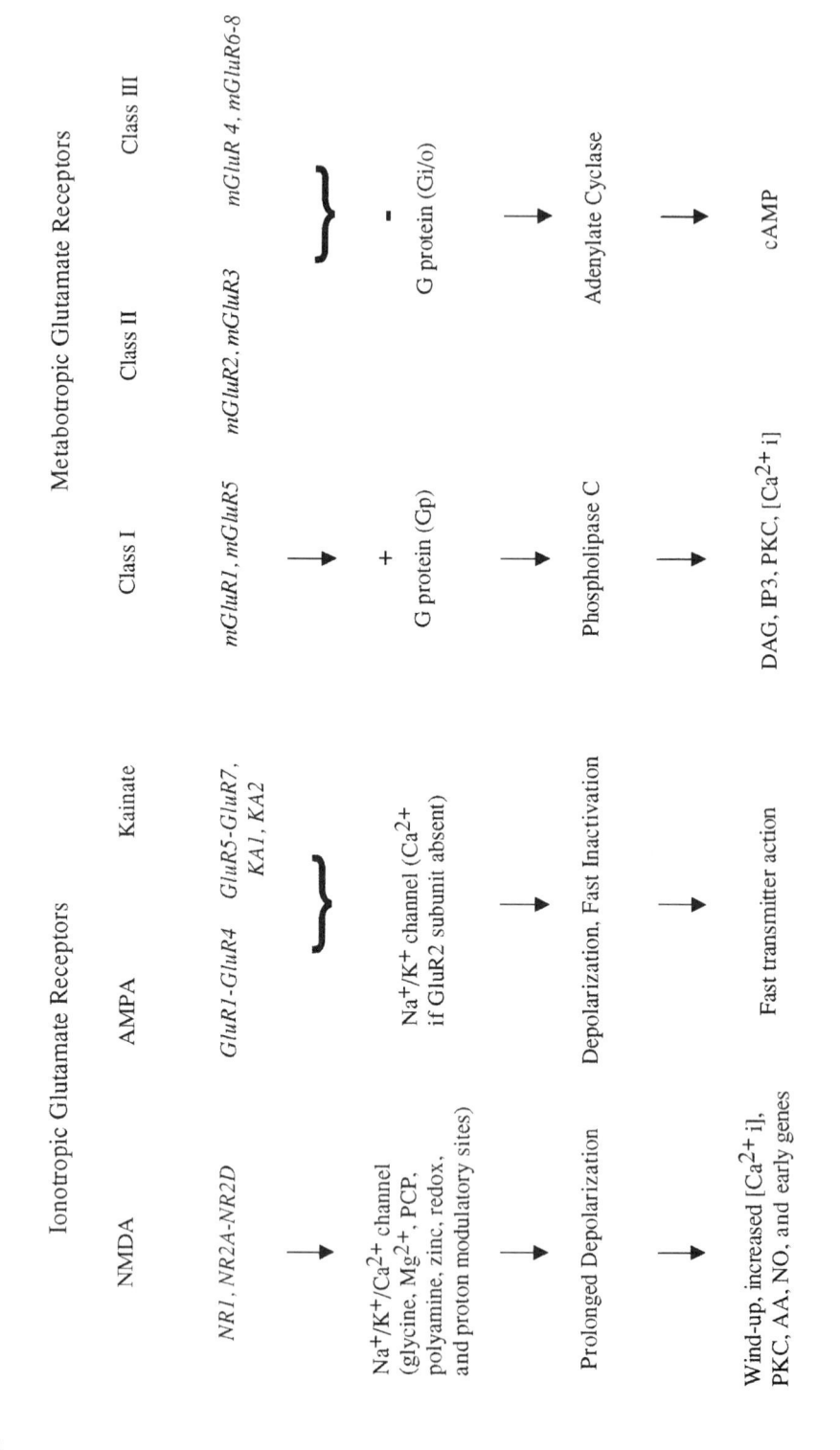

Ionotropic Glutamate Receptors

NMDA	AMPA	Kainate
NR1, NR2A-NR2D	*GluR1-GluR4*	*GluR5-GluR7, KA1, KA2*

NMDA:
$Na^+/K^+/Ca^{2+}$ channel (glycine, Mg^{2+}, PCP, polyamine, zinc, redox, and proton modulatory sites)
→ Prolonged Depolarization
→ Wind-up, increased $[Ca^{2+} i]$, PKC, AA, NO, and early genes

AMPA / Kainate:
Na^+/K^+ channel (Ca^{2+} if GluR2 subunit absent)
→ Depolarization, Fast Inactivation
→ Fast transmitter action

Metabotropic Glutamate Receptors

Class I	Class II	Class III
mGluR1, mGluR5	*mGluR2, mGluR3*	*mGluR 4, mGluR6-8*

Class I:
→ + G protein (Gp)
→ Phospholipase C
→ DAG, IP3, PKC, $[Ca^{2+} i]$

Class II / Class III:
− G protein (Gi/o)
→ Adenylate Cyclase
→ cAMP

164

Figure 8.1 The endogenous excitatory amino acids (EAAs) glutamate and aspartate act nonselectively at two types of EAA receptors—ionotropic glutamate receptors (iGluRs), which regulate ion channel activity, and metabotropic glutamate receptors (mGluRs), which regulate intracellular signaling. iGluRs are further broken down into three classes: N-methyl-D-aspartate (NMDA), ($\pm$)-α-amino-3-hydroxy-5-methylisoxazole-4-propionic acid (AMPA), and kainate, named after the synthetic agents to which they are selectively sensitive. NMDA receptors reflect a co-assembly of NR1 and NR2 subunits, and are distinguished by the permeability of their channels to calcium (Ca^{2+}), as well as sodium (Na^+) and potassium (K^+). The NMDA receptor has binding sites for glycine, magnesium (Mg^{2+}), phencyclidine-like drugs (PCP), polyamines, protons, and zinc, as well as a redox site, all of which modulate channel activity. A voltage-dependent blockade by Mg^{2+} causes the NMDA receptor to function only after the cell has been depolarized and underlies its importance in conditions of excess activity. Furthermore, its permeability to Ca^{2+} ensures that the NMDA receptor is capable of producing long-term effects; it is associated with prolonged and cumulative depolarizations, wind-up, and the production of various intracellular messengers, including protein kinase C (PKC), arachidonic acid (AA), and nitric oxide (NO), and proto-oncogenes such as c-fos and c-jun. AMPA and kainate receptors composed of subunit assemblies of GluR1–4 and GluR5–7, KA1–2, respectively, are often referred to as non-NMDA receptors. Their permeability is normally restricted to Na^+ and K^+, although AMPA receptors that do not contain a GluR2 subunit are also permeable to Ca^{2+}. Because they are not susceptible to a Mg^{2+} block, AMPA and kainate receptors are easily depolarized, and this, coupled with a fast inactivation, means that these receptors normally mediate fast transmitter actions. mGluRs are also broken down into three classes. Class I, including mGluR1 and 5, are positively coupled by a G protein (Gp) to phosphatidylinositol hydrolysis, whereby phospholipase C catalyzes the hydrolysis of phosphatidylinositol 4,5-bisphosphate (PIP_2), producing diacylglycerol (DAG) and inositol 1,4,5-trisphosphate (IP3), which in turn enhance the production of PKC and the release of Ca^{2+} from internal stores. Class II (mGluR2 and 3) and Class III (mGluR4, 6-8) are negatively coupled by a G protein (Gi/o) to adenylate cyclase and inhibit this enzyme's ability to catalyze the conversion of adenosine 5' triphosphate (ATP) to cyclic adenosine 3',5' monophosphate (cAMP). Through their effects on various intracellular messengers, mGluRs have the potential to produce long-term effects on cellular function and activity.

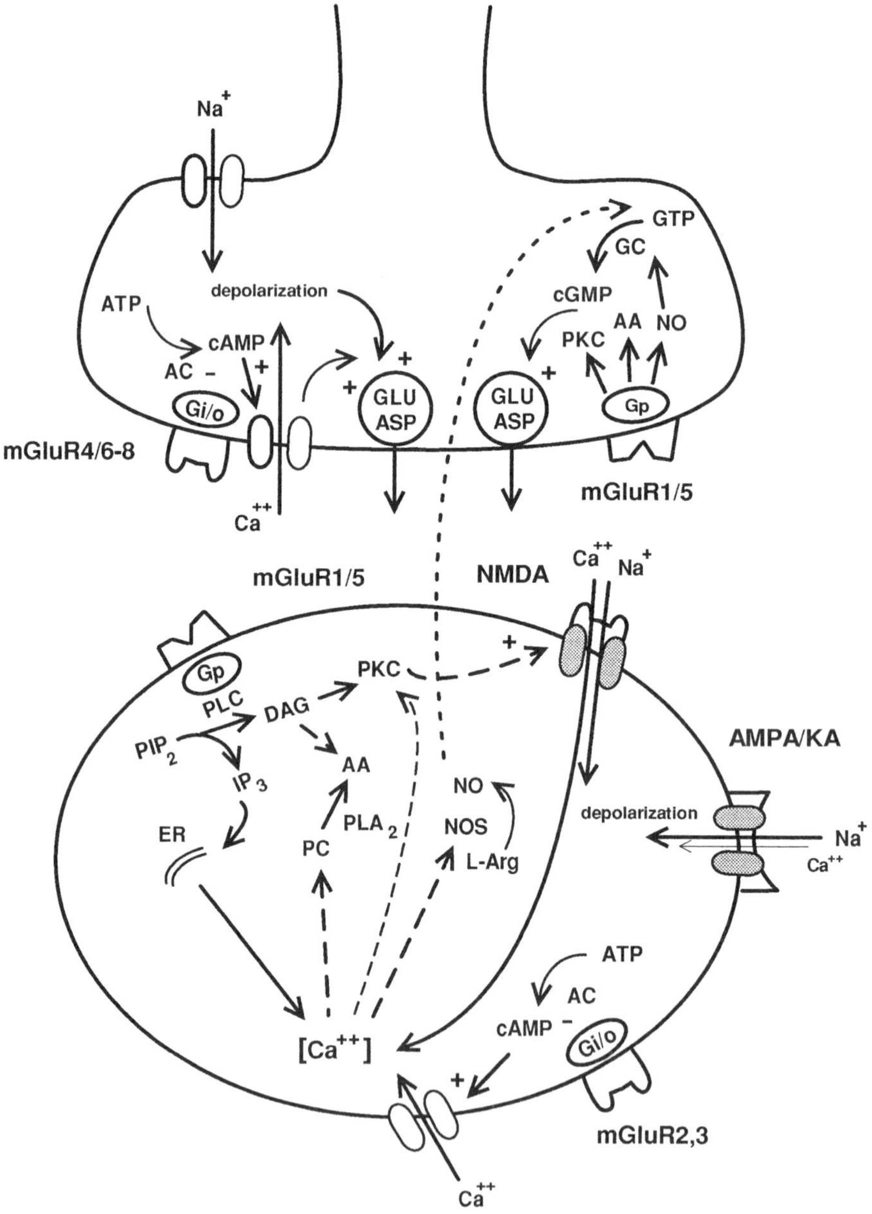

Na+
ATP
depolarization
cAMP
AC
Gi/o
+
GLU
ASP
GTP
GC
cGMP
AA
NO
PKC
Gp
mGluR4/6-8
Ca++
mGluR1/5
mGluR1/5
NMDA
Ca++ Na+
Gp
PLC
DAG
PKC
PIP2
IP3
AA
NO
ER
PLA2
PC
NOS
L-Arg
AMPA/KA
depolarization
Na+
Ca++
ATP
AC
cAMP
Gi/o
[Ca++]
mGluR2,3
Ca++

implicating mGluRs in these responses. Our recent studies also point to a specific role of spinal mGluR1 in nociception, because intrathecal administration of the mGluR1/5 agonist (R,S)-DHPG produces spontaneous nociceptive behaviors, as well as thermal and mechanical hyperalgesia, which are very pronounced and of long duration, whereas intrathecal administration of the reportedly selective mGluR5 agonist, *trans*-azetidine-2,4-dicarboxylic acid, fails to produce any nociceptive behaviors even at doses 100 times greater than the doses of (R,S)-DHPG used (Coderre and Fisher, 1996; Fisher and Coderre, 1996a).

The possibility that mGluRs might influence the development of thermal and mechanical hyperalgesia prompted us to examine the possible role of these

Figure 8.2 Schematic diagram indicating possible mechanisms by which excitatory amino acids may produce long-term effects that contribute to sensitization of spinal cord dorsal horn neurons and result in persistent nociception. High levels of afferent input cause the release of aspartate and glutamate within the dorsal horn. Repetitive fast-transmitter activity of aspartate and glutamate at AMPA/kainate receptors produces a membrane depolarization which would counter a voltage-dependent blockade of the NMDA receptor by Mg^{2+}. A further action of aspartate and glutamate at NMDA and mGluR1,5 receptors, respectively, would produce an influx of Ca^{2+} (through NMDA receptor-operated Ca^{2+} channels), and the activation of phospholipase C (PLC) by Gp. PLC catalyzes the hydrolysis of phosphatidylinositol 4,5-bisphosphate (PIP_2), producing ionositol trisphosphate (IP_3) and diacyclglycerol (DAG). The production of IP_3 causes the release of Ca^{2+} from intracellular stores within the endoplasmic reticulum (ER). The increases in intracellular Ca^{2+} produced by the influx of Ca^{2+} through NMDA receptor-operated channels, and by the release of Ca^{2+} from internal stores, stimulates the nitric oxide (NO) synthase-induced conversion of L-arginine to NO, and the phospholipase A_2 (PLA_2)-induced release of arachidonic acid (AA). The production of DAG further stimulates AA release and induces the translocation and activation of protein kinase C (PKC), which is activated during high rates of Ca^{2+} influx. Activation of NO, AA, and PKC induces sustained alterations in the cellular membrane, affecting membrane permeability for prolonged periods. NO is also able to diffuse to the presynaptic terminal and enhance the release of glutamate and aspartate by activating guanylate cyclase (GC), which stimulates the conversion of GTP to cGMP. PKC is capable of phosphorylating the NMDA receptor, resulting in an enhancement of NMDA channel currents. PKC also interacts with Ca^{2+} to stimulate increases in the expression of the proto-oncogenes c-*fos* and c-*jun* (not shown). The protein products of these proto-oncogenes participate in the regulation of mRNA encoding various peptides in spinal cord, and can influence long-term changes in cellular function. Finally, aspartate and glutamate will have actions at mGluR2,3 (normally postsynaptic) or mGluR4/6-8 (normally presynaptic) that are coupled to Gi/o and inhibit adenylate cyclase (AC), thereby blocking the conversion of ATP to cAMP. This would result in the inhibition of Ca^{2+} influx through voltage-gated calcium channels, and thus have an inhibitory influence both postsynaptically and presynaptically, where it would reduce Ca^{2+} stimulation of glutamate and aspartate release.

receptors in the development of pathological pain following injury of the sciatic nerve. We found that intrathecal pretreatment with an mGluR1/5 antagonist or mGluR1 antireceptor antibodies was able to produce a significant reduction of either cold hyperalgesia or mechanical allodynia that is normally expressed 4–16 days after nerve injury (Fisher et al., 1998; Fundytus et al., 1998). Together, these findings suggest that mGluRs, in particular mGluR1, contribute significantly to the development of pathological pain following nerve injury.

INTERACTION BETWEEN iGluRS and mGluRS IN NOCICEPTION

It is now well documented that mGluR activity potentiates L-glutamate, NMDA, AMPA, or kainate responses in spinal cord both *in vitro* and *in vivo* (Bleakman et al., 1992; Cerne and Randic, 1992; Bond and Lodge, 1995). These findings paralleled our observation that an intrathecal combination of NMDA and *trans*-ACPD produced a significantly greater increase in nociceptive scores in the formalin test than did twice the doses of either agonist alone (Coderre and Melzack, 1992). Furthermore, it has been shown that intrathecal co-administration of AMPA and *trans*-ACPD produced mechanical hyperalgesia, that is not produced by either agent alone (Meller et al., 1993). In addition, the enhancement of formalin-induced nociception, as well as spontaneous nociception induced by intrathecal administration of mGluR agonists, are attenuated by nonanalgesic doses of the NMDA antagonist D-AP5 (Fisher and Coderre, 1996a,b). Together, these findings suggest there are interactive effects of iGluRs and mGluRs in nociceptive processing. It is possible that the activation of presynaptic mGluR1/5 leads to an increase in aspartate and/or glutamate release, and that stimulation of postsynaptic mGluR1/5 increases NMDA and AMPA channel activity, resulting in a prolonged facilitation of iGluR-mediated dorsal horn neuronal responses. This hypothesis is supported by observations that mGluRs linked to presynaptic phosphatidylinositol hydrolysis facilitate glutamate release (Herrero et al., 1992) and the demonstration that protein kinase C, produced in response to mGluR1/5 activation, potentiates NMDA-induced currents postsynaptically (Chen and Huang, 1992) and stimulates the release of aspartate and glutamate in spinal cord slices (Gerber et al., 1989). These interactive effects may be critical to the long-term consequences of glutamate receptor activation on nociceptive processing (see Fig. 8.2). Furthermore, the realization that mGluRs play a significant role in nociceptive processing provides the opportunity for new treatment options that may lack the serious consequences associated with many NMDA antagonists.

ACKNOWLEDGMENTS

The author wishes to acknowledge the support of the Medical Research Council of Canada, Fonds de la recherche en santé du Québec, Institut de recherche en santé et sécurité du travail du Québec, and the Montreal Astra Research Center. TJC holds the IRSST-Quebec chair in Pain Research at the Clinical Research Institute of Montreal and is an MRC scientist.

REFERENCES

Aanonsen LM, Wilcox GL (1987): Nociceptive action of excitatory amino acids in the mouse: effects of spinally administered opioids, phencyclidine and σ agonists. J Pharmacol Exp Ther 243:9–19.

Aanonsen LM, Lei S, Wilcox GL (1990): Excitatory amino acid receptors and nociceptive neuro-transmission in rat spinal cord. Pain 41:309–321.

Abe T, Sugihara H, Nawa H, Shigemoto R, Mizuno N, Nakanishi S (1992): Molecular characterization of a novel metabotropic glutamate receptor mGluR5 coupled to inositol phosphate/Ca^{2+} signal transduction. J Biol Chem 267:13361–13368.

Andersen OK, Felsby S, Nicolaisen L, Bjerring P, Jensen TS, Arendtnielsen L (1996): The effect of ketamine on stimulation of primary and secondary hyperalgesic areas induced by capsaicin—a double-blind, placebo-controlled, human experimental study. Pain 66:51–62.

Aramori I, Nakanishi S (1992): Signal transduction, pharmacological characteristics of a metabotropic glutamate receptor, mGluR1, in transfected CHO cells. Neuron 8: 757–765.

Arendtnielsen L, Petersenfelix S, Fischer M, Bak P, Bjerring P, Zbinden AM (1995): The effect of N-methyl-D-aspartate antagonist (ketamine) on single and repeated nociceptive stimuli—a placebo-controlled experimental human study. Anesth Analg 81:63–68.

Ault B, Hildebrand LM (1993a). Activation of nociceptive reflexes by peripheral kainate receptors. J Pharmacol Exp Ther 265:927–932.

Ault B, Hildebrand LM (1993b): L-Glutamate activates peripheral nociceptors. Agents Actions 39(Suppl. C):C142–C144.

Backonja M, Arndt G, Gombar KA, Check B, Zimmermann M (1994): Response of chronic neuropathic pain syndromes to ketamine: a preliminary study. Pain 56:51–57.

Banos JE, Verdu E, Buti M, Navarro X (1994). Effects of dizocilpine on autotomy behaviour after nerve section in mice. Brain Res 636:107–110.

Björkman R, Hallman KM, Hedner J, Hedner T, Henning M (1994): Acetaminophen blocks spinal hyperalgesia induced by NMDA and substance P. Pain 57:259–264.

Bleakman D, Rusin KI, Chard PS, Glaum SR, Miller RJ (1992): Metabotropic glutamate receptors potentiate ionotropic glutamate responses in the rat dorsal horn. Mol Pharmacol 42:192–196.

Bond A, Lodge D (1995): Pharmacology of metabotropic glutamate receptor-mediated enhancement of responses to excitatory and inhibitory amino acids on rat spinal neurones *in vivo*. Neuropharmacol 34:1015–1023.

Boxall SJ, Thompson SWN, Dray A, Dickenson AH, Urban L (1996): Metabotropic glutamate receptor activation contributes to nociceptive reflex activity in the rat spinal cord *in vitro*. Neuroscience 74:13–20.

Brambilla A, Prudentino A, Grippa N, Borsini F (1996): Pharmacological characterization of AMPA-induced biting behaviour in mice. Eur J Pharmacol 305:115–117.

Cahusac PMB, Evans RH, Hill RG, Rodriquez RE, Smith DAS (1984): The behavioural effects of an N-methylaspartate receptor antagonist following application to the lumbar spinal cord of conscious rats. Neuropharmacol 23:719–724.

Carlton SM, Hargett GL (1995): Treatment with the NMDA antagonist memantine attenuates nociceptive responses to mechanical stimulation in neuropathic rats. Neurosci Lett 198:115–118.

Carlton SM, Hargett GL, Coggeshall RE (1995): Localization and activation of glutamate receptors in unmyelinated axons of rat glabrous skin. Neurosci Lett 197:25–28.

Carter CJ, Lloyd KG, Zivkovic B, Scatton B (1990): Ifenprodil, SL 82.0715 as cerebral antiischemic agents. III. Evidence for antagonistic effects at the polyamine modulatory site within the N-methyl-D-aspartate receptor complex. J Pharmacol Exp Ther 253:475–482.

Cerne R, Randic M (1992): Modulation of AMPA and NMDA responses in rat spinal dorsal horn neurons by trans-1-aminocyclopentane-1,3-dicarboxylic acid. Neurosci Lett 144:180–184.

Chaplan SR, Malmberg AB, Yaksh TL (1997): Efficacy of spinal NMDA receptor antagonism in formalin hyperalgesia and nerve injury evoked allodynia in the rat. J Pharmacol Exp Ther 280:829–838.

Chapman V, Dickenson AH (1995): Time-related roles of excitatory amino acid receptors during persistent noxiously evoked responses of rat dorsal horn neurones. Brain Res 703:45–50.

Chen L, Huang L-YM (1992): Protein kinase C reduces Mg^{2+} block of NMDA-receptor channels as a mechanism of modulation. Nature 356:521–523.

Cherry DA, Plummer JL, Gourlay GK, Coates KR, Odgers CL (1995): Ketamine as an adjunct to morphine in the treatment of pain. Pain 62:119–121.

Coderre TJ (1993): The role of excitatory amino acid receptors and intracellular messengers in persistent nociception after tissue injury in rats. Mol Neurobiol 7:229–246.

Coderre TJ, Fisher K (1996): Mechanical and thermal allodynia induced by intrathecal administration of (RS)-3,5-dihydroxyphenylglycine ((RS)-(R,S)-DHPG). Abstracts of the VIIIth World Congress on Pain, p. 243.

Coderre TJ, Melzack R (1991): Central neural mediators of secondary hyperalgesia following heat injury in rats: neuropeptides and excitatory amino acids. Neurosci Lett 131:71–74.

Coderre TJ, Melzack R (1992): The contribution of excitatory amino acids to central sensitization and persistent nociception after formalin-induced tissue injury. J Neurosci 12:3665–3670.

Coderre TJ, Van Empel I (1994a): The utility of excitatory amino acid (EAA) antagonists as analgesic agents. I. Comparison of the antinociceptive activity of various classes of EAA antagonists in mechanical, thermal and chemical nociceptive tests. Pain 59:345–352.

Coderre TJ, Van Empel I (1994b): The utility of excitatory amino acid (EAA) antagonists as analgesic agents. II. Assessment of the antinociceptive activity of combinations of competitive and non-competitive NMDA antagonists with agents acting at allosteric-glycine and polyamine receptor sites. Pain 59:353–359.

Coutinho SV, Meller ST, Gebhart GF (1996): Intracolonic zymosan produces visceral hyperalgesia in the rat that is mediated by spinal NMDA and non-NMDA receptors. Brain Res 736:7–15.

Cumberbatch MJ, Herrero JF, Headley PM (1994): Exposure of rat spinal neurones to NMDA, AMPA and kainate produces only short-term enhancements of responses to noxious and non-noxious stimuli. Neurosci Lett 181:98–102.

Curtis DR, Phillips JW, Watkins JC (1959): Chemical excitation of spinal neurons. Nature 183:611–612.

Davar G, Hama A, Deykin A, Vos B, Maciewicz R (1991): MK-801 blocks the development of thermal hyperalgesia in a rat model of experimental painful neuropathy. Brain Res 553:327–330.

Davidson EM, Coggeshall RE, Carlton SM (1997): Peripheral NMDA and non-NMDA glutamate receptors contribute to nociceptive behaviours in the rat formalin test. Neuroreport 8:941–946.

Davies SN, Lodge D (1987): Evidence for involvement of N-methylaspartate receptors in "wind-up" of class 2 neurones in the dorsal horn of the rat. Brain Res 424: 402–406.

Dickenson AH (1994): NMDA receptor antagonists as analgesics. In Fields HL, Liebeskind JC (eds): *Progress in Pain Research and Management*, Vol. 1. Seattle: IASP Press, pp. 173–187.

Dickenson AH, Aydar E (1991): Antagonism at the glycine site on the NMDA receptor reduces spinal nociception in the rat. Neurosci Lett 121:263–266.

Dickenson AH, Sullivan AF (1987): Evidence for a role of the NMDA receptor in the frequency dependent potentiation of deep rat dorsal horn nociceptive neurones following C fibre stimulation. Neuropharmacology 26:1235–1238.

Domino EF, Chodof P, Corssen G (1965): Pharmacologic effects of CI,581, a new dissociative anesthetic, in man. Clin Pharmacol Ther 6:279–291.

Dougherty PM, Willis WD (1991): Enhancement of spinothalamic neuron responses to chemical and mechanical stimuli following combined microiontophoretic application of N-methyl-D-aspartic acid and substance P. Pain 47:85–93.

Dougherty PM, Willis WD (1992): Enhanced responses of spinothalamic tract neurons to excitatory amino acids accompany capsaicin-induced sensitization in the monkey. J Neurosci 12:883–894.

Dougherty PM, Palecek J, Paleckova V, Sorkin LS, Willis WD (1992): The role of NMDA and non-NMDA excitatory amino acid receptors in the excitation of primate spinothalamic tract neurons by mechanical, thermal and electrical stimuli. J Neurosci 12:3025–3041.

Eide PK, Jørum E, Stubhaug A, Bremnes J, Breivik H (1994): Relief of post-herpetic neuralgia with N-methyl-D-aspartic acid receptor antagonist ketamine: a doubleblind, cross-over comparison with morphine and placebo. Pain 58:347–354.

Eide PK, Stubhaug A, Oye I (1995a): The NMDA-antagonist ketamine for prevention and treatment of acute and chronic post-operative pain. Baillieres Clin Anaesthesiol 9:539–554.

Eide PK, Stubhaug A, Stenehjem AE (1995b): Central dysesthesia pain after traumatic spinal cord injury is dependent on N-methyl-D-aspartate receptor activation. Neurosurgery 37:1080–1087.

Eisenberg E, LaCross S, Strassman AM (1994): The effects of the clinically tested NMDA receptor antagonist memantine on carrageenan-induced thermal hyperalgesia in rats. Eur J Pharmacol 255:123–129.

Eisenberg E, LaCross S, Strassman AM (1995): The clinically tested N-methyl-D-aspartate receptor antagonist memantine blocks and reverses thermal hyperalgesia in a rat model of painful mononeuropathy. Neurosci Lett 187:17–20.

Eisenberg E, Vos BP, Strassman AM (1993): The NMDA antagonist memantine blocks pain behaviour in a rat model of formalin-induced facial pain. Pain 54:301–307.

Elliott KJ, Brodsky M, Hynansky AD, Foley KM, Inturrisi CE (1995): Dextromethorphan suppresses both formalin-induced nociceptive behaviour and the formalin-induced increase in spinal cord c-*fos* mRNA. Pain 61:401–409.

Felsby S, Nielsen J, Arendtnielsen L, Jensen TS (1996): NMDA receptor blockade in chronic neuropathic pain—a comparison of ketamine and magnesium chloride. Pain 64:283–291.

Fisher K, Coderre TJ (1996a): Comparison of nociceptive effects produced by intrathecal administration of mGluR agonists. Neuroreport 7:2743–2747.

Fisher K, Coderre TJ (1996b): The contribution of metabotropic glutamate receptors (mGluRs) to formalin-induced nociception. Pain 68:255–263.

Fisher K, Fundytus ME, Cahill CM, Coderre TJ (1998): Intrathecal administration of the mGluR compound, (S)-4CPG, attenuates hyperalgesia and allodynia associated with sciatic nerve constriction injury in rats. Pain 77:259–266.

Fundytus ME, Fisher K, Dray A, Henry JL, Coderre TJ (1998): *In vivo* antinociceptive activity of anti-rat mGluR1 and mGluR5 antibodies in rats. Neuroreport 9:731–735.

Gerber G, Kangrga I, Ryu PD, Larew JSA, Randic M (1989): Multiple effects of phorbol esters in the rat spinal dorsal horn. J Neurosci 9:3606–3617.

Graham LT, Shank PR, Werman R, Aprison MH (1967): Distribution of some synaptic transmitter suspects in cat spinal cord. J Neurochem 14:465–472.

Greenamyre JT, Young AB, Penny JB (1984): Quantitative autoradiographic distribution of L-[^{3}H]glutamate-binding sites in the rat central nervous system. J Neurosci 4: 2133–2144.

Hao JX, Xu XJ (1996): Treatment of a chronic allodynia-like response in spinally injured rats—effects of systemically administered excitatory amino acid receptor antagonists. Pain 66:279–285.

Hargreaves RJ, Rigby M, Smith D (1991): L-687,414 (+)cis-4-methyl-HA-966, an NMDA receptor antagonist acting at the glycine site, does not alter glucose metabolism or neuronal morphology at neuroprotective dose levels. J Cereb Blood Flow 11(Suppl. 2):S301.

Herrero I, Miras-Portugal MT, Sánchez-Prieto J (1992): Positive feedback of glutamate exocytosis by metabotropic presynaptic receptor stimulation. Nature 360:163–166.

Hoffmann V, Coppejans H, Vercauteren M, Adriaensen H (1994): Successful treatment of postherpetic neuralgia with oral ketamine. Clin J Pain 10:240–242.

Hopkin J, Neal MJ (1971): Effect of electrical stimulation and high potassium concentrations on the efflux of ^{14}C-glycine from slices of spinal cord. Br J Pharmacol 42: 215–223.

Hori Y, Endo K, Takahashi T (1992): Presynaptic inhibitory action of enkephalin on excitatory transmission in superficial dorsal horn of the rat spinal cord. J Physiol 450:673–685.

Hunter JC, Singh L (1994): Role of excitatory amino acid receptors in the mediation of nociceptive response to formalin in the rat. Neurosci Lett 174:217–221.

Ilkjaer S, Petersen KL, Brennum J, Wernberg M, Dahl JB (1996): Effect of systemic N-methyl-D-aspartate receptor antagonist (ketamine) on primary and secondary hyperalgesia in humans. Br J Anaesth 76:829–834.

Jackson DL, Graff CB, Durnett-Richardson J, Hargreaves KM (1995): Glutamate participates in the peripheral modulation of thermal hyperalgesia in rats. Eur J Pharmacol 284:321–325.

Jane DE, Jones PLStJ, Pook PC-K, Tse H-W, Watkins JC (1994): Actions of two new antagonists showing selectivity for different sub-types of metabotropic glutamate receptor in the neonatal rat spinal cord. Br J Pharmacol 112:809–816.

Jansen KL, Faull RL, Dragunow M, Waldvogel H (1990): Autoradiographic localisation of NMDA, quisqualate and kainic acid receptors in human spinal cord. Neurosci Lett 108:53–57.

Johnson, JL (1978): The excitant amino acids glutamate and aspartic acid as transmitter candidates in the vertebrate central nervous system. Prog Neurobiol 10:155–202.

Johnson JW, Ascher P (1987): Glycine potentiates the NMDA responses in cultured mouse brain neurons. Nature 325:529–532.

Kauppila T, Gronroos M, Pertovaara A (1995): An attempt to attenuate experimental pain in humans by dextromethorphan, an NMDA receptor antagonist. Pharmacol Biochem Behav 52:641–644.

Kishimoto N, Kato J, Suzuki T, Arakawa H, Ogawa S, Suzuki H (1995): A case of RSD with complete disappearance of symptoms following intravenous ketamine infusion combined with stellate ganglion block and continuous epidural block. Masui—Jap J Anesthesiol 44:1680–1684.

Kolhekar R, Gebhart GF (1994): NMDA and quisqualate modulation of visceral nociception in the rat. Brain Res 651:215–226.

Kolhekar R, Meller ST, Gebhart GF (1994): N-methyl-D-aspartate receptor-mediated changes in thermal nociception: Allosteric modulation at glycine and polyamine recognition sites. Neuroscience 63:925–936.

Kristensen JD, Svensson B, Gordh T-Jr (1992): The NMDA-receptor antagonist CPP abolishes 'wind-up pain' after intrathecal administration in humans. Pain 51:249–253.

Kristensen JD, Karlsten R, Gordh T, Berge O-G (1994): The NMDA antagonist 3-(2-carboxypiperazin-4-yl)propyl-1-phosphonic acid (CPP) has antinociceptive effect after intrathecal injection in the rat. Pain 56:59–67.

Liu XG, Sandkuhler J (1995): Long-term potentiation of c-fiber-evoked potentials in the rat spinal dorsal horn is prevented by spinal N-methyl-D-aspartic acid receptor blockage. Neurosci Lett 191:43–46.

Lutfy K, Weber E (1996): Attenuation of nociceptive responses by ACEA-1021, a competitive NMDA receptor glycine site antagonist, in mice. Brain Res 743:17–23.

Ma QP, Woolf CJ (1995): Noxious stimuli induce an N-methyl-D-aspartate receptor-dependent hypersensitivity of the flexion withdrawal reflex to touch—implications for the treatment of mechanical allodynia. Pain 61:383–390.

Malmberg AB, Yaksh TL (1993): Spinal nitric oxide synthesis inhibition blocks NMDA-induced thermal hyperalgesia and produces antinociception in the formalin test in rats. Pain 54:291–300.

Mao J, Price DD, Hayes RL, Lu J, Mayer DJ (1992a): Differential roles of NMDA and non-NMDA receptor activation in induction and maintenance of thermal hyperalgesia in rats with painful peripheral mononeuropathy. Brain Res 598:271–278.

Mao J, Price DD, Mayer DJ, Lu J, Hayes RL (1992b): Intrathecal MK-801 and local nerve anesthesia synergistically reduce nociceptive behaviours in rats with experimental peripheral mononeuropathy. Brain Res 576:254–262.

Mao J, Price DD, Hayes RL, Lu J, Mayer DJ, Frenk H (1993): Intrathecal treatment with dextrorphan or ketamine potently reduces pain-related behaviours in a rat model of peripheral mononeuropathy. Brain Res 605:164–168.

Masu M, Tanabe Y, Ysuchida K, Shigemoto R, Nakanishi S (1991): Sequence and expression of a metabotropic glutamate receptor. Nature 349:760–765.

Mathisen LC, Skjelbred P, Skoglund LA, Oye I (1995): Effect of ketamine, an NMDA receptor inhibitor, in acute and chronic orofacial pain. Pain 61:215–220.

Maurset A, Skoglund LA, Hustveit O, Oye I (1989): Comparison of ketamine and pethidine in experimental and postoperative pain. Pain 36:37–41.

Max MB, Byassmith MG, Gracely RH, Bennett GJ (1995): Intravenous infusion of the NMDA antagonist, ketamine, in chronic posttraumatic pain with allodynia—a double-blind comparison to alfentanil and placebo. Clin Neuropharmacol 18:360–368.

McQuay HJ, Carroll D, Jadad AR, Glynn CJ, Jack T, Moore RA, Wiffen PJ (1994): Dextromethorphan for the treatment of neuropathic pain: a double-blind randomised controlled crossover trial with integral n-of-1 design. Pain 59:127–133.

Meldrum BS (1985): Possible therapeutic applications of antagonists of excitatory amino acid neurotransmitters. Clin Sci 68:113–122.

Meller ST (1996): Ketamine—relief from chronic pain through actions at the NMDA receptor. Pain 68:435–436.

Meller ST, Dykstra CL, Gebhart GF (1993): Acute mechanical hyperalgesia is produced by coactivation of AMPA and metabotropic glutamate receptors. Neuroreport 4:879–882.

Meller ST, Dykstra CL, Gebhart GF (1996): Acute thermal hyperalgesia in the rat is produced by activation of N-methyl-D-aspartate receptors and protein kinase C and production of nitric oxide. Neuroscience 71:327–335.

Mercadante S, Lodi F, Sapio M, Calligara M, Serretta R (1995): Long-term ketamine subcutaneous continuous infusion in neuropathic cancer pain. J Pain Symptom Management 10:564–568.

Millan MJ, Seguin L (1994): Chemically-diverse ligands at the glycine B site coupled to N-methyl-D-aspartate (NMDA) receptors selectively block the late phase of formalin-induced pain in mice. Neurosci Lett 178:139–143.

Miller KE, Clements JR, Larson AA, Beitz AJ (1988): Organization of glutamate-like immunoreactivity in the rat superficial dorsal horn: light and electron microscopic observations. J Comp Neurol 277:28–36.

Monaghan DT, Cotman CW (1985): Distribution of N-methyl-D-aspartate-sensitive L-[^{3}H]glutamate-binding sites in rat brain. J Neurosci 5:2909–2919.

Murray CW, Cowan A, Larson AA (1991): Neurokinin and NMDA antagonists (but not a kainic acid antagonist) are antinociceptive in the mouse formalin model. Pain 44: 179–185.

Näsström J, Karlsson U, Post C (1992): Antinociceptive actions of different classes of excitatory amino acid receptor antagonists in mice. Eur J Pharmacol 212:21–29.

Neugebauer V, Kornhuber J, Lucke T, Schaible HG (1993): The clinically available NMDA receptor antagonist memantine is antinociceptive on rat spinal neurones. Neuroreport 4:1259–1262.

Neugebauer V, Lucke T, Schaible HG (1994): Requirement of metabotropic glutamate receptors for the generation of inflammation-evoked hyperexcitability in rat spinal cord neurons. Eur J Neurosci 6:1179–1186.

Nicolodi M, Sicuteri F (1995): Exploration of NMDA receptors in migraine: therapeutic and theoretic implications. Int J Clin Pharmacol Res 15:181–189.

Nikolajsen L, Hansen CL, Nielsen J, Keller J, Arendtnielsen L, Jensen TS (1996): The effect of ketamine on phantom pain—a central neuropathic disorder maintained by peripheral input. Pain 67:69–77.

Olney JW (1990): Excitotoxic amino-acids and neuropsychiatric disorders. Ann Rev Pharm Toxicol 30:47–71.

Onaka M, Minami T, Nishihara I, Ito S (1996): Involvement of glutamate receptors in strychnine- and bicuculline-induced allodynia in conscious mice. Anesthesiology 84: 1215–1222.

Oshima E, Tei K, Kayazawa H, Urabe N (1990): Continuous subcutaneous injection of ketamine for cancer pain. Can J Anaesth 37:385–392.

Oye I, Paulsen O, Maurset A (1992): Effects of ketamine on sensory perception: Evidence for a role of N-methyl-D-aspartate receptors. J Pharmacol Exp Ther 260:1209–1213.

Oye I, Rabben T, Fagerlund TH (1996): Analgesic effect of ketamine in a patient with neuropathic pain. Tidsskrift Den Norske Laegeforening 116:3130–3131.

Palecek J, Palečková V, Dougherty PM, Willis WD (1994): The effect of *trans*-ACPD, a metabotropic excitatory amino acid receptor agonist, on the responses of primate spinothalamic tract neurons. Pain 56:261–269.

Park KM, Max MB, Robinovitz E, Gracely RH, Bennett GJ (1995): Effects of intravenous ketamine, alfentanil, or placebo on pain, pinprick hyperalgesia, and allodynia produced by intradermal capsaicin in human subjects. Pain 63:163–172.

Perrault G, Morel E, Joly D, Sanger DJ, Zivkovic B (1990): Differential neuropsychopharmacological profiles of NMDA antagonists: Ifenprodil-like, PCP-like and CPP-like compounds. Eur J Pharmacol 183:942.

Persson J, Axelsson G, Hallin RG, Gustafsson LL (1995): Beneficial effects of ketamine in a chronic pain state with allodynia, possibly due to central sensitization. Pain 60: 217–222.

Price DD, Mao J, Frenk H, Mayer DJ (1994): The N-methyl-D-aspartate receptor antagonist dextromethorphan selectively reduces temporal summation of second pain in man. Pain 59:165–174.

Qian J, Brown SD, Carlton SM (1996): Systemic ketamine attenuates nociceptive behaviours in a rat model of peripheral neuropathy. Brain Res 715:51–62.

Randic M, Jiang MC, Cerne R (1993): Long-term potentiation and long-term depression of primary afferent neurotransmission in the rat spinal cord. J Neurosci 13:5228–5241.

Ransom RW, Stec NL (1988): Cooperative modulation of [^{3}H]MK-801 binding to the N-methyl-D-aspartate receptor-ion channel complex by L-glutamate, glycine, and polyamines. J Neurochem 51:830–836.

Ren K, Dubner R (1993): NMDA receptor antagonists attenuate mechanical hyperalgesia in rats with unilateral inflammation of the hindpaw. Neurosci Lett 163:22–26.

Ren K, Hylden JLK, Williams GM, Ruda MA, Dubner R (1992): The effects of a non-competitive NMDA receptor antagonist, MK-801, on behavioural hyperalgesia and dorsal horn neuronal activity in rats with unilateral inflammation. Pain 50:331–344.

Rice ASC, McMahon SB (1994): Pre-emptive intrathecal administration of an NMDA receptor antagonist (AP-5) prevents hyper-reflexia in a model of persistent visceral pain. Pain 57:335–340.

Schaible H-G, Grubb BD, Neugebauer V, Oppmann M (1991): The effects of NMDA antagonists on neuronal activity in cat spinal cord evoked by acute inflammation in the knee joint. Eur J Neurosci 3:981–991.

Seltzer Z, Cohn S, Ginzburg R, Beilin BZ (1991): Modulation of neuropathic pain behaviour in rats by spinal disinhibition and NMDA receptor blockade of injury discharge. Pain 45:69–75.

Shaw PJ, Ince PG, Johnson M, Perry EK, Candy J (1991): The quantitative autoradiographic distribution of [^{3}H] MK-801 binding sites in the normal human spinal cord. Brain Res 539:164–168.

Skilling SR, Smullin DH, Larson AA (1988): Extracellular amino acid concentrations in the dorsal spinal cord of freely moving rats following veratridine and nociceptive stimulation. J Neurochem 51:127–132.

Sluka KA, Westlund KN (1992): An experimental arthritis in rats: Dorsal horn aspartate and glutamate increases. Neurosci Lett 145:141–144.

Smith GD, Harrison SM, Birch PJ (1995): Peri-administration of clonidine or MK801 delays but does not prevent the development of mechanical hyperalgesia in a model of mononeuropathy in the rat. Neurosci Lett 192:33–36.

Sorensen J, Bengtsson A, Backman E, Henriksson KG, Bengtsson M (1995): Pain analysis in patients with fibromyalgia—effects of intravenous morphine, lidocaine, and ketamine. Scand J Rheumatol 24:360–365.

Sorkin LS, Puig S (1996): Neuronal model of tactile allodynia produced by spinal strychnine—effects of excitatory amino acid receptor antagonists and a mu-opiate receptor agonist. Pain 68:283–292.

Stannard CF, Porter GE (1993): Ketamine hydrochloride in the treatment of phantom limb pain. Pain 54:227–230.

Sun X, Larson AA (1991): Behavioural sensitization to kainic acid and quisqualic acid in mice: Comparison to NMDA and substance P responses. J Neurosci 11:3111–3123.

Suzuki T, Kato J, Saeki S, Ogawa S, Suzuki H (1996): Analgesic effect of dextromethorphan for postherpetic neuralgia. Masui—Jap J Anesthesiol 45:629–633.

Tal M, Bennett GJ (1994): Neuropathic pain sensations are differentially sensitive to dextrorphan. Neuroreport 5:1438–1440.

Thompson SWN, Gerber G, Sivilotti LG, Woolf CJ (1992): Long duration ventral root potentials in the neonatal rat spinal cord *in vitro*; The effects of ionotropic and metabotropic excitatory amino acid receptor antagonists. Brain Res 595:87–97.

Ueda M, Kuraishi Y, Sugimoto K, Satoh M (1994): Evidence that glutamate is released from capsaicin-sensitive primary afferent fibers in rats: study with on-line continuous monitoring of glutamate. Neurosci Res 20:231–237.

Ueda M, Sugimoto K, Oyama T, Kuraishi Y, Satoh M (1995): Opioidergic inhibition of capsaicin-evoked release of glutamate from rat spinal dorsal horn slices. Neuropharmacology 34:303–308.

Vaccarino AL, Marek P, Kest B, Weber E, Keane JFW, Liebeskind JC (1993): NMDA receptor antagonists, MK-801 and ACEA-1011, prevent the development of tonic pain following subcutaneous formalin. Brain Res 615:331–334.

Warncke T, Jorum E, Stubhaug A (1997): Local treatment with the N-methyl-D-aspartate receptor antagonist ketamine, inhibits development of secondary hyperalgesia in man by a peripheral action. Neurosci Lett 227:1–4.

Willetts J, Balster RL, Leander JD (1990): The behavioural pharmacology of NMDA receptor antagonists. Trends Pharmacol Sci 11:423–428.

Williams K, Romano C, Molinoff PB (1989): Effects of polyamines on the binding of [^{3}H] MK-801 to the N-methyl-D-aspartate receptor: Pharmacological evidence for the existence of a polyamine recognition site. Mol Pharmacol 36:575–581.

Woolf CJ, Thompson SWN (1991): The induction and maintenance of central sensitization is dependent on N-methyl-D-aspartic acid receptor activation: implications for post-injury pain hypersensitivity states. Pain 44:293–299.

Xiao W-H, Bennett GJ (1994): Magnesium suppresses neuropathic pain responses in rats via a spinal site of action. Brain Res 666:168–172.

Xu XJ, Hao JX, Seiger A, Wiesenfeld-Hallin Z (1993): Systemic excitatory amino acid receptor antagonists of the alpha-amino-3-hydroxy-5-methyl-4-isoxazolepropionic acid (AMPA) receptor and of the N-methyl-D-aspartate (NMDA) receptor relieve mechanical hypersensitivity after transient spinal cord ischemia in rats. J Pharmacol Exp Ther 267:140–144.

Yamamoto T, Yaksh TL (1992a): Comparison of the antinociceptive effects of pre- and post-treatment with intrathecal morphine and MK-801, an NMDA antagonist, on the formalin test in the rat. Anesthesiology 77:757–763.

Yamamoto T, Yaksh TL (1992b): Spinal pharmacology of thermal hyperesthesia induced by constriction injury of sciatic nerve. II. Excitatory amino acid antagonists. Pain 49:121–128.

Yang LC, Marsala M, Yaksh TL (1996): Characterization of time course of spinal amino acids, citrulline and PGE$_2$ release after carrageenan/kaolin-induced knee joint inflammation—a chronic microdialysis study. Pain 67:345–354.

Young MR, Fleetwood-Walker M, Mitchell R, Munro FE (1994): Evidence for a role of metabotropic glutamate receptors in sustained nociceptive inputs to rat dorsal horn neurons. Neuropharmacol 33:141–144.

Young MR, Fleetwood-Walker M, Mitchell R, Dickenson T (1995): The involvement of metabotropic glutamate receptors and their intracellular signalling pathways in sustained nociceptive transmission in rat dorsal horn neurons. Neuropharmacol 34: 1033–1041.

Zhou ST, Bonasera L, Carlton SM (1996): Peripheral administration of NMDA, AMPA or KA results in pain behaviours in rats. Neuroreport 7:895–900.

CHAPTER 9

ALPHA-2 ADRENERGIC AGONISTS AS ANALGESICS

TONY L. YAKSH
University of California, San Diego
La Jolla, California

Sympathomimetic agonists have long been known to alter nociceptive transmission and to attenuate the behavioral response to an otherwise noxious stimulus, that is, produce analgesia. Weber (1904) demonstrated in unanesthetized rabbits that injection of an extract from the adrenal medulla (Adrenalinstöffe) would block the thermally evoked hindpaw withdrawal. Subsequent investigations with systemically delivered agents also demonstrated a potent effect in humans (Kiessig and Orzechowski, 1941; Burrill et al., 1961) and animals (Kroneberg et al., 1967; Schmitt et al., 1974a,b). These early observations laid the groundwork that foreshadowed the present interest in the clinical implementation of alpha-2 adrenoceptor agonists as analgesics. Various aspects of the mechanisms and actions of the antinociceptive effects of alpha-2 adrenergic agonists are considered here. Particular focus is placed on the role of the spinal cord in these actions.

ALPHA-2 ADRENERGIC RECEPTOR AND SUBTYPES

Early work led to the appreciation that sympathomimetic agonists could exert their effects by several subclasses of receptors. The first separation of receptor type was alpha versus beta (Ahlquist, 1948). Subsequently, studies examining the effects of various agents on the release of norepinephrine led to the appreciation that adrenergic agonists could inhibit the release of noradrenaline from sympathetic terminals; this developed into the concept that a specific adrenergic receptor could be sympatholytic by blocking the terminal release of noradrenaline. Such work has culminated in the development of agents that can selec-

Novel Aspects of Pain Management: Opioids and Beyond, Edited by Jana Sawynok and Alan Cowan
ISBN 0-471-180173 Copyright © 1999 by Wiley-Liss, Inc.

tively activate and antagonize α-adrenergic receptors; several of these are listed in Table 9.1.

In the early 1980s, it was further appreciated that the α_2 adrenergic receptor might possess additional subtypes. The existence of at least three distinct subtypes—α_{2A}, α_{2B} and α_{2C}—has been proposed on the basis of several lines of convergent evidence: (*a*) differential association with chromosomes 10 (Kobilka et al., 1987), 2 (Regan et al., 1988), and 4 (Lomasney et al., 1990); (*b*) isolation and cloning of receptor message (Aantaa et al., 1995); (*c*) definition of distinctive bioassay profiles (see Bylund, 1995). Species differences have been identified. Thus an α_{2D} receptor was found in the rat and was subsequently thought to be the rodent homologue of the α_{2A} receptor found in humans (MacKinnon et al., 1994). Characteristics of the receptor subtypes are summarized in Table 9.1.

The α_2 receptor, once sequenced, was found to be a member of the superfamily of G-protein-coupled receptors. It thus has seven transmembrane spanning regions and displays considerable sequence homology with other such receptors.

TABLE 9.1 Summary of the Properties of α_2 Receptor Subtypes

	α_2 Receptor Subtypes		
	α_{2A}	α_{2B}	α_{2C}
Receptor Property[a]			
Location on chromosome	C10	C2	C4
Receptor structure			
Number of amino acids	450	450	461
Transmembrane domains	7	7	7
Second messenger	Gi/o	Gi/o	Gi/o
Pharmacology[b]			
Agonists			
Dexmedetomidine	+++	++	+
Clonidine	+++	++	+
UK14304	+++	+	+
Oxymetazoline	+++	0	+
Antagonists			
WB4101	+++	+	+
Atipamezole	+++	+++	+++
Idazoxan	++	++	++
Yohimbine	++	+++	+++
Prazosin	0	++	++
Imiloxan	0	++	++

[a]See MacDonald et al., 1997; Marjamaki et al., 1993; Jansson et al., 1994.
[b]Affinity: K_d +++ < 10; ++ <100; + <1000; 0 >1000 nM.

Functional Coupling of α_2 Receptors

Biochemical studies have revealed that agonist activation of this receptor suppresses adenylate cyclase activity. This receptor was coupled to Gi/o protein and exerted many of the effects that were attendant to such coupling, notably increasing K^+ conductance leading to a hyperpolarization of excitable membranes and inhibiting the opening of voltage-sensitive calcium channels and thereby reducing transmitter release in several systems, including the sympathetic terminal and the terminals of small primary afferents (see North et al., 1987; Holz et al., 1989; Maze and Tranquilli, 1991).

ADRENOCEPTOR MODULATION OF NOCICEPTION

Spinal Adrenoceptors in Physiological Systems Regulating Nociceptive Processing

As noted previously, some classic observations have emphasized that adrenoceptor agonists can exert potent antinociceptive effects after systemic and spinal delivery. Anden et al. (1966) showed that systemic L-dopa, which increases the release of noradrenaline from spinal terminals in acutely spinal transsected cats, can suppress ventral root activity otherwise evoked by small afferents. These effects were reversed by phenoxybenzamine, an adrenergic receptor antagonist (Anden et al., 1966). It was later demonstrated that microinjection of mu opioid agonists into the brainstem, or electrical stimulation in the brainstem, would suppress spinal nociceptive reflexes and produce a behaviorally defined analgesia (see Yaksh and Rudy, 1978 for review). Subsequent work demonstrated that supraspinal manipulations blocking spinal reflexes would (*a*) evoke the release of noradrenaline from the spinal cord (Hammond et al., 1985); (*b*) be blocked at the spinal level by antagonism of α-noradrenergic receptors of the α_2 receptor type (Yaksh, 1979; Kuraishi et al., 1979a; Jensen and Yaksh, 1986) (see Fig. 9.1), and (*c*) that the antinociceptive effects of supraspinal manipulations were mimicked by spinal delivery of noradrenaline and other α_2 adrenoceptor agonists (Kuraishi et al., 1979b; Reddy et al., 1980). These findings emphasized the physiological importance of bulbospinal projections and demonstrated the role played by adrenergic systems and the spinal α_2 receptor in this control.

Antinociceptive Effects of Spinal α_2 Adrenoceptor Agonists

Subsequent preclinical work emphasized the general relevance of this spinal antinociceptive action arising from the activation of spinal adrenergic receptors.

Species. Systemic and spinal injections of α_2 adrenoceptor agonists in frogs (Brenner et al., 1994; Craig Stevens, personal communication), mice (Hylden and Wilcox, 1983; Ossipov et al., 1989), rats (Reddy et al., 1980; Howe et al.,

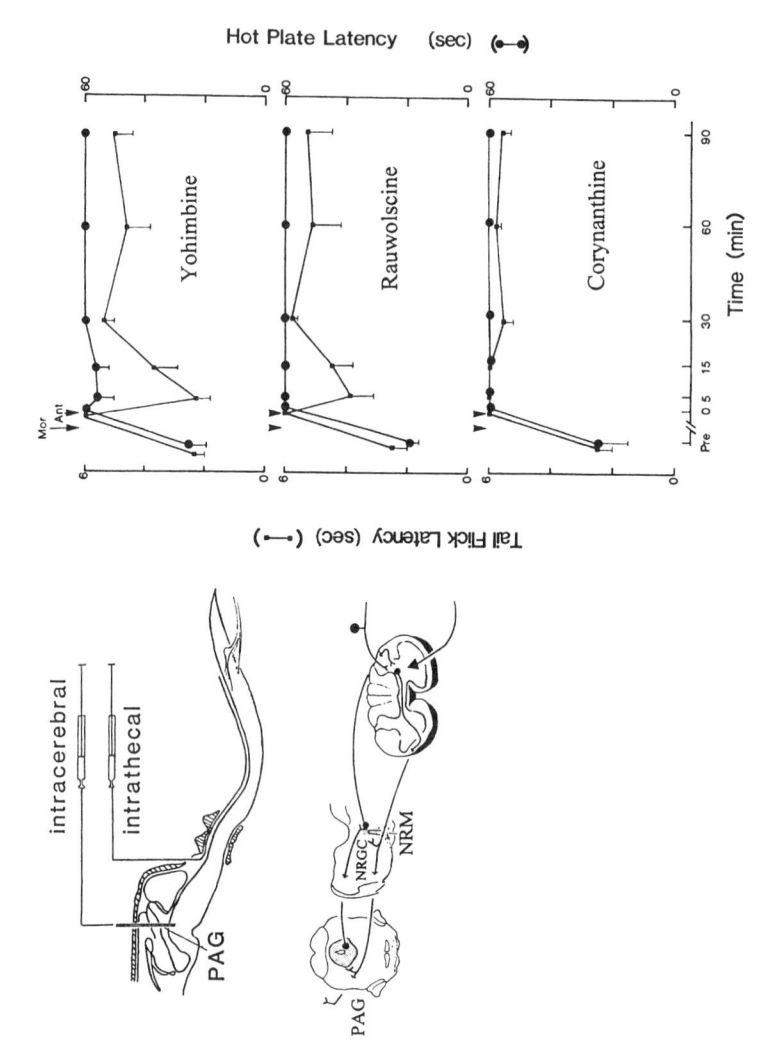

Figure 9.1 (Left) Schematic indicating the experimental paradigm in which the rat is prepared with a chronic intrathecal catheter and an indwelling microinjection guide cannula in the periaqueductal gray. The microinjection of morphine is believed to result in the activation of a bulbospinal pathway that regulates spinal nociceptive reflexes. (Right) The delivery of morphine (5 μg/0.5 μl) in the PAG results in an increase in the tail flick response latency (left), and the intrathecal injection of yohimbine or rauwolscine, but not corynanthine (all in doses of 30 μg/10 μl), results in a reversal of the anti-reflexive action of PAG–morphine. Similar results were observed with intrathecal prazosin (data not shown) (from Camarata and Yaksh, 1985).

1983; Sherman et al., 1988), dogs (Sabbe et al., 1994), sheep (Waterman et al., 1988; Eisenach et al., 1989a), ponies (Fikes et al., 1989; Skarda and Muir, 1996) or primates (Yaksh and Reddy, 1981) result in powerful, dose-dependent increases in the level of noxious stimulation that the animal will tolerate as measured by (*a*) increases in the threshold mechanical or thermal stimulus necessary to evoke an escape response; (*b*) increase of the latency with which an animal responds to a given stimulus; (*c*) increase in the index of responding that reflects the intensity of the stimulus (e.g., number of flinches). Importantly, these effects occur at doses that fail to alter either normal motor behavior or the response to non-noxious stimuli. Thus, in the primate, intrathecal clonidine at doses that produced a powerful analgesic action failed to alter the ability of the animal to recognize low-threshold tactile stimuli applied to regions rendered analgesic (Yaksh and Reddy, 1981).

Antinociceptive Models. Preclinical studies emphasized that the activation of α_2 adrenoceptors can exert an antinociceptive effect in a wide variety of nociceptive models involving (*a*) pain/escape behavior evoked by an acute high-intensity somatic (hot plate, tail flick, tail dip) (see Fig. 9.2) or visceral (colonic distention) stimulus; (*b*) facilitated states of nociceptive processing evoked by tissue injury (formalin, carrageenan-evoked thermal and mechanical hyperalgesia); (*c*) post nerve injury pain models (thermal hyperalgesia; tactile allodynia) (see Fig. 9.3) (for review of models see Yaksh, 1997). The antinociceptive effect of spinal adrenoceptor agonists has been demonstrated in a wide variety of animal models. A brief summary of several representative models that were examined are presented in Table 9.2.

A consideration of the physiological substrate underlying several classes of nociceptive processing has led to the broad appreciation that they represent distinct underlying mechanisms (see Yaksh, 1997 for extensive discussion of preclinical models). Importantly, where examined, these effects are believed to be mediated by an action on α_2 receptors. The pharmacological criteria for that assertion is typically based on (*a*) the effects of defined α_2 agonists (such as dexmedetomidine, clonidine, ST-91), but not α_1 (methoxamine, cirazoline) or β (isoproterenol) agonists, and (*b*) the ability to antagonize the actions of the putative α_2 agonists by agents considered to have selective affinity for α_2 sites (e.g., yohimbine, rauwolscine, atipamezole) (see Figs. 9.2 and 9.3).

In all cases, where examined, these antinociceptive actions have been characterized by a specific pharmacology that is defined by a consistent agonist and antagonist structure–activity relationship. The activity observed in a variety of models is summarized in Table 9.2. Several important elements should be extracted from this table: (*a*) In terms of the rank ordering of agonist activity, in models of acute nociception (hot plate), facilitated processing (formalin test), and neuropathic pain (Chung model-tactile allodynia) in rodents, as well as across species (rat thermal escape versus primate thermal escape), there are no differences with respect to the agonists examined. (*b*) Considering antagonist potency, the ability of four intrathecally delivered antagonists (yohimbine, pra-

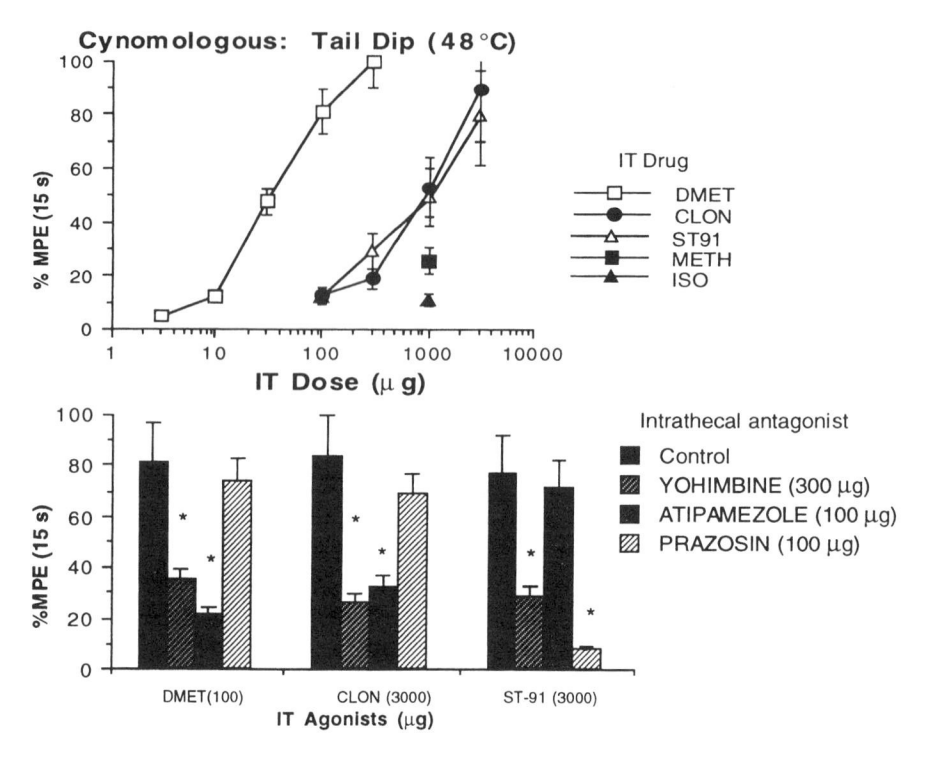

Figure 9.2 (Top) Dose effect curve for intrathecal dexmedetomidine (DMET), clonidine (CLON), ST-91, methoxamine (METH), or isoproterenol (ISO) in blocking the withdrawal response of the tail of primates evoked by tail immersion in 48°C water. (Bottom) Effects of intrathecal pretreatment with saline (control), yohimbine, atipamezole, or prazosin on the increased tail dip response latency otherwise evoked by intrathecal DMET, CLON, or ST-91 (Yaksh, unpublished observations).

zosin, rauwolscine, and corynanthine) to reverse the effect of exogenous adrenoceptor agonists or to reverse the antinociceptive effects of morphine given into the periaqueductal gray is no different. These observations suggest that the pharmacology of the α_2 receptor mediating the effects of several exogenous agonists, as well as endogenously released noradrenaline from the bulbospinal pathway activated by supraspinal morphine, is indistinguishable. The potent effects of prazosin may reflect upon an α_1 adrenoceptor effect. However, this alternative is considered unlikely, because intrathecal α_1 agonists such as methoxamine or cirazoline are not antinociceptive (Howe et al., 1983; Takano and Yaksh, 1992) and prazosin, although it is a good α_1 antagonist, also has significant affinity for the α_{2nonA} receptor (see Table 9.3).

The identity of the receptor subtype that regulates nociceptive processing is currently the subject of great interest. Takano and colleagues demonstrated that the intrathecal action of dexmedetomidine, clonidine, and ST-91 were all readily reversed by yohimbine (Takano et al., 1992; Takano and Yaksh, 1992).

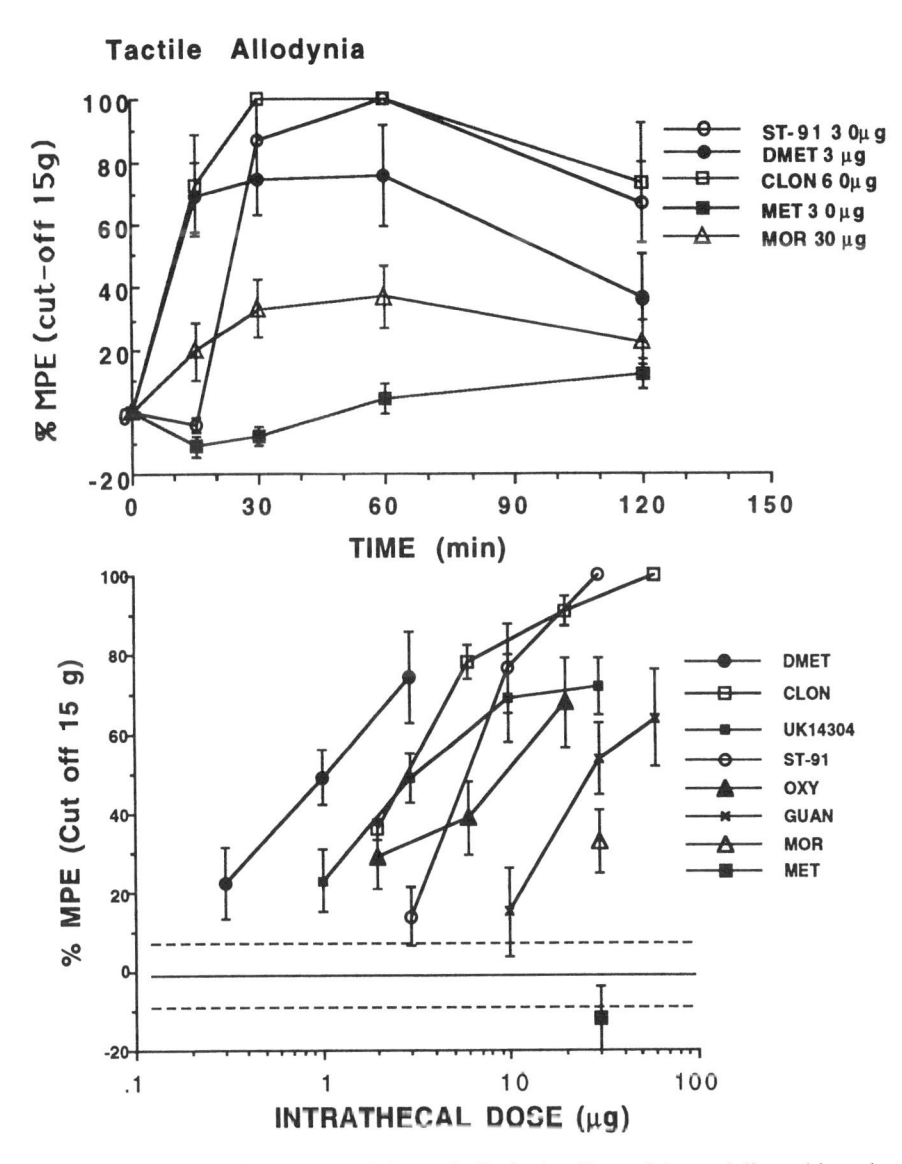

Figure 9.3 (Top) Time course of the anti-allodynic effect of drugs delivered intrathecally in rats rendered allodynic by L5/L6 nerve ligation. Each line presents the mean and S.E.M. of four to six rats. Doses shown in micrograms are those that produce a maximum effect or represent the maximum usable doses. (Bottom) Dose–response curves plotting the peak effect (% of the maximum possible effect, %MPE) observed within 60 min after the intrathecal injection versus the intrathecal drug dose in rats prepared with L5/L6 nerve ligations to be allodynic. Each point presents the mean and S.E.M. for four to six rats (CLON, clonidine; DMET, dexemedetomidine; GUAN, guanafacine; MET, methoxamine; MOR, morphine; OXY, oxymetazoline) (from Yaksh et al., 1995).

TABLE 9.2 Antinociceptive Effects of Spinal α_2 Agonists

Class of Test	Test Model	References
Acute nociceptive stimulus		
Thermal	Hot plate	Reddy et al., 1980; Kuraishi et al., 1985; Kalso et al., 1991
	Tail flick	Takano and Yaksh, 1992; Horvath et al., 1997
	Evoked autonomic response	Nagasaka and Yaksh, 1990; Saeki and Yaksh, 1992
Mechanical	Tail compression	Kuraishi et al., 1985
Cutaneous shock	Foot shock titration	Yaksh and Reddy, 1981
Visceral-mechanical	Colonic distention	Ness and Gebhart, 1989; Danzebrink and Gebhart, 1990
Tissue injury/inflammation		
Visceral-irritant	Writhing	Yaksh, 1985
Cutaneous-irritant	Formalin test	Malmberg and Yaksh, 1992
Nerve injury		
Nerve section	Autotomy	Puke et al., 1991
Bennett model	Thermal hyperalgesia	Yamamoto and Yaksh, 1991
Chung model	Tactile allodynia	Yaksh et al., 1995
Spinal ischemia-focal	Allodynia	Xu et al., 1992
Spinal ischemia-global	Tactile allodynia	Marsala and Yaksh, unpublished

However, although the effects of intrathecal clonidine and dexmedetomidine were reversed by atipamezole, the effects of ST-91 were not (see Fig. 4). Conversely, intrathecal prazosin reversed the effects of ST-91, but not clonidine or atipamezole. Given the affinity of prazosin for the α_{2nonA} site, it was speculated that at least a component of the yohimbine sensitive receptors that regulated nociceptive transmissions were α_{2nonA} in character. This argument is supported additionally by the observation that the effects of ST-91 are reversed by imiloxan, an α_2 nonpreferring antagonist (see Table 9.1). In these studies, there is clearly the likelihood of two sites, reflecting actions mediated by α_{2A} and α_{2nonA} elements. The possibility of two sites is consistent with the observation of a differential cross-tolerance in rats receiving chronic spinal delivery of dexmedetomidine and ST-91 (Takano and Yaksh, 1993). Although all types of α_2 receptors have been identified at the spinal level, their absolute levels differ (Uhlen and Wikberg, 1991; Rosin et al., 1993; Smith et al., 1995; Rosin et al., 1996). Studies utilizing a systemic route of administration also have addressed the issue of the α_2 receptor subtype involved in antinociception. Thus mice with aberrant α_{2A} sites showed a reduced antinociception in response to systemic dexmedetomidine, whereas those deficient in α_{2B} and α_{2C} sites were not

TABLE 9.3 ID$_{50}$ Values for Effects of Adrenergic Antagonists on the Antinociceptive Effects Produced by Periaqueductal Gray Morphine or Norepinephrine, ST-91, Dexmedetomidine, or Clonidine[a]

Test Drug	MI-PAG Morphine (5 μg) TF	NE (10 μg i.t.) TF	ST-91 (10 μg i.t.) TF	ST-91 (20 μg i.t.) HP	Dexmedetomidine (10 μg i.t.) HP	Clonidine (100 μg i.t.) HP
Phentolamine	38	26	18			
Yohimbine	4.9	43	1.1	23	24	14
Rauwolscine	14	39	2.3			
Corynanthine	140	98	249			
Prazosin	5.6	2.4	10	11	>33	>33
Propranolol	>386	>386	>386			

[a]ID$_{50}$ values represent the dose (in nM) of intrathecally administered antagonists that produced a 50% reduction in the antinociceptive effects of PAG morphine (Camarata and Yaksh 1985) or intrathecally administered norepinephrine or ST-91 on the tail flick test (TF) (Yaksh, 1985) and ST-91, dexmedetomidine, and clonidine on the hot plate test (HP) (Takano and Yaksh, 1992). In all work, the intrathecal agent was administered 5–15 min after the PAG morphine or 5–10 min after the intrathecal alpha agonist. Each entry presents the mean ID$_{50}$ calculated from the regression equation and the 95% dose confidence interval.
>: No reversal of the response inhibition was observed at this dose.

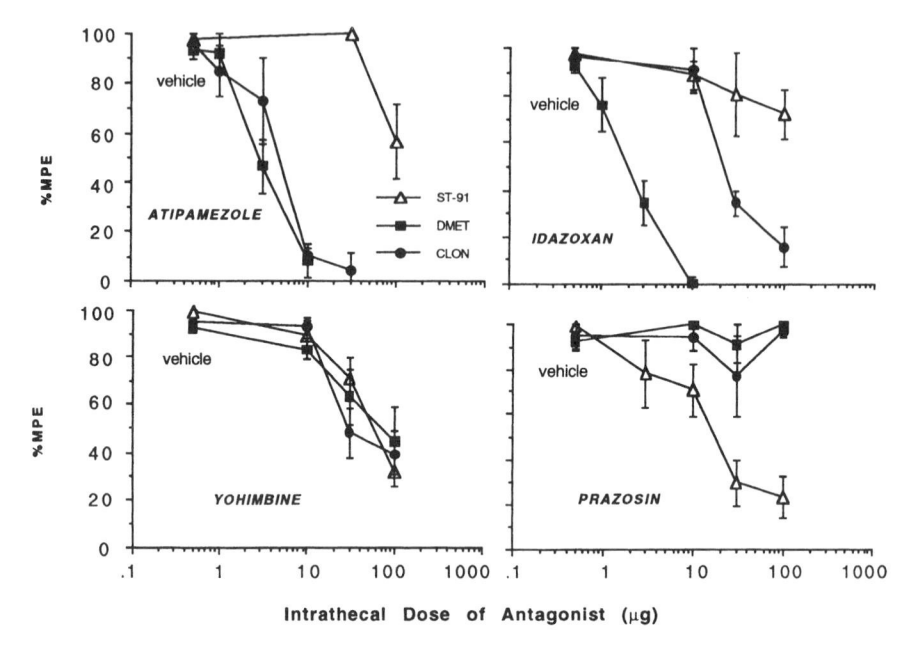

Figure 9.4 Antagonist dose–response curves (maximum %MPE vs. log dose) for atipamezole (top left), yohimbine (bottom left), idazoxan (upper right), and prazosin (lower right) carried out in each case with a maximally effective dose of ST-91 (20 mg), DMET (10 mg), or CLON (100 mg). The left end point of each dose–response curve represents %MPE data of each agonist administration with respective vehicle (VEH) for antagonist injected at proper time (from Takano and Yaksh, 1992).

(Hunter et al., 1997). Millan et al. (1994) had previously compared the activity of a structural series of agents when given systemically to the mouse with different affinity for the several α_2 binding sites. Although motor effects appeared to correlate with α_{2A} affinity, the activity in tail flick and writhing tests was in fact comparable across $\alpha_{2A,B,C}$ receptor types. These approaches, although important, employ systemic delivery and thus say little about the nature of the spinal systems that are relevant to the spinal α_2 receptor systems related to regulation of nociceptive processing.

Mechanisms of α_2 Adrenoceptor-Mediated Antinociceptive Actions

As noted above, early studies indicated that the spinal delivery of adrenaline would result in a powerful antinociceptive action in animal models, and this finding has been widely confirmed. In the following sections, mechanisms that may impact upon the several classes of nociceptive processing at different potential loci of action are summarized.

Peripheral Actions. Although considerable attention has been focused on central actions of α_2 agonists (see below), there is also evidence that α_2 agonists may exert a direct effect upon the sensitivity of the peripheral terminal of the sensory afferent that is innervating injured or inflamed tissue. Previous work has demonstrated that following local tissue injury, there is the generation of spontaneous activity in small primary afferents, an increase in the slope of the stimulus–response relationship (reflecting a sensitization of the peripheral terminal), and the appearance of a behaviorally defined hyperalgesia (see Schaible and Grubb, 1993; Dray, 1997). After nerve injury, α_2 preferring receptors may be involved in the activation of sensory afferents by peripheral noradrenaline release from sympathetic terminals (Sato and Perl, 1991). Khasar and colleagues (1995) demonstrated that locally applied α_2 agonists, such as clonidine or WB14304, may suppress the hyperalgesia otherwise induced by the local cutaneous injection of prostaglandin E_2. Considering the relative potency of antagonists believed to vary in affinity for the α_2 receptor subtype, it was argued that the effects may be mediated by an α_{2nonA} site. Though their observations are based on only moderately selective compounds, they have in fact argued that the pharmacology supports the hypothesis that α_{2B} receptors are on sympathetic nerve terminals and α_{2C} receptors are on the primary afferent terminals. These data suggest that under certain circumstances, α_2 agonists may regulate the excitability of the peripheral terminal. The mechanisms of this regulation, and whether it is directly upon the terminals or upon adjacent inflammatory cells that are otherwise releasing cytokines, is not at present known.

Spinal Actions. The mechanisms of the effect of spinal α_2 agonists are believed to be associated with a spinal modulation of small afferent transmission at sites pre- and postsynaptic to the small primary afferent. This thinking is based on several properties. Identification of α_2 adrenoceptor binding sites as defined by the binding of [^{3}H]rauwolscine has been shown to be highest within the dorsal horn of the spinal cord; rhizotomies reduce this binding, suggesting that these sites are in part located on the terminals of primary afferents (Howe et al., 1987). It is appreciated that the depolarization of small afferents (C fibers) results in the spinal release of substance P and calcitonin gene-related peptide (CGRP) (see Wilcox and Seybold, 1997). Accordingly, the ability of α_2 adrenoceptor agonists to reduce the afferent-evoked (Go and Yaksh, 1987) or capsaicin-evoked release of substance P and CGRP (Takano et al., 1993) from spinal slices is considered to support the hypothesis that these agents exert a direct effect upon small afferent terminals (Calvillo and Ghignone, 1986) (see Fig. 9.5). These observations are consistent with the ability of spinal α_2 agonists to suppress somatic and viscerosomatic spinal reflexes preferentially (Downie and Bialik, 1988; Downie et al., 1991); the excitation of dorsal horn neurons evoked by C, but not by Aβ, afferent activity is also suppressed (Fleetwood-Walker et al., 1985; Murata et al., 1989; Sullivan et al., 1992; Hamalainen and Pertovaara, 1995). In addition, the ability of locally delivered α_2 adrenoceptor agonists to suppress the direct excitation evoked by the iontophoretically de-

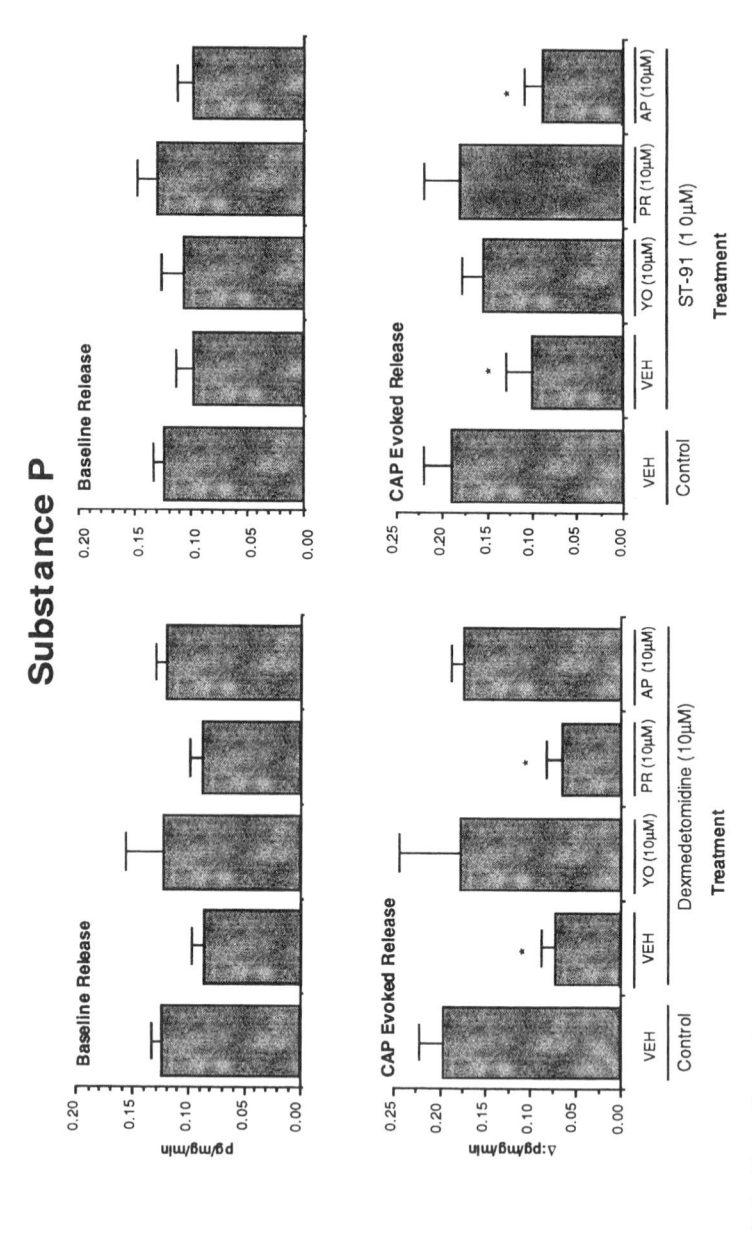

Figure 9.5 The effect of α_2 agonists dexmedetomidine (10 μM; left panels) and ST-91 (10 μM, right panels) on the resting (top) and capsaicin-evoked (bottom) release of substance P when given alone (vehicle: VEH) or in the presence of the α_2 antagonist yohimbine (YO, 10 μM); prazosin (PR, 10 μM); or atipamezole (AP, 10 μM). Each histogram presents the mean and S.E.M. of the resting release (baseline release: pg/mg/min) or the difference between levels measured prior to capsaicin subtracted from the levels measured with capsaicin (CAP, evoked release, pg/mg/min). Each drug effect is based on data from 6 to 20 experiments. (Note different ordinate scales for top and bottom histograms.) (From Takano et al., 1993.)

livered glutamate (Fleetwood-Walker et al., 1985) is believed to be consistent with the ability of α_2 receptors to hyperpolarize dorsal horn neurons by an increase in potassium conductance through a Gi-coupled protein (North and Yoshimura, 1984; North et al., 1987).

Previous work has shown that the facilitation of dorsal horn neurons generated by repetitive afferent activation depends upon the activation of small (C-fiber) primary afferents. The observation that α_2 receptor activation can inhibit the release of afferent transmitters is thus consistent with the ability of spinally delivered α_2 agents to produce a potent blockade of dorsal horn wind up and the corresponding facilitation (Sullivan et al., 1992).

The ability of spinal α_2 agonists to diminish the thermal hyperalgesia observed following compression injury of the sciatic nerve (Bennett and Xie, 1988) is consistent with the possibility that small afferent thermal nociceptors may be modulated by spinal α_2 receptors. However, the mechanism by which intrathecally delivered α_2 agonists reduce the tactile allodynia observed after tight ligation of the L5/L6 nerve roots (Kim and Chung, 1992) is not certain. It has been reported that the tactile allodynia in this model is mediated in part by sympathetic nerve activity (Kim et al., 1993). In this regard, as is noted below, spinal α_2 adrenoceptor agonists can reduce sympathetic outflow secondary to a direct inhibitory effect on the preganglionic sympathetic neurons. In this manner, depending on the sympathetic dependency of the pain model, spinal α_2 agonists could reduce the tactile allodynia observed in the Chung model. It should be noted that the tactile allodynia observed after the spinal delivery of strychnine is not diminished by intrathecal α_2 agonists (Yaksh, 1989), indicating that the effects in the Chung model are not strictly due to some unanticipated action upon large (low-threshold) afferent input.

Supraspinal Actions. Although considerable evidence has focused upon the spinal action of α_2 agents in altering nociceptive responses, direct microinjection of α_2 agonists, such as dexmedetomidine, into the locus coeruleus has been shown to produce a dose-dependent increase in the tail flick latency. This effect was blocked by α_2 antagonists (Guo et al., 1996). Although α_2 agonists are known to produce sedation by a supraspinal action, this effect on a spinal reflex may represent the activation of a bulbospinal projection that regulates dorsal horn function. Whether this effect has relevance to the processing of a nociceptive stimulus remains to be seen. The potent sedative effects produced by such supraspinal actions (see below) make specific assessment of antinociception difficult to evaluate.

Non-antinociceptive Actions of α_2 Agonists

Sedation. Aside from their antinociceptive action, α_2 agonists produce a dose-dependent sedation that is associated with high voltage, slow wave electroencephalogram activity (synchronization). The mechanisms of this effect are poorly understood, but intracranial drug delivery studies suggest that this outcome may be mediated in part by an action on α_2 receptors within the dorsal brainstem, perhaps the locus coeruleus (De Sarro et al., 1988).

Respiration. Although systemic and spinally delivered α_2 agonists produce sedation, they produce only mild respiratory depression as compared to opiates. Thus, assessment of CO_2 responsivity in animals and humans after systemic (Bloor et al., 1989; Bailey et al., 1991; Jarvis et al., 1992; Smith et al., 1992, Sabbe et al., 1994) or spinal (Penon et al., 1991; Filos et al., 1992; Sabbe et al., 1994) delivery of α_2 agonists typically shows only a modest reduction in the CO_2-ventilation slope.

Autonomic Outflow. The systemic delivery of α_2 adrenoceptor agonists generally elicits a hypertensive component and a hypotensive component. The latter effect is produced by a reduction in tonic sympathetic activity. Mice deficient in functional α_{2B} receptors display a reduced hypertensive response to α_2 agonists; but mice with a mutation of the α_{2A} receptor display a loss of the hypotensive effect (Link et al., 1996; MacMillan et al., 1996). There were no effects of α_{2C} receptor deficiencies on α_2-agonist-induced changes in blood pressure.

The organization of this effect was considered initially to be mediated by α_2 receptors located preterminally on sympathetic efferents to reduce nerve terminal catecholamine release. Subsequent work demonstrated a supraspinal action of these agents mediated by receptors that were believed to suppress excitatory drive to the intermediolateral preganglionic neurons (Head, 1992). This depression led to a reduction in bulbospinal-mediated excitation of spinal preganglionic neurons located in the intermediolateral cell column outflow (Lopachin and Rudy, 1981; Sundaram et al., 1991). It has also been demonstrated that spinal adrenergic agonists will reduce splanchnic nerve and adrenal secretion (Gaumann et al., 1990). It has been confirmed subsequently that α_2 agonists can reduce sympathetic outflow by a direct action at the spinal level on preganglionic outflow (Eisenach and Tong, 1991).

Antinociceptive Activity of α_2 Agonists in Human Pain States

α_2 adrenergic agonists that have been used in humans have been limited to clonidine and, to a lesser extent, dexmedetomidine. Preclinical safety studies indicate that acute spinal administration of clonidine has no deleterious effects upon spinal cord blood flow in pigs and sheep (Gordh et al., 1986a; Eisenach and Grice, 1988), and systematic 7–14-day intrathecal exposure in rats (Gordh et al., 1986b) or chronic (28-day) epidural infusion in dogs (Yaksh et al., 1994) are without histopathological consequence. Clonidine has recently received FDA approval for epidural delivery (marketed initially under the name of Duraclon in a concentration of 100 μg/mL). Two principal areas of application have been those related to postoperative pain and those associated with neuropathic disorders. An extensive review of the clinical use of clonidine has been published (Eisenach, et al., 1996).

Postoperative Pain. Acute systemic administration of α_2-adrenergic agonists has resulted in antinociception in several clinically relevant human pain states. Thus systemic delivery of α_2-adrenergic agonists (clonidine or dexmedetomidine) causes a reduction in postoperative analgesia requirements (Porchet et al., 1990; Jaakola et al., 1991, but see Striebel et al., 1993). Additionally, oral administration followed by transdermal clonidine in applications sufficient to maintain plasma clonidine concentrations (1–2 ng/mL) in patients receiving general anesthesia for abdominal surgery displayed a postoperative morphine use that was reduced by 40–50%, as compared to placebo control (Segal et al., 1991). Intravenous delivery of clonidine and dexmedetomidine for postoperative pain demonstrates a modest, short-lasting analgesia. In either case, the doses of systemic α_2 agonists are limited by side effects, notably sedation, bradycardia, and hypotension (see Bernard et al., 1991; Segal et al., 1991; De Kock et al., 1992).

In addition to the systemic effects of clonidine, epidural delivery produces a dose-dependent analgesia in postoperative patients, as indicated by pain report, duration of complete analgesia, and reduction in supplemental morphine use (Eisenach et al., 1989a,b; Mendez et al., 1990; Huntoon et al., 1992). Epidural clonidine analgesia is brief in comparison to morphine, requiring continuous infusion for sustained analgesia. Several studies have examined clonidine infusion rates of 10–40 µg/hr and demonstrated rate-dependent reduction in supplemental postoperative morphine (Mendez et al., 1990; Huntoon et al., 1992). These infusions are reported not to cause sedation, respiratory depression, or clinically significant hypotension and bradycardia.

Neuropathic Pain. Systemic clonidine has modest effects upon neuropathic pain states at clinically usable doses (Kingery, 1997). Max et al. (1988) reported moderate oral efficacy in postherpetic neuralgia.

As noted above, systemic and spinal α_2 agonists can cause sympatholysis. Accordingly, it is thus likely that a local action of clonidine in the periphery might diminish sympathetically maintained pain states. Transdermal clonidine has been reported to yield pain relief in the area surrounding the patch in patients with pain otherwise diminished by sympathetic blockade (Davis et al., 1991; Byas-Smith et al., 1995). Transdermal clonidine provides some relief in diabetic neuropathy (Zeigler et al., 1992).

Epidural clonidine has been employed in humans for the relief of protracted pain states with a neuropathic component (Glynn et al., 1986, 1988; Rauck et al., 1993). Neuropathic pain in humans may be relatively "opioid insensitive," requiring larger doses of opioids than non-neuropathic pain. A double-blind, placebo-controlled trial of epidural clonidine for intractable cancer pain has been completed (Eisenach et al., 1995). In that study, patients with severe cancer pain not responding to large doses of epidural morphine were randomized to receive epidural clonidine by continuous infusion. The efficacy of epidural clonidine depended on the nature of the pain. Approximately 40% of patients had pain of the somatic type, and clonidine was no more effective than saline in these patients. In contrast, the success rate of epidural clonidine in the remaining patients, all of whom had neuropathic pain, was significantly higher than the success rate in the placebo-treated group.

CONCLUSION

There is considerable evidence that α_2 adrenoceptors in the periphery, at spinal, and perhaps at supraspinal loci can regulate the response of the animal and human to strong and otherwise aversive stimuli. The mechanism of this effect appears to reflect several distinct mechanisms, but commonly reflects the ability of α_2 receptors to modulate the excitability of nerve terminals and to hyperpolarize cell bodies by an increase in potassium conductance. At the spinal level, it seems certain that antinociceptive actions are mediated by a reduction in the release of small-diameter afferent transmitters. The actions of α_2 receptor agonists in neuropathic pain states, particularly those possessing allodynic components, are not clearly understood, but may reflect upon the sympatholytic actions expressed at all levels of the neuraxis and in the periphery. An exciting element is the growing appreciation of the possible role played by different subtypes of the α_2 receptor. Current developments suggest that several of the "side effects" of α_2 agonists as related to their use as analgesics (e.g., sedation and/or hypotension) may be mediated by discrete receptor subtypes. The relationship of subtype and physiological action is not completely understood and awaits the development of appropriately selective agonists and antagonists. The current progress in synthetic chemistry suggests that this will indeed occur.

Several properties suggest that α_2 agonists, particularly those delivered spinally, may have importance in human pain therapy. (1) These agents have therapeutic efficacy in pain states affected by opiates (postoperative) and those in which opiates are believed to be less effective (e.g., neuropathic pain). (2) α_2 agonists and opiates have nonoverlapping side-effect profiles (e.g., respiratory depression by opiates versus hypotension by α_2 agonists). (3) Preclinical work has shown that long-term use of α_2 agonists results in a minimal cross-tolerance that has been reported between opioids and α_2 agonists (Solomon and Gebhart, 1988; Stevens et al., 1988, but see Kalso et al., 1993). Although not systematically examined in humans, the analgesic potency of epidural clonidine in cancer patients receiving large doses of opioid is no different from that required in postoperative, opioid-naive patients (see Eisenach et al., 1996). (4) Considerable evidence emphasizes that the spinal α_2 system can synergize with opioid systems with respect to analgesic action (Yaksh and Reddy, 1981; Loomis et al., 1988; Monasky et al., 1990). This interaction may provide an additional example of some virtues of combination therapy focusing on different pharmacological targets that jointly regulate the processing of nociceptive information.

Finally, it should be noted that of the "novel" nonopiate mechanisms, α_2 agonists represent the first class of agents defined by preclinical models to produce a marketed product for pain. This occurrence provides support for the contention that the preclinical models serve as a useful vehicle for the development of novel analgesic agents.

REFERENCES

Aantaa R, Marjamaki A, Scheinin M (1995): Molecular pharmacology of alpha 2-adrenoceptor subtypes. Ann Med 27:439–449.

Ahlquist RP (1948): A study of the adrenotrophic receptor. Am J Physiol 153:586–600.

Anden N-E, Jukes MGM, Lundberg A (1966): The effect of DOPA on the spinal cord. 2. A pharmacological analysis. Acta Physiol Scand 67:387–397.

Bailey PL, Sperry RJ, Johnson GK, Eldredge SJ, East KA, East TD, Pace NL, Stanley TH (1991): Respiratory effects of clonidine alone and combined with morphine in humans. Anesthesiology 74:43–48.

Bennett GJ, Xie YK (1988): A peripheral mononeuropathy in rat that produces disorders of pain sensation like those seen in man. Pain 33:87–107.

Bernard J-M, Hommeril J-L, Passuti N, Pinaud M (1991): Postoperative analgesia by intravenous clonidine. Anesthesiology 75:577–582.

Bloor B, Abdul-Rasool I, Temp J, Jenkins S, Valcke C, Ward D (1989): The effects of medetomidine, an α_2-adrenergic agonist, on ventilatory drive in the dog. Acta Vet Scand 85:65–70.

Brenner GM, Klopp AJ, Deason LL, Stevens CW (1994): Analgesic potency of alpha adrenergic agents after systemic administration in amphibians. J Pharmacol Exp Ther 270:540–545.

Burrill DY, Goetzl FR, Ivy AC (1961): The pain threshold raising effects of amphetamines. J Dent Res 12:478–485.

Byas-Smith MG, Max MB, Muir J, Kingman A (1995): Transdermal clonidine compared to placebo in painful diabetic neuropathy using a two-stage 'enriched enrollment' design. Pain 60:267–274.

Bylund DB (1995): Pharmacological characteristics of alpha-2 adrenergic receptor subtypes. Ann NY Acad Sci 763:1–7.

Calvillo O, Ghignone M (1986): Presynaptic effect of clonidine on unmyelinated afferent fibers in the spinal cord of the cat. Neurosci Lett 64:335–339.

Camarata PJ, Yaksh TL (1985): Characterization of the spinal adrenergic receptors mediating the spinal effects produced by the microinjection of morphine into the periaqueductal gray. Brain Res 336:133–142.

Danzebrink RM, Gebhart GF (1990): Antinociceptive effects of intrathecal adrenoceptor agonists in a rat model of visceral nociception. J Pharmacol Exp Ther 253:698–705.

Davis KD, Treede RD, Raja SN, Meyer RA, Campbell JN (1991): Topical application of clonidine relieves hyperalgesia in patients with sympathetically maintained pain. Pain 47:309–317.

De Kock MF, Pichon G, Scholtes J-L (1992): Intraoperative clonidine enhances postoperative morphine patient-controlled analgesia. Can J Anaesth 39:537–544.

De Sarro GB, Bagetta G, Ascioti C, Libri V, Nistico G (1988): Microinfusion of clonidine and yohimbine into locus coeruleus alters EEG power spectrum: effects of aging and reversal by phosphatidylserine. Br J Pharmacol 95:1278–1286.

Downie JW, Bialik GJ (1988): Evidence for a spinal site of action of clonidine on somatic and viscerosomatic reflex activity evoked on the pudendal nerve in cats. J Pharmacol Exp Ther 246:352–358.

Downie JW, Espey MJ, Gajewski JB (1991): Alpha 2-adrenoceptors not imidazole receptors mediate depression of a sacral spinal reflex in the cat. Eur J Pharmacol 195: 301–304.

Dray A (1997): Pharmacology of peripheral afferent terminals. In Yaksh TL, Lynch III C, Zapol WM, Maze M, Biebuyck JF, Saidman LJ (eds): *Anesthesia: Biologic Foundations.* Philadelphia: Lippincott-Raven, pp. 543–556.

Eisenach JC, Grice SC (1988): Epidural clonidine does not decrease blood pressure or spinal cord blood flow in awake sheep. Anesthesiology 68:335–340.

Eisenach JC, Tong C (1991): Site of hemodynamic effects of intrathecal 2-adrenergic agonists. Anesthesiology 74:766–771.

Eisenach JC, Castro MI, Dewan DM, Rose JC (1989a): Epidural clonidine analgesia in obstetrics: sheep studies. Anesthesiology 70:51–56.

Eisenach JC, Lysak SZ, Viscomi CM (1989b): Epidural clonidine analgesia following surgery: Phase I. Anesthesiology 71:640–646.

Eisenach JC, DuPen S, Dubois M, Miguel R, Allin D (1995): Study Group. Epidural clonidine analgesia for intractable cancer pain. Pain 61:391–399.

Eisenach JC, De Kock M, Klimscha W (1996): Alpha(2)-adrenergic agonists for regional anesthesia. A clinical review of clonidine (1984–1995). Anesthesiology 85: 655–674.

Fikes LW, Lin HC, Thurmon JC (1989): A preliminary comparison of lidocaine and xylazine as epidural analgesics in ponies. Vet Surg 18:85–86.

Filos KS, Goudas LC, Patroni O, Polyzou V (1992): Intrathecal clonidine as a sole analgesic for pain relief after cesarean. Anesthesiology 77:267–274.

Fleetwood-Walker SM, Mitchell R, Hope PJ, Molony V, Iggo A (1985): An alpha 2 receptor mediates the selective inhibition by noradrenaline of nociceptive responses of identified dorsal horn neurones. Brain Res 334:243–254.

Gaumann DM, Yaksh TL, Tyce GM (1990): Effects of intrathecal morphine, clonidine, and midazolam on the somato-sympathoadrenal reflex response in halothane-anesthetized cats. Anesthesiology 73:425–432.

Glynn CJ, Teddy PJ, Jamous MA, Moore RA, Lloyd JW (1986): Role of spinal noradrenergic system in transmission of pain in patients with spinal cord injury. Lancet ii:1249–1250.

Glynn C, Dawson D, Sanders R (1988): A double-blind comparison between epidural morphine and epidural clonidine in patients with chronic non-cancer pain. Pain 34: 123–128.

Go VLW, Yaksh TL (1987): Release of substance P from the cat spinal cord. J Physiol 391:141–167.

Gordh T Jr, Feuk U, Norlen K (1986a): Effect of epidural clonidine on spinal cord blood flow and regional and central hemodynamics in pigs. Anesth Analg 65: 1312–1318.

Gordh T Jr, Post C, Olsson Y (1986b): Evaluation of the toxicity of subarachnoid clonidine, guanfacine, and a substance P-antagonist on rat spinal cord and nerve roots: Light and electron microscopic observations after chronic intrathecal administration. Anesth Analg 65:1303–1311.

Guo TZ, Jiang JY, Buttermann AE, Maze M (1996): Dexmedetomidine injection into the locus coeruleus produces antinociception. Anesthesiology 84:873–881.

Hamalainen MM, Pertovaara A (1995): The antinociceptive action of an alpha 2-adrenoceptor agonist in the spinal dorsal horn is due to a direct spinal action and not to activation of descending inhibition. Brain Res Bull 37:581–587.

Hammond DL, Tyce GM, Yaksh TL (1985): Efflux of 5-hydroxytryptamine and noradrenaline into spinal cord superfusates during stimulation of the rat medulla. J Physiol 359:151–162.

Head GA(1992): Central monoamine neurons and cardiovascular control. Kidney International 37:S8–S13.

Holz GG IV, Kream RM, Spiegel A, Dunlap K (1989): G proteins couple alpha-adrenergic and $GABA_b$ receptors to inhibition of peptide secretion from peripheral sensory neurons. J Neurosci 9:657–666.

Horvath G, Dobos I, Liszli P, Klimscha W, Szikszay M, Benedek G (1997): Antinociceptive effects of the hydrophilic alpha2-adrenoceptor agonist ST-91 in different test circumstances after intrathecal administration to Wistar rats. Pharmacol Res 35: 561–568.

Howe JR, Wang J-Y, Yaksh TL (1983): Selective antagonism of the antinociceptive effect of intrathecally applied α-adrenergic agonists by intrathecal prazosin and intrathecal yohimbine. J Pharmacol Exp Ther 224:552–558.

Howe JR, Yaksh TL, Go VLW (1987): The effect of unilateral dorsal root ganglionectomies or ventral rhizotomies on $α_2$-adrenoceptor binding to, and the substance P, enkephalin, and neurotensin content of, the cat lumbar spinal cord. Neuroscience 21: 385–394.

Hunter JC, Fontana DJ, Hedley I R, Jasper JR, Lewis R, Link RE, Secchi R, Sutton J, Eglen RM (1997): Assessment of the role of alpha2-adrenoceptor subtypes in the antinociceptive, sedative and hypothermic action of dexmedetomidine in transgenic mice. Br J Pharmacol 122:1339–1344.

Huntoon M, Eisenach JC, Boese P (1992): Epidural clonidine after cesarean section: Appropriate dose and effect of prior local anesthetic. Anesthesiology 76:187–193.

Hylden J, Wilcox GL (1983): Pharmacological characterization of substance P induced nociception in the mouse: Modulation by opioid adrenergic agonists at the spinal level. J Pharmacol Exp Ther 226:398–404.

Jaakola M-L, Salonen M, Lehtinen R, Scheinin H (1991): The analgesic action of dexmedetomidine—a novel alpha-2-adrenoceptor agonist—in healthy volunteers. Pain 46:281–285.

Jansson CC, Marjamaki A, Luomala K, Savola JM, Scheinin M, Akerman KE (1994): Coupling of human alpha 2-adrenoceptor subtypes to regulation of cAMP production in transfected S115 cells. Eur J Pharmacol 266:165–174.

Jarvis DA, Duncan SR, Segal IS, Maze M (1992): Ventilatory effects of clonidine alone and in the presence of alfentanil, in human volunteers. Anesthesiology 76:899–905.

Jensen TS, Yaksh TL (1986): II. Examination of spinal monoamine receptors through which brain stem opiate-sensitive systems act in the rat. Brain Res 363:114–127.

Kalso EA, Poyhia R, Rosenberg PH (1991): Spinal antinociception by dexmedetomidine, a highly selective alpha 2-adrenergic agonist. Pharmacol Toxicol 68:140–143.

Kalso EA, Sullivan AF, McQuay HJ, Dickenson AH, Roques BP (1993): Cross-tolerance between mu opioid and alpha-2 adrenergic receptors, but not between mu and delta opioid receptors in the spinal cord of the rat. J Pharmacol Exp Ther 265:551–558.

Khasar SG, Green PG, Chou B, Levine JD (1995): Peripheral nociceptive effects of alpha 2-adrenergic receptor agonists in the rat. Neuroscience 66:427–532.

Kiessig HJ, Orzechowski G (1941): Untersuchungen uber die wirkungweise der sympathomimetic. Naunyn-Schmiedeberg's Arch Exp Pathol Pharmacol 197:391–404.

Kim SH, Chung JM (1992): An experimental model for peripheral neuropathy produced by segmental spinal nerve ligation in the rat. Pain 50:355–363.

Kim SH, Na HS, Sheen K, Chung JM (1993): Effects of sympathectomy on a rat model of peripheral neuropathy. Pain 55:85–92.

Kingery WS (1997): A critical review of controlled clinical trials for peripheral neuropathic pain and complex regional pain syndromes. Pain 73:123–139.

Kobilka BK, Matsui H, Kobilka TS, Yang-Feng TL, Francke U, Caron MG, Lefkowitz RJ, Regan JW (1987): Cloning, sequencing, and expression of the gene coding for the human platelet alpha 2-adrenergic receptor. Science 238:650–656.

Kroneberg G, Oberdorf A, Hoffmeister F, Wirth W (1967): Zur pharmakologie von 2-(2,6-dimethyl-phenylamino)-4H-5,6-dihydro-1,3thiazin (Bayer 1470), eines hemmstoffes adrenergischer und cholinergischer neurone. Naunyn-Schmiedeberg's Arch Exp Pathol Pharmacol 256:257–280.

Kuraishi Y, Harada Y, Satoh M, Takagi H (1979a): Antagonism by phenoxybenzamine of the analgesic effect of morphine injected into the nucleus reticularis gigantocellularis. Neuropharmacology 18:107–110.

Kuraishi Y, Harqada Y, Takagi H (1979b): Noradrenaline regulation of pain transmission in the spinal cord mediated by alpha adrenoceptors. Brain Res 174:333–336.

Kuraishi Y, Hirota N, Sato Y, Kaneko S, Satoh M, Takagi H (1985): Noradrenergic inhibition of the release of substance P from the primary afferent in the rabbit spinal dorsal horn. Brain Res 359:177–182.

Link RE, Desai K, Hein L, Stevens ME, Chruscinski A, Bernstein D, Barsh GS, Kobilka BK (1996): Cardiovascular regulation in mice lacking alpha2-adrenergic receptor subtypes b and c. Science 273:803–805.

Lomasney JW, Lorenz W, Allen LF, King K, Regan JW, Yang-Feng TL, Caron MG, Lefkowitz RJ (1990): Expansion of the alpha 2-adrenergic receptor family: cloning and characterization of a human alpha 2-adrenergic receptor subtype, the gene for which is located on chromosome 2. Proc Natl Acad Sci USA 87:5094–5098.

Loomis CW, Milne B, Cervenko FW (1988): A study of the interaction between clonidine and morphine on analgesia and blood pressure during continuous intrathecal infusion in the rat. Neuropharmacology 27:191–199.

Lopachin RM, Rudy TA (1981): The effects of intrathecal sympathomimetic agents on neural activity in the lumbar sympathetic chain of rats. Brain Res 224:195–198.

MacDonald E, Kobilka B, Scheinin, M (1997): Gene targeting-homing in on alpha 2 receptor-subtype function. Trends Pharmacol Sci 18:211–219.

MacKinnon AC, Spedding M, Brown CM (1994): Alpha 2-adrenoceptors: more subtypes but fewer functional differences. Trends Pharmacol Sci 15:119–123.

MacMillan LB, Hein L, Smith MS, Piascik MT, Limbird LE (1996): Central hypotensive effects of the alpha-2a-adrenergic receptor subtype. Science 273:801–803.

Malmberg AB, Yaksh TL (1993): Pharmacology of the spinal actions of ketorolac, morphine, ST-91, U50488 and L-PIA on the formalin test and an isobolographic analysis of the NSAID interaction. Anesthesiology 79:270–281.

Marjamaki A, Luomala K, Ala-Uotila S, Scheinin M (1993): Use of recombinant human alpha 2-adrenoceptors to characterize subtype selectively of antagonist binding. Eur J Pharmacol 246:219–226.

Max MB, Schafer SC, Culnane M, Dubner R, Gracely RH (1988): Association of pain relief with drug side effects in postherpetic neuralgia: A single-dose study of clonidine, codeine, ibuprofen, and placebo. Clin Pharmacol Ther 43:363–371.

Maze M, Tranquilli W (1991): Alpha-2 adrenoceptor agonists: defining the role in clinical anesthesia. Anesthesiology 74:581–605.

Mendez R, Eisenach JC, Kashtan K (1990): Epidural clonidine analgesia after caesarean section. Anesthesiology 73:848–852.

Millan MJ, Bervoets K, Rivet JM, Widdowson P, Renouard A, LeMarouille-Girardon S, Gobert A (1994): Multiple alpha2-adrenergic receptor subtypes. II. Evidence for a role of rat Rα2A-ARs in the control of nociception, motor behaviour and hippocampal synthesis of noradrenaline. J Pharmacol Exp Ther 270:958–972.

Monasky MS, Zinsmeister AR, Stevens CW, Yaksh TL (1990): Interaction of intrathecal morphine and ST-91 on antinociception in the rat: dose-response analysis, antagonism and clearance. J Pharmacol Exp Ther 254:383–392.

Murata K, Nakagawa I, Kumeta Y, Kitahata LM, Collins JG (1989): Intrathecal clonidine suppresses noxiously evoked activity of spinal wide dynamic range neurons in cats. Anesth Analg 69:185–191.

Nagasaka H, Yaksh TL (1990): Pharmacology of intrathecal adrenergic agonists: cardiovascular and nociceptive reflexes in halothane-anesthetized rats. Anesthesiology 73:1198–1207.

Ness TJ, Gebhart GF (1989): Differential effects of morphine and clonidine on visceral and cutaneous spinal nociceptive transmission in the rat. J Neurophysiol 62:220–230.

North RA, Yoshimura M (1984): The actions of noradrenaline on neurones of the rat substantia gelatinosa in vitro. J Physiol 349:43–55.

North RA, Williams JT, Suprenant A, Christie MJ (1987): Mu and delta opioid receptors belong to a family of receptors that are coupled to potassium channels. Proc Natl Acad Sci USA 84:5487–5491.

Ossipov MH, Suarez LJ, Spaulding TC (1989): Antinociceptive interactions between alpha 2-adrenergic and opiate agonists at the spinal level in rodents. Anesth Analg 68:194–200.

Penon C, Ecoffey C, Cohen SE (1991): Ventilatory response to carbon dioxide after epidural clonidine injection. Anesth Analg 72:761–764.

Porchet HC, Piletta P, Dayer P (1990): Objective assessment of clonidine analgesia in man and influence of naloxone. Life Sci 46:991–998.

Puke MJ, Xu XJ, Wiesenfeld-Hallin Z (1991): Intrathecal administration of clonidine suppresses autotomy, a behavioral sign of chronic pain in rats after sciatic nerve section. Neurosci Lett 133:199–202.

Rauck RL, Eisenach JC, Jackson K, Young LD, Southern J (1993): Epidural clonidine treatment for refractory reflex sympathetic dystrophy. Anesthesiology 79:1163–1169.

Reddy SVR, Maderdrut JL, Yaksh TL (1980): Spinal cord pharmacology of adrenergic agonist-mediated antinociception. J Pharmacol Exp Ther 213:525–533.

Regan JW, Kobilka TS, Yang-Feng TL, Caron MG, Lefkowitz RJ, Kobilka BK (1988): Cloning and expression of a human kidney cDNA for an alpha 2-adrenergic receptor subtype. Proc Natl Acad Sci USA 85:6301–6305.

Rosin DL, Zeng D, Stornetta RL, Norton FR, Riley T, Okusa MD, Guyenet PG, Lynch KR (1993): Immunohistochemical localization of alpha 2A-adrenergic receptors in catecholaminergic and other brainstem neurons in the rat. Neuroscience 56:139–155.

Rosin DL, Talley EM, Lee A, Stornetta RL, Gaylinn BD, Guyenet PG, Lynch KR (1996): Distribution of alpha 2C-adrenergic receptor-like immunoreactivity in the rat central nervous system. J Comp Neurol 372:135–165.

Sabbe MB, Penning JP, Ozaki GT, Yaksh TL (1994): Spinal and systemic action of the α_2 receptor agonist dexmedetomidine in dogs: Antinociception and carbon dioxide response. Anesthesiology 80:1057–1072.

Saeki S, Yaksh TL (1992): Suppression by spinal alpha-2 agonists of motor and autonomic responses evoked by low- and high-intensity thermal stimuli. J Pharmacol Exp Ther 260:795–802.

Sato J, Perl ER (1991): Adrenergic excitation of cutaneous pain receptors induced by peripheral nerve injury. Science 251:1608–1610.

Schaible HG, Grubb BD (1993): Afferent and spinal mechanisms of joint pain. Pain 55:5–54.

Schmitt H, LeDouarec JC, Petillot N (1974a): Antagonisms of the antinociceptive action of xylazine, an alpha sympathomimetic by adrenoceptor and cholinoceptor blocking agents. Neuropharmacology 13:295–303.

Schmitt H, LeDouarec JC, Petillot N (1974b): Antinociceptive effects of some alpha sympathomimetic agents. Neuropharmacology 13:289–294.

Segal IS, Jarvis DJ, Duncan SR, White PF, Maze M (1991): Clinical efficacy of oral-transdermal clonidine combinations during the perioperative period. Anesthesiology 74:220–225.

Sherman SE, Loomis CW, Milne B, Cervenko FW (1988): Intrathecal oxymetazoline produces analgesia via spinal alpha-adrenoceptors and potentiates spinal morphine. Eur J Pharmacol 148:371–380.

Skarda RT, Muir WW 3rd (1996): Comparison of antinociceptive, cardiovascular, and respiratory effects, head ptosis, and position of pelvic limbs in mares after caudal epidural administration of xylazine and detomidine hydrochloride solution. Am J Vet Res 57:1338–1345.

Smith BD, Baudendistel LJ, Gibbons JJ, Schweiss JF (1992): A comparison of two epidural alpha 2-agonists, guanfacine and clonidine, in regard to duration of antinociception, and ventilatory and hemodynamic effects in goats. Anesth Analg 74: 712–718.

Smith MS, Schambra UB, Wilson KH, Page SO, Hulette C, Light AR, Schwinn DA (1995): Alpha 2-Adrenergic receptors in human spinal cord: specific localized expression of mRNA encoding alpha 2-adrenergic receptor subtypes at four distinct levels. Brain Res Mol Brain Res 34:109–117.

Solomon RE, Gebhart GF (1988): Intrathecal morphine and clonidine: antinociceptive tolerance and cross-tolerance and effects on blood pressure. J Pharmacol Exp Ther 245:444–454.

Stevens CW, Monasky MS, Yaksh TL (1988): Spinal infusion of opiate and 2-agonists in rats: tolerance and cross-tolerance studies. J Pharmacol Exp Ther 244:63–70.

Striebel WH, Koenigs DI, Krämer JA (1993): Intravenous clonidine fails to reduce postoperative meperidine requirements. J Clin Anesth 5:221–225.

Sullivan AF, Kalso EA, McQuay HJ, Dickenson AH (1992): The antinociceptive actions of dexmedetomidine on dorsal horn neuronal responses in the anaesthetized rat. Eur J Pharmacol 215:127–133.

Sundaram K, Murugaian J, Sapru H (1991): Microinjections of norepinephrine into the intermediolateral cell column of the spinal cord exert excitatory as well as inhibitory effects on the cardiac function. Brain Res 544:227–234.

Takano M, Takano Y, Yaksh TL (1993): Release of calcitonin gene-related peptide (CGRP), substance P (SP), and vasoactive intestinal polypeptide (VIP) from rat spinal cord: Modulation by alpha-2 agonists. Peptides 14:371–378.

Takano Y, Yaksh TL (1992): Characterization of the pharmacology of intrathecally administered alpha-2 agonists and antagonists in rats. J Pharmacol Exp Ther 261: 764–772.

Takano Y, Yaksh TL (1993): Chronic spinal infusion of dexmedetomidine, ST-91 and clonidine: Spinal alpha$_2$ adrenoceptor subtypes and intrinsic activity. J Pharmacol Exp Ther 264:327–335.

Takano Y, Takano M, Yaksh TL (1992): The effect of intrathecally administered imiloxan and WB4101: possible role of a2-adrenoceptor subtypes in the spinal cord. Eur J Pharmacol 219:465–468.

Uhlen S, Wikberg JE (1991): Rat spinal cord alpha 2-adrenoceptors are of the alpha 2A-subtype: comparison with alpha 2A- and alpha 2B-adrenoceptors in rat spleen, cerebral cortex and kidney using ^{3}H-RX821002 ligand binding. Pharmacol Toxicol 69:341–350.

Waterman A, Livingston A, Bouchenafa O (1988): Analgesic effects of intrathecally-applied alpha 2-adrenoceptor agonists in conscious, unrestrained sheep. Neuropharmacology 27:213–216.

Weber HU (1904): Anasthesie durch adrenalin. Verhandlungen der Deutschen Gesellschaft fur Inn Medizin 21:616–619.

Wilcox GL, Seybold V (1997): Pharmacology of afferent processing. In Yaksh TL, Lynch III C, Zapol WM, Maze M, Biebuyck JF, Saidman LJ (eds.): *Anesthesia: Biologic Foundations*. Philadelphia: Lippincott-Raven, pp. 557–576.

Xu XJ, Hao JX, Aldskogius H, Seiger A, Wiesenfeld-Hallin Z (1992): Chronic pain-related syndrome in rats after ischemic spinal cord lesion: a possible animal model for pain in patients with spinal cord injury. Pain 48:279–290.

Yaksh TL (1979): Direct evidence that spinal serotonin and noradrenaline terminals mediate the spinal antinociceptive effects of morphine in the periaqueductal gray. Brain Res 160:180–185.

Yaksh TL (1985): Pharmacology of spinal adrenergic systems which modulate spinal nociceptive processing. Pharmacol Biochem Behav 22:845–858.

Yaksh TL (1989): Behavioral and autonomic correlates of the tactile evoked allodynia produced by spinal glycine inhibition: effects of modulatory receptor systems and excitatory amino acid antagonists. Pain 37:111–123.

Yaksh TL (1997): Preclinical models of nociception. In Yaksh TL, Lynch III C, Zapol WM, Maze M, Biebuyck JF, Saidman LJ (eds): *Anesthesia: Biologic Foundations*. Philadelphia: Lippincott-Raven, pp. 685–718.

Yaksh TL, Reddy SVR (1981): Studies in the primate on the analgesic effects associated with intrathecal actions of opiate, a-adrenergic agonists and baclofen. Anesthesiology 54:451–467.

Yaksh TL, Rudy TA (1978): Narcotic analgesics: CNS sites and mechanisms of action as revealed by intracerebral injection techniques. Pain 4:299–359.

Yaksh TL, Rathbun M, Jage J, Mirzai T, Grafe M, Hiles RA (1994): Pharmacology and toxicology of chronically infused epidural clonidine HCl in dogs. Fundam Appl Toxicol 23:319–335.

Yaksh TL, Pogrel JW, Lee YW, Chaplan SR (1995): Reversal of nerve ligation-induced allodynia by spinal *alpha*-2 adrenoceptor agonists. J Pharmacol Exp Ther 272:207–214.

Yamamoto T, Yaksh TL (1991): Spinal pharmacology of thermal hyperesthesia induced by incomplete ligation of sciatic nerve. 1. Opioid and nonopioid receptors. Anesthesiology 75:817–826.

Zeigler D, Lynch SA, Muir J, Benjamin J, Max MB (1992): Transdermal clonidine versus placebo in painful diabetic neuropathy. Pain 48:403–408.

CHAPTER 10

SEROTONIN AND ITS RECEPTORS IN PAIN CONTROL

MICHEL HAMON and SYLVIE BOURGOIN
INSERM U288
Faculté de Médecine Pitié-Salpêtrière
Paris, France

Serotonin (5-hydroxytryptamine, 5-HT) has been known for several decades to be a key neurohormone in the control of pain mechanisms. At the periphery, it is one of the active components of the so-called "inflammatory soup," which is present in the extracellular space of injured (inflamed) tissues (Alstergren and Kopp, 1997), where it directly participates in the injury (inflammation)-associated pain. Thus injection of 5-HT, either intravenously or intradermally, has been shown reproducibly to potentiate pain induced by inflammatory mediators such as prostaglandins or algogenic compounds such as bradykinin. In contrast, when directly injected in the central nervous system (CNS), and especially into the intrathecal space at the spinal level, 5-HT exerts clear-cut antinociceptive effects, although with variable potency, depending on the nociceptive stimuli applied to reveal these effects (Bardin et al., 1997a). Like that observed at the periphery, the centrally mediated action of 5-HT on pain mechanisms is physiologically relevant because it can be reproduced through the release of endogenous 5-HT at the spinal level, notably in response to direct electrical stimulation of bulbospinal serotoninergic neurons (see Cesselin et al., 1994). Such dual actions of 5-HT, algesic at the periphery and analgesic in the central nervous system, emphasize the complexity of its implication in the neurobiological mechanisms of nociception. Indeed, 5-HT is known to act at multiple specific receptors, from which it can evoke a wide variety of responses on its target cells, including neurons that are concerned with the triggering, transfer, and modulation of nociceptive messages. Accordingly, much more than only an excitatory influence at the periphery and an inhibitory influence in the central nervous system, 5-HT can exert multiple effects at the various

Novel Aspects of Pain Management: Opioids and Beyond, Edited by Jana Sawynok and Alan Cowan
ISBN 0-471-180173 Copyright © 1999 by Wiley-Liss, Inc.

levels of nociceptive circuits by acting at these numerous receptors. The objective of this chapter is to analyze the respective roles of these various receptor types in the pro- or anti-nociceptive actions of 5-HT, in an attempt to define which 5-HT-related compounds might possibly be of interest as novel non-opioid analgesics in humans.

THE BULBOSPINAL SEROTONINERGIC SYSTEM INVOLVED IN PAIN CONTROL

As clearly shown by the potent antinociceptive effect of direct electrical stimulation of serotoninergic neurons in the caudal part of the raphe complex in the bulb-mesencephalon (see Le Bars, 1988), the bulbospinal 5-HT systems participate in pain control mechanisms in the rat. Serotoninergic neurons projecting specifically to the dorsal horn, where peripheral nociceptive messages are addressed, are located in the rostroventromedial medulla and caudal pons, especially in the nucleus raphe magnus, the nucleus paragigantocellularis, and the ventral portion of the nucleus gigantocellularis (Kwiat and Basbaum, 1992). Although there is a contralateral contribution, 5-HT fibers projecting within the dorsal horn are mainly located in the ipsilateral dorsolateral funiculus of the spinal cord (Bullitt and Light, 1989).

Within the dorsal horn of the spinal cord, serotoninergic fibers and nerve endings specifically labeled by anti-5-HT antibodies have been visualized in all laminae, with the highest densities in laminae I, II, IV, V, and X (Ruda et al., 1986). Although some targets of 5-HT terminals have been identified (spinothalamic neurons in laminae I and V, lamina IV neurons, and enkephalin immunoreactive neurons; see Ruda et al., 1986), only one-fifth of all 5-HT immunoreactive profiles apparently contribute to differentiated synapses within the dorsal horn (Ridet et al., 1993).

At least at the lumbar level, 5-HT terminals appear to have an exclusive supraspinal origin, because transection of the thoracic spinal cord leads to an extensive depletion of 5-HT and the disappearance of 5-HT immunoreactivity in the lumbar segments (Oliveras et al., 1977; Ruda et al., 1986). There is some evidence for a few intrinsic 5-HT cells in restricted portions of the spinal cord in monkeys (LaMotte et al., 1982), but their contribution to the spinal 5-HT fiber plexus is likely to be small.

In addition to 5-HT, several neuropeptides are also present in the descending projections that innervate the spinal cord. Indeed, several of these peptides (substance P, somatostatin, enkephalin, thyrotropin-releasing hormone) have been shown to be co-localized with 5-HT in the same neurons within the medullary raphe nuclei (Bowker and Abbott, 1990). Accordingly, all effects due to the stimulation (electrical, chemical, or physiological) of serotoninergic neurons in the nucleus raphe magnus can probably not be attributed solely to the release of 5-HT within the dorsal horn of the spinal cord (see Sorkin et al., 1993). Co-release of a given neuropeptide or other neuroactive molecule might well result in some modulation of the effects of 5-HT, and contribute to either the enhancement or the reduction in the analgesic action of the indoleamine in response to the stimulation of specific 5-HT receptors.

SEROTONIN RECEPTORS INVOLVED IN PAIN MECHANISMS

Heterogeneity of Central Serotonin Receptors

The existence of multiple receptors for 5-HT is now well established (Boess and Martin, 1994; Hoyer et al., 1994; Uphouse, 1997; Table 10.1) and very probably accounts for the great variety of 5-HT actions on various cell types both in the central nervous system and at the periphery. 5-HT receptors can be divided into seven main classes, namely, 5-HT$_1$ (with five different subclasses: 5-HT$_{1A}$, 5-HT$_{1B}$, 5-HT$_{1D}$, 5-HT$_{1E}$, 5-HT$_{1F}$), 5-HT$_2$ (which comprises the 5-HT$_{2A}$, 5-HT$_{2B}$ and 5-HT$_{2C}$ subtypes), 5-HT$_3$ (with its two variants, 5-HT$_{3A}$L and 5-HT$_{3A}$S, due to alternative splicing of the primary transcript), 5-HT$_4$ (which is also characterized by a short and a long isoform), 5-HT$_{5A}$ and 5-HT$_{5B}$, 5-HT$_6$, and 5-HT$_7$ (Table 10.1). All but the 5-HT$_3$ receptor are G-protein-coupled receptors. Another distinction concerns their respective affinities for 5-HT, because 5-HT$_1$ receptor subtypes are characterized by K_d values in the nanomolar range, whereas the other classes generally exhibit a lower affinity for the indoleamine. Among the G-protein-coupled 5-HT receptors, the 5-HT$_{1A}$, 5-HT$_{1B}$, 5-HT$_{1D}$, 5-HT$_{1E}$, and 5-HT$_{1F}$ subtypes exert their cellular actions through the inhibition of adenylyl cyclase and/or, at least for some of them, the opening of K$^+$ channels (Boess and Martin, 1994). Conversely, activation of 5-HT$_{2(A,B,C)}$ receptors results in the closure of K$^+$ channels and the stimulation of phospholipase C, and activation of 5-HT$_4$, 5-HT$_6$, and 5-HT$_7$ receptors produces an increase in adenylyl cyclase activity (Boess and Martin, 1994). On the other hand, the 5-HT$_3$ receptor is a 5-HT-gated cation channel, whose activation triggers an increased conductance for Na$^+$ and K$^+$ (and to a lesser extent Ca^{2+}) ions, leading to plasma membrane depolarization in cell types expressing this receptor (Yakel et al., 1990). Finally, little is known to date about the transduction mechanisms of the two 5-HT$_5$ receptor subtypes, although a recent report provided evidence for a negative coupling of the 5-HT$_{5A}$ subtype with adenylyl cyclase in astrocytes (Carson et al., 1996).

All the 5-HT receptors identified to date apparently exist in all mammalian species, but a given receptor type can have different pharmacological properties from one species to another. This is notably the case for the 5-HT$_{1B}$ receptor, which is recognized by some β-adrenoceptor antagonists in rodents but not in human and other mammals. Conversely, the human 5-HT$_{1B}$ receptor has a relatively high affinity (in the inframicromolar range) for some α2 adrenoceptor antagonists, in contrast to the rodent 5-HT$_{1B}$ receptor, which does not bind these compounds (Hoyer et al., 1994).

TABLE 10.1 5-HT Receptor Subtypes—Main Properties and Expression in the Dorsal Horn of the Spinal Cord and Dorsal Root Ganglia

Receptor Type	Agonists	Antagonists	G Protein	Transduction Mechanism	Dorsal Horn of the Spinal Cord (Protein)[a]	Dorsal Root Ganglia (mRNA)[a]
5-HT$_{1A}$	8-OH-DPAT alnespirone	WAY 100635 NAD-299	Gi/o	cAMP↘	+++	−?
5-HT$_{1B}$	CP 93129 sumatriptan	GR 55562 SB 242289	Gi/o	cAMP↘	++	+
5-HT$_{1D}$	GR 46611 L-694,247	GR 127935	Gi/o	cAMP↘	+	++
5-HT$_{1E}$	—	—	Gi/o	cAMP↘	+	−
5-HT$_{1F}$	LY 334370 sumatriptan	—	Gi/o	cAMP↘	+	+
5-HT$_{2A}$	α-Me-5-HT DOI	ketanserin MDL 100,907	Gq/11	PLC↗	(+)	+
5-HT$_{2B}$	α-Me-5-HT BW 723686	SB 206553 LY 266097	Gq/11	PLC↗	(+)	−?
5-HT$_{2C}$	α-Me-5-HT MK 212	SB 206553 SB 221284	Gq/11	PLC↗	(+)	+
5-HT$_4$	RS 67333 RS 67506	GR 113808 LY 297582	Gs	cAMP↗	+	+
5-HT$_{5A}$	—	—	Gi	cAMP↘	+	++
5-HT$_{5B}$	—	—	?	?	+	++
5-HT$_6$	—	Ro 04-6790	Gs	cAMP↗	+	−
5-HT$_7$	—	—	Gs	cAMP↗	+	+
5-HT$_3$	m-Cl-phenyl-biguanide SR 57227 A	ondansetron granisetron	None	Na$^+$, K$^+$ channel	++	++

[a] +++, ++, +, (+): graded levels of expression. —: no expression. ?: unknown.

Serotonin Receptors in the Spinal Cord

A number of selective or preferential 5-HT receptor agonists and antagonists (see Table 10.1) have been radiolabeled, and have proved to be useful for the visualization and quantification of the various 5-HT receptor types using autoradiographic and membrane binding techniques. At the spinal level, quantitative analysis of high affinity [^{3}H]5-HT binding (5-HT$_1$ receptors) revealed specific binding throughout the gray matter, with the highest levels of binding sites in laminae I and II of the dorsal horn, and the lowest in lamina VII of the ventral horn (Daval et al., 1987; Marlier et al., 1991; Pubols et al., 1992). Interestingly, a relatively good correspondence exists between the degree of [^{3}H]5-HT specific binding and the density of 5-HT-containing fibers and terminals within the dorsal horn (Oliveras et al., 1977; Daval et al., 1987).

Both autoradiographic experiments using a selective radioligand ([^{3}H]8-OH-DPAT) and immunohistochemical studies with specific anti-5-HT$_{1A}$ receptor antibodies showed that 5-HT$_{1A}$ receptors (which contribute to about half of all 5-HT$_1$ sites in the spinal cord) are concentrated within two superficial layers in the dorsal horn (Marlier et al., 1991; Radja et al., 1991; Thor et al., 1993; Laporte et al., 1995; Kia et al., 1996). Variations in 5-HT$_{1A}$ receptor density can be observed along the rostrocaudal axis. Thus, several groups reported that 5-HT$_{1A}$ binding sites are more numerous at the lumbar and sacral levels than at the cervical and thoracic levels (Marlier et al., 1991; Thor et al., 1993). Similarly, in humans, 5-HT$_{1A}$ sites specifically labeled by [^{3}H]8-OH-DPAT within the superficial layers of the dorsal horn are more abundant in the lumbar cord than in cervicothoracic segments (Laporte et al., 1996).

Like 5-HT$_{1A}$ receptors, the 5-HT$_{1B}$ receptors are also concentrated within the superficial layers (laminae I, III, and IV in the rat; Thor et al., 1993; Laporte et al., 1995) of the dorsal horn at the cervical, thoracic, and lumbar levels of the rat spinal cord. However, the density of 5-HT$_{1B}$ sites is relatively low, being about 35–40% of that of 5-HT$_{1A}$ sites all along the spinal cord (Daval et al., 1987; Thor et al., 1993). Furthermore, no clear-cut rostrocaudal gradient exists regarding the density of 5-HT$_{1B}$ sites in the rat spinal cord (Thor et al., 1993; Laporte et al., 1995). Similarly, in humans, 5-HT$_{1B}$ receptors are relatively abundant within the superficial layers of the dorsal horn, notably in the substantia gelatinosa (Laporte et al., 1996; Castro et al., 1997). In addition, using [^{3}H]sumatriptan as a radioligand, Castro et al. (1997) recently found that the 5-carboxamidotryptamine-insensitive 5-HT$_{1F}$ receptors are also present at a high density in this subregion of the spinal cord in humans.

Evidence for the presence of 5-HT$_{2A}$, 5-HT$_{2B}$, and 5-HT$_{2C}$ receptors in the rat spinal cord has been obtained through mRNA detection (Julius et al., 1990; Helton et al., 1994) and receptor binding studies (Lyon et al., 1987; Marlier et al., 1991; Thor et al., 1993). In contrast to 5-HT$_{1A}$ and 5-HT$_{1B}$ sites, 5-HT$_{2A}$ and 5-HT$_{2C}$ sites are not concentrated in the superficial layers of the dorsal horn, but are diffusely distributed throughout the gray matter, with some enrichment within the ventral motor neuron area in the case of 5-HT$_{2A}$ receptors

(Thor et al., 1993). Nevertheless, the density of 5-HT$_{2A}$ sites within the rat spinal cord is very low, and several groups even concluded that binding studies with appropriate radioligands ([^{3}H]ketanserin, [^{125}I]DOI) do not allow the detection of these receptors (Blackshear et al., 1981; Leysen et al., 1982; Monroe and Smith, 1983). Similarly, investigations in the human spinal cord showed that [^{3}H]ketanserin specific binding to 5-HT$_{2A}$ receptors could not be found in thoracic and lumbar segments, and only a low density of such receptor sites could be labeled within the cervical cord (Laporte et al., 1996). In contrast, 5-HT$_{2C}$ sites could be labeled by [^{3}H]mesulergine at all levels of the human spinal cord. Their density is two to four times higher in the dorsal horn than in the ventral horn all along the rostrocaudal axis. However, even in the dorsal horn, absolute values of the density (B$_{max}$) of 5-HT$_{2C}$ sites are only ~20% of those for 5-HT$_{1A}$ receptors (Laporte et al., 1996).

The specific binding of [^{3}H]zacopride (Hamon et al., 1989; Laporte et al., 1995) and immunocytochemical labeling with anti-5-HT$_3$ receptor antibodies (Kia et al., 1995) showed that 5-HT$_3$ receptors are even more restricted to the superficial layers (mainly the lamina 1) of the spinal cord than are 5-HT$_1$ sites, in both rats and humans (see Laporte et al., 1996). 5-HT$_3$ receptors are also present in the spinal trigeminal nucleus (equivalent, for the face, to the superficial layers of the dorsal horn for the rest of the body) (Waeber et al., 1988; Reynolds et al., 1991; Laporte et al., 1992).

5-HT$_4$ receptors, specifically labeled by [^{3}H]GR 113808, exist in the spinal cord, with a marked enrichment within the superficial layers 1 and 2 of the dorsal horn as compared to the ventral horn (Waeber et al., 1994). In addition, expression of functional 5-HT$_4$ receptors by capsaicin-sensitive primary afferent sensory fibers that convey nociceptive messages has been demonstrated (Cardenas et al., 1997). Such locations would suggest that 5-HT$_4$ receptors, like the other receptor types already cited, are also possibly involved in 5-HT modulatory action on pain (see below). To date, few studies have addressed this question. In particular, Romanelli et al. (1993) reported that some 5-HT$_4$ receptor agonists can exert potent antinociceptive effects in relevant algesic tests in rodents.

Evidence for the presence of 5-HT$_{5A}$ and 5-HT$_{5B}$, 5-HT$_6$, and 5-HT$_7$ receptors within the dorsal horn of the spinal cord has occasionally been reported (see Table 10.1), but almost nothing is known yet about their functions, notably with regard to nociception, because of the lack of selective agonists and antagonists.

Cell Types Expressing Serotonin Receptors in the Spinal Cord

Lesion studies have been performed in order to gain information about the localization of 5-HT receptors on neurochemically identified neuronal elements in the dorsal horn of the spinal cord. In particular, the selective degeneration of descending serotoninergic pathways in rats treated with the neurotoxin 5,7-dihydroxytryptamine (5,7-DHT) was shown to produce no decrease in the density of 5-HT$_1$ binding sites in the spinal cord, indicating that these sites are probably located on postsynaptic targets of bulbospinal 5-HT neurons (Brown et al., 1989; Laporte et al., 1995). In fact, an increased density of 5-HT$_{1A}$ receptors has even been observed after such a lesion, notably in the superficial layers of the dorsal lumbar cord ($\sim$+40%, Laporte et al., 1995), leading to the suggestion that postsynaptic targets of descending serotoninergic neurons adapt to the loss of 5-HT input by developing supersensitivity to 5-HT$_{1A}$ receptor ligands. Indeed, several groups (Sawynok and Reid, 1990; Eide et al., 1992) confirmed that 5,7-DHT-treated rats are supersensitive to the antinociceptive effects of 5-HT and 5-HT$_{1A}$ receptor agonists administered directly into the intrathecal space. Alternatively, the changes in 5-HT$_{1A}$ receptors in these animals might reflect neuronal alterations more complex than only some kind of denervation-induced upregulation, for the selective lesion of descending noradrenergic systems by the alkylating agent DSP-4 [N-(2-chloroethyl)-N-ethyl-2-bromobenzylamine] also led to a significant enhancement in the density of 5-HT$_{1A}$ receptors in the superficial layers of the lumbar cord in rats (Laporte et al., 1995).

The fact that the selective lesion of descending serotoninergic pathways by 5,7-DHT does not reduce the density of a given receptor type is not enough to exclude completely the location of this particular receptor at the presynaptic level. Indeed, only a very small or even no change in the density of spinal 5-HT$_{1B}$ sites has been reported in 5,7-DHT-treated rats (Brown et al., 1989; Laporte et al., 1995), in spite of the clear-cut demonstration of the existence of presynaptic 5-HT$_{1B}$ autoreceptors on 5-HT terminals in the rat spinal cord (Brown et al., 1988; Murphy and Zemlan, 1988; Matsumoto et al., 1992). Accordingly, it can be concluded that the proportion of presynaptic 5-HT$_{1B}$ autoreceptors with respect to postsynaptic 5-HT$_{1B}$ receptors is probably very small (i.e., less than 10%). Furthermore, an upregulation of the latter receptors might also occur in 5,7-DHT-treated rats, thus masking any decrease expected from the disappearance of 5-HT$_{1B}$ autoreceptors located on serotoninergic terminals. Although some behavioral studies (Archer et al., 1986, 1987; Post et al., 1986; Sawynok and Reid, 1996) concluded that the antinociceptive effects of intrathecally administered 5-HT and related agonists might involve some excitatory action of these ligands at noradrenergic terminals within the dorsal horn, data from lesion studies excluded the existence of 5-HT$_{1B}$ (and 5-HT$_{1A}$; see above) receptors on these terminals. Indeed, rather than a decrease, which would be expected from such a location, Laporte et al. (1995) observed a significant increase (+18–30%) in the density of 5-HT$_{1B}$ receptors within the superficial laminae of the dorsal horn in rats whose spinal noradrenergic terminals had been lesioned by DSP-4.

It has been assumed that part of the 5-HT$_{1A}$ and 5-HT$_{1B}$ sites in the dorsal horn are probably located on the terminals of primary afferent fibers, because dorsal rhizotomy or neonatal administration of capsaicin (which preferentially destroys the unmyelinated C fibers that convey nociceptive messages) produces a 20–25% decrease in their density within the superficial layers of the dorsal horn in rats (Daval et al., 1987; Laporte et al., 1995). In agreement with this conclusion, mRNAs encoding 5-HT$_{1B}$ and 5-HT$_{1A}$ receptors were reported to be present in neurons of the rat dorsal root and trigeminal ganglia using in situ hybridization histochemistry (Bruinvels et al., 1992; Pompeiano et al., 1992; Doucet et al., 1995). Subsequent reverse transcription–polymerase chain reaction (RT-PCR) studies fully confirmed the presence of 5-HT$_{1B}$ receptor mRNAs in these ganglia (Pierce et al., 1996; Chen et al., 1998) but did not support such a conclusion about 5-HT$_{1A}$ receptor mRNA (Pierce et al., 1996; Chen et al., 1998). This discrepancy further stresses that interpretation of changes in binding sites after lesion must be extremely cautious. Indeed, the slight loss of [^{3}H]8-OH-DPAT binding sites that was observed in the dorsal horn ipsilateral to the sectioned roots (Daval et al., 1987; Laporte et al., 1995; but see Croul et al., 1995) more probably reflected plastic phenomena at the postsynaptic level following the degeneration of primary afferent fibers (Laporte et al., 1995), rather than the disappearance of 5-HT$_{1A}$ receptors that would be located on these fibers. Accordingly, it can be concluded that, in the rat, 5-HT$_{1A}$ receptors in the dorsal horn of the spinal cord are located exclusively on neurons situated postsynaptically with regard to primary afferent fibers.

Messenger RNAs coding for 5-HT$_3$ receptors have also been visualized in neurons of the rat dorsal root ganglia as well as in the dorsal horn of the spinal cord (Tecott et al., 1993; Kia et al., 1995). This is congruent with the finding that dorsal rhizotomy or neonatal capsaicin treatment leads to a 50–80% decrease in the density of 5-HT$_3$ receptor binding sites in the superficial layers of the dorsal horn (Hamon et al., 1989; Kidd et al., 1993; Laporte et al., 1995). Indeed, there is presently no doubt that a large part of spinal 5-HT$_3$ receptors are located on primary afferent fibers entering the dorsal horn of the spinal cord. Nevertheless, 5-HT$_3$ receptor binding sites located postsynaptically with regard to these fibers also exist within the superficial laminae of the dorsal horn (Hamon et al., 1989; Kidd et al., 1993; Laporte et al., 1995).

With regard to the possible presence of other 5-HT receptor subtypes on primary afferent fibers projecting within the superficial layers of the dorsal horn of the spinal cord, important progress has recently been made by using the RT-PCR method to demonstrate synthesis of corresponding mRNAs in dorsal root ganglion cells. Thus Pierce et al. (1996) provided clear-cut evidence for the presence in the rat of not only the 5-HT$_{1B}$ and 5-HT$_3$ receptor mRNAs, but also of the 5-HT$_{1D}$, 5-HT$_{2A}$, 5-HT$_{2C}$, and 5-HT$_7$ receptor mRNAs in these cells. Using a similar approach applied to isolated dorsal root ganglia neurons in culture, Chen et al. (1998) partially confirmed and extended these findings by showing that 5-HT$_{1F}$, 5-HT$_4$, 5-HT$_{5A}$, and 5-HT$_{5B}$ mRNAs are also expressed in these cells. In contrast, transcripts encoding 5-HT$_{1A}$ and 5-HT$_{1E}$ receptors, and probably those encoding 5-HT$_{2B}$ receptors, were absent in dorsal root ganglion cells (Pierce et al., 1996; Chen et al., 1998).

The RT-PCR technique has also been applied to human dorsal root ganglia for the detection of transcripts encoding various 5-HT receptor subtypes. Although the data showed striking similarities with those found in the rat, differences were also noted. Thus, as in the rat, mRNAs encoding 5-HT$_{1B}$, 5-HT$_{1D}$, 5-HT$_{1F}$, 5-HT$_{2A}$, and 5-HT$_7$ receptors were found in human dorsal root ganglia (Pierce et al., 1997). In contrast, 5-HT$_{1E}$ mRNA was detected in humans but not in the rat (see above), and conversely, 5-HT$_{2C}$ mRNA could not be detected in humans although its presence in the rat was clearly demonstrated (Pierce et al., 1996, 1997; Chen et al., 1998). Finally, some ambiguity still persists in the case of the 5-HT$_{1A}$ receptor because its encoding mRNA was found in only one of the four subjects from which postmortem dorsal root ganglia were investigated (Pierce et al., 1997).

Serotonin Receptors in the Trigeminal Complex

Of particular interest with regard to pain associated with migraine are studies concerning the trigeminal ganglion from which originate the fibers projecting to the spinal trigeminal nucleus. Clearly, both 5-HT$_{1B}$ and 5-HT$_{1D}$ receptor mRNAs are expressed by trigeminal ganglion cells, but the 5-HT$_{1D}$ receptor subtype appears to be the most abundant in both the guinea pig and human (Rebeck et al., 1994; Bouchelet et al., 1996; Bonaventure et al., 1998a). Interestingly, double hybridization histochemistry allowed the demonstration that these receptors are in fact differentially distributed in the ganglia. Thus, using this approach, Bonaventure et al. (1998b) reported that 5-HT$_{1B}$ receptor mRNA is present in both calcitonin gene-related peptide (CGRP)- and substance P-containing neurons, whereas 5-HT$_{1D}$ receptor mRNA exists only in the latter neurons. On the other hand, functional 5-HT$_{2A}$ and 5-HT$_3$ receptors mediating excitatory actions of 5-HT do exist on neurons in the spinal trigeminal nucleus (Ebersberger et al., 1995).

In conclusion, almost all of the 5-HT receptors that have been cloned so far are present within the dorsal horn of the spinal cord (Table 10.1) and (also probably) the trigeminal complex, where the nociceptive messages generated at the periphery are processed to be transferred to brain areas. However, studies on their possible implications in pain mechanisms are still limited to only a few of these receptors, namely those for which selective, or at least preferential, agonists and antagonists are available. For this reason, we mainly focus our review of the relevant literature on the 5-HT$_{1A}$, 5-HT$_{1B/1D}$, 5-HT$_{2A}$, 5-HT$_{2C}$, and 5-HT$_3$ receptors.

PHARMACOLOGICAL EVIDENCE OF SEROTONIN RECEPTOR-MEDIATED CONTROL OF NOCICEPTION

Depending on the dose, route of administration, species under study, and experimental procedures used to assess sensitivity to nociceptive stimuli, 5-HT may either facilitate or inhibit nociceptive transmission. The availabilty of selective ligands of the 5-HT receptor subtypes cloned to date (Table 10.1) allowed investigations of their differential involvement in these multiple actions of the indoleamine. However, such investigations were limited because of the lack of appropriate ligands for studies on several of these receptors, particularly the 5-HT$_{5A}$, 5-HT$_{5B}$, 5-HT$_6$, and 5-HT$_7$ receptors (Table 10.1).

Numerous studies have shown that intrathecal administration of 5-HT itself produces an antinociceptive effect, as shown, for instance, in the tail flick test in mice and rats (Yaksh and Wilson, 1979; Hylden and Wilcox, 1983; Solomon and Gebhart, 1988; Advokat, 1993; Xu et al., 1994), and the paw pressure test in rats (Alloui et al., 1996). Several receptors probably mediate this effect because it can be blocked by various antagonists injected via the same route (Yaksh and Wilson, 1979; Solomon and Gebhart, 1988; Alloui et al., 1996).

In line with this hypothesis, evidence for the involvement of 5-HT$_{1A}$, 5-HT$_{1B}$, 5-HT$_2$, and/or 5-HT$_3$ receptors in the modulation of spinal nociceptive reflexes by 5-HT has been reported. Thus the antinociceptive effects of intrathecally administered 5-HT against a visceral stimulus (colorectal distension) appear to be mediated by all these receptors in the rat (Danzebrink and Gebhart, 1991a). In addition, the stimulation of both spinal 5-HT$_{1A}$ and 5-HT$_{1B}$ receptors by specific agonists is able to increase the tail flick latency in rats (Xu et al., 1994). This suggests that several receptor subtypes may be necessary for 5-HT to exert its antinociceptive action. In line with this conclusion, evidence has been reported that antinociception elicited by the direct electrical stimulation of the periaqueductal gray could be prevented by the pharmacological blockade of 5-HT$_{1A}$ receptors (by S-propranolol; Lin et al., 1996) and 5-HT$_3$ receptors (by ondansetron; Peng et al., 1996) at the spinal level in rats.

A major difficulty in identifying the various receptor subtypes responsible for the modulatory actions of 5-HT on nociception is that variable effects can be obtained with selective agonists, depending on the test used for assessing sensitivity to nociceptive stimuli. For instance, the 5-HT$_{1A}$ receptor agonist 8-OH-DPAT was shown to decrease tail flick latency when given intrathecally to rats (Solomon and Gebhart, 1988; Crisp et al., 1991; Xu et al., 1994). However, using a modified test, adjusted for skin temperature, it was shown that neither 8-OH-DPAT nor the 5-HT$_{1A/1B}$ receptor agonist RU 24969 [5-methoxy-3-(1,2,3,6-tetrahydropyridin-4-yl)-1H-indole succinate], administered via the same route, were active on tail flick latency in rats (Eide and Tjolsen, 1988; Mjellem et al., 1992). Indeed, spinal 5-HT is involved, not only in nociception, but also in non-nociceptive functions, such as motor control, and this may affect the response in nociceptive testing. In particular, spontaneous tail flicks can be elicited by the systemic administration of 8-OH-DPAT, which acts on postsynaptic 5-HT$_{1A}$ receptors at the spinal level in rats (Bervoets et al., 1993). This effect probably reflects an increased excitability of motoneurons, as demonstrated after intravenous administration of this 5-HT$_{1A}$ receptor agonist in rats (Jackson and White, 1990).

5-HT$_{1A}$ and 5-HT$_{1B}$ Receptors

Experiments in spinal rats showed that stimulation of 5-HT$_{1A}$ and 5-HT$_{1B}$ receptors by systemic administration of selective agonists produces opposite effects on nociceptive reflexes (Murphy and Zemlan, 1990). Thus the 5-HT$_{1A}$ receptor agonists, 8-OH-DPAT and buspirone, increased the receptive field area of a spinal nociceptive ventroflexion reflex after noxious levels of mechanical stimulation, whereas the 5-HT$_{1B}$ receptor agonists, m-chlorophenylpiperazine (m-CPP) and trifluoromethylphenylpiperazine, produced the opposite effect. In support of antinociceptive properties of 5-HT$_{1B}$ receptor agonists, Zemlan et al. (1988) reported that iontophoretic application of m-CPP inhibited the glutamic acid-induced firing of dorsal horn wide-dynamic-range nociceptive units, as well as their response to noxious peripheral stimulation. Similarly, El-Yassir et al. (1988) found that the 5-HT$_{1B}$ receptor agonist, RU 24969, selectively inhibited the response of wide-dynamic-range spinal units to noxious stimulation.

In contrast with the complex data obtained after their systemic administration (Millan, 1994), 5-HT$_{1A}$ receptor agonists are generally found to exert marked antinociceptive effects when injected intrathecally in rats (Gjerstad et al., 1996; Lin et al., 1996). Furthermore, via the latter route of injection, these compounds also exert a potent inhibitory influence on the electrical activity of nociceptive neurons in the rat dorsal horn (Gjerstad et al., 1996; Lin et al., 1996). According to some authors, analgesia consecutive to social conflict (Canto de Souza et al., 1997; De Souza et al., 1997) or psychological stress (Tokuyama et al., 1993) would be mediated through serotonin, acting (notably) at 5-HT$_{1A}$ receptors.

5-HT$_2$ Receptors

The involvement of 5-HT$_{2A/2C}$ receptors in the spinal antinociceptive action of 5-HT (Solomon and Gebhart, 1988) has received little support; Eide and Hole (1991a) and Kjørsvik et al. (1997) even concluded that the stimulation of spinal 5-HT$_{2A/2C}$ receptors facilitates the transmission of nociceptive information. Indeed, subcutaneous administration of the selective 5-HT$_{2A}$ receptor antagonist, ketanserin, produces antinociception in the hot plate and acetic acid-induced writhing tests in mice, but not in the tail flick test. However, this effect could involve supraspinal 5-HT$_{2A}$ receptors, because their stimulation may produce an inhibition of descending (including aminergic) control pathways (Barber et al., 1989; Alhaider, 1991). In addition, the peripheral blockade of 5-HT$_{2A}$ receptors also probably contributed to the antinociceptive effect of ketanserin, as these receptors clearly participate in the sensitization of nociceptors excited by algogenic agents (Meller et al., 1991a; Abbott et al., 1996, 1997; Germonpré et al., 1997). Indeed, evidence has been reported that 5-HT, released from mast cells and platelets in inflamed tissues, activates 5-HT$_{2A}$ receptors on nociceptors, thereby triggering nociceptive messages in Aδ and C fibers projecting into the dorsal horn of the spinal cord (Fig. 10.1). This sequence probably occurs for the biphasic pain response to intraplantar formalin, because 5-HT$_{2A}$ receptor antagonists such as ketanserin, ritanserin, and spiperone efficiently reduce this response in rats (Abbott et al., 1996, 1997). Accordingly, 5-HT$_{2A}$ receptor antagonists can be proposed as peripheral analgesics for the reduction of pain

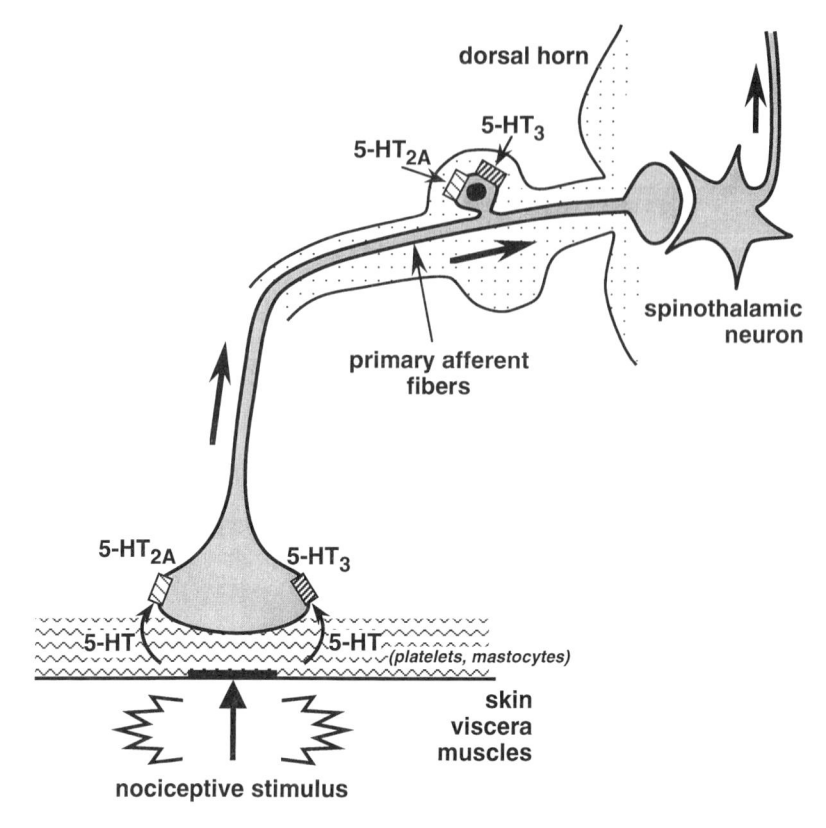

Figure 10.1 Involvement of 5-HT receptors in the generation of nociceptive messages at peripheral nociceptors. Tissue injury (inflammation) results in the local release of 5-HT from mastocytes and platelets, thereby activating excitatory 5-HT$_{2A}$ and 5-HT$_3$ receptors on nociceptors. The resulting sensitization to algogenic molecules (bradykinin, ATP, protons) triggers nerve impulse flow in primary afferent fibers, ending with pain sensation through message transfer to supraspinal centers. Blockade of peripheral 5-HT$_{2A}$ and 5-HT$_3$ receptors is efficient in reducing pain associated with tissue inflammation and acute injury (see text).

associated with local 5-HT release, such as that occurring during inflammation and acute tissue injury.

5-HT$_3$ Receptors

According to Glaum et al. (1988, 1990) and Bardin et al. (1997b), spinal 5-HT$_3$ receptors mediate the antinociceptive effect of intrathecally administered 5-HT (see Fig. 10.2); this possibly occurs via the local release of γ-aminobutyric acid (GABA; Alhaider et al., 1991). However, the involvement of 5-HT$_3$ receptors in the transfer and/or control of nociception is not limited to this

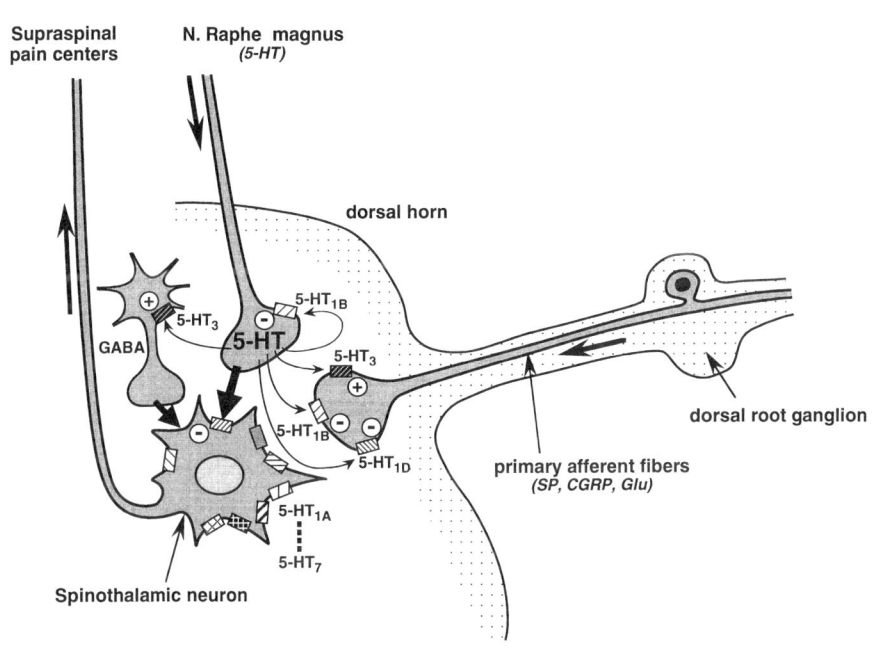

PHARMACOLOGICAL EVIDENCE OF SEROTONIN RECEPTOR-MEDIATED CONTROL   215

Figure 10.2 Pre- and postsynaptic 5-HT control of nociceptive messages in the dorsal horn of the spinal cord. 5-HT, released from descending bulbospinal projections (originating mainly in the nucleus raphe magnus), acts both at receptors located presynaptically on the terminals of primary afferent fibers, and postsynaptically at receptors expressed by interneurons (notably GABAergic neurons) and spinothalamic neurons. Thus 5-HT$_{1B/1D}$ receptor agonists inhibit the transfer of pain messages notably through a presynaptic blockade of substance P- and CGRP-containing primary afferent fibers (Arvieu et al., 1996). As analgesics at the spinal level, 5-HT$_{1A}$ receptor agonists act postsynaptically through a direct hyperpolarization of (spinothalamic) nociceptive neurons, whereas 5-HT$_3$ receptor agonists activate first GABAergic interneurons, which exert a secondary inhibitory influence on the spinothalamic neurons (Alhaider et al., 1991).

effect, as the stimulation of receptors of the 5-HT$_3$ type located on peripheral sensory nerves has—in contrast—been shown to induce pain in humans (Richardson and Buchheit, 1988) and to produce pain-related behavior in rats (Meller et al., 1991a,b, 1992). Indeed, at the periphery, 5-HT$_3$ receptors act in concert with 5-HT$_{2A}$ receptors to mediate the pain-triggering action of the indoleamine (Fig. 10.1; Grubb et al., 1988; Giordano and Rogers, 1989; Guilbaud et al., 1989; Meller et al., 1991a,1992; Taiwo and Levine, 1992). In particular, in addition to 5-HT$_2$ receptors, 5-HT$_3$ receptors have been reported to be involved in 5-HT-induced activation of nociceptive afferent fibers in inflamed tissues such as an arthritic joint (Grubb et al., 1988; Giordano and Rogers, 1989). Accordingly, opposite modulations of nociception may occur through 5-HT$_3$ receptor stimulation, depending on the location of these receptors. Indeed, within the spinal cord, Alhaider et al. (1991) provided clear-cut evidence that only the 5-HT$_3$ receptors located postsynaptically with respect to primary afferent fibers mediate the antinociceptive action of 5-HT and 5-HT$_3$ receptor agonists (Fig. 10.2). In contrast, the 5-HT$_3$ receptors located on the terminals of these fibers within the dorsal horn, like those on the peripheral sensory fibers (Fig. 10.1), might mediate an excitatory action of 5-HT leading to the release of neuropeptides ensuring the transfer of nociceptive messages, such as substance P and CGRP (Saria et al., 1990; Hua and Yaksh, 1993; Inoue et al., 1997). However, systemic injection of 5-HT$_3$ antagonists prevents only the behavioral responses to chemical noxious stimuli, not those to mechanical or thermal noxious stimuli in rats (Sufka and Giordano, 1991), thus suggesting that 5-HT$_3$ receptors on peripheral sensory fibers participate only in inflammatory pain (Eschalier et al., 1989; Giordano and Dyche, 1989; Giordano and Rogers, 1989). For the same reason as that explained for 5-HT$_{2A}$ receptors, 5-HT$_3$ receptor antagonists might therefore be of interest for the reduction of pain associated with inflammation and acute tissue injury (Kishibayashi et al., 1993; Langlois et al., 1996). Indeed, like that previously noted for 5-HT$_{2A}$ receptor antagonists (Abbott et al., 1996, 1997), 5-HT$_3$ receptor antagonists such as tropisetron and ondansetron were found to reduce nociceptive behavior normally triggered by injection of formalin or collagenase into a hindpaw in rats (Damas et al., 1997; Doak and Sawynok, 1997).

POSSIBLE MECHANISMS INVOLVED IN SEROTONIN RECEPTOR-MEDIATED MODULATION OF NOCICEPTION

Interactions between 5-HT and other neuroactive substances, such as substance P and adenosine, have been shown to exist at the spinal level (Eide and Hole, 1991b; Sawynok and Reid, 1991), but much emphasis has been placed on noradrenaline (NA) (Sawynok and Reid, 1996). In particular, Archer and co-workers reported that NA depletion, owing to the systemic or intrathecal administration of neurotoxins, blocks the antinociceptive effect of intrathecally injected 5-HT in the tail flick test, and that NA injected via the same route restored the antinociceptive effect of the potent 5-HT$_1$ receptor agonist 5-methoxy-N,N-dimethyltryptamine in NA-depleted rats (Minor et al., 1985, 1988; Archer et al., 1986; Post et al., 1986). This could not be due to some toxin-induced decrease in spinal 5-HT receptor densities, because the selective lesion of the noradrenergic system by DSP-4 actually enhances the density of both 5-HT$_{1A}$ and 5-HT$_{1B}$ sites (Laporte et al., 1995). However, if the net effect of intrathecally administered 5-HT on nociception results from a balance between a pronociceptive effect due to 5-HT$_{1A}$ receptor stimulation and an antinociceptive effect due to 5-HT$_{1B}$ receptor stimulation (Murphy and Zemlan, 1990; Alhaider and Wilcox, 1993), it is possible that the lack of analgesic action of 5-HT after NA depletion may be due to a 5-HT$_{1A}$ receptor-mediated effect that is relatively higher than in intact animals. Other mechanisms can also be proposed. Thus DeLander and Hopkins (1987) reported that intrathecally injected NA and 5-HT potentiate each other as antinociceptive agents in the tail flick test in mice. Similarly, Danzebrink and Gebhart (1991b) found that the intrathecal co-administration of the α2 adrenoceptor agonist, clonidine, with 5-HT receptor agonists produces supra-additive visceral antinociception in the rat. Conversely, α2 adrenoceptor blockade by yohimbine has been shown to prevent the inhibitory effect of intrathecally administered 5-HT on noxious-evoked activity of wide-dynamic-range neurons in the cat dorsal horn (Nakagawa et al., 1990). Finally, evidence has been reported that 5-methoxy-*N,N*-dimethyltryptamine facilitates NA release from rat spinal cord slices (Reinmann and Schneider, 1993). Hence, all of these observations point to a NA mediation of the antinociceptive effect of spinal 5-HT that probably involves both pre- and postsynaptic mechanisms with respect to noradrenergic terminals. Although the 5-HT receptor(s) that interact(s) with NA receptors (α_2 adrenoceptors) on the postsynaptic targets of noradrenergic terminals has (have) not yet been identified, those responsible for the stimulatory effect of 5-HT on NA release from presynaptic noradrenergic terminals probably belong to the 5-HT_{2C} subtype (Sawynok and Reid, 1992).

Relatively little is known yet about the cellular mechanisms underlying 5-HT modulation of dorsal horn activity. Local administration of the indoleamine generally produces an inhibition of nociceptive neurons, although excitatory effects on deep dorsal horn neurons were also observed. Serotonin has diverse actions on frog dorsal horn neurons (depolarization, hyperpolarization, and biphasic responses), which appear to be mediated by at least three receptor subtypes: depolarization is triggered by the stimulation of $5\text{-HT}_{2A/2C}$ receptors in some cells and by that of 5-HT_3 receptors in others; hyperpolarization apparently results from the stimulation of 5-HT_{1A} receptors (Tan and Miletic, 1992). Some data suggest that 5-HT fibers may participate in axo-axonic synapses in the dorsal horn. In particular, 5-HT receptors exist on primary afferent fibers (Table 10.1, Fig. 10.2), and it has been shown that iontophoretic application of 5-HT increases the threshold for antidromic activation of such fibers in the cat (Carstens et al., 1981). More complex data were obtained on frog primary afferent fibers, as Holohean et al. (1990) described both hyperpolarizations and depolarizations of these fibers upon local application of 5-HT. Thus the indoleamine could either decrease the amplitude of primary afferent-evoked excitatory postsynaptic potential or increase the electrical stimulation threshold for primary afferent-evoked action potentials, as expected of an action on the primary afferent fibers themselves (Tan and Miletic, 1992). Several types of 5-HT receptors are potentially involved in these actions in light of their proven expression in dorsal root ganglion cells (Table 10.1).

In fact, 5-HT does cause a variety of membrane responses in cell bodies of primary afferent neurons (Holz et al., 1986; Morita and Katayama, 1987; Tan and Miletic, 1992). 5-HT_{2A} and 5-HT_3 receptors have been implicated in the 5-HT-induced depolarization of dorsal root ganglion cells (Todorovic and Anderson, 1990; Robertson and Bevan, 1991). In contrast, 5-HT hyperpolarizes capsaicin-sensitive C-type sensory neurons probably by activating 5-HT$_1$ receptors (Todorovic and Anderson, 1992). Similarly, clear-cut evidence has been reported that 5-HT$_{1B/1D}$ receptor agonists such as sumatriptan and its analogues (zolmitriptan, rizatriptan, naratriptan) prevent the excitation of spinal trigeminal nucleus neurons evoked by direct electrical stimulation of the superior sagittal sinus or neurogenic inflammation of the meninges (Nozaki et al., 1992; Goadsby and Knight, 1997). This effect very probably accounts for the efficiency of these drugs to reduce pain associated with migraine.

As expected from their location on sensory fibers conveying nociceptive messages (Fig. 10.2), 5-HT$_{1B/1D}$ and 5-HT$_3$ receptors have been shown to mediate modulatory effects of 5-HT on the release of neurotransmitters contained in these fibers. In particular, Arvieu et al. (1996) provided the first direct demonstration of a neuronal action of sumatriptan by showing that this 5-HT$_{1B/1D/1F}$ agonist (Castro et al., 1997) significantly reduces the spinal release of both substance P and CGRP evoked by the electrical stimulation of primary afferent fibers. Further studies with various agonists and antagonists showed that this effect, in fact, results from the activation of presynaptic 5-HT$_{1B}$ receptors by sumatriptan (Arvieu et al., 1996; Bourgoin, unpublished observations). In addition, electrophysiological data suggested that sumatriptan, also via the activation of presynaptic 5-HT$_{1B/1D}$ receptors, probably inhibits the release of glutamate from primary afferent terminals in the spinal trigeminal nucleus (Travagli and Williams, 1996). In contrast, 5-HT$_{1A}$ receptor stimulation in the dorsal horn does not affect substance P release (Nobrega et al., 1995) in agreement with its probably exclusive postsynaptic location with regard to primary afferent fibers (see above).

In line with the peripheral excitatory effect of 5-HT via the stimulation of 5-HT$_3$ receptors, it has been shown that the indoleamine enhances the release of CGRP evoked by capsaicin from C fibers in the rat trachea, and that this effect can be blocked by the potent 5-HT$_3$ receptor antagonist, tropisetron, but not by 5-HT$_1$ or 5-HT$_2$ receptor antagonists (Hua and Yaksh, 1993). Such an excitatory effect of 5-HT$_3$ receptor stimulation on CGRP-containing terminals of primary afferent fibers within the dorsal horn has also been reported by Saria et al. (1990). However, the latter effect is probably unrelated to the modulatory action of 5-HT$_3$ receptor agonists on nociception at the spinal level, because Alhaider et al. (1991) convincingly showed that only the postsynaptic 5-HT$_3$ receptors, that is, those located downstream of (CGRP-containing) primary afferent fibers, participate in the analgesic action of intrathecally administered 5-HT.

CONCLUSION AND PERSPECTIVES

Considerable progress has been made in recent years in the knowledge of the various receptors that mediate the multiple actions of 5-HT. With regard to nociception, clear-cut evidence has been obtained in support of the idea that

5-HT$_{1A}$, 5-HT$_{1B}$, 5-HT$_{1D}$, 5-HT$_{2A/2C}$, and 5-HT$_3$ receptors participate in the modulatory effects of 5-HT either in the central nervous system or at the periphery. Among the drugs that have been developed for the selective activation or blockade of 5-HT receptors, only 5-HT$_{1B/1D}$ agonists such as sumatriptan and its derivatives have revealed a therapeutic value thanks to their remarkable efficacy in reducing pain associated with migraine. In contrast, no analgesic has yet been developed on the basis of extensive studies devoted to the other receptor types. Nevertheless, promising data suggest that antagonists acting at peripheral 5-HT$_{2A}$ and 5-HT$_3$ receptors should be of value in reducing local pain associated with tissue injury, especially inflammation. In addition, further investigations on the mechanisms of action of sumatriptan (Waeber and Moskowitz, 1995; Castro et al., 1997) and its derivatives recently led to the synthesis of selective 5-HT$_{1F}$ receptor agonists as novel antimigraine drugs (Johnson et al., 1997). If such drugs prove to be really active for this indication, their development will represent a real progress because 5-HT$_{1F}$ agonists, in contrast to 5-HT$_{1B/1D}$ agonists, should be devoid of any secondary vasoconstrictor effects, notably on coronary arteries. Other developments might also concern neuropathic pain, on which spinal 5-HT has recently been shown to exert a strong inhibitory influence in a relevant animal model (chronic constriction injury of the sciatic nerve in rats) (Eaton et al., 1997). However, the receptors involved in this effect of the indoleamine (Sanchez et al., 1995) are still poorly characterized. Finally, it has to be emphasized that the most recently discovered 5-HT receptors of the 5-HT$_{2B}$, 5-HT$_4$, 5-HT$_{5A}$, 5-HT$_{5B}$, 5-HT$_6$, and 5-HT$_7$ subtypes are also located within the strategic area for the 5-HT control of nociceptive messages at the spinal level. To date, however, these receptors have been the matter of only very limited—or even no—studies regarding their possible involvement in this function. Selective ligands for such studies are therefore eagerly needed.

ACKNOWLEDGMENT

We are grateful to Claude Sais for her excellent secretarial assistance.

REFERENCES

Abbott FV, Hong Y, Blier P (1996): Activation of 5-HT$_{2A}$ receptors potentiates pain produced by inflammatory mediators. Neuropharmacology 35:99–110.

Abbott FV, Hong Y, Blier P (1997): Persisting sensitization of the behavioural response to formalin-induced injury in the rat through activation of serotonin$_{2A}$ receptors. Neuroscience 77:575–584.

Advokat A (1993): Intrathecal coadministration of serotonin and morphine differentially modulates the tail-flick reflex of intact and spinal rats. Pharmacol Biochem Behav 45:871–879.

Alhaider AA (1991): Antinociceptive effect of ketanserin in mice: involvement of supraspinal 5-HT$_2$ receptors in nociceptive transmission. Brain Res 543:335–340.

Alhaider AA, Wilcox GL (1993): Differential roles of 5-hydroxytryptamine$_{1A}$ and 5-hydroxytryptamine$_{1B}$ receptor subtypes in modulating spinal nociceptive transmission in mice. J Pharmacol Exp Ther 265:378–385.

Alhaider AA, Lei SZ, Wilcox GL (1991): Spinal 5-HT$_3$ receptor-mediated antinociception: possible release of GABA. J Neurosci 11:1881–1888.

Alloui A, Pelissier T, Dubray C, Lavarenne J, Eschalier A (1996): Tropisetron inhibits the antinociceptive effect of intrathecally administered paracetamol and serotonin. Fundam Clin Pharmacol 10:406–407.

Alstergren P, Kopp S (1997): Pain and synovial fluid concentration of serotonin in arthritic temporomandibular joints. Pain 72:137–143.

Archer T, Danysz W, Jonsson G, Minor BG, Post C (1986): 5-methoxy-N-N-dimethyl-tryptamine-induced analgesia is blocked by α-adrenoreceptor antagonists in rats. Br J Pharmacol 89:293–298.

Archer T, Arweström E, Minor BG, Persson ML, Post C, Sundstrom E, Jonsson G (1987): (+)-8-OH-DPAT and 5-MeODMT-induced analgesia is antagonized by noradrenaline depletion. Physiol Behav 39:95–102.

Arvieu L, Mauborgne A, Bourgoin S, Oliver C, Feltz P, Hamon M, Cesselin F (1996): Sumatriptan inhibits the release of CGRP and substance P from the rat spinal cord. NeuroReport 7:1973–1976.

Barber A, Harting J, Wolf HP (1989): Antinociceptive effects of the 5-HT$_2$ antagonist ritanserin in rats: evidence for an activation of descending monoaminergic pathways in the spinal cord. Neurosci Lett 99:234–238.

Bardin L, Bardin M, Lavarenne J, Eschalier A (1997a): Effect of intrathecal serotonin on nociception in rats: Influence of the pain test used. Exp Brain Res 113:81–87.

Bardin L, Jourdan D, Alloui A, Lavarenne J, Eschalier A (1997b): Differential influence of two serotonin 5-HT$_3$ receptor antagonists on spinal serotonin-induced analgesia in rats. Brain Res 765:267–272.

Bervoets K, Rivet JM, Millan MJ (1993): 5-HT$_{1A}$ receptors and the tail-flick response. IV. Spinally localized 5-HT$_{1A}$ receptors postsynaptic to serotoninergic neurones mediate spontaneous tail-flicks in the rat. J Pharmacol Exp Ther 264:95–104.

Blackshear MA, Steranka LR, Sanders-Bush E (1981): Multiple serotonin receptors: regional distribution and effects of raphe lesions. Eur J Pharmacol 76:326–334.

Boess FG, Martin JL (1994): Molecular biology of 5-HT receptors. Neuropharmacology 33:275–317.

Bonaventure P, Voorn P, Luyten WHML, Jurzak M, Schotte A, Leysen JE (1998a): Detailed mapping of serotonin 5-HT$_{1B}$ and 5-HT$_{1D}$ receptor messenger RNA and ligand binding sites in guinea-pig brain and trigeminal ganglion: clues for function. Neuroscience 82:469–484.

Bonaventure P, Voorn P, Luyten WHML, Leysen JE (1998b): 5-HT$_{1B}$ and 5-HT$_{1D}$ receptor mRNA differential co-localization with peptide mRNA in the guinea pig trigeminal ganglion. NeuroReport 9:641–645.

Bouchelet I, Cohen Z, Case B, Seguela P, Hamel E (1996): Differential expression of sumatriptan-sensitive 5-hydroxytryptamine receptors in human trigeminal ganglia and cerebral blood vessels. Mol Pharmacol 50:219–223.

Bowker RM, Abbott LC (1990): Quantitative re-evaluation of descending serotonergic and non-serotonergic projections from the medulla of the rodent: evidence for extensive co-existence of serotonin and peptides in the same spinally projecting neurons, but not from the nucleus raphe magnus. Brain Res 512:15–25.

Brown L, Amedro J, Williams GM, Smith D (1988): A pharmacological analysis of the rat spinal cord serotonin (5-HT) autoreceptor. Eur J Pharmacol 145:163–171.

Brown LM, Smith DL, Williams GM, Smith DJ (1989): Alterations in serotonin binding after 5,7-dihydroxytryptamine treatment in the rat spinal cord. Neurosci Lett 102: 103–107.

Bruinvels AT, Landwehrmeyer BL, Moskowitz MA, Hoyer D (1992): Evidence for the presence of 5-HT$_{1B}$ receptor messenger RNA in neurons of the rat trigeminal ganglia. Eur J Pharmacol—Mol Pharmacol Sect 227:357–359.

Bullitt E, Light AR (1989): Intraspinal course of descending serotoninergic pathways innervating the rodent dorsal horn and Lamina X. J Comp Neurol 286:231–242.

Canto de Souza A, Nunes de Souza RL, Pelà IR, Graeff FG (1997): High intensity social conflict in the swiss albino mouse induces analgesia modulated by 5-HT$_{1A}$ receptors. Pharmacol Biochem Behav 56:481–486.

Cardenas CG, DelMar LP, Cooper BY, Scroggs RS (1997): 5-HT$_4$ receptors couple positively to tetrodotoxin-insensitive sodium channels in a subpopulation of capsaicin-sensitive rat sensory neurons. J Neurosci 17:7181–7189.

Carson MJ, Thomas EA, Danielson PE, Sutcliffe JG (1996): The 5-HT$_{5A}$ serotonin receptor is expressed predominantly by astrocytes in which it inhibits cAMP accumulation: a mechanism for neuronal suppression of reactive astrocytes. Glia 17:317–326.

Carstens E, Klumpp D, Randic M, Zimmermann M (1981): Effect of iontophoretically applied-5-hydroxytryptamine on the excitability of single primary afferent C- and A-fibers in the cat spinal cord. Brain Res 220:151–158.

Castro ME, Pascual J, Romon T, Del Arco C, Del Olmo E, Pazos A (1997): Differential distribution of [^{3}H]sumatriptan binding sites (5-HT$_{1B}$, 5-HT$_{1D}$ and 5-HT$_{1F}$ receptors) in human brain: Focus on brainstem and spinal cord. Neuropharmacology 36:535–542.

Cesselin F, Laporte AM, Miquel MC, Bourgoin S, Hamon M (1994): Serotonergic mechanisms of pain control. In Gebhart GF, Hammond DL, Jensen TS (eds): *Proceedings of the 7th World Congress on Pain*, Vol. 2. Seattle: IASP Press, pp. 669–695.

Chen JJ, Vasko MR, Wu X, Staeva TP, Baez M, Zgombick JM, Nelson DL (1998): Multiple subtypes of serotonin receptors are expressed in rat sensory neurons in culture. J Pharmacol Exp Ther 287:1119–1127.

Crisp T, Stafinsky JL, Spanos LJ, Uram M, Perni V, Donepudi HB (1991): Analgesic effects of serotonin and receptor-selective serotonin agonists in the rat spinal cord. Gen Pharmacol 22:247–251.

Croul S, Sverstiuk A, Radzievsky A, Murray M (1995): Modulation of neurotransmitter receptors following unilateral L1-S2 deafferentation: NK1, NK3, NMDA, and 5-HT$_{1a}$ receptor binding autoradiography. J Comp Neurol 361:633–644.

Damas J, Liégeois JF, Bourdon V (1997): Involvement of 5-hydroxytryptamine and bradykinin in the hyperalgesia induced in rats by collagenase from Clostridium histolyticum. Naunyn-Schmiedeberg's Arch Pharmacol 355:566–570.

Danzebrink RM, Gebhart GF (1991a): Evidence that 5-HT_1, 5-HT_2 and 5-HT_3 receptor subtypes modulate responses to noxious colorectal distension in the rat. Brain Res 538:64–75.

Danzebrink RM, Gebhart GF (1991b): Intrathecal coadministration of clonidine with serotonin receptor agonists produces supra-additive visceral antinociception in the rat. Brain Res 555:35–42.

Daval G, Vergé D, Basbaum AI, Bourgoin S, Hamon M (1987): Autoradiographic evidence of serotonin$_1$ binding sites on primary afferent fibres in the dorsal horn of the rat spinal cord. Neurosci Lett 83:71–76.

DeLander GE, Hopkins CJ (1987): Interdependence of spinal adenosinergic, serotonergic and noradrenergic systems mediating antinociception. Neuropharmacology 26:1791–1794.

DeSouza AC, deSouza RLN, Pela IR, Graeff FG (1997): High intensity social conflict in the Swiss albino mouse induces analgesia modulated by 5-HT_{1A} receptors. Pharmacol Biochem Behav 56:481–486.

Doak GJ, Sawynok J (1997): Formalin-induced nociceptive behavior and edema: Involvement of multiple peripheral 5-hydroxytryptamine receptor subtypes. Neuroscience 80:939–949.

Doucet E, Pohl M, Fattaccini CM, Adrien J, El Mestikawy S, Hamon M (1995): In situ hybridization evidence for the synthesis of 5-HT_{1B} receptor in serotoninergic neurons of anterior raphe nuclei in the rat brain. Synapse 19:18–28.

Eaton MJ, Santiago DI, Dancausse HA, Whittemore SR (1997): Lumbar transplants of immortalized serotonergic neurons alleviate chronic neuropathic pain. Pain 72:59–69.

Ebersberger A, Anton F, Tolle TR, Zieglgansberger W (1995): Morphine, 5-HT_2 and 5-HT_3 receptor antagonists reduce c-fos expression in the trigeminal nuclear complex following noxious chemical stimulation of the rat nasal mucosa. Brain Res 676:336–342.

Eide PK, Hole K (1991a): Different role of 5-HT_{1A} and 5-HT_2 receptors in spinal cord in the control of nociceptive responsiveness. Neuropharmacology 30:727–731.

Eide PK, Hole K (1991b): Interactions between serotonin and substance P in the spinal regulation of nociception. Brain Res 550:225–230.

Eide PK, Tjolsen A (1988): Effects of serotonin receptor antagonists and agonists on the tail flick response in mice involve altered tail-skin temperature. Neuropharmacology 27:889–893.

Eide PK, Hole K, Broch OJ (1992): Supersensitivity to the antinociceptive effect of a 5-HT_1 receptor agonist after lesion of raphe-spinal serotonergic neurones. Pharmacol Toxicol 71:62–64.

El-Yassir N, Fleetwood-Walker SM, Mitchell R (1988): Heterogeneous effects of serotonin in the dorsal horn: the involvement of 5-HT_1 receptor subtypes. Brain Res 456:147–158.

Eschalier A, Kayser V, Guilbaud G (1989): Influence of a specific 5-HT_3 antagonist on carrageenan-induced hyperalgesia in rats. Pain 36:249–255.

Germonpré PR, Joos GF, Mekeirele K, Pauwels RA (1997): Role of the 5-HT receptor in neurogenic inflammation in Fisher 344 rat airways. Eur J Pharmacol 324:249–255.

Giordano J, Dyche J (1989): Differential analgesic actions of serotonin 5-HT$_3$ receptor antagonists in the mouse. Neuropharmacology 28:423–427.

Giordano J, Rogers LV (1989): Peripherally administered serotonin 5-HT$_3$ receptor antagonists reduce inflammatory pain in rats. Eur J Pharmacol 170:83–86.

Gjerstad J, Tjolsen A, Hole K (1996): The effect of 5-HT$_{1A}$ receptor stimulation on nociceptive dorsal horn neurones in rats. Eur J Pharmacol 318:315–321.

Glaum SR, Proudfit HK, Anderson EG (1988): Reversal of the antinociceptive effects of intrathecally administered serotonin in the rat by a selective 5-HT$_3$ receptor antagonist. Neurosci Lett 95:313–317.

Glaum SR, Proudfit HK, Anderson EG (1990): 5-HT$_3$ receptors modulate spinal nociceptive reflexes. Brain Res 510:12–16.

Goadsby PJ, Knight Y (1997): Inhibition of trigeminal neurones after intravenous administration of naratriptan through an action of 5-hydroxytryptamine (5-HT$_{1B/1D}$) receptors. Br J Pharmacol 122:918–922.

Grubb BD, McQueen DS, Iggo A, Birrell GJ, Dutia MB (1988): A study of 5-HT receptors associated with afferent nerves located in normal and inflamed rat ankle joints. Agents Actions 25:216–218.

Guilbaud G, Benoist JM, Eschalier A, Gautron M, Kayser V (1989): Evidence for peripheral serotonergic mechanisms in the early sensitization after carrageenan-induced inflammation: electrophysiological studies in the ventrobasal complex of the rat thalamus using a specific antagonist of peripheral 5-HT receptors. Brain Res 502: 187–197.

Hamon M, Gallissot MC, Ménard F, Gozlan H, Bourgoin S, Vergé D (1989): 5-HT$_3$ receptor binding sites are on capsaicin-sensitive fibres in the rat spinal cord. Eur J Pharmacol 164:315–322.

Helton LA, Thor KB, Baez M (1994): 5-Hydroxytryptamine$_{2A}$, 5-hydroxytryptamine$_{2B}$, and 5-hydroxytryptamine$_{2C}$ receptor mRNA expression in the spinal cord of rat, cat, monkey and human. NeuroReport 5:2617–2620.

Holohean AM, Hackman JC, Davidoff RA (1990): An in vitro study of the effects of serotonin on frog primary afferent terminals. Neurosci Lett 113:175–180.

Holz GG, Shefner SA, Anderson EG (1986): Serotonin decreases the duration of action potentials recorded from tetraethylammonium-treated bullfrog dorsal root ganglion cells. J Neurosci 6:620–626.

Hoyer D, Clarke DE, Fozard JR, Hartig PR, Martin GR, Mylecharane EJ, Saxena PR, Humphrey PPA (1994): VII. International Union of Pharmacology classification of receptors for 5-hydroxytryptamine (serotonin). Pharmacol Rev 46.157–203.

Hua XY, Yaksh TL (1993): Pharmacology of the effects of bradykinin, serotonin, and histamine on the release of calcitonin gene-related peptide from C-fiber terminals in the rat trachea. J Neurosci 13:1947–1953.

Hylden JL, Wilcox GL (1983): Intrathecal serotonin in mice: analgesia and inhibition of a spinal action of substance P. Life Sci 33:789–795.

Inoue A, Hashimoto T, Hide I, Nishio H, Nakata Y (1997): 5-Hydroxytryptamine-facilitated release of substance P from rat spinal cord slices is mediated by nitric oxide and cyclic GMP. J Neurochem 68:128–133.

Jackson DA, White SR (1990): Receptor subtypes mediating facilitation by serotonin of excitability of spinal motoneurons. Neuropharmacology 29:787–797.

Johnson KW, Schaus JM, Durkin MM, Audia JE, Kaldor SW, Flaugh ME, Adham N, Zgombick JM, Cohen ML, Branchek TA, Phebus LA (1997): 5-HT$_{1F}$ receptor agonists inhibit neurogenic dural inflammation in guinea pigs. NeuroReport 8:2237–2240.

Julius D, Huang KN, Livelli TJ, Axel R, Jessell TM (1990): The 5-HT$_2$ receptor defines a family of structurally distinct but functionally conserved serotonin receptors. Proc Natl Acad Sci USA 87:928–932.

Kia HK, Miquel MC, McKernan RM, Laporte AM, Lombard MC, Bourgoin S, Hamon M, Vergé D (1995): Localization of 5-HT$_3$ receptors in the rat spinal cord: immunohistochemistry and in situ hybridization. NeuroReport 6:257–261.

Kia HK, Miquel MC, Brisorgueil MJ, Daval G, Riad M, El Mestikawy S, Hamon M, Vergé D (1996): Immunocytochemical localization of serotonin$_{1A}$ receptors in the rat central nervous system. J Comp Neurol 365:289–305.

Kidd EJ, Laporte AM, Langlois X, Fattaccini CM, Doyen C, Lombard MC, Gozlan H, Hamon M (1993): 5-HT$_3$ receptors in the rat central nervous system are mainly located on nerve fibres and terminals. Brain Res 612:289–298.

Kishibayashi N, Miwa Y, Hayashi H, Ishii A, Ichikawa S, Nonaka H, Yokoyama T, Susuki F (1993): 5-HT$_3$ receptor antagonists. 3. Quinoline derivatives which may be effective in the therapy of irritable bowel syndrome. J Med Chem 36:3286–3292.

Kjørsvik A, Størkson R, Tjølsen A, Hole K (1997): Differential effects of activation of lumbar and thoracic 5-HT$_{2A/2C}$ receptors on nociception in rats. Pharmacol Biochem Behav 56:523–527.

Kwiat GC, Basbaum AI (1992): The origin of brainstem noradrenergic and serotonergic projections to the spinal cord dorsal horn of the rat. Somatosensory Motor Res 9:157–173.

LaMotte CC, Johns DR, DeLanerolle NC (1982): Immunohistochemical evidence of indolamine neurons in monkey spinal cord. J Comp Neurol 206:359–370.

Langlois A, Pascaud X, Junien JL, Dahl SG, Riviere PJM (1996): Response heterogeneity of 5-HT$_3$ receptor antagonists in a rat visceral hypersensitivity model. Eur J Pharmacol 318:141–144.

Laporte AM, Doyen C, Nevo IT, Chauveau J, Hauw JJ, Hamon M (1996): Autoradiographic mapping of serotonin 5-HT$_{1A}$, 5-HT$_{1D}$, 5-HT$_{2A}$, and 5-HT$_3$ receptors in the aged human spinal cord. J Chem Neuroanat 11:67–75.

Laporte AM, Koscielniak T, Ponchant M, Vergé D, Hamon M, Gozlan H (1992): Quantitative autoradiographic mapping of 5-HT$_3$ receptors in the rat CNS using [^{125}I]iodozacopride and [^{3}H]zacopride as radioligands. Synapse 10:271–281.

Laporte AM, Fattaccini CM, Lombard MC, Chauveau J, Hamon M (1995): Effects of dorsal rhizotomy and selective lesion of serotonergic and noradrenergic systems on 5-HT$_{1A}$, 5-HT$_{1B}$ and 5-HT$_3$ receptors in the rat spinal cord. J Neural Transm [Gen Sect] 100:207–223.

Le Bars D (1988): Serotonin and pain. In Osborne NN, Hamon M (eds): *Neuronal Serotonin*. Chichester: John Wiley & Sons, pp. 171–229.

Leysen JE, Niemegeers CJE, Van Nueten JM, Laduron PM (1982): [^{3}H]ketanserin (R 41 468), a selective ^{3}H-ligand for serotonin$_2$ receptor binding sites. Binding properties, brain distribution, and functional role. Mol Pharmacol 21:301–314.

Lin Q, Peng YB, Willis WD (1996): Antinociception and inhibition from the periaqueductal gray are mediated in part by spinal 5-hydroxytryptamine$_{1A}$ receptors. J Pharmacol Exp Ther 276:958–967.

Lyon RA, Davis KH, Titeler M (1987): ^{3}H-DOB labels a guanylnucleotide-sensitive state of 5-HT$_2$ receptor. J Pharmacol Exp Ther 31:194–199.

Marlier L, Teilhac JR, Cerruti C, Privat A (1991): Autoradiographic mapping of 5-HT$_1$, 5-HT$_{1A}$, 5-HT$_{1B}$, and 5-HT$_2$ receptors in the rat spinal cord. Brain Res 550:15–23.

Matsumoto I, Combs MR, Jones DJ (1992): Characterization of 5-hydroxytryptamine$_{1B}$ receptors in rat spinal cord via [^{125}I]iodocyanopindolol binding and inhibition of [^{3}H]-5-hydroxytryptamine release. J Pharmacol Exp Ther 260:614–626.

Meller ST, Lewis SJ, Brody MJ, Gebhart GF (1991a): The peripheral nociceptive actions of intravenously administered 5-HT in the rat requires dual activation of both 5-HT$_2$ and 5-HT$_3$ receptor subtypes. Brain Res 561:61–68.

Meller ST, Lewis SJ, Ness TJ, Brody MJ, Gebhart GF (1991b): Neonatal capsaicin treatment abolishes the nociceptive responses to intravenous 5-HT in the rat. Brain Res 542:212–218.

Meller ST, Lewis SJ, Brody MJ, Gebhart GF (1992): Vagal afferent-mediated inhibition of a nociceptive reflex by i.v. serotonin in the rat. II. Role of 5-HT receptor subtypes. Brain Res 585:71–86.

Millan MJ (1994): Serotonin and pain: evidence that activation of 5-HT$_{1A}$ receptors does not elicit antinociception against noxious thermal, mechanical and chemical stimuli in mice. Pain 58:45–61.

Minor BG, Post C, Archer T (1985): Blockade of intrathecal 5-hydroxytryptamine-induced antinociception in rats by noradrenaline depletion. Neurosci Lett 54:39–44.

Minor BG, Persson ML, Post C, Jonsson G, Archer T (1988): Intrathecal noradrenaline restores 5-methoxy-N,N-dimethyltryptamine-induced antinociception abolished by intrathecal 6-hydroxydopamine. J Neural Transm 72:107–120.

Mjellem N, Lundt A, Eide PK, Storkson R, Tjølsen A (1992): The role of 5-HT$_{1A}$ and 5-HT$_{1B}$ receptors in spinal transmission and in the modulation of NMDA-induced behaviour. NeuroReport 3:1061–1064.

Monroe PJ, Smith DJ (1983): Characterization of multiple [^{3}H]5-hydroxytryptamine binding sites in rat spinal cord tissue. J Neurochem 41:349–355.

Morita K, Katayama Y (1987): 5-hydroxytryptamine effects on the soma of bullfrog primary afferent neurons. Neuroscience 21:1007–1018.

Murphy RM, Zemlan FP (1988): Selective 5-HT$_{1B}$ agonists identify the 5-HT autoreceptor in lumbar spinal cord of rat. Neuropharmacology 27:37–42.

Murphy RM, Zemlan FP (1990): Selective serotonin1A/1B agonists differentially affect spinal nociceptive reflexes. Neuropharmacology 29:463–468.

Nakagawa I, Omote K, Kitahata LM, Collins JG, Murata K (1990): Serotonergic mediation of spinal analgesia and its interaction with noradrenergic systems. Anesthesiology 73:474–478.

Nobrega ACL, Meintjes AF, Ally A, Wilson LB (1995): Modulation of reflex pressor response to contraction and effect on substance P release by spinal 5-HT$_{1A}$ receptors. Am J Physiol 268:H1577–H1585.

Nozaki K, Moskowitz MA, Boccalini P (1992): CP-93,129, sumatriptan, dihydroergotamine block c-fos expression within rat trigeminal nucleus caudalis caused by chemical stimulation of the meninges. Br J Pharmacol 106:409–415.

Oliveras JL, Bourgoin S, Héry F, Besson JM, Hamon M (1977): The topographical distribution of serotoninergic terminals in the spinal cord of the cat: biochemical mapping by the combined use of microdissection and microassay procedures. Brain Res 138:393–406.

Peng YB, Lin Q, Willis WD (1996): The role of 5-HT$_3$ receptors in periaqueductal gray-induced inhibition of nociceptive dorsal horn neurons in rats. J Pharmacol Exp Ther 276:116–124.

Pierce PA, Xie GX, Levine JD, Peroutka SJ (1996): 5-hydroxytryptamine receptor subtype messenger RNAs in rat peripheral sensory and sympathetic ganglia: a polymerase chain reaction study. Neuroscience 70:553–559.

Pierce PA, Xie GX, Meuser T, Peroutka SJ (1997): 5-hydroxytryptamine receptor subtype messenger RNAs in human dorsal root ganglia: a polymerase chain reaction study. Neuroscience 81:813–819.

Pompeiano M, Palacios JM, Mengod G (1992): Distribution and cellular localization of mRNA coding for 5-HT$_{1A}$ receptor in the rat brain: correlation with receptor binding. J Neurosci 12:440–453.

Post C, Minor BG, Davies M, Archer T (1986): Analgesia induced by 5-hydroxytryptamine receptor agonists is blocked or reversed by noradrenaline-depletion in rats. Brain Res 363:18–27.

Pubols LM, Bernau NA, Kane LA, Dawson SD, Burleigh AL, Polans AS (1992): Distribution of 5-HT$_1$ binding sites in the cat spinal cord. Neurosci Lett 142:111–114.

Radja F, Laporte AM, Daval G, Vergé D, Gozlan H, Hamon M (1991): Autoradiography of serotonin receptor subtypes in the central nervous system. Neurochem Int 18:1–15.

Rebeck GW, Maynard KI, Hyman BT, Moskowitz MA (1994): Selective 5-HT$_{1D\alpha}$ serotonin receptor gene expression in trigeminal ganglia: implications for antimigraine drug development. Proc Natl Acad Sci USA 91:3666–3669.

Reinmann W, Schneider F (1993): The serotonin receptor agonist 5-methoxy-N,N-dimethyltryptamine facilitates noradrenaline release from rat spinal cord slices and inhibits monoamine oxidase activity. Gen Pharmacol 24:449–453.

Reynolds DJM, Leslie RA, Grahame-Smith DG, Harvey JM (1991): Autoradiographic localization of 5-HT$_3$ receptor ligand binding in the cat brainstem. Neurochem Int 18:69–73.

Richardson BP, Buchheit KH (1988): The pharmacology, distribution and function of 5-HT$_3$ receptors. In Osborne NN, Hamon M (eds): *Neuronal Serotonin*. Chichester: John Wiley & Sons, pp. 465–506.

Ridet JL, Rajaofetra N, Teilhac JR, Geffard M, Privat A (1993): Evidence for non-synaptic serotonergic and noradrenergic innervation of the rat dorsal horn and possible involvement of neuron-glia interactions. Neuroscience 52:143–157.

Robertson B, Bevan S (1991): Properties of 5-hydroxytryptamine$_3$ receptor-gated currents in adult rat dorsal root ganglion neurones. Br J Pharmacol 102:272–276.

Romanelli MN, Ghelardini C, Dei S, Matucci R, Mori F, Scapecchi S, Teodori E, Bartolini A, Galli A, Giotti A, Gualtieri F (1993): Synthesis and biological activity of a series of aryl tropanyl esters and amides chemically related to 1H-indole-3-carboxylic acid and endo-8-methyl-8-azabicyclo[3.2.1]oct-3-yl ester—Development of a 5-HT$_4$ agonist endowed with potent antinociceptive activity. Arzneim Forsch (Drug Res) 43:913–918.

Ruda MA, Bennett GJ, Dubner R (1986): Neurochemistry and neural circuitry in the dorsal horn. In Emson PC, Rossor M, Tohyama M (eds): *Progress in Brain Research*, Vol. 66. Amsterdam: Elsevier, pp. 219–268.

Sanchez A, Niedbala B, Feria M (1995): Modulation of neuropathic pain in rats by intrathecally injected serotonergic agonists. NeuroReport 6:2585–2588.

Saria A, Javorsky F, Humpel C, Gamse R (1990): 5-HT$_3$ receptor antagonists inhibit sensory neuropeptide release from the rat spinal cord. NeuroReport 1:104–106.

Sawynok J, Reid A (1990): Supersensitivity to intrathecal 5-hydroxytryptamine, but not noradrenaline, following depletion of spinal 5-hydroxytryptamine by 5,7-dihydroxytryptamine administered into various sites. Naunyn-Schmiedeberg's Arch Pharmacol 342:1–8.

Sawynok J, Reid A (1991): Noradrenergic and purinergic involvement in spinal antinociception by 5-hydroxytryptamine and 2-methyl-5-hydroxytryptamine. Eur J Pharmacol 204:301–309.

Sawynok J, Reid A (1992): Noradrenergic mediation of spinal antinociception by 5-hydroxytryptamine: characterization of receptor subtypes. Eur J Pharmacol 223:49–56.

Sawynok J, Reid A (1996): Interactions of descending serotonergic systems with other neurotransmitters in the modulation of nociception. Behav Brain Res 73:63–68.

Solomon RE, Gebhart GF (1988): Mechanisms of effects of intrathecal serotonin on nociception and blood pressure in rats. J Pharmacol Exp Ther 245:905–911.

Sorkin LS, McAdoo DJ, Willis WD (1993): Raphe magnus stimulation-induced antinociception in the cat is associated with release of amino acids as well as serotonin in the lumbar dorsal horn. Brain Res 618:95–108.

Sufka KJ, Giordano J (1991): Analgesic effects of S and R isomers of the novel 5-HT$_3$ receptor antagonists ADR-851 and ADR-882 in rats. Eur J Pharmacol 204:117–119.

Taiwo YO, Levine JD (1992): Serotonin is a directly-acting hyperalgesic agent in the rat. Neuroscience 48:485–490.

Tan H, Miletic V (1992): Diverse actions of 5-hydroxytryptamine on frog spinal dorsal horn neurons in vitro. Neuroscience 49:913–923.

Tecott LH, Maricq AV, Julius D (1993): Nervous system distribution of the serotonin 5-HT$_3$ receptor mRNA. Proc Natl Acad Sci USA 90:1430–1434.

Thor KB, Blitz-Siebert A, Helke CJ (1993): Autoradiographic localization of 5-hydroxytryptamine$_{1A}$, 5-hydroxytryptamine$_{1B}$, and 5-hydroxytryptamine$_{1C/2}$ binding sites in the rat spinal cord. Neuroscience 55:235–252.

Todorovic S, Anderson EG (1990): 5-HT$_2$ and 5-HT$_3$ receptors mediate two distinct depolarizing responses in rat dorsal root ganglion neurons. Brain Res 511:71–79.

Todorovic S, Anderson EG (1992): Serotonin preferentially hyperpolarizes capsaicin-sensitive C-type sensory neurons by activating 5-HT$_{1A}$ receptors. Brain Res 585:212–218.

Tokuyama S, Takahashi M, Kaneto H (1993): Involvement of serotonergic receptor subtypes in the production of antinociception by psychological stress in mice. Jpn J Pharmacol 61:237–242.

Travagli RA, Williams JT (1996): Endogenous monoamines inhibit glutamate transmission in the spinal trigeminal nucleus of the guinea-pig. J Physiol Lond 491:177–185.

Uphouse L (1997): Multiple serotonin receptors: Too many, not enough, or just the right number? Neurosci Biobehav Rev 21:679–698.

Waeber C, Moskowitz MA (1995): [^{3}H]sumatriptan labels both 5-HT$_{1D}$ and 5-HT$_{1F}$ receptor binding sites in the guinea pig brain: an autoradiographic study. Naunyn-Schmiedeberg's Arch Pharmacol 352:263–275.

Waeber C, Dixon K, Hoyer D, Palacios JM (1988): Localization by autoradiography of neuronal 5-HT$_3$ receptors in the mouse CNS. Eur J Pharmacol 151:351–352.

Waeber C, Sebben M, Nieoullon A, Bockaert J, Dumuis A (1994): Regional distribution and ontogeny of 5-HT$_4$ binding sites in rodent brain. Neuropharmacology 33:527–541.

Xu W, Qiu XC, Han JS (1994): Serotonin receptor subtypes in spinal antinociception in the rat. J Pharmacol Exp Ther 269:1182–1189.

Yakel JL, Shao XM, Jackson MB (1990): The selectivity of the channel coupled to the 5-HT$_3$ receptor. Brain Res 533:46–52.

Yaksh TL, Wilson PR (1979): Spinal serotonin terminal system mediates antinociception. J Pharmacol Exp Ther 208:446–453.

Zemlan FP, Behbehani MM, Murphy RM (1988): Serotonin receptor subtypes and the modulation of pain transmission. In Fields HL, Besson JM (eds): *Progress in Brain Research*, Vol. 77. Amsterdam: Elsevier, pp. 349–355.

CHAPTER 11

PURINES: POTENTIAL FOR DEVELOPMENT AS ANALGESIC AGENTS

JANA SAWYNOK and ANTHONY POON
Dalhousie University
Halifax, Nova Scotia, Canada

Adenosine and adenine nucleotides can exert both facilitatory and inhibitory influences on the transmission of pain, depending on the specific location of the receptor in relation to pain pathways and the nature of the receptor activated. Although such actions have been recognized for some time, the past decade has been the most active for developing an understanding of these diverse actions as the role of purines in nociception has been addressed from a number of points of view. This chapter reviews concepts underlying the development of this field—the multiple peripheral and central effects of adenosine A_1, A_2, and A_3 receptors, indirectly acting adenosine agents (inhibitors of adenosine kinase and adenosine deaminase), and effects of P_2 purinoceptor agonists on pain transmission—and considers the therapeutic potential for development of purinergic agents as pharmaceuticals for treatment of pain.

Pain initiating or algogenic actions for adenosine 5'-triphosphate (ATP) were initially demonstrated on the human blister base (Keele and Armstrong, 1964). This action received further attention when ATP was identified as the agent released from red blood cells that activated sensory afferents (Bleehen et al., 1976); adenosine, adenosine 5'-diphosphate (ADP), and ATP all were demonstrated to produce a similar response (Bleehen and Keele, 1977). A particular interest in algogenic actions of adenosine was generated when it was demonstrated that a bolus intravenous (i.v.) administration of adenosine could provoke an angina-pectoris like pain in human subjects, and it was suggested that adenosine contributed to ischemic cardiac pain (Sylvén et al., 1986). This peripheral pronociceptive action of adenosine and the adenosine receptors mediating this response have received close attention in both the basic and clinical sciences

---

Novel Aspects of Pain Management: Opioids and Beyond, Edited by Jana Sawynok and Alan Cowan
ISBN 0-471-180173   Copyright © 1999 by Wiley-Liss, Inc.

since the early 1990s. The role of adenosine as a chemical mediator of the pain of angina in humans has been reviewed recently (Crea and Gaspardone, 1997).

Antinociceptive or analgesic actions of adenosine analogues initially were noted in the early 1970s as a part of screening behavioral effects (Vapaatalo et al., 1975), and modulatory effects of adenosine and adenine nucleotides on analgesia by morphine were examined in the context of examining a role for cyclic adenosine 5′-monophosphate (cyclic AMP) in the action of morphine (Gourley and Beckner, 1973; Ho et al., 1973). Attention shifted to the spinal cord following the introduction of techniques that allowed for the direct delivery of drugs to spinal sites via acute percutaneous lumbar puncture injections or chronically implanted intrathecal cannulas. It was then demonstrated that the spinal administration of adenosine analogues produced an intrinsic antinociception (Post, 1984; Sawynok et al., 1986; DeLander and Hopkins, 1986) that probably accounted for the antinociception observed following systemic administration of these agents (Holmgren et al., 1986), and that adenosine release might mediate a component of analgesia produced by morphine when it is administered spinally (Jurna, 1984; DeLander and Hopkins, 1986; Sweeney et al., 1987). The latter issue has since been addressed in greater detail (cf. DeLander and Keil, 1994; Cahill et al., 1995). The involvement of release of endogenous adenosine in the pharmacological actions of other agents is reviewed elsewhere (Sawynok, 1997).

PERIPHERAL EFFECTS OF PURINES ON PAIN TRANSMISSION

Adenosine and ATP are released endogenously under conditions of hypoxia/ischemia and in inflammatory states, and may subsequently exert local regulatory functions under such conditions. Adenosine is released from both cardiac and neural tissue following hypoxia/ischemia and may then play a protective role (Van Wylen et al., 1991; Ely and Berne, 1992). In inflammatory states, ATP can be released or co-released from a variety of cell types by exocytotic release from granule stores, from cytosolic sites by using specific transporter molecules, or nonspecifically following cell lysis (cf. Dubyak and El-Moatassim, 1993). Adenosine can be formed extracellularly by the subsequent action of ecto-ATPases, or it could be released directly from certain cell types following its intracellular production (cf. Cronstein, 1995). Adenosine inhibits a number of aspects of inflammatory cell function by activating adenosine A_{2A} receptors, and has been proposed to be a local anti-inflammatory autacoid (Cronstein, 1994). Activation of adenosine A_3 receptors on mast cells can provoke mediator release from mast cells, which then contributes to inflammation (Linden, 1994). ATP exerts a number of influences on the inflammatory process by interacting with a variety of P_2 purinoceptors on neutrophils, monocytes, macrophages, mast cells, platelets, and vascular endothelial cells (Dubyak and El-Moatassim, 1993). Both adenosine and ATP may also interact with their respective receptors either directly on sensory nerve terminals or indirectly on cells adjacent to the nerve terminal to release endogenous mediators, which then interact with the nerve terminal to modulate the pain signal generated under ischemic and inflammatory conditions.

Adenosine A_1 Receptors

Activation of adenosine A_1 receptors on peripheral sensory nerve terminals produces a local antinociceptive action. This has been demonstrated following peripheral administration of selective adenosine A_1 agonists in a rodent model of mechanical hyperalgesia (Taiwo and Levine, 1990) and in the formalin test (Karlsten et al., 1991; Doak and Sawynok, 1995). Antinociception has been attributed to an interaction of adenosine with G proteins and subsequent inhibition of adenylate cyclase (Khasar et al., 1995). Repeated administration of N^6-cyclopentyladenosine (CPA) produces tolerance to antinociception (Aley et al., 1995), and CPA exhibits both cross-tolerance and cross-dependence with a μ opioid agonist (Aley et al., 1995). Antinociception by CPA is blocked by a selective adenosine A_1 receptor antagonist, as well as by yohimbine (but not naloxone), and the peripheral adenosine A_1 receptor was proposed to occur as part of an adenosine A_1—α_2-adrenergic—μ opioid multireceptor complex on the sensory nerve terminal (Aley and Levine, 1997).

Adenosine A_1 receptors have not been visualized directly on sensory afferent nerve terminals but a number of observations support such a localization. These include (a) the interactions between adenosine A_1 receptors and μ opioid receptor systems noted above as μ opioid receptors are known to be localized on sensory afferents (Hassan et al., 1993), and (b) the observations that adenosine A_1 agonists have inhibitory effects on cell bodies of dorsal root ganglion cells (Dolphin et al., 1986) while central terminals of afferent neurons contain inhibitory adenosine A_1 receptors (Santicioli et al., 1993); it is likely that adenosine A_1 receptors produced by the cell body are transported to both peripheral and central aspects of the afferent neuron.

Adenosine A_2 Receptors

The pain initiating or algogenic actions of adenosine are mediated by adenosine A_{2A} receptors in rodents. Thus the local administration of selective adenosine A_{2A} receptor agonists produces hyperalgesia in a mechanical threshold test (Taiwo and Levine, 1990) and enhances nociceptive behaviors in the formalin test (Karlsten et al., 1992a; Doak and Sawynok, 1995). Hyperalgesia has been attributed to interactions with a G protein and increased cyclic AMP activity in the sensory nerve terminal (Taiwo and Levine, 1991; Khasar et al., 1995).

Adenosine A_3 Receptors

The existence of the adenosine A_3 receptor has been recognized only recently (Linden, 1994). The local peripheral administration of the adenosine A_3 receptor selective agonist N^6-benzyl-5'-N-ethylcarboxamidoadenosine (N^6-benzyl-NECA) into the rat hindpaw produces an intrinsic nociceptive behavior and augments the response to formalin (Sawynok et al., 1997). The intrinsic response is blocked by the histamine H_1 receptor antagonist mepyramine and the 5-hydroxytryptamine$_2$ (5-HT$_2$) receptor antagonist ketanserin, indicating that behaviors result from release of histamine and 5-HT from mast cells. An earlier study demonstrated that intraperitoneal injection of another adenosine A_3 agonist produced scratching behavior that was blocked by an antihistamine (Jacobson et al., 1993).

Indirectly Acting Adenosine Agents

Extracellular adenosine levels can be regulated by the actions of adenosine kinase and adenosine deaminase (reviewed Geiger et al., 1997). Local concentrations of adenosine are increased by the inflammatory process (Cronstein et al., 1995), and anti-inflammatory effects of some clinically effective agents are proposed to be mediated in part by adenosine (Cronstein et al., 1993). Inhibitors of adenosine kinase produce anti-inflammatory actions mediated by adenosine A_{2A} receptor activation (Rosengren et al., 1995). In addition, it has recently been demonstrated that peripheral administration of the adenosine kinase inhibitor 5'-amino-5'-deoxyadenosine (NH$_2$dAD) produces a local antinociceptive action due to adenosine A_1 receptor activation in the formalin test; co-administration of an adenosine deaminase inhibitor significantly enhances this effect (Sawynok et al., 1998). There is evidence for a peripheral tonic modulatory influence on the pain signal by the adenosine released under inflammatory conditions (Doak and Sawynok, 1995).

Algogenic Actions in Humans

Pain initiating effects of adenosine have been observed in humans in a number of studies following the intravenous administration of adenosine. Adenosine given as an intravenous bolus or short duration infusion (2 min) produces pain that is indistinguishable from angina pectoris in healthy volunteers (Sylvén et al., 1986; Crea et al., 1990) or in subjects with ischemic heart disease (Sylvén et al., 1988a; Crea et al., 1990). When injected into the brachial artery, adenosine generates pain and discomfort in the arm that is similar to that provoked by ischemic work (Sylvén et al., 1988b). Chest pain produced by intravenous adenosine was reduced by aminophylline and potentiated by dipyridamole (Sylvén et al., 1988a; Crea et al., 1990). Aminophylline also reduced exercise-induced muscle and chest pain (Jonzon et al., 1989; Crea et al., 1990) providing support for a participation of endogenous adenosine in ischemic pain. The pain induced by adenosine is augmented by substance P (Gaspardone et al., 1994) and nicotine (Sylvén et al., 1990). Adenosine-induced chest pain is not seen following cardiac denervation (Bertolet et al., 1993) and has been attributed to the ability of adenosine to activate cardiac afferent neurons (Biaggioni et al., 1991; Dibner-Dunlap et al., 1993; Huang et al., 1995).

The adenosine receptor subtype mediating pain enhancing properties in humans has been suggested to be an adenosine A_1 receptor on the basis of the ability of bamiphylline to block cutaneous, muscular, and cardiac pain provoked by adenosine (Pappagallo et al., 1993; Gaspardone et al., 1995). This conclusion is in direct contradiction to that obtained in rodents, where adenosine A_{2A} receptors have been implicated in pronociceptive actions of adenosine. It should be noted that both adenosine A_1 and A_2 receptors have been implicated in stimulation of cardiac afferents in dogs (Dibner-Dunlap et al., 1993; Huang et al., 1995), such that a species difference may contribute to the difference in receptor profile. This important issue requires a clear resolution, as there are definite implications for the development of potential therapeutic agents.

ATP Receptors

The algogenic actions of ATP have been known for some time, being demonstrated both in the human blister base preparation (Keele and Armstrong, 1964; Bleehen and Keele, 1977) and a rodent behavioral model (Collier et al., 1966). ATP was subsequently shown to depolarize sensory neurons directly by activating a nonspecific cation channel in dorsal root ganglion neurons (Krishtal et al., 1983; Jahr and Jessell, 1983; Bean, 1990), and this action was considered to account for the algogenic response. The receptor mediating this electrophysiological response has been cloned and characterized as a P_{2x} receptor heteromer (Chen et al., 1995; Lewis et al., 1995). Additional pronociceptive actions also may occur by interactions with inflammatory mediators, for coadministration of ATP and α,β-methylene-ATP with formalin augments nociceptive behaviors (Sawynok and Reid, 1997). Whereas the interactions of ATP with inflammatory cells to promote mediator release directly, or to facilitate the actions of other agents to release mediators, are likely mediated by other P_2 receptor subtypes (Dubyak and El-Moatassim, 1993), mediators could subsequently interact with P_{2x} receptors on the sensory nerve terminal. Thus both direct and indirect actions of ATP at sensory nerve terminals are possible.

Neuropathic pain results from injury to peripheral nerves, nerve roots, the spinal cord, and in some cases, the central nervous system. Certain forms of damage to peripheral nerves provoke sprouting of sympathetic nerve fibers, resulting in sympathetic-sensory coupling and a form of pain dependent on the sympathetic nervous system (reflex sympathetic dystrophy, causalgia, sympathetically maintained pain) (Portenoy, 1991). ATP is co-released with noradrenaline (NA) from sympathetic nerve terminals and may act in concert with NA and contribute to the initiation of pain under such conditions (Burnstock and Wood, 1996). Sympathetic nerve activity also contributes to inflammatory pain and ATP–NA interactions may be involved in these pain states as well (Levine et al., 1987).

SPINAL EFFECTS OF PURINES ON PAIN TRANSMISSION

Adenosine and Adenosine Analogues

A number of early studies observed antinociceptive properties with systemically administered adenosine analogues (Vapaatalo et al., 1975; Crawley et al., 1981; Holmgren et al., 1983), and this was subsequently attributed primarily to a spinal site of action (Holmgren et al., 1986). The direct spinal administration of adenosine analogues produces antinociception in a range of nociceptive test systems. These include the tail flick and hot plate thermal tests (Post, 1984; Sawynok et al., 1986; DeLander and Hopkins, 1987; Sosnowski et al., 1989; Karlsten et al., 1990), the writhing test (Sosnowski et al., 1989; Sierralta and Miranda, 1993), intrathecal substance P, capsaicin, or N-methyl-D-aspartate (NMDA) behavioral tests (Hunskaar et al., 1986; Doi et al., 1987; DeLander and Wahl, 1988), the formalin test (Malmberg and Yaksh, 1993; Poon and Sawynok, 1995), and the carrageenan hyperalgesia test (Poon and Sawynok, 1996). The intrathecal administration of adenosine itself produces only a weak effect (DeLander and Hopkins, 1987); this most likely is due to cellular uptake and metabolic inactivation, because the effects of adenosine can be markedly enhanced by co-administration of inhibitors of adenosine metabolism (Keil and DeLander, 1994). Antinociceptive activity for spinally administered adenosine analogues has also been observed in tests for neuropathic pain, including the intrathecal strychnine or prostaglandin E_2 allodynia models (Sosnowski and Yaksh, 1989; Sosnowski et al., 1989; Minami et al., 1992), the sciatic nerve loose ligation model (Yamamoto and Yaksh, 1991; Sjölund et al., 1996; Cui et al., 1997), and the dorsal root tight ligation model (Lee and Yaksh, 1996).

Although earlier studies implicated both adenosine A_1 and A_2 receptors in antinociception, the involvement of adenosine A_2 receptors was based primarily on the activity of 5'-N-ethylcarboxamidoadenosine (NECA), which actually has a comparable activity at both receptors. More recent studies examined the activity of selective adenosine A_1 receptor agonists and antagonists and concluded that spinal antinociception by adenosine analogues is due to activation of adenosine A_1 rather than A_2 receptors (Karlsten et al., 1991; Lee and Yaksh, 1996).

A number of the studies mentioned above noted motor deficits resulting from the intrathecal administration of adenosine analogues, particularly at higher doses, but only a few quantified the motor response and determined a potency comparison between doses required to produce the two effects. For R-phenylisopropyladenosine (R-PIA), there is an order of magnitude difference in doses required to produce antinociception and motor effects in rats (Karlsten et al., 1990; Lee and Yaksh, 1996), although less difference was noted in mice (DeLander and Hopkins, 1987). Although antinociception is attributed to adenosine A_1 receptor activation, and adenosine A_2 receptors in motor effects (Lee and Yaksh, 1996), a recent electrophysiological study has suggested that both sensory and motor responses result from adenosine A_1 receptor activation, but different doses are required to elicit the two effects (Nakamura et al., 1997).

Adenosine A$_1$ receptors have been identified in the superficial layers of the dorsal spinal cord (Goodman and Snyder, 1982; Geiger et al., 1984; Choca et al., 1987). These receptors are located predominantly on neurons postsynaptic to primary afferent nerve terminals and to descending projection neurons (Geiger et al., 1984; Choca et al., 1988). Electrophysiological studies have provided evidence for a postsynaptic hyperpolarization of projection neurons due to an enhanced K$^+$ conductance contributing to antinociceptive properties of adenosine (Salter et al., 1993). Accordingly, blockers of ATP-sensitive K$^+$ channels block antinociception by adenosine A$_1$ analogues (Ocaña and Baeyens, 1994). In behavioral experiments, the ability of adenosine analogues to inhibit responses produced by substance P and NMDA (Doi et al., 1987; DeLander and Wahl, 1988) has been attributed to inhibitory actions of the adenosine on projection neurons. Some electrophysiological studies note properties that may be due to actions on interneurons as well as projection neurons (Li and Perl, 1994; Reeve and Dickenson, 1995). (The ability of γ-aminobutyric acid antagonists to inhibit antinociception by systemically administered adenosine analogues (Sabetkasai and Zarrindast, 1993) would be consistent with an action on interneurons if this interaction occurs at the spinal level.) Adenosine A$_1$ receptor activation produces inhibitory actions on dorsal root ganglion cell bodies (MacDonald et al., 1986; Dolphin et al., 1986), and inhibits electrically evoked release of substance P and calcitonin gene-related peptide from sensory afferents in the spinal cord (Santicioli et al., 1993), indicating some actions at sites presynaptic to afferent nerve terminals. Pertussis toxin-sensitive G proteins and a reduction in cyclic AMP levels are implicated in the spinal actions of adenosine A$_1$ receptor agonists (Sawynok and Reid, 1988).

Indirectly Acting Adenosine Agents

Within the spinal cord, there is evidence for the existence of an endogenous tonic regulation of nociceptive activity by adenosine. Thus the spinal administration of methylxanthines produces hyperalgesia in rats (Jurna, 1984; Sawynok et al., 1986), and in mice, elicits behaviors suggesting nociceptive activation (Nagaoka et al., 1993; Keil and DeLander, 1996). In biochemical studies, there is a basal tone of adenosine release from dorsal spinal cord preparations; this release is enhanced by depolarization with K$^+$ or capsaicin, with evoked release originating from a capsaicin-sensitive source (Sweeney et al., 1989). Release of adenosine from the spinal cord is enhanced by inhibitors of both adenosine kinase and adenosine deaminase (Golembiowska et al., 1995, 1996). In behavioral experiments, the intrathecal administration of adenosine kinase inhibitors produces antinociception in the tail flick and hot plate tests (Keil and DeLander, 1992; Kowaluk et al., 1996), the intrathecal NMDA and substance P tests (Keil and DeLander, 1996), and the formalin and carrageenan thermal hyperalgesia inflammatory tests (Poon and Sawynok, 1995, 1998). Antinociception in the latter test is enhanced by co-administration of an adenosine deaminase inhibitor (Poon and Sawynok, 1998). In these studies, antinociception occurred in the absence of motor effects, but such effects can occur if doses are elevated (Keil and DeLander, 1992, 1994; Poon and Sawynok, 1995). The activity of adenosine kinase inhibitors in inflammatory tests is of particular interest in view of the suggestion that spinal purine metabolism may be enhanced by chronic inflammation (Weil-Fugazza et al., 1986).

ATP, ATP Analogues, and Antagonists

When administered directly to the spinal cord, ATP can produce both pain facilitatory effects due to activation of P_2 receptors and pain inhibitory effects due to activation of adenosine A_1 receptors following breakdown to adenosine. In electrophysiological experiments, these dual excitatory and inhibitory effects are readily demonstrated (Salter and Henry, 1985; Salter et al., 1993). In behavioral experiments, the intrathecal administration of α,β-methylene-ATP and 2-methylthio-ATP produces hyperalgesia whereas P_2 purinoceptor antagonists produce antinociception in the tail flick and formalin tests (Driessen et al., 1994). When ATP, ADP, or AMP is administered spinally, it can be converted to adenosine and produce a methylxanthine-sensitive antinociception in the intrathecal substance P test (Doi et al., 1987). When ATP is administered intravenously, it produces antinociception, which is likely mediated by breakdown to adenosine (Gomaa, 1987). However, whether the adenosine acts at peripheral or spinal sites to produce this effect is not entirely clear. The systemic administration of the P_2 purinoceptor antagonist, suramin, produces antinociception in the hot plate, writhing (Ho et al., 1992), and formalin tests (Sawynok and Reid, 1997), most likely reflecting a spinal action of suramin (Driessen et al., 1994).

There are also some clinical reports of analgesia mediated by AMP and ATP. The intramuscular administration of AMP produces pain-relieving properties in humans with viral-mediated neuralgia (Sklar et al., 1985), and this effect likely results from breakdown to adenosine with subsequent peripheral and/or spinal actions. Analgesia resulting from transcutaneous electrical nerve stimulation in humans is inhibited by caffeine (Marchand et al., 1995); this phenomenon is proposed to result from the release of ATP from large-diameter sensory afferents, with the subsequent breakdown to adenosine producing analgesic properties (Salter and Henry, 1987; Salter et al., 1993).

Adenosine and Adenosine Analogues in Human Studies

There is one report of the spinal administration of R-PIA alleviating allodynia evoked by touch and vibration in humans (Karlsten and Gordh, 1995). R-PIA had been shown to produce no adverse effects on heart rate or blood pressure (Sosnowski et al., 1989) or on blood flow to the spinal cord (Karlsten et al., 1992b; Kristensen et al., 1993), or any morphological changes that could be considered to reflect a neurotoxic action (Karlsten et al., 1993) prior to this evaluation in humans. In other studies, the intravenous infusion of adenosine has been reported to produce analgesia in experimental pain in healthy volunteers (Ekblom et al., 1995; Segerdahl et al., 1994, 1995) and to alleviate spontaneous and stimulus-evoked pain in subjects with neuropathic pain resulting from peripheral nerve injury (Belfrage et al., 1995; Sollevi et al., 1995).

A number of features of pain relief produced by adenosine infusions in neuropathic pain states require comment. (*a*) *Pain relief rather than pain induction occurs following intravenous adenosine infusions.* It had previously been reported that intravenous administration of bolus doses of adenosine provoked pain resembling ischemic cardiac pain (see Peripheral Effects section). In studies where pain relief is reported, adenosine was given as an infusion of 50–80 µg/kg/hr for 45–60 min. Because of the short half-life of adenosine in blood (seconds) (Möser et al., 1989), it is difficult to compare paradigms directly. However, two studies provide comparative data. Lagerqvist et al. (1992) demonstrated that each of a bolus intracoronary injection, an intravenous bolus or an intravenous infusion with adenosine could provoke cardiac pain, with the lowest intravenous infusion dose producing pain being 0.347 µmol/kg/min (92.6 µg/kg/min). When Ekblom et al. (1995) examined effects of infusion of adenosine 50, 70, and 80 µg/kg/min for 10 min in healthy volunteers, chest oppression was noted at the 70 and 80 µg/kg/min infusion doses but not at the 50 µg/kg/min dose. The difference in outcome seems to depend on dose, with pain relief occurring with a lower dose, and perhaps on rate, for pain results from sudden exposure by bolus. (*b*) *Site of action.* Although the studies observing analgesic properties in humans conclude that these actions are likely exerted within the spinal cord, in view of antinociceptive actions resulting from adenosine A_1 receptor activation at peripheral nerve terminals, a peripheral action of adenosine could well be involved. It is not clear to what extent adenosine crosses the blood–brain barrier and gains access to spinal sites, because although there is a transporter system for adenosine in brain capillary endothelial cell membranes, adenosine is metabolized rapidly in blood, in the endothelial cell itself, and in nervous tissue, such that there is effectively a "metabolic blood–brain barrier" to adenosine (Pardridge et al., 1994). (*c*) *Duration of action.* In human experimental pain paradigms, the analgesic actions were noted during adenosine infusions (Ekblom et al., 1995; Segerdahl et al., 1994). In the cases of neuropathic pain, pain relief persisted 4–6 hr following intravenous adenosine infusion (Sollevi et al., 1995; Belfrage et al., 1995), and up to 6 months following intrathecal R-PIA (Karlsten and Gordh, 1995). This may indicate a selective interruption of central sensitization processes involved in neuropathic pain. Alternatively, there may be some redress of a metabolic or neurochemical imbalance that occurs during neuropathic pain, for it has recently been reported that subjects with neuropathic pain have decreased plasma and cerebrospinal fluid levels of adenosine (Guieu et al., 1996). In view of the long-lasting nature of the relief of neuropathic pain following adenosine infusions, and the recent report of the relative deficiency of adenosine in subjects with neuropathic pain, this area requires further attention to explore the therapeutic potential of this modality for this condition.

ANALGESIC PROPERTIES OF CAFFEINE

Caffeine is an antagonist at both adenosine A_1 and A_2 receptors, exhibiting a comparable affinity for both sites. Caffeine has been a constituent of analgesic formulations containing aspirin and acetaminophen for some time, but it is only relatively recently that adjuvant analgesic properties for caffeine in human pain paradigms have been established (Laska et al., 1984). In animal studies, caffeine produces both intrinsic analgesic properties, as well as adjuvant analgesic properties in combination with other analgesics (Sawynok and Yaksh, 1993; Sawynok, 1996). The mechanisms by which caffeine produces these actions must be considered in terms of the multiple effects that adenosine has on pain transmission. Although blockade of peripheral pronociceptive effects of adenosine is appealing as a hypothesis to account for such properties, local antinociceptive properties for caffeine have not been demonstrated (Doak and Sawynok, 1995). Within the spinal cord, methylxanthines produce hyperalgesia (Jurna, 1984; Sawynok et al., 1986) rather than analgesia, so an action at this site is unlikely. Supraspinal actions of caffeine have been implicated in analgesic properties of caffeine on the basis of manipulation of analgesia by lesions to discrete central aminergic pathways (Sawynok and Reid, 1996) and also on the basis of the potency of caffeine when administered directly into the cerebral ventricles (Ghelardini et al., 1997). Although such an action may appear paradoxical in view of the observation that the supraspinal administration of adenosine agonists also can produce antinociception (Yarbrough and McGuffin-Clineschmidt, 1981; Herrick-Davis et al., 1989), supraspinal caffeine antinociception may involve inhibition of presynaptic adenosine A_1 receptors on cholinergic nerve terminals (Ghelardini et al., 1997), whereas supraspinal adenosine analogues act postsynaptically at other sites to produce antinociception. A comprehensive understanding of the effects of caffeine on pain transmission at multiple sites is required to understand both adjuvant actions of caffeine when it is included in analgesic formulations, as well as potential interactions of dietary caffeine with pain-relieving regimens whether pharmacological (e.g., morphine) or physiological (e.g., transcutaneous electrical nerve stimulation) in nature.

THERAPEUTIC IMPLICATIONS

Both adenosine and ATP exert complex effects on pain transmission depending on the site of action (peripheral, spinal, supraspinal) and the receptor subtype activated (A_1, A_2, A_3, or P_2). This complexity of action must be clearly appreciated in the pursuit of therapeutic agents that may recruit purine systems. In view of the wide spectrum of antinociceptive properties produced by the systemic and spinal administration of adenosine/adenosine analogues and of adenosine kinase inhibitors in a variety of test systems, there is considerable interest in the possible development of both directly and indirectly acting adenosine agents as therapeutic targets for the relief of pain. Adenosine A_1 receptor agonists have the potential to exert both peripheral and central antinociceptive properties, but this approach may be limited by sedative and other potential side effects (e.g., cardiovascular), for adenosine is a ubiquitous agent with effects on multiple organ systems. There is, however, a prominent effect of low doses of adenosine in neuropathic pain states in particular, and if this can be understood, there may be a particular benefit to be derived in such conditions. Also, in view of the presence of peripheral sites of action for pain relief, a local route of administration (e.g., cream or patch application) might provide a selective local high concentration with minimal side effects mediated by systemic absorption. Finally, this class of agents may find a particular utility in combination with other agents in both inflammatory and neuropathic states, whereby lower and more selective doses can be used. Adenosine kinase inhibitors, which augment levels of adenosine especially under conditions of enhanced production (e.g., inflammatory states), may produce peripheral antinociception via adenosine A_1 receptors, peripheral anti-inflammatory effects via adenosine A_2 receptors, and spinal antinociception via adenosine A_1 receptors. Sedative and cardiovascular effects may be lesser in these cases, but the potential for such actions to occur still requires attention. In situations where peripheral inflammation is a particularly prominent feature, the development of agents that do not have access to central compartments or of formulations that express an action primarily at a local site might be of particular benefit. Any development of either directly or indirectly acting agents must recognize the potential for caffeine, which is widely consumed in the diet, to interfere with therapeutic efficacy. P_{2x} purinoceptor antagonists also exhibit a potential for development, exerting analgesic actions both at the peripheral nerve terminal and within the spinal cord. One concern here may be side effects mediated by blockade of other P_2 receptor subtypes on other cellular structures if antagonists cannot adequately discriminate the appropriate receptor variant. Within the purine system, there are clearly multiple targets that exhibit a potential for development as pharmaceuticals for the relief of pain.

ACKNOWLEDGMENTS

Work cited from this laboratory has been supported by the Medical Research Council of Canada.

REFERENCES

Aley KO, Levine JD (1997): Multiple receptors involved in peripheral α_2, μ, and A_1 antinociception, tolerance and withdrawal. J Neurosci 17:735–744.

Aley KO, Green PG, Levine JD (1995): Opioid and adenosine peripheral antinociception are subject to tolerance and withdrawal. J Neurosci 15:8031–8038.

Bean BP (1990): ATP-activated channels in rat and bullfrog sensory neurons: concentration dependence and kinetics. J Neurosci 10:1–10.

Belfrage M, Sollevi A, Segerdahl M, Sjölund K-F, Hansson P (1995): Systemic adenosine infusion alleviates spontaneous and stimulus evoked pain in patients with peripheral neuropathic pain. Anesth Analg 81:713–717.

Bertolet B, Belardinelli L, Hill JA (1993): Absence of adenosine-induced chest pain after total cardiac afferent denervation. Am J Cardiol 72:483–484.

Biaggioni I, Killian TJ, Mosqueda-Garcia R, Robertson RM, Robertson D (1991): Adenosine increases sympathetic nerve traffic in humans. Circulation 83:1668–1675.

Bleehen T, Keele CA (1977): Observations on the algogenic actions of adenosine compounds on the human blister base preparation. Pain 3:367–377.

Bleehen T, Hobbiger F, Keele CA (1976): Identification of algogenic substances in human erythrocytes. J Physiol 262:131–149.

Burnstock G, Wood JN (1996): Purinergic receptors: their role in nociception and primary afferent neurotransmission. Curr Opinion Neurobiol 6:526–532.

Cahill CM, White TD, Sawynok J (1995): Spinal opioid receptors and adenosine release: neurochemical and behavioural characterization of opioid subtypes. J Pharmacol Exp Ther 275:84–93.

Chen C-C, Akoplan AN, Sivilotti N, Colquhoun D, Burnstock G, Wood JN (1995): A P2X purinoceptor expressed by a subset of sensory neurons. Nature 377:428–431.

Choca JI, Proudfit HK, Green RG (1987) Identification of A_1 and A_2 adenosine receptors in the rat spinal cord. J Pharmacol Exp Ther 242:905–910.

Choca JI, Green RD, Proudfit HK (1988): Adenosine A_1 and A_2 receptors of the substantia gelatinosa are located predominantly on intrinsic neurons: an autoradiographic study. J Pharmacol Exp Ther 247:757–764.

Collier HOJ, James GWL, Schneider C (1966): Antagonism by aspirin and fenamates of bronchoconstriction and nociception induced by adenosine 5′-triphosphate. Nature 5060:411–412.

Crawley JN, Patel J, Marangos PJ (1981): Behavioral characterization of two long-lasting adenosine analogs: sedative properties and interaction with diazepam. Life Sci 29:2623–2630.

Crea F, Gaspardone A (1997) New look to an old symptom: angina pectoris. Circulation 96:3766–3773.

Crea F, Pupita G, Galassi AR, El-Tamimi H, Kaski JC, Davies G, Maseri A (1990): Role of adenosine in pathogenesis of anginal pain. Circulation 81:164–172.

Cronstein BN (1994): Adenosine, an endogenous anti-inflammatory agent. J Appl Physiol 76:5–13.

Cronstein BN (1995): A novel approach to the development of anti-inflammatory agents: adenosine release at inflamed sites. J Invest Med 43:50–57.

Cronstein BN, Naime D, Ostad E (1993): The antiinflammatory mechanism of methotrexate. Increased adenosine release at inflamed sites diminishes leucocyte accumulation in an in vivo model of inflammation. J Clin Invest 92:2675–2682.

Cronstein BN, Naime D, Firestein G (1995): The antiinflammatory effects of an adenosine kinase inhibitor are mediated by adenosine. Arthritis Rheum 38:1040–1045.

Cui J-G, Sollevi A, Linderoth B, Meyerson BA (1997): Adenosine receptor activation suppresses hypersensitivity and potentiates spinal cord stimulation in mononeuropathic rats. Neurosci Lett 223:173–176.

DeLander GE, Hopkins CJ (1986): Spinal adenosine modulates descending antinociceptive pathways stimulated by morphine. J Pharmacol Exp Ther 239:88–93.

DeLander GE, Hopkins CJ (1987): Involvement of A_2 adenosine receptors in spinal mechanisms of antinociception. Eur J Pharmacol 139:215–223.

DeLander GE, Keil GJ (1994): Antinociception induced by intrathecal coadministration of selective adenosine receptor and selective opioid receptor agonists. J Pharmacol Exp Ther 268:943–951.

DeLander GE, Wahl JJ (1988): Behavior induced by putative nociceptive neurotransmitters is inhibited by adenosine or adenosine analogs coadministered intrathecally. J Pharmacol Exp Ther 246:565–570.

Dibner-Dunlap ME, Kinugawa T, Thames MD (1993): Activation of cardiac sympathetic afferents: effects of exogenous adenosine and adenosine analogues. Am J Physiol 265:H395–H400.

Doak GJ, Sawynok J (1995): Complex role of peripheral adenosine in the genesis of the response to subcutaneous formalin in the rat. Eur J Pharmacol 281:311–318.

Doi T, Kuzuna S, Maki Y (1987): Spinal antinociceptive effects of adenosine compounds in mice. Eur J Pharmacol 137:227–231.

Dolphin AC, Forda SR, Scott RH (1986): Calcium-dependent currents in cultured rat dorsal root ganglion neurons are inhibited by an adenosine analogue. J Physiol (London) 373:47–61.

Driessen B, Reimann W, Selve N, Friderichs E, Bültmann R (1994): Antinociceptive effect of intrathecally administered P_2-purinoceptor antagonists in rats. Brain Res 666:182–188.

Dubyak GR, El-Moatassim C (1993): Signal transduction via P_2-purinergic receptors for extracellular ATP and other nucleotides. Am J Physiol 265:C577–C606.

Ekblom A, Segerdahl M, Sollevi A (1995): Adenosine increases the cutaneous heat pain threshold in healthy volunteers. Acta Anaesthesiol Scand 39:717–722.

Ely SW, Berne RM (1992): Protective effects of adenosine in myocardial ischemia. Circulation 85:893–904.

Gaspardone A, Crea F, Tomai F, Iamele M, Crossman DC, Pappagallo M, Versaci F, Chiariello L, Giottrè PA (1994): Substance P potentiates the algogenic effects of intraarterial infusion of adenosine. J Am Coll Cardiol 24:477–482.

Gaspardone A, Crea F, Tomai F, Versaci F, Iamele M, Gioffrè G, Chiariello L, Gioffrè PA (1995): Muscular and cardiac adenosine-induced pain is mediated by A_1 receptors. J Am Coll Cardiol 25:251–257.

Geiger JD, LaBella FS, Nagy JI (1984): Characterization and localization of adenosine receptors in rat spinal cord. J Neurosci 4:2303–2310.

Geiger JD, Parkinson FE, Kowaluk EA (1997): Regulators of endogenous adenosine levels as therapeutic agents. In Jacobson KA, Jarvis MF (eds): *Purinergic Approaches in Experimental Therapeutics*. New York: Wiley-Liss, pp. 55–84.

Ghelardini C, Galeotti N, Bartolini A (1997) Caffeine induces central cholinergic analgesia. Naunyn-Schmiedeberg's Arch Pharmacol 356:590–595.

Golembiowska K, White TD, Sawynok J (1995): Modulation of adenosine release from rat spinal cord by adenosine deaminase and adenosine kinase inhibitors. Brain Res 699:315–320.

Golembiowska K, White TD, Sawynok J (1996): Adenosine kinase inhibitors augment release of adenosine from spinal cord slices. Eur J Pharmacol 307:157–162.

Gomaa AA (1987): Characteristics of analgesia induced by adenosine triphosphate. Pharmacol Toxicol 61:199–202.

Goodman RG, Snyder SH (1982) Autoradiographic localization of adenosine receptors in rat brain using [^{3}H]cyclohexyladenosine. J Neurosci 2:1230–1241.

Gourley DRH, Beckner SK (1973): Antagonism of morphine analgesia by adenine, adenosine, and adenine nucleotides. Proc Soc Exp Biol Med 144:774–778.

Guieu R, Peragut JC, Roussel P, Hassani H, Sampieri F, Bechis G, Gola R, Rochat H (1996): Adenosine and neuropathic pain. Pain 68:271–274.

Hassan AHS, Ableitner A, Stein C, Herz A (1993): Inflammation of the rat paw enhances axonal transport of opioid receptors in the sciatic nerve and increases their density in the inflamed tissue. Neuroscience 55:185–195.

Herrick-Davis K, Chippari S, Luttinger D, Ward SJ (1989) Evaluation of adenosine agonists as potential analgesics. Eur J Pharmacol 162:365–369.

Ho BT, Huo YY, Lu JG, Newman RA, Levin VA (1992): Analgesia activity of anti-cancer agent suramin. Anti-Cancer Drugs 3:91–94.

Ho IK, Loh HH, Leong Way E (1973): Cyclic adenosine monophosphate antagonism of morphine analgesia. J Pharmacol Exp Ther 185: 336–346.

Holmgren M, Hednar T, Nordberg G, Mellstrand T (1983): Antinociceptive effects in the rat of an adenosine analogue, N^6-phenylisopropyladenosine. J Pharm Pharmacol 35:679–680.

Holmgren M, Hedner J, Mellstrand T, Nordberg G, Hedner T (1986): Characterization of the antinociceptive effects of some adenosine analogues in the rat. Naunyn-Schmiedeberg's Arch Pharmacol 334:290–293.

Huang MH, Sylvén C, Horackova M, Armour JA (1995): Ventricular sensory neurons in canine dorsal root ganglia: effects of adenosine and substance P. Am J Physiol 269 (Regulatory Integrative Comp Physiol 38):R318–R324.

Hunskaar S, Post C, Fasmer OB, Arwestrom E (1986): Intrathecal injection of capsaicin can be used as a behavioural nociceptive test in mice. Neuropharmacol 25:1149–1153.

Jacobson KA, Nikodijević O, Shi D, Gallo-Rodriguez C, Olah ME, Stiles GL, Daly JW (1993): A role for central A_3-adenosine receptors in mediation of behavioural depressant effects. FEBS 336:57–60.

Jahr CE, Jessell TM (1983): ATP excites a subpopulation of rat dorsal horn neurones. Nature 304:730–733.

Jonzon B, Sylvén C, Kaijser L (1989): Theophylline decreases pain in the ischaemic forearm test. Cardiovasc Res 9:807–809.

Jurna I (1984): Cyclic nucleotides and aminophylline produce different effects on nociceptive motor and sensory responses in the rat spinal cord. Naunyn-Schmiedeberg's Arch Pharmacol 327:23–30.

Karlsten R, Gordh T (1995): An A_1-selective adenosine agonist abolishes allodynia elicited by vibration and touch after intrathecal injection. Anesth Analg 50:844–847.

Karlsten R, Gordh T, Hartvig P, Post C (1990): Effects of intrathecal injection of the adenosine receptor agonists R-phenylisopropyl-adenosine and N-ethylcarboxamide-adenosine on nociception and motor function in the rat. Anesth Analg 71:60–64.

Karlsten R, Post C, Hide I, Daly JW (1991): The antinociceptive effect of intrathecally administered adenosine analogs in mice correlates with the affinity for the A_1-adenosine receptor. Neurosci Lett 121:267–270.

Karlsten R, Gordh T, Post C (1992a): Local antinociceptive and hyperalgesic effects in the formalin test after peripheral administration of adenosine analogues in mice. Pharmacol Toxicol 70:434–438.

Karlsten R, Kristensen JD, Gordh T (1992b): R-phenylisopropyl-adenosine increases spinal cord blood flow after intrathecal injection in the rat. Anesth Analg 75:972–976.

Karlsten R, Gordh T, Svensson BA (1993): A neurotoxicological evaluation of the spinal cord after chronic intrathecal injection of R-phenylisopropyl adenosine (R-PIA) in the rat. Anesth Analg 77:731–736.

Keele CA, Armstrong D (1964): *Substances Producing Pain and Itch*. Baltimore: Williams and Wilkins, pp. 124–151.

Keil GJ II, DeLander GE (1992): Spinally-mediated antinociception is induced in mice by an adenosine kinase-, but not by an adenosine deaminase-, inhibitor. Life Sci 51:171–176.

Keil GJ, DeLander GE (1994): Adenosine kinase and adenosine deaminase inhibition modulate spinal adenosine- and opioid agonist-induced antinociception in mice. Eur J Pharmacol 271:37–46.

Keil GJ, DeLander GE (1996): Altered sensory behaviours in mice following manipulation of endogenous spinal adenosine neurotransmission. Eur J Pharmacol 312:7–14.

Khasar SG, Wang J-F, Taiwo YO, Heller PH, Green PG, Levine JD (1995): Mu-opioid agonist enhancement of prostaglandin-induced hyperalgesia in the rat: a G-protein βγ subunit-mediated effect? Neuroscience 67:189–195.

Kowaluk EA, Bannon A, Gunther K, Kohlhaas K, Lynch J, Jarvis MF (1996): The effects of adenosine kinase (AK) inhibitors on acute thermal nociception. Soc Neurosci Abst 22:1568.

Krishtal OA, Marchenko SM, Pidoplichko VI (1983): Receptor for ATP in the membrane of mammalian sensory neurones. Neurosci Lett 35:41–45.

Kristensen JD, Karlsten R, Gordh T (1993): Spinal cord blood flow after intrathecal injection of a N-methyl-D-aspartate receptor antagonist or an adenosine receptor agonist in rats. Anesth Analg 76:1279–1283.

Lagerqvist B, Sylvén C, Theodorsen E, Kaijser L, Helmius G, Waldenström A (1992): Adenosine induced chest pain—a comparison between intracoronary bolus injection and steady state infusion. Cardiovasc Res 26:810–814.

Laska EM, Sunshine A, Mueller F, Elvers WB, Siegel C, Rubin A (1984): Caffeine as an analgesic adjuvant. JAMA 251:1711–1718.

Lee Y-W, Yaksh TL (1996): Pharmacology of the spinal adenosine receptor which mediates the antiallodynic action of intrathecal adenosine agonists. J Pharmacol Exp Ther 277:1642–1648.

Levine JD, Goetzl EJ, Basbaum AI (1987): Contribution of the nervous system to the pathophysiology of rheumatoid arthritis and other polyarthritides. Rheum Dis North Am 13:369–383.

Lewis C, Neldhart S, Holy C, North RA, Buell G, Suprenant A (1995): Coexpression of $P2X_2$ and $P2X_3$ receptor subunits can account for ATP-gated currents in sensory neurons. Nature 377:432–435.

Li J, Perl ER (1994): Adenosine inhibition of synaptic transmission in the substantia gelatinosa. J Neurophysiol 72:1611–1621.

Linden J (1994): Cloned adenosine A_3 receptors; pharmacological properties, species differences and receptor functions. Trends Pharmacol Sci 15:298–306.

MacDonald RL, Skerritt JH, Werz MA (1986): Adenosine agonists reduce voltage-dependent calcium conductance of mouse sensory neurons in cell culture. J Physiol (London) 370:75–90.

Malmberg AB, Yaksh TL (1993): Pharmacology of the spinal action of ketorolac, morphine, ST-91, U50488H, and L-PIA on the formalin test and an isobolographic analysis of the NSAID interaction. Anesthesiology 79:270–281.

Marchand S, Li J, Charest J (1995): Effects of caffeine on analgesia from transcutaneous electrical nerve stimulation. New Engl J Med 333:325–326.

Minami T, Uda R, Horiguchi S, Ito S, Hyodo M, Hayashi O (1992): Allodynia evoked by intrathecal administration of prostaglandin $F_{2\alpha}$ to conscious mice. Pain 50:223–229.

Möser GH, Schrader J, Deussen A (1989): Turnover of adenosine in plasma of human and dog blood. Am J Physiol 256 (Cell Physiol 25):C799–C806.

Nagaoka H, Sakurada S, Sakurada T, Takeda S, Nakagawa Y, Kisara K, Arai Y (1993): Theophylline-induced nociceptive behavioral response in mice: possible indirect interaction with spinal *N*-methyl-D-aspartate receptors. Neurochem Int 22:69–74.

Nakamura I, Ohta Y, Kemmotsu O (1997): Characterization of adenosine receptors mediating spinal sensory transmission related to nociceptive information in the rat. Anesthesiology 87:577–584.

Ocaña M, Baeyens JM (1994): Role of ATP-sensitive K^+ channels in antinociception induced by R-PIA, an adenosine A_1 receptor agonist. Naunyn-Schmiedeberg's Arch Pharmacol 350:57–62.

Pappagallo M, Gaspardone A, Tomai F, Iamele M, Crea F, Gioffré PA (1993): Analgesic effect of bamiphylline on pain induced by intradermal injection of adenosine. Pain 53:199–204.

Pardridge WM, Yoshikawa T, Kang Y-S, Miller LP (1994): Blood-brain barrier transport and brain metabolism of adenosine and adenosine analogs. J Pharmacol Exp Ther 268:14–18.

Poon A, Sawynok J (1995): Antinociception by adenosine analogs and an adenosine kinase inhibitor: dependence on formalin concentration. Eur J Pharmacol 286:177–184.

Poon A, Sawynok J (1998): Antinociception by adenosine analogs and inhibitors of adenosine metabolism in an inflammatory thermal hyperalgesia model. Pain 74:235–245.

Portenoy RK (1991): Issues in the management of neuropathic pain. In Basbaum AI, Besson J-M (eds): *Towards a New Pharmacotherapy of Pain*. New York: Wiley & Sons, pp. 393–414.

Post C (1984): Antinociceptive effects in mice after intrathecal injection of 5'-N-ethyl-carboxamide adenosine. Neurosci Lett 51:325–330.

Reeve AJ, Dickenson AH (1995): The roles of spinal adenosine receptors in the control of acute and more persistent nociceptive responses of dorsal horn neurones in the anaesthetized rat. Br J Pharmacol 116:2221–2228.

Rosengren S, Bong GW, Firestein GS (1995): Anti-inflammatory effects of an adenosine kinase inhibitor. Decreased neutrophil accumulation and vascular leakage. J Immunol 154:5444–5451.

Sabetkasai M, Zarrindast MR (1993): Antinociception: interaction between adenosine and GABA systems. Arch Int Pharmacodyn 322:14–22.

Salter MW, Henry JL (1985): Effects of adenosine 5'-monophosphate and adenosine 5'-triphosphate on functionally identified units in the cat spinal dorsal horn. Evidence for a differential effect of adenosine 5'-triphosphate on nociceptive vs nonnociceptive units. Neuroscience 15:815–825.

Salter MW, Henry JL (1987): Evidence that adenosine mediates the depression of spinal dorsal horn neurons induced by peripheral vibration in the cat. Neuroscience 22:631–650.

Salter MW, De Koninck Y, Henry JL (1993): Physiological roles for adenosine and ATP in synaptic transmission in the spinal dorsal horn. Prog Neurobiol 41:125–156.

Santicioli P, Del Bianco E, Maggi CA (1993): Adenosine A_1 receptors mediate the presynaptic inhibition of calcitonin gene-related peptide release by adenosine in the rat spinal cord. Eur J Pharmacol 231:139–142.

Sawynok J (1996): Caffeine: biochemistry, pharmacology and adjuvant effects. Royal Society of Medicine, International Congress and Supplement Series 218:35–42.

Sawynok J (1997): Purines and nociception. In Jacobson KA, Jarvis MF (eds): *Purinergic Approaches in Experimental Therapeutics*. New York: Wiley-Liss, pp. 495–513.

Sawynok J, Reid A (1988): Role of G-proteins and adenylate cyclase in antinociception produced by intrathecal purines. Eur J Pharmacol 156:25–34.

Sawynok J, Reid A (1996): Neurotoxin-induced lesions to central serotonergic, noradrenergic and dopaminergic systems modify caffeine-induced antinociception in the formalin test and locomotor stimulation in rats. J Pharmacol Exp Ther 277:646–653.

Sawynok J, Reid A (1997): Peripheral adenosine 5'-triphosphate enhances nociception in the formalin test via activation of a purinergic P_{2X} receptor. Eur J Pharmacol 330:115–121.

Sawynok J, Sweeney MI, White TD (1986): Classification of adenosine receptors mediating antinociception in the rat spinal cord. Br J Pharmacol 88:923–930.

Sawynok J, Yaksh TL (1993): Caffeine as an analgesic adjuvant: a review of pharmacology and mechanisms of action. Pharmacol Rev 45:43–85.

Sawynok J, Reid A, Poon A (1998): Peripheral antinociceptive effect of an adenosine kinase inhibitor, with augmentation by an adenosine deaminase inhibitor, in the rat formalin test. Pain 74:75–81.

Sawynok J, Zarrindast M-R, Reid AR, Doak GJ (1997): Adenosine A_3 receptor activation produces nociceptive behaviour and edema by release of histamine and 5-hydroxytryptamine. Eur J Pharmacol 333:1–7.

Segerdahl M, Ekblom A, Sollevi A (1994): The influence of adenosine, ketamine and morphine on experimentally induced ischemic pain in healthy volunteers. Anesth Analg 79:787–791.

Segerdahl M, Ekblom A, Sandelin K, Wickman M, Sollevi A (1995): Peroperative adenosine infusion reduces the requirements for isoflurane and postoperative analgesics. Anesth Analg 80:1145–1149.

Sierralta F, Miranda HF (1993): Adenosine modulates the antinociceptive action of benzodiazepines. Gen Pharmacol 24:891–894.

Sjölund K-F, Sollevi A, Segerdahl M, Hansson P, Lundeberg T (1996): Intrathecal and systemic R-phenylisopropyladenosine reduces scratching behaviour in a rat mononeuropathy model. Neuroreport 7:1856–1860.

Sklar SH, Blue WT, Alexander EJ, Bodian CA (1985): Herpes zoster: The treatment and prevention of neuralgia with adenosine monophosphate. JAMA 253:1427–1430.

Sollevi A, Belfrage M, Lundeberg T, Segerdahl M, Hansson P (1995): Systemic adenosine infusion: a new treatment modality to alleviate neuropathic pain. Pain 61:155–158.

Sosnowski M, Yaksh TL (1989): Role of spinal adenosine receptors in modulating the hyperesthesia produced by spinal glycine receptor antagonism. Anesth Analg 69: 587–592.

Sosnowski M, Stevens CW, Yaksh TL (1989): Assessment of the role of A_1/A_2 adenosine receptors mediating the purine antinociception, motor and autonomic function in the rat spinal cord. J Pharmacol Exp Ther 250:915–922.

Sweeney MI, White TD, Sawynok J (1987): Involvement of adenosine in the spinal antinociceptive effects of morphine and noradrenaline. J Pharmacol Exp Ther 243: 657–665.

Sweeney MI, White TD, Sawynok J (1989): Morphine, capsaicin and K^+ release purines from capsaicin-sensitive primary afferent nerve terminals in the spinal cord. J Pharmacol Exp Ther 248:447–454.

Sylvén C, Beermann B, Jonzon B, Brandt R (1986): Angina pectoris-like pain provoked by intravenous adenosine in healthy volunteers. Brit Med J 293:227–230.

Sylvén C, Beermann B, Edlund A, Lewander R, Jonzon B, Mogensen L (1988a): Provocation of chest pain in patients with coronary insufficiency using the vasodilator adenosine. Eur Heart J 9(Suppl. N):6–10.

Sylvén C, Jonzon B, Fredholm BB, Kaijser L (1988b): Adenosine injection into the brachial artery produces ischemia like pain or discomfort in the forearm. Cardiovasc Res 22:674–678.

Sylvén C, Beermann B, Kaijser L, Jonzon B (1990): Nicotine enhances angina pectoris-like pain and atrioventricular blockade provoked by intravenous bolus of adenosine in healthy volunteers. J Cardiovasc Pharmacol 16:962–965.

Taiwo YO, Levine JD (1990): Direct cutaneous hyperalgesia induced by adenosine. Neuroscience 38:757–762.

Taiwo YO, Levine JD (1991): Further confirmation of the role of adenyl cyclase and of cAMP-dependent protein kinase in primary afferent hyperalgesia. Neuroscience 44:131–135.

Van Wylen DGL, Sciotti VM, Winn HR (1991): Adenosine and the regulation of cerebral blood flow. In Phillis JW (ed): *Adenosine and Adenine Nucleotides as Regulators of Cellular Function.* Boca Raton, FL: CRC Press, pp. 191–202.

Vapaatalo H, Onken D, Neuvonen PJ, Westermann E (1975): Stereospecificity in some central and circulatory effects of phenylisopropyl-adenosine (PIA). Arzneim-Forsch (Drug Res) 25:407–410.

Weil-Fugazza J, Godefroy F, Manceau V, Besson JM (1986): Increased norepinephrine and uric acid levels in the spinal cord of arthritic rats. Brain Res 374:190–194.

Yamamoto T, Yaksh TL (1991): Spinal pharmacology of thermal hyperesthesia induced by incomplete ligation of sciatic nerve. Anesthesiology 75:817–826.

Yarbrough GC, McGuffin-Clineschmidt JC (1981): In vivo behavioral assessment of central nervous system purinergic receptors. Eur J Pharmacol 76:137–144.

CHAPTER 12

γ-AMINOBUTYRIC ACID AND PAIN

NORMAN G. BOWERY
University of Birmingham
Birmingham, United Kingdom

MARZIA MALCANGIO
UMDS, St Thomas's Campus
London, United Kingdom

PRESENCE, LOCALIZATION, AND FUNCTION OF GABA IN PAIN PATHWAYS

Any painful stimulus perceived in the periphery (skin, muscle, viscera) is conveyed to the spinal cord by unmyelinated and thinly myelinated primary afferent fibers (nociceptors), transmitted to the higher centers by ascending pathways and modulated by descending pathways. The periaqueductal gray (PAG) and nucleus raphe magnus (NRM) regions together with descending pathways and spinal cord neuronal circuits are regarded as part of an endogenous antinociceptive system. In fact, stimulation of both segmental and supraspinal descending nociceptive systems is used to alleviate pain in humans (see Meyerson, 1990).

The dorsal horn of the spinal cord constitutes the area in which nociceptive fibers (C and Aδ) terminate and spinothalamic tract (STT) cells are localized. These cells are considered a major somatosensory pathway that conveys primary nociceptive information from the spinal cord to the brain, signalling location and encoding the character of the nociceptive input. In the superficial layers of the dorsal horn, γ-aminobutyric acid (GABA) (with or without glycine) is contained in intrinsic interneurons (stalked cells in lamina II) and in the terminals of descending fibers originating from the medulla (Millhorn et al., 1988; Blessing, 1990; Reichling and Basbaum, 1990; Jones et al., 1991; Antal et al., 1996; Todd, 1996). GABAergic interneurons make presynaptic contacts onto primary afferent nerve terminals (Barber et al., 1978; Merighi et

---

Novel Aspects of Pain Management: Opioids and Beyond, Edited by Jana Sawynok and Alan Cowan
ISBN 0-471-180173   Copyright © 1999 by Wiley-Liss, Inc.

al., 1989; Todd and Lochhead 1990; Alvarez et al., 1992) and postsynaptic contacts on dendrites and cell bodies (Barber et al., 1978; Magoul et al., 1987; Merighi et al., 1989; Spike and Todd, 1992) of STT cells (Lekan and Carlton, 1995).

This anatomical distribution of GABAergic neurons suggests that GABA is involved in the modulation of pain at the segmental level by inhibiting the transmission of nociceptive information. A variety of experimental evidence supports this concept and it has been recently suggested that there is a tonic release of GABA within the dorsal horn to modulate the functional activity of dorsal horn neurons (Lin et al., 1996).

Intrathecally injected $GABA_A$ and $GABA_B$ receptor agonists induce antinociception in rodents and primates (Yaksh and Reddy, 1981; Aanonsen and Wilcox, 1989; Hammond and Drower, 1984; Sawynok and Dickson, 1985). By contrast, intrathecal application of $GABA_A$ and $GABA_B$ receptor antagonists induces allodynia (innocuous stimuli are perceived as painful) (Yaksh, 1989; Hao et al., 1994). GABA, $GABA_A$, and $GABA_B$ receptor agonists can depress spinal cord neuronal firing after primary afferent fiber stimulation (Curtis et al., 1968; Kangrga et al., 1991) and can inhibit the release of substance P (SP) and glutamate from these fiber terminals (Kangrga et al., 1991; Malcangio and Bowery, 1993; Teoh et al., 1996a). Furthermore, iontophoretically applied GABA reduces spontaneous firing of STT cells and inhibits the activity evoked by either glutamate application or noxious stimulation (pinching of the skin) (Willcockson et al., 1984). GABA-mediated antinociception in the rat can be induced by electrical stimulation of PAG, NRM, or spinal cord (Lin et al., 1994; Linderoth et al., 1994; Stiller et al., 1995). Spinal cord stimulation causes an increase in the extracellular concentration of GABA in the dorsal horn (Stiller et al., 1996), thus potentiating endogenous segmental antinociception. Electrical stimulation of the two endogenous antinociceptive systems in the PAG and NRM appears to cause release of GABA in the spinal cord. GABA would then inhibit STT cell activity via activation of $GABA_A$ receptors or reduce release of neurotransmitters from primary afferent fibers via $GABA_B$ receptors (McGowan and Hammond, 1993; Lin et al., 1994, 1996). Evidence that GABAergic fibers, which are independent of serotoninergic systems, descend from NRM to the spinal cord has been obtained recently (Antal et al., 1996). They terminate on glutamatergic neurons, which can make synaptic contacts on STT cells (Lekan and Carlton, 1995); GABA can thus reduce glutamate-induced excitation of STT cells, resulting in inhibition of their activity. A scheme of these neuronal pathways is outlined in Figure 12.1.

GABA CHANGES IN CHRONIC PAIN MODELS

In recent years, the plastic changes that occur within the spinal cord during development of chronic pain of either inflammatory or neuropathic origin have received much attention. Both types of pain are characterized by an increased

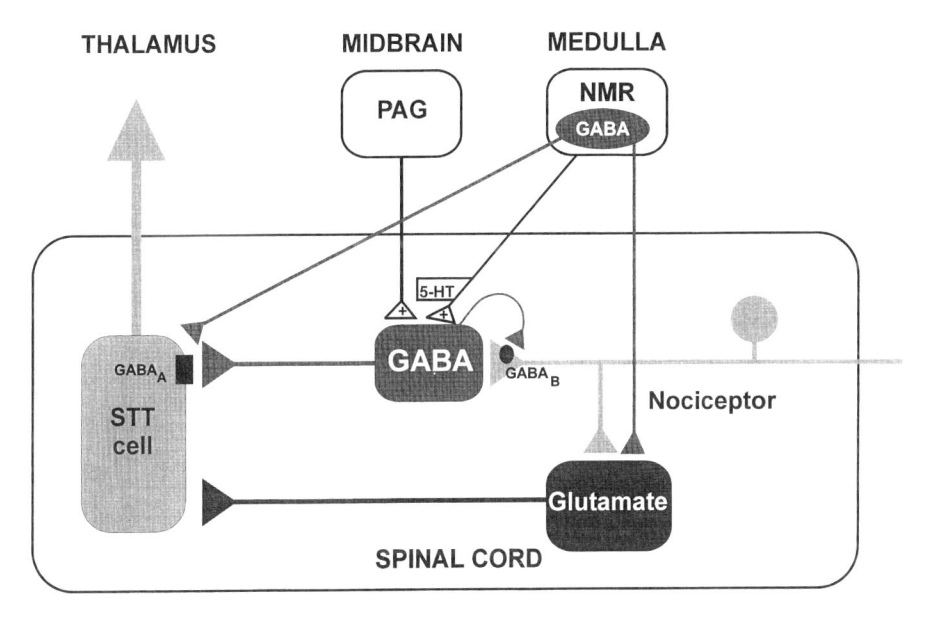

Figure 12.1 GABA-mediated segmental antinociception. Activation of interneuronal GABA in the spinal cord can produce analgesia (1) by inhibiting the release of neurotransmitters/neuromodulators from primary afferent fibers (via $GABA_B$ receptor activation), and (2) by reducing spinothalamic tract (STT) cells input to the thalamus (via activation of $GABA_A$ receptors). The interneuronal pool of GABA can be released by stimulation of either supraspinal descending inhibitory sites, periaqueductal gray matter (PAG) and nucleus raphe magnus (NRM), or spinal cord stimulation.

activity of nociceptive fibers that induces an increased excitability and discharge frequency of dorsal horn neurons (wind-up) (see Chapter 1). In this context, the role played by the segmental GABAergic system may be essential.

During development of inflammatory pain, an increase in neuropeptide (SP and calcitonin gene-related peptide, CGRP) content in primary afferent neurons and SP release in the spinal cord occurs (Kar et al., 1991; Malcangio and Bowery, 1994). These changes are concomitant with an increase in glutamate release from the same fibers (Sluka and Westlund, 1993). GABA content in interneurons is also increased, probably to support its role as an endogenous antinociceptive agent counteracting the nociception consequent to an increased activity of nociceptive fibers (Malcangio and Bowery, 1994). A different picture emerges in the spinal cord during neuropathic pain. Neuropeptide (SP and CGRP) content and release from nociceptive fibers is reduced (M. Malcangio, unpublished results) in contrast to glutamate release, which is probably increased (see Dickenson and Sullivan, 1990). GABA content in dorsal horn neurons is also reduced (Castro-Lopes et al., 1993; Ibuki et al., 1997), thus possibly exacerbating glutamate excitotoxicity (Laird and Bennett, 1992). By contrast to inflammatory pain, in neuropathic pain the loss of the GABAergic endogenous antinociceptive system (i.e., disinhibition occurs) contributes to the ongoing pain and touch-evoked allodynia (Sivilotti and Woolf, 1994). It has been proposed that spinal cord stimulation-induced release of GABA could be used to alleviate pain in patients with peripheral neuropathies (Stiller et al., 1996).

GABA RECEPTORS

GABA receptors in the CNS can be broadly classified into fast and slow types. The fast ionotropic $GABA_A$-type receptor incorporates a chloride channel, mediates rapid synaptic transmission, can be antagonized by bicuculline, and is modulated by a variety of ligands such as benzodiazepines and barbiturates (Burt and Kamatchi, 1990). Other forms of "fast" GABA receptors, namely, $GABA_C$ receptors, have been described (Bormann and Feigenspan, 1995). The "slow" receptor, a metabotropic $GABA_B$ receptor, which is coupled to G proteins (guanine nucleotide binding protein) and modulates synaptic transmission either by opening of K^+ channels or via inhibition of Ca^{2+} channel opening events (Bowery and Brown, 1997), has recently been cloned (Kaupmann et al., 1997). There is a specific agonist for the $GABA_B$ receptor, baclofen, and several antagonists have been described (Bowery, 1993).

PHARMACOLOGICAL ASPECTS

Much attention has been devoted to the involvement of central GABA receptors in nociception and there seems little doubt that endogenous GABA mechanisms are implicated at the spinal cord level as well as in higher centers (Sawynok, 1987; Bowery, 1993; Lin et al., 1996). Can this physiological, or even pathological, role be exploited pharmacologically? Some attempts have been made to recruit these systems, although there is no current pain therapy based on the activation of GABA systems. Agonists selective for either $GABA_A$ or $GABA_B$ receptors produce antinociceptive effects in animal models. Moreover, drugs that facilitate the action of GABA at $GABA_A$ receptors, the benzodiazepines, neurosteroids, and barbiturates, have variously been shown to exert an antinociceptive effect, although some pro-nociceptive activity has been reported for barbiturates. Antinociception produced by baclofen, the $GABA_B$ receptor agonist, in animal models is also well documented, and this can be blocked by $GABA_B$ receptor antagonists. Some studies have been reported with compounds that interfere with the inactivation processes for GABA (Buckett, 1980; Sawynok, 1987), and inhibition of GABA uptake also can produce an antinociceptive effect (Zorn and Enna, 1985).

GABA$_A$ Receptor Agonists

Among the directly acting GABA$_A$ receptor agonists, probably muscimol and its stable analogue, THIP (4,5,6,7-tetrahydroisoxazolo[5,4-c]pyridin-3-ol), are the two most studied for their analgesic properties. Muscimol (up to 1mg/kg i.p.) delays the paw lick response in mice in the hot plate test (Laviola et al., 1992). However, after systemic injection only a very small amount of unchanged muscimol reaches the brain, suggesting that this antinociception is probably due to the combined action of muscimol and a derivative (Maggi and Enna, 1979). Nevertheless, GABA$_A$ systems in the forebrain may be more important than spinal GABA$_A$ mechanisms (Krogsgaard-Larsen et al., 1997). When muscimol is administered intracerebroventricularly, it produces antinociception (Liebman and Pastor, 1980), whereas intrathecal injection is ineffective in acute pain models such as the hot plate and tail flick tests (Hammond and Drower, 1984). However, intrathecally administered muscimol is effective in reducing caudally directed biting and scratching behavior in mice caused by excitatory amino acid injections (Aanonsen and Wilcox, 1989) and can suppress the protracted nociceptive response to formalin in rats (Dirig and Yaksh, 1995).

THIP is more potent than muscimol in a variety of animal models as well as in man (Hill et al, 1981; Hammond and Drower, 1984; Krogsgaard-Larsen et al., 1984, 1985, 1988). In fact, THIP is reported to be equipotent with morphine in certain animal species (Krogsgaard-Larsen et al., 1997) but unlike morphine, its action is not blocked by naloxone. Interestingly, it has been considered that the analgesia that accompanies prolonged treatment of rats with naloxone might be mediated via the GABA$_A$ receptor system. However, Rochford and Stewart (1992) have shown that neither the GABA$_A$ agonist, muscimol, nor the antagonist, bicuculline, affect the paw lick latencies of rats injected daily for 8 days with 10 mg/kg naloxone in a standard hot plate test. It has been reported that the acute analgesic action of THIP can be reduced by muscarinic cholinoceptor antagonism and enhanced by the anticholinesterase agent physostigmine (Zorn and Enna, 1987). This would suggest a possible involvement with cholinergic mechanisms but the nature of this interaction has yet to be clarified.

GABA$_A$ Receptor Modulators

The activation of GABA$_A$ receptor systems can be enhanced by a variety of compounds. The most well established among these are the benzodiazepines and related drugs, but in addition there is clear evidence that the neurosteroids and barbiturates, which also act at sites on the GABA$_A$ receptor complex and which are distinct from the benzodiazepine receptor, can exert an analgesic effect in animal models. The overwhelming evidence that the benzodiazepines exert an analgesic effect stems from studies performed at the level of the spinal cord (Edwards et al., 1990; Yanez et al., 1990; Boulter et al., 1991; Serrao et al., 1991; Clavier et al., 1992; Miyamoto et al., 1992) and higher centers of the brain (Behbenhani et al., 1990), but even after systemic administration an antinociceptive response, presumably mediated in the brain, can be observed (Bianchi et al., 1993; Bartusch et al., 1996). However, in the rat formalin test, diazepam (0.5–5 mg/kg) given systemically failed to suppress the nociceptive response and even attenuated the reduction in nociception that normally occurs between the two characteristic phases of nociception in this model (Franklin and Abbott, 1993). Dirig and Yaksh (1995) also showed that midazolam, administered intrathecally in this model, failed to suppress the two phases of nociception but found no evidence for any diminution in the quiescent period between phase 1 and 2. These authors point out that the level of endogenous GABA in the spinal cord is too low for a GABA potentiator such as midazolam to exert any antinociceptive activity following intrathecal administration. However, this may depend upon the type of pain and the nature of the GABA potentiator. Although a "benzodiazepine-type" potentiator might be inactive, because it acts only via the $GABA_A$ receptor system, an inhibitor of GABA uptake could increase the extracellular GABA levels and this would be available to activate $GABA_B$ as well as $GABA_A$ receptors (see below). In fact, GABA uptake inhibitors have been reported to induce a greater antinociceptive response in the mouse than other GABAergic drugs (Zorn and Enna, 1985).

There exists little or no evidence for the benzodiazepine receptor antagonist, flumazenil, exerting any direct analgesic activity although it has been reported to reverse the antinociceptive action of chlordiazepoxide (Boulter et al., 1991) and, perhaps surprisingly, that of melatonin (Golombek et al., 1992) which presumably mediates its effect via GABA.

Benzodiazepines may also modify the development of tolerance to morphine (Yanez et al., 1990). Thus diazepam can suppress the delay in tolerance to the antinociceptive response to morphine in the formalin model (Rahman et al., 1994). Flumazenil prevented this effect of diazepam.

Barbiturates are a well-established group of drugs that enhance GABA-mediated inhibition, and this effect is believed to be responsible for their anxiolytic and sedative properties. However, despite their similarity to the benzodiazepines in behavioral outcome, their antinociceptive activity is not so predictable. In fact, the barbiturates are considered to be without analgesic activity and can even elicit hyperalgesia in man (Hobbs et al., 1996). Pentobarbitone has also been reported to be without effect in the rat formalin model (Franklin and Abbott, 1993; Gilron and Coderre, 1996). A hyperalgesic enhancement of motor responses to noxious stimulation has been described for thiopentone (Archer et al., 1996) but the authors concluded that this is not mediated via the $GABA_A$ receptor complex.

In contrast to the above observations reporting lack of activity, Goto et al. (1994) reported that pentobarbitone could suppress the second phase of formalin-induced hyperalgesia. Jewett and colleagues (1992) also demonstrated an apparent antinociceptive effect of pentobarbitone on the monosynaptic reflex in rat spinal cord. They suggest that the observed effects are consistent with an analgesic action of the drug. The reason for the apparent discrepancy in outcome with the barbiturates is unclear but overall, particularly with reference to man, it has to be concluded that they are of little significance as analgesics (Hobbs et al., 1996).

A group of $GABA_A$ receptor modulators that has emerged more recently is the neurosteroids, which act at nongenomic receptors within the $GABA_A$ receptor complex. The steroids are endogenous in mammals, although synthetic derivatives have been developed. A notable example is the anesthetic alphaxalone, which, like the benzodiazepines and barbiturates, enhances the functional activity of $GABA_A$ receptors. It can transiently suppress the second phase of formalin-induced nociception in rats and this action can be antagonized by the $GABA_A$ antagonist, picrotoxin (Gilron and Coderre, 1996). Involvement of the $GABA_A$ receptor complex in the antinociceptive action of neurosteroids is also supported by structure–activity studies performed by Frye and Duncan (1994) in the radiant heat tail flick test in rats. The antinociceptive activity of seven progestogens was compared following intracerebroventricular injection. The activity of each compound was consistent with their known activity at the $GABA_A$ receptor complex

$GABA_A$ Receptor Antagonism

Although the reversal of alphaxalone antinociception by picrotoxin supports a $GABA_A$ receptor-mediated action, there exists evidence that picrotoxin alone can produce "pain-like" behavior in rats (Oliveras and Montagne-Clavel, 1994). If picrotoxin is microinjected into the thalamic reticular nucleus, a behavioral response occurs whereby the contralateral hindpaw is repetitively raised. This effect is not produced following injection into the ventrobasal complex. It is assumed that the action of picrotoxin depends on the presence of a "GABA-tone" in the reticular nucleus.

Intrathecal injection of bicuculline into the spinal cord of mice and rats can also induce allodynia (Yaksh, 1989; Onaka et al., 1996), which is consistent with an antinociceptive action of GABA. Intrathecal administration of bicuculline also enhances the thermal hyperalgesia that follows sciatic nerve constriction in rats (Yamamoto and Yaksh, 1993). However, the situation with GABA receptor antagonism appears to be complex, because bicuculline-induced antinociception has been reported (Heinricher and Kaplan, 1991; see Krogsgaard-Larsen et al., 1997). For example, Malcangio et al. (1992) have shown that bicuculline can produce an increase in the latency of paw licking in the hot plate test in mice. This effect may be produced by a facilitation of the action of GABA at the metabotropic receptor, $GABA_B$, which has been strongly implicated in pain mechanisms, as the selective $GABA_B$ antagonist, CGP 35348, blocked the antinociceptive effect of bicuculline.

$GABA_B$ Receptor Mechanisms

Baclofen, the selective $GABA_B$ receptor agonist, has long been known to produce an antinociceptive action in a variety of models of acute pain in rodents including the hot plate, tail flick, and acetic acid writhing tests (Cutting and Jordan, 1975; Levy and Proudfit, 1979; Sawynok and LaBella, 1982; Malcangio et al., 1991; Rochford and Stewart, 1992; Serrano et al., 1992) at doses below that which produces motor impairment. Although strong evidence for a supraspinal site of action for baclofen has been provided (Levy and Proudfit, 1979; Liebman and Pastor, 1980; Thomas et al., 1995), there is no doubt that an action within the spinal cord contributes to the antinociceptive effect (Wilson and Yaksh, 1978; Smith, 1984; Sawynok and Dickson, 1985; Hammond and Washington, 1993; Dirig and Yaksh, 1995; Buritova et al., 1996; Thomas et al., 1996). The contribution of spinal cord mechanisms to the antinociceptive action of baclofen appears to stem from activation of $GABA_B$ receptors on pain fibre terminals in the dorsal horn (Figure 12.1). At least 50% of $GABA_B$ receptor binding sites detected in laminae I–III of the rat spinal cord are located on small-diameter primary afferent terminals (Price et al., 1984; 1987). Activation of these receptors suppresses the evoked release of sensory transmitters including SP and glutamate (Kangrga et al., 1991; Malcangio and Bowery, 1993; Teoh et al., 1996b) in isolated preparations of rat spinal cord. This decrease in release probably accounts for at least part of the acute antinociceptive action of systemically administered baclofen and certainly the full action following intrathecal administration. $GABA_B$ receptor antagonists reverse the action of GABA and baclofen on these release processes and block their antinociceptive activity. By comparison, $GABA_A$ receptor activation did not suppress the release of SP, and bicuculline failed to modify the suppressant action of GABA (Malcangio and Bowery, 1993).

Although this effect of baclofen may account for its acute antinociceptive effect, it does not explain its reduced efficacy in models of chronic pain (Hansson and Kinnman, 1996). Nevertheless, baclofen has been successfully used in humans to treat trigeminal neuralgia in which it reduces the number of painful paroxysms (Fromm, 1994; Sidebottom and Maxwell, 1995). However, the effect of baclofen seems to vary with the model. In a neuropathic pain model involving ligation of the sciatic nerve in rats, the antinociceptive response to baclofen appeared to increase (Smith et al., 1994), whereas in inflammatory pain models, the response to baclofen was either unchanged (Smith et al., 1994) or reduced (Malcangio and Bowery, 1994). In the latter case, this is probably due to the increase in GABA levels within the dorsal horn that occurs during the inflammatory process (Castro-Lopes et al., 1992). The excess GABA increases the presynaptic inhibition to the primary afferent terminals to decrease sensory input. In support of this hypothesis, we have shown that $GABA_B$ receptor antagonist superfused over spinal cord slices obtained from monoarthritic rats induces a significant increase in the evoked release of SP (Malcangio and Bowery, 1994). This would suggest that an increase in GABA tone, which would reduce the evoked release of SP, has been removed by the $GABA_B$ antagonist. Moreover, when the antagonist was administered *in vivo* to rats with monoarthritis, a marked and significant decrease in paw withdrawal latency occurred (Malcangio and Bowery, 1994). By comparison, in naive rats the same antagonist produced no change in the paw withdrawal latency to a heat stimulus. Hao et al. (1994) have also observed that the GABA$_B$ antagonist CGP 35348, administered intrathecally, has no effect in the hot plate test in naive rats. However, the antagonist did produce a painlike response to innocuous mechanical stimulation. They suggested that the input of low-threshold afferent fibers innervating mechanoceptors is tonically inhibited by GABA$_B$ receptor activation even under normal physiological conditions.

The apparent increase in GABA tone during monoarthritis would suggest that GABA can also become an endogenous pathological antinociceptive substance. The change in GABA tone during pathological events may, in part, explain why baclofen is inactive in chronic pain due to a strong, or even maximal, preexisting GABA$_B$ receptor activation. However, this may not be the only reason for the inactivity of baclofen. Following prolonged and repeated administration of baclofen, a tolerance to its action occurs and this can be readily observed, for example, in spinal cord and olfactory cortex where a decrease in the number of GABA$_B$ receptor binding sites and responses to baclofen has been noted (Malcangio et al., 1993, 1995).

GABA Derivatives

The synthesis of some GABA derivatives as potential new antiepileptic drugs has been successful in providing clinicians with vigabatrin and gabapentin (Satzinger, 1994). Gabapentin has been anecdotally reported to exert an analgesic effect in postherpetic neuralgia (Segal and Rodorf, 1996) and reflex sympathetic dystrophy (Mellick and Mellicy, 1995). However, even though gabapentin prevents allodynia in neuropathic rats, this effect is not prevented by either GABA$_A$ or GABA$_B$ antagonists excluding any direct involvement of GABA systems (Hwang and Yaksh, 1997).

FUTURE POTENTIAL

There seems little doubt that GABA-ergic mechanisms play a major role in sensory processing and that drugs that affect GABA-mediated events can influence the nociceptive process. There seem to be two possible targets for future consideration: (1) enhancement of the synaptic activation of GABA by blocking the uptake and degradation processes or by selective block of GABA$_B$ autoreceptors if such drugs emerge and (2) development of a selective GABA$_B$ agonist that produces little or no tolerance. This latter idea may prove to be impossible but at present it remains as a viable alternative because we do not know whether receptor subtypes may eventually provide a basis for differentiating between effects. A selective focus on the spinal cord may prove to be a better target, particularly because it is known already that low-dose intrathecal infusion of baclofen for spasticity produces little or no tolerance (Penn et al., 1989; Malcangio and Bowery, 1996). Production of effective analgesia by intrathecal infusion of baclofen in man has just recently been reported by two groups (Taira et al 1995; Loubses and Akman 1996).

REFERENCES

Aanonsen LM, Wilcox GL (1989): Muscimol, γ-aminobutyric acid$_A$ receptors and excitatory amino acids in the mouse spinal cord. J Pharmacol Exp Ther 248:1034–1038.

Alvarez FJ, Kavookjian AM, Light AR (1992): Synaptic interactions between GABA-immunoreactive profiles and the terminals of functionally defined myelinated nociceptors in the monkey and cat spinal cord. J Neurosci 12:2901–2917.

Antal M, Petko M, Polgar E, Heizmann CW, Storm-Mathisen J (1996): Direct evidence of an extensive GABAergic innervation of the spinal dorsal horn by fibres descending from rostral ventromedial medulla. Neuroscience 73:509–518.

Archer DP, Ewen A, Froelich J, Roth SH, Samanani N (1996): Thiopentone induced enhancement of somatic motor responses to noxious stimulation: influence of GABA$_A$ receptor modulation. Can J Anaesth 43:503–510.

Barber RP, Vaughn JE, Saito K, McLaughin BJ, Roberts E (1978): GABAergic terminals are presynaptic to the primary afferent terminals in the substantia gelatinosa of the rat spinal cord. Brain Res 141:35–55.

Bartusch SL, Sanders BJ, D'Alessio JG, Jernigan JR (1996): Clonazepam for the treatment of lancinating phantom limb pain. Clin J Pain 12:59–62.

Behbehani MM, Jiang MR, Chandler SD, Ennis M (1990): The effect of GABA and its antagonists on midbrain periaqueductal gray neurons in the rat. Pain 40:195–204.

Bianchi M, Mantegazza P, Tammiso R, Zonta N, Zambotti F (1993): Peripherally administered benzodiazepines increase morphine-induced analgesia in the rat. Effect of RO 15-3505 and FG 7142. Arch Int Pharmacodyn Ther 322:5–13.

Blessing WW (1990): Distribution of glutamate decarboxylase-containing neurons in rabbit medulla oblongata with attention to intramedullary and spinal projections. Neuroscience 37:171–185.

Bormann J, Feigenspan A (1995): GABA$_C$ receptors. Trends Neurosci 18:515–519.

Boulter N, Serrao JM, Gent JP, Goodchild CS (1991): Spinally mediated antinociception following intrathecal chlordiazepoxide—further evidence for a benzodiazepine spinal analgesic effect. Eur J Anaesth 8:407–411.

Bowery NG (1993): GABA$_B$ receptor pharmacology. Ann Rev Pharmacol Toxicol 33:109–147.

Bowery NG, Brown DA (1997): The cloning of GABA receptors. Nature 386:223–224.

Buckett WR (1980): Irreversible inhibitors of GABA transaminase induced antinociceptive effects and potentiate morphine. Neuropharmacology 19:715–722.

Buritova J, Chapman V, Honore P, Besson J-M (1996): The contribution of GABA$_B$ receptor-mediated events to inflammatory pain processing: carrageenan oedema and associated spinal c-Fos expression in the rat. Neuroscience 73:487–496.

Burt DR, Kamatchi GL (1990): GABA$_A$ receptor subtypes: from pharmacology to molecular biology. FASEB J 5:2916–2923.

Castro-Lopes JM, Tavares I, Tolle TR, Coito A, Coimbra A (1992): Increase in GABAergic cells and GABA levels in the spinal cord in unilateral inflammation of the hindlimb of the rat. Neuroscience 4:763–773.

Castro-Lopes JM, Tavares I, Coimbra A (1993): GABA decreases in the spinal cord dorsal horn after peripheral neurectomy. Brain Res 620:287–291.

Clavier N, Lombard MC, Besson JM (1992): Benzodiazepines and pain: effects of midazolam on the activities of nociceptive non-specific dorsal horn neurons in the rat spinal cord. Pain 48:61–71.

Curtis DR, Hosli L, Johnston GAR (1968): A pharmacological study of the depression of spinal neurones by glycine and related amino acids. Exp Brain Res 6:1–18.

Cutting DA, Jordan CC (1975): Alternative approaches to analgesia: baclofen as a model compound. Br J Pharmacol 54:171–179.

Dickenson AH, Sullivan AF (1990): Differential effects of excitatory amino acid antagonists on dorsal horn nociceptive neurones in the rat. Brain Res 506:31–39.

Dirig DM, Yaksh TL (1995): Intrathecal baclofen and muscimol, but not midazolam, are antinociceptive using the rat-formalin model. J Pharmacol Exp Ther 275:219–227.

Edwards M, Serrao JM, Gent JP, Goodchild CS (1990): On the mechanism by which midazolam causes spinally mediated analgesia. Anaesthesiology 73:273–277.

Franklin KB, Abbott FV (1993): Pentobarbital, diazepam, and ethanol abolish the interphase diminution of pain in the formalin test: evidence for pain modulation by GABA$_A$ receptors. Pharmacol Biochem Behav 46:661–666.

Fromm GH (1994): Baclofen as an adjuvant analgesic. J Pain Symptom Manage 9:500–509.

Frye CA, Duncan JE (1994): Progesterone metabolites, effective at the GABA$_A$ receptor complex, attenuate pain sensitivity in rats. Brain Res 643:194–203.

Gilron I, Coderre TJ (1996): Preemptive analgesic effects of steroid anesthesia with alphaxalone in the rat formalin test. Evidence for differential GABA(A) receptor modulation in persistent nociception. Anaesthesiology 84:572–579.

Golombek DA, Escolar E, Burin LJ, De Brito Sanchez MG, Fernandez Duque D, Cardinali DP (1992): Chronopharmacology of melatonin: inhibition by benzodiazepine antagonism. Chronobiol Int 9:124–131.

Goto T, Marota JJ, Crosby G (1994): Pentobarbitone, but not propofol, produces preemptive analgesia in the rat formalin model. Br J Anaesthesia 72:662–667.

Hammond DL, Drower EJ (1984): Effect of intrathecally administered THIP and muscimol on nociceptive threshold. Eur J Pharmacol 103:121–125.

Hammond DL, Washington JD (1993): Antagonism of L-baclofen-induced antinociception by CGP 35348 in the spinal cord of the rat. Eur J Pharmacol 234:255–262.

Hansson P, Kinnman E (1996): Unmasking mechanisms of peripheral neuropathic pain in a clinical perspective. Pain Rev 3:272–292.

Hao J-X, Xu X-J, Wiesenfeld-Hallin Z (1994): Intrathecal γ-aminobutyric acid$_B$ (GABA$_B$) receptor antagonist CGP 35348 induces hypersensitivity to mechanical stimuli in the rat. Neurosci Lett 182:299–302.

Heinricher MM, Kaplan HJ (1991): GABA-mediated inhibition in rostral ventromedial medulla: role in nociceptive modulation in the light anesthetized rat. Pain 47:105–113.

Hill RC, Maurer R, Buescher HH, Roemer D (1981): Analgesic properties of the GABA-mimetic THIP. Eur J Pharmacol 69:221–224.

Hobbs WR, Rall TW, Verdoorn TA (1996): Hypnotics and sedatives. In Hardman JG, Gilman AG, Limbird LE (eds): Goodman & Gilman's *The Pharmacological Basis of Therapeutics*, 9th ed. New York: McGraw-Hill, pp. 361–396.

Hwang JH, Yaksh TL (1997): Effect of subarachnoid gabapentin on tactile-evoked allodynia in a surgically induced neuropathic pain model in the rat. Reg Anesth 22:249–256.

Ibuki T, Hama AT, Wang X-T, Pappas GD, Sagen J (1997): Loss of GABA-immunoreactivity in the spinal dorsal horn of rats with peripheral nerve injury and promotion of recovery by adrenal medullary grafts. Neuroscience 76:845–858.

Jewett BA, Gibbs LM, Tarasiuk A, Kendig JJ (1992): Propofol and barbiturate depression of spinal nociceptive neurotransmission. Anaesthesiology 77:1148–1154.

Jones BE, Holmes CJ, Rodrignez-Vega E, Mainville L (1991): GABA-synthesizing neurones in the medulla: their relationship to serotonin-containing and spinally projecting neurones in the rat. J Comp Neurol 313:349–367.

Kangrga I, Jang M, Randic M (1991): Actions of (-)baclofen on rat dorsal horn neurons. Brain Res 562:265–275.

Kar S, Gibson SJ, Rees RG, Jura WGZO, Brewerton DA, Polak JM (1991): Increased calcitonin gene-realted peptide (CGRP), substance P and enkephalin immunoreactivities in dorsal spinal cord and loss of CGRP-immunoreactive motoneurones in arthritic rats depend on intact peripheral nerve supply. J Mol Neurosci 3:7–18.

Kaupmann K, Huggel K, Heid J, Flor P J, Bischoff S, Mickel S J, McMaster G, Angst C, Bittiger H, Froestl W, Bettler B (1997): Expression cloning of $GABA_B$ receptors uncovers similarity to metabotropic glutamate receptors. Nature 386:239–246.

Krogsgaard-Larsen P, Falch E, Christensen AV (1984): Chemistry and pharmacology of the GABA agonists THIP (Gaboxadol) and isoguvacine. Drugs Fut 9:597–618.

Krogsgaard-Larsen P, Falch E, Hjeds H (1985): Heterocyclic analogues of GABA: chemistry, molecular pharmacology and therapeutic aspects. Prog Med Chem 22:67–120.

Krogsgaard-Larsen P, Hjeds H, Falch E, Jørgensen FS, Nielsen L (1988): Recent advances in GABA agonists, antagonists and uptake inhibitors: structure-activity relationships and therapeutic potential. Adv Drug Res 17:381–456.

Krogsgaard-Larsen P, Frølund B, Ebert B (1997): $GABA_A$ receptor agonists, partial agonists and antagonists. In Enna SJ, Bowery NG (eds): "The GABA Receptors." Totowa, NJ, Humana Press, pp. 37–81.

Laird JM, Bennett GJ (1992): Dorsal root potentials and afferent input to the spinal cord in rats with an experimental peripheral neuropathy. Brain Res 584:181–190.

Laviola G, Chiarotti F, Alleva E (1992): Development of GABAergic modulation of mouse locomotor activity and pain sensitivity after prenatal benzodiazepine exposure. Neurotoxicol Teratol 14:1–5.

Lekan HA, Carlton SM (1995): Glutamatergic and GABAergic input to rat spinothalamic tract cells in the superficial dorsal horn. J Comp Neurol 361:417–428.

Levy RA, Proudfit HK (1979): Analgesia produced by microinjection of baclofen and morphine at brain stem sites. Eur J Pharmacol 57:43–55.

Liebman JM, Pastor G (1980): Antinociceptive effects of baclofen and muscimol upon intraventricular administration. Eur J Pharmacol 61:225–230.

Lin Q, Peng YB, Willis WD (1994): Glycine and GABA$_A$ antagonists reduce the inhibition of primate spinothalamic tract neurones produced by stimulation in periaqueductal gray. Brain Res 654:286–302.

Lin Q, Peng YB, Willis WD (1996): Role of GABA receptor subtypes in inhibition of primate spinothalamic tract neurons: difference between spinal and periaqueductal gray inhibition. J Neurophysiol 75:109–123.

Linderoth B, Stiller C-O, Gunasekera L, O'Connor WT, Ungerstedt U, Brodin E (1994): Gamma-aminobutyric acid is released in the dorsal horn by electrical spinal cord stimulation: an in vivo microdialysis study in the rat. Neurosurgery 34:484–489.

Loubser PG, Akman NM (1996): Effects of intrathecal baclofen on chronic spinal cord injury pain. J Pain Symptom Manage 12:241–247.

Maggi A, Enna SJ (1979): Characteristics of muscimol accumulation in mouse brain after systemic administration. Neuropharmacology 18:361–366.

Magoul R, Onteniente B, Geffard M, Calas A (1987): Anatomical distribution and ultrastructural organization of the GABAergic system in the spinal cord. An immunocytochemical study using anti-GABA antibodies. Neuroscience 20:1001–1009.

Malcangio M, Bowery NG (1993): Gamma-aminobutyric acid$_B$, but not gamma-aminobutyric acid$_A$ receptor activation, inhibits electrically evoked substance P-like immunoreactivity release from the rat spinal cord *in vitro*. J Pharmacol Exp Ther 266:1490–1496.

Malcangio M, Bowery NG (1994): Spinal cord SP release and hyperalgesia in monoarthritic rats: involvement of the GABA$_B$ receptor system. Br J Pharmacol 113:1561–1566.

Malcangio M, Bowery NG (1996): GABA and its receptors in the spinal cord. Trends Pharmacol Sci 17:457–462.

Malcangio M, Ghelardini C, Giotti A, Malmberg-Aiello P, Bartolini A (1991): CGP 35348, a new GABA$_B$ antagonist, prevents antinociception and muscle-relaxant effect induced by baclofen. Br J Pharmacol 103:1303–1308.

Malcangio M, da Silva H, Bowery NG (1993): Plasticity of GABA$_B$ receptor in rat spinal cord detected by autoradiography. Eur J Pharmacol 250:153–156.

Malcangio M, Malmberg-Aiello P, Giotti A, Ghelardini C, Bartolini A (1992): Desensitization of GABA$_B$ receptors and antagonism by CGP 35348 prevent bicuculline—and picrotoxin—induced antinociception. Neuropharmacology 31:783–791.

Malcangio M, Libri V, Teoh H, Constanti A, Bowery NG (1995): Chronic (-)baclofen or CGP36742 alters GABA$_B$ receptor sensitivity in rat brain and spinal cord. Neuroreport 6:399–403.

McGowan MK, Hammond DL (1993): Antinociception produced by microinjection of L-glutamate in the ventrolateral medulla of the rat: mediation by spinal GABA$_A$ receptors. Brain Res 620:89–96.

Mellick GA, Mellicy LB (1995): Gabapentin in the management of reflex sympathetic dystrophy. J Pain Symptom Manage 10:265–266.

Merighi A, Polak JM, Fumagalli G, Theodosis DT (1989): Ultrastructural localization of neuropeptides and GABA in rat dorsal horn: a comparison of different immunogold labeling techniques. J Histochem Cytochem 37:529–540.

Meyerson BA (1990): Electric stimulation of the spinal cord and brain. In Bonica JJ, Loeser JD, Chapman RC, Fordyce WE (eds): *The Management of Pain*. Philadelphia: Lea & Febiger, pp. 1862–1877.

Millhorn DE, Hokfelt T, Seroogy K, Verhofstad AAJ (1988): Extent of colocalization of serotonin and GABA in neurons of the ventral medulla oblungata in rat. Brain Res 461:169–174.

Miyamoto K, Wakita K, Okuda T, Fuji K, Suekane K (1992): Suppressant efforts of midazolam on responses of spinal dorsal horn neurones in rabbits. Neuropharmacology 31:49–53.

Oliveras JL, Montagne-Clavel J (1994): The $GABA_A$ receptor antagonist picrotoxin induces a 'pain-like' behavior when administered into the thalamic reticular nucleus of the behaving rat: a possible model for 'central' pain? Neurosci Lett 179:21–24.

Onaka M, Miniami T, Nishihara I, Ito S (1996): Involvement of glutamate receptors in strychnine-and bicuculline-induced allodynia in conscious mice. Anaesthesiology 84:1215–1222.

Penn RD, Savoy SM, Corcos D, Latash M, Gottlieb G, Parke B, Kroin K (1989): Intrathecal baclofen for severe spinal spasticity. New Engl J Med 320:1517–1521.

Price GW, Wilkin GP, Turnbull MJ, Bowery NG (1984): Are baclofen-sensitive $GABA_B$ receptors present on primary afferent terminals of the spinal cord? Nature 307:376–380.

Price GW, Kelly JS, Bowery NG (1987): The location of $GABA_B$ receptor binding sites in mammalian spinal cord. Synapse 1:530–538.

Rahman AF, Takahashi M, Kaneto H (1994): Involvement of pain associated anxiety in the development of morphine tolerance in formalin treated mice. Jap J Pharmacol 65:313–317.

Reichling DB, Basbaum AI (1990): Contribution of brainstem GABAergic circuitry to descending antinociceptive control. I. GABA-immunoreactive projection neurons in the periaqueductal gray and nucleus raphe magnus. J Comp Neurol 302:370–377.

Rochford J, Stewart J (1992): Naloxone-induced hypoalgesia: lack of involvement of the GABA-benzodiazepine receptor complex. Pharmacol Biochem Behav 43:321–328.

Satzinger G (1994): Antiepileptics from gamma-aminobutyric acid. Arzneimittelforschung 44:261–266.

Sawynok J (1987): GABAergic mechanism of analgesia: an update. Pharmacol Biochem Behav 26:463–474.

Sawynok J, Dickson C (1985): D-baclofen is an antagonist at baclofen receptor mediating antinociception in the spinal cord. Pharmacology 31:248–259.

Sawynok J, LaBella FS (1982): On the involvement of GABA in the analgesia produced by baclofen, muscimol and morphine. Neuropharmacology 21:397–404.

Segal AZ, Rodorf G (1996): Gabapentin as a novel treatment for post-herpetic neuralgia. Neurology 46:1175–1176.

Serrano I, Ruiz RM, Serrano JS, Fernandez A (1992): GABAergic and cholinergic mediation in the antinociceptive action of homotaurine. Gen Pharmacol 23:421–426.

Serrao JM, Goodchild CS, Gent JP (1991): Reversal by naloxone of spinal antinociceptive effects of fentanyl, ketocyclazocine and midazolam. Eur J Anaesthesiol 8: 401–406.

Sidebottom A, Maxwell S (1995): The medical and surgical management of trigeminal neuralgia. J Clin Pharm Ther 20:31–35.

Sivilotti L, Woolf CJ (1994): The contribution of $GABA_A$ and glycine receptors to central sensitization: disinhibition and touch-evoked allodynia in the spinal cord. J Neurophysiol 72:169–179.

Sluka KA, Westlund KN (1993): Spinal cord amino acid release and content in an arthititis model: the effects of pretreatment with non-NMDA, NMDA, NK1 receptor antagonists. Brain Res 627:89–103.

Smith DF (1984): Stereoselectivity of spinal neurotransmission: effects of baclofen enantiomers on tail flick reflex in rats. J Neural Trans 60:63–67.

Smith GD, Harrison SM, Birch PJ, Elliott PJ, Malcangio M, Bowery NG (1994): Increased sensitivity to the antinociceptive activity of ($\pm$) baclofen in an animal model of chronic neuropathic, but not chronic inflammatory hyperalgesia. Neuropharmacology 33:1103–1108.

Spike RC, Todd AJ (1992): Ultrastructural and immunocytochemical study of lamina II islet cells in rat spinal dorsal horn. J Comp Neurol 323:359–369.

Stiller C-O, Linderoth B, O'Connor WT, Franck J, Falkenberg T, Ungerstedt U, Brodin E (1995): Repeated spinal cord stimulation decreases the extracellular level of γ-aminobutyric acid in the periaqueductal gray matter of freely moving rats. Brain Res 699:231–241.

Stiller C-O, Cui J-G, O'Connor WT, Brodin E, Meyerson BA, Linderoth B (1996): Release of γ-aminobutyric acid in the dorsal horn and suppression of tactile allodynia by spinal cord stimulation in mononeuropathic rats. Neurosurgery 39:367–375.

Taira T, Kawamura H, Tanikawa T, Iseki H, Kawabatake H, Takakura K (1995): A new approach to control central deafferentation pain: spinal intrathecal baclofen. Stereotactic Funct Neurosurgery 65:101–105.

Teoh H, Malcangio M, Bowery NG (1996a): GABA, glutamate and substance P-like immunoreactivity release: effects of novel $GABA_B$ antagonists. Br J Pharmacol 118: 1153–1160.

Teoh H, Malcangio M, Fowler LJ, Bowery NG (1996b): Evidence for release of glutamic acid, aspartic acid and substance P but not γ-amino butyric acid from primary afferent fibres in rat spinal cord. Eur J Pharmacol 302:27–36.

Thomas DA, McGowan MK, Hammond DL (1995): Microinjection of baclofen in the ventromedial medulla of the rat produces antinociception or hyperalgesia. J Pharmacol Exp Ther 275:274–284.

Thomas DA, Navarette IM, Graham BA, McGowan MK, Hammond DL (1996): Antinociception produced by systemic R(+)-baclofen hydrochloride is attenuated by CGP 35348 administered to the spinal cord or ventromedial medulla of rats. Brain Res 718:129–137.

Todd AJ (1996): GABA and glycine in synaptic glomeruli of the rat spinal dorsal horn. Eur J Neurosci 8:2492–2498.

Todd AJ, Lochhead V (1990): GABA-like immunoreactivity in type I glomeruli of rat substantia gelatinosa. Brain Res 514:171–174.

Willcockson WS, Chung JM, Hori Y, Lee KH, Willis WD (1984): Effects of iontophoretically released amino acids and amines on primate spinothalamic tract cells. J Neurosci 4:732–740.

Wilson PR, Yaksh TL (1978): Baclofen is antinociceptive in the spinal intrathecal space of animals. Eur J Pharmacol 51:323–330.

Yaksh TL (1989): Behavioral and autonomic correlates of the tactile evoked allodynia produced by spinal glycine: effects of modulatory receptor systems and excitatory amino acid antagonists. Pain 37:111–123.

Yaksh TL, Reddy SV (1981): Studies in the primate on the analgesic effect associated with intrathecal actions of opiates, α-adrenergic agonists and baclofen. Anaesthesiology 54:451–467.

Yamamoto T, Yaksh TL (1993): Effects of intrathecal strychnine and bicuculline on nerve compression-induced thermal hyperalgesia and selective antagonism by MK-801. Pain 54:79–84.

Yanez A, Sabbe MB, Stevens CW, Yaksh TL (1990): Interaction of midazolam and morphine in the spinal cord of the rat. Neuropharmacology 29:359–364.

Zorn SH, Enna SJ (1985): GABA uptake inhibitors produce a greater antinociceptive response in the mouse tail-immersion assay than other types of GABAergic drugs. Life Sci 37:1901–1912.

Zorn SH, Enna SJ (1987): The GABA agonist THIP attenuates antinociception in the mouse of modifying central cholinergic transmission. Neuropharmacology 26:433–437.

CHAPTER 13

CHOLINERGIC AGONISTS AS ANALGESICS

EDGAR T. IWAMOTO
University of Kentucky College of Medicine
Lexington, Kentucky

The most conspicuous feature about the enigma of cholinergic agonists as analgesics has been the absence of a therapeutically useful cholinergic drug for the management of acute and chronic pain states. The current flurry of activity by the drug industry and pain researchers to target cholinergic agonists as analgesics began relatively recently. Many factors may have militated against the development of cholinergic analgesics. The endogenous opioid networks and classical biogenic amine pathways have long dominated the pain research field. Central cholinergic systems have been associated more with "aversive," "avoidance," "tonic immobility," sleep, memory, or extrapyramidal functions than with pain mechanisms. Morphine was known to inhibit the release of acetylcholine in a variety of classical preparations. Finally, the troublesome side effects produced by cholinergic agonists via the neuromuscular junction and autonomic ganglia were sure to hinder serious commercial development of this group of agents. However, the search for a selective analgesic that produces few side effects and possesses no addiction liability continues to drive preclinical pain research. This chapter presents the current status of cholinergic mechanisms of analgesia. As an aid to the reader, a list of cholinergic agents mentioned in this chapter and their putative mechanisms of action can be found in Table 13.1.

BACKGROUND

The early literature on the modulation of nociceptive reactions by cholinergic agents has been surveyed extensively by Pert (1987) and by Hartvig et al.

Novel Aspects of Pain Management: Opioids and Beyond, Edited by Jana Sawynok and Alan Cowan
ISBN 0-471-180173 Copyright © 1999 by Wiley-Liss, Inc.

TABLE 13.1   Cholinergic Agents[a] and Their Putative Mechanism of Action

ABT-418	Tertiary nicotinic receptor agonist
ABT-594	Secondary nicotinic receptor agonist
AFDX 116	Tertiary competitive M2 muscarinic receptor antagonist
Arecoline	Muscarinic and nicotinic cholinergic receptor agonist
Atropine	Tertiary competitive muscarinic receptor antagonist
α-Bungarotoxin	Polypeptide neuromuscular nicotinic receptor antagonist
κ-Bungarotoxin	Polypeptide neuronal nicotinic receptor antagonist
Butylthio[2.2.2]	Tertiary M1 agonist; M2 and M3 partial agonist and/or antagonist
Carbachol	Muscarinic and nicotinic receptor agonist
Chlorisondamine	Quaternary long-lasting ganglionic nicotinic receptor antagonist
Cytisine	Tertiary nicotinic receptor agonist
4-DAMP	Quaternary competitive muscarinic receptor antagonist, M1 = M3 > M2
4-DAMP mustard	Tertiary irreversible M3 muscarinic receptor antagonist
DBO-83	Secondary nicotinic receptor agonist
Dihydro-β-erythroidine	Tertiary competitive nicotinic receptor antagonist
Echothiophate	Quaternary organophosphorus cholinesterase inhibitor
Edrophonium	Short-acting quaternary reversible cholinesterase inhibitor
Epibatidine	Secondary nicotinic receptor agonist
Epiboxidine	Secondary nicotinic receptor agonist
Hemicholinium-3	Quaternary inhibitor of choline uptake by presynaptic nerve terminals
Hexamethonium	Quaternary competitive ganglionic nicotinic receptor antagonist
Lobeline	Tertiary nicotinic receptor agonist
Mecamylamine	Secondary noncompetitive ganglionic nicotinic receptor antagonist
Methoctramine	Secondary competitive M2 muscarinic receptor antagonist
N-Methylcarbachol	Quaternary nicotinic receptor agonist
cis-Methyldioxolane	Quaternary muscarinic receptor agonist
Neostigmine	Quaternary reversible cholinesterase inhibitor
Nicotine	Tertiary nicotinic receptor agonist
Oxotremorine	Tertiary muscarinic receptor agonist
Physostigmine	Tertiary reversible cholinesterase inhibitor
Pilocarpine	Tertiary muscarinic receptor agonist
Pirenzepine	Tertiary competitive M1 muscarinic receptor antagonist
Scopolamine	Tertiary competitive muscarinic receptor antagonist
SM-21	Tertiary competitive M2 muscarinic receptor antagonist
SM-32	Tertiary competitive M2 muscarinic receptor antagonist
Tetrahydroacridine	Tertiary reversible cholinesterase inhibitor
Vesamicol	Tertiary inhibitor of synaptic vesicular acetylcholine storage

[a]Secondary, tertiary, or quaternary ionizable amino groups of each agent are indicated.
ABT-418: (S)-3-methyl-5-(1-methyl-2-pyrrolidinyl) isoxazole.
ABT-594: (R)-5-(2-azetidinylmethoxy)-2-chloropyridine.
AFDX 116: 11,2-(diethylamino)methyl-1-piperidinylacetyl-5,11-dihydro-6H-pyrido[2,3-b]1,4-benzodiazepine-6-one.
Butylthio[2.2.2]: (+)-(S)-3-(4-butylthio-1,2,5-thiadiazol-3-yl)-1-azabicyclo[2.2.2]octane.
DBO-83: 3-(6-chloro-pyridazin-3-yl)diazabicyclo[3.2.1]octane.
SM-21: 3-α-tropanyl-(2-chloro)-acid phenoxybutyrate.
SM-32: (±)-2-phenylthiobutyric acid α-tropyl ester oxalate.

(1989). Numerous anecdotal reports suggested that smoking was analgesic. Subsequent studies showed that nicotine and the acetylcholinesterase inhibitors physostigmine and neostigmine not only elicited antinociception but also potentiated the antinociception produced by narcotic analgesics in animals and humans. Results indicated that the antinociception produced by cholinergic drugs such as nicotine, oxotremorine, arecoline, and pilocarpine probably had a central site of origin and may act through central serotonin, catecholamine, or endogenous opioid systems. However, data interpretation was confounded by the side effects, such as excess salivation, muscular twitching, tremor, muscular weakness, rigidity, and behavioral depression, caused by these agents. The cholinergic *antagonists* atropine and scopolamine *also* produced antinociception in animals and humans. Pert (1987) cited many issues that needed clarification. Was the antinociception produced by cholinergic drugs caused by interference with the expression of the nociceptive end points? Where were the sites of action of the cholinergic analgesics within the central nervous system? Did cholinergic analgesia involve enhancement of descending inhibitory pathways to the spinal cord? Where was the site of action of cholinergic analgesia in humans: central, peripheral, or both? A number of these issues were addressed over the next decade.

MUSCARINIC MECHANISMS OF CHOLINERGIC ANALGESIA

Research Strategies in Muscarinic Cholinergic Analgesia

Parenterally Administered Postsynaptic Muscarinic Agonists. Significant progress has been made recently in identifying lead cholinergic analgesics. Butylthio[2.2.2], a new antinociceptive muscarinic agent (Olesen et al., 1996), exhibits mixed M1 agonistic, and possibly partial agonist and/or antagonist pharmacological effects at M2 and M3 muscarinic receptors (Shannon et al., 1997). Butylthio[2.2.2] possesses nanomolar affinity for central muscarinic binding sites with much lower affinity at nicotinic, noncholinergic, and transporter sites. Because the median effective oral doses of butylthio[2.2.2] for producing parasympathetic side effects in mice are much greater than the median antinociceptive doses, and because it is equieffective and more potent than morphine, its clinical usefulness appears promising (Swedberg et al., 1997). Because agonistic activity at M1 receptors is not a requirement for antinociception (Sheardown et al., 1997), the precise identity of the muscarinic receptor mediating butylthio[2.2.2]-induced antinociception is unclear. Aside from a report that the calcium channel blocker nifedipine diminishes oxotremorine antinociception (Pavone et al., 1993), there is little information on postreceptor events of parenterally administered, postsynaptic, muscarinic antinociceptive agents.

Parenterally Administered Presynaptic Muscarinic Antagonists. Progress has also been made in identifying cholinergic analgesics that act presynaptically. Low, μg/kg doses of atropine produced antinociception in mice and rats in the hot plate, tail flick, and writhing assays, which was antagonized by central administration of the M1 antagonist pirenzepine and by centrally administered hemicholinium-3 (Ghelardini et al., 1990). Central or peripheral administration of M1 agonists induced antinociception in mice using chemical, thermal, and mechanical noxious stimuli (Bartolini et al., 1992). SM-21, a new M2 antagonist, at 30 mg/kg intraperitoneally was equieffective to 8 mg/kg of morphine intraperitoneally in the mouse hot plate test and was active in three other antinociceptive tests, but showed little activity in rota rod and hole board tests (Ghelardini et al., 1997b). SM-32, another M2 antagonist, was antinociceptive in mice and did not disrupt spontaneous locomotion (Ghelardini et al., 1997c). R-(+)-Hyoscyamine (atropine), but not its enantiomer, increased acetylcholine release in vitro and in vivo at doses below those that block postsynaptic muscarinic receptors (Gualtieri et al., 1994; Ghelardini et al., 1997d). These data strongly suggest that low doses of cholinergic antagonists block presynaptic M2 receptors and enhance acetylcholine release on to M1 postsynaptic sites to produce antinociception. This mechanism also has been invoked for part of the efficacy of the antimigraine drug, sumatriptan (Ghelardini et al., 1996).

NICOTINIC MECHANISMS OF CHOLINERGIC ANALGESIA

Epibatidine

Discovery and Early Characterization. Perhaps the most exciting new development in the field of cholinergic analgesics was the discovery of the alkaloid epibatidine in skin extracts from a certain colony of the inch-long, Ecuadoran poison arrow frog, *Epipedobates tricolor*. A fascinating account of the history of the isolation, early pharmacological assays, loss of the supply of frogs, microchemistry, identification, total synthesis, and stereochemistry has been given (Spande et al., 1992; Badio et al., 1994). Initially, the skin extract was thought to contain an opioid-like analgesic because, like morphine, it induced the Straub tail reaction in mice. However, because this response was not antagonized by the opioid antagonist naloxone and the structure–activity of epibatidine related more with nicotine, a cholinergic focus was embarked upon.

Pharmacology. The pharmacology of epibatidine was soon characterized by the relative nonstereoselectivity of its enantiomers. Natural (+)-epibatidine was slightly more potent than its enantiomer in the 55°C mouse hot plate test with a median effective dose of about 1.5 μg after intraperitoneal injection (Badio and Daly, 1994). After subcutaneous administration, the median effective dose was approximately 6 μg/kg in the mouse tail flick test (Damaj et al., 1994a). In the 53°C hot plate-evoked paw lick test, the magnitude of the antinociception produced by epibatidine was approximately two-thirds of that produced by 32 mg/kg of morphine after subcutaneous administration (Bonhaus et al., 1995). Epibatidine antinociception was antagonized by the nicotinic blockers mecamylamine, dihydro-β-erythroidine, and chlorisondamine, but not by blockers of opioid, muscarinic, or biogenic aminergic receptors (Badio and Daly, 1994; Damaj et al., 1994a; Rupniak et al., 1994; Sullivan et al., 1994; Badio et al., 1995). Both epibatidine enantiomers had very high affinity at nicotinic binding sites in rat brain membranes, but extremely low affinity at opioid receptors.

Adverse Effects. At antinociceptive doses, both (+)- and (−)-epibatidine dramatically reduced core body temperature by 3–4°C, and also greatly diminished spontaneous locomotor activity (Damaj et al., 1994a; Sullivan et al., 1994). Mice injected with 2 μg/kg of epibatidine oxalate exhibited hypoactivity with labored breathing, prostration, and seizures. Spontaneous locomotor activity was depressed by epibatidine in two studies but mixed results were obtained in the rota rod test (Sullivan et al., 1994; Bannon et al., 1995a). Epiboxidine, an epibatidine analogue, produced less lethality in mice than epibatidine at equi-antinociceptive doses (Badio et al., 1997). Thus, although epibatidine may represent a new addition to the pharmacopoeia of centrally acting nicotinic agonists, its side effects and toxicity raise worrying issues of safety.

Research Strategies of Nicotinic Cholinergic Analgesia

Structure–Activity Relationships. A structure–activity relationship study of a series of 52 aminopyridine, nicotine, and epibatidine derivatives demonstrated that nicotinic binding affinity correlated with nicotine-produced antinociception (Damaj et al., 1996a). In contrast, a bridged-nicotine analogue was synthesized that, like nicotine, produced antinociception in mice, but unlike nicotine, did not appear to act at central nicotinic binding sites (Damaj et al., 1997a). This latter compound may be the first of a new class of antinociceptive agents.

Stereoenantiomers. Pharmacological differences often exist between stereoenantiomers. For example, (−)-nicotine is many times more antinociceptive than (+)-nicotine in the rat tail flick test, and there is evidence that (+)-nicotine may have partial agonistic activity (Rao et al., 1996). In contrast, such a differential does not exist between (+)- and (−)-epibatidine. A potentially advantageous characteristic of (+)-epibatidine, in contrast to the enantiomers of nicotine, is the lack of development of antinociceptive tolerance after repeated injections in mice (Damaj and Martin, 1996).

Cross-tolerance. Tolerance develops to the antinociceptive effects of nicotine after acute and repeated injection in mice (Damaj and Martin, 1996; Damaj et al., 1996b) and after chronic infusion in rats (Yang et al., 1992). Cross-tolerance to the antinociceptive effects of nicotine occurred in mice with (−)- but not with (+)-epibatidine (Damaj and Martin, 1996). Thus differences exist between the epibatidine enantiomers with respect to chronic actions at nicotinic receptors. In contrast to rodents, a recent report showed that acute tolerance to the analgesic effects of nicotine did not develop in humans. A trend toward sensitization, that is, greater thermal antinociception, was observed when multiple doses of 20 µg/kg of nicotine were administered in five doses over 2.5 hr to 16 subjects (Perkins et al., 1995).

Signal Transducers. It was reported that a calcium chelator enhanced, and parenterally administered calcium chloride diminished, the antinociceptive effects of nicotine in rats (Chin et al., 1993). Nicotine-induced antinociception and hypomotility in mice was potentiated by the calcium agonist Bay K 8644 and reduced by calcium channel blockers nifedipine and nimodipine but not verapamil (Damaj and Martin, 1993). These data indicated that an L-type calcium channel was involved in nicotine-induced antinociception (Damaj et al., 1993). The antinociception produced by racemic epibatidine was potentiated by the calcium channel agonist (−)-Bay K 8644 and attenuated by the calcium channel antagonist (+)-Bay K 8644 (Bannon et al., 1995b). Calcium-dependent mechanisms also appear to play an important role in nicotine-tolerant mice (Damaj, 1997). In a study employing the intrathecal administration of pertussis toxin, forskolin, and cyclic AMP analogues, results indicated that a G-protein/cyclic AMP system mediated nicotinic antinociception in mice (Damaj et al., 1994b).

Nicotinic Receptor Subtypes. The neuronal nicotinic receptor is an acetylcholine-gated sodium (and calcium) ion channel composed of five subunits that span the membrane bilayer and surround the internal channel. There are two types of central neuronal nicotinic acetylcholine receptor (colorfully illustrated in Stroud et al., 1990; Lindstrom et al., 1995). The α4β2 subtype, which is probably composed of two α4 and three β2 subunits, does not bind α-bungarotoxin and accounts for more than 90% of the high-affinity nicotine binding sites in mammalian brain membranes. The α7 subtype of nicotinic acetylcholine receptor is probably a homo-oligomer of five α7 subunits with one α-bungarotoxin-binding site (Chen and Patrick, 1997). Epibatidine and nicotine displace [^{3}H](−)-nicotine or [^{3}H](−)-cytisine binding with K_i values of 0.05 and 1 nM, respectively (Badio and Daly, 1994; Sullivan et al., 1994). Because the predominant nicotinic site in rodent brain is the α4β2 subtype, the antinociceptive actions of nicotine may be initiated at this site. However, epibatidine and nicotine both bind the α-bungarotoxin binding site, but with 5000-fold lower affinity (Sullivan et al., 1994). What is the functional significance of the neuronal α7 nicotinic receptor subtype in rodent brain? Based on studies utilizing methyllycaconitine, a putative antagonist of α-bungarotoxin-sensitive nicotinic acetylcholine receptors, the α-bungarotoxin binding site does not appear to play a role in nicotinic antinociception using the tail-flick assay (Rao et al., 1996). In the electroplax preparation, which contains the α,β1,δ,γ, nicotinic receptor, a subtype also found at the neuromuscular junction, nicotine weakly displaced [^{125}I]α-bungarotoxin binding with a K_i value greater than 20 μM whereas epibatidine had a K_i value of 2.7 nM (Sullivan et al., 1994). The significance of this 7400-fold difference between nicotine and epibatidine is not known.

Questions Regarding Nicotinic Receptors and Antinociception. Is the nicotinic receptor that mediates antinociception presynaptic, postsynaptic, or both (McGehee et al., 1995; Wonnacott, 1997)? Can selective nicotinic agents be developed that activate one type and not the rest of the population of nicotinic receptors? Do the presynaptic and/or postsynaptic neuronal nicotinic receptors that mediate antinociception desensitize? Which of the presynaptic neuronal nicotinic receptors that regulate the release of norepinephrine, dopamine, serotonin, GABA, glutamate, and acetylcholine (McGehee and Role, 1995) are involved in nicotinic antinociception? Are the nicotinic analgesic mechanisms that are operative in brain different from those active in the spinal cord, and if so, are these differences caused by dissimilar nicotinic receptor subtypes? Are the neuronal nicotinic receptors that bind κ-bungarotoxin (Grant et al., 1997) involved in nicotinic antinociception? Are nicotine and epibatidine receptor sites distinct? Does epibatidine produce physical dependence? What is its abuse potential? If acetylcholine stimulated the flare axon reflex after peripheral administration in humans which was antagonized by hexamethonium (Benarroch and Low, 1991), and if the peripherally acting nicotinic antagonist chlorisondamine blocked nicotine antinociception in a tail withdrawal test but not in a paw withdrawal test (Caggiula et al., 1995), is nociception mediated by peripheral nicotinic receptors? Are peripheral nicotinic receptors useful therapeutic targets? What are the post-receptor signaling mechanisms that transduce antinociception? What is the molecular subunit structure of the nicotinic receptor that mediates antinociception? Because strain dependence with respect to the antinociceptive potency of nicotine in mice has recently been demonstrated (Seale et al., 1996), will transgenic mice that underexpress or overexpress α2β2, α4β2, α3, α5, α7, αβ1δγ, or α1β1δγε nicotinic receptors respond to cholinergic analgesics differently? Answers to some of these questions are necessary in order to characterize fully new antinociceptive nicotinic agents, such as ABT-418 and DBO-83, that will continue to appear (Damaj et al., 1995; Ghelardini et al., 1997a). In summary, the ideal nicotinic analgesic of the future will activate selectively the central neuronal nicotinic acetylcholine receptor that transduces antinociception but not the receptors responsible for cholinergic adverse effects.

ABT-594. Recently, a novel nicotinic agent, ABT-594, demonstrated potent antinociceptive activity in an acute thermal nociceptive test and antihyperalgesic activity in the formalin test after intraperitoneal administration in rats (Bannon et al., 1998). These antinociceptive responses were diminished or blocked by mecamylamine but not by naltrexone. ABT-594 also showed antiallodynic activity (which was antagonized by mecamylamine) in the Chung model of neuropathic pain. Like epibatidine, ABT-594 bound tritiated cytisine binding sites in rat brain with high affinity. In contrast, ABT-594 had 4000-fold less affinity for neuromuscular nicotinic binding sites than epibatidine. Like nicotine, microinjections of ABT-594 into the rostral ventral medulla in rats produced antinociception to noxious thermal stimuli. Finally, abrupt withdrawal of ABT-594 in chronically treated rats was not accompanied by a decrease in food intake that was associated with abrupt morphine abstinence. Thus these promising findings suggest that ABT-594 produces antinociception via a nicotinic, nonopioid, nonepibatidine-like manner.

SUPRASPINAL MECHANISMS OF CHOLINERGIC ANALGESIA

Subcortical Brain Sites and Mechanisms of Action

Dorsal Parabrachial Region. Studies examining the neural mechanisms of desynchronized sleep in the 1950s revealed that microinjections of cholinergic drugs into the rostral pontine tegmentum elicited postural atonia and a diminished responsiveness to external stimuli. Katayama et al. (1984) further showed that responses to heat and pinch were selectively suppressed for at least 60 min in cats microinjected bilaterally with 400 ng of carbachol into the nearby dorsal parabrachial region. This antinociception was antagonized by atropine but not by mecamylamine or naloxone; morphine injections into the same site were without effect (Katayama et al., 1984). Carbachol injections into adjacent areas including the cuneiform nucleus disrupted postural and eye-opening responses, EEG pattern, and cardiovascular function, but did not induce antinociception. Microinjections of carbachol into the dorsal parabrachial region of guinea pigs elicited atropine-reversible antinociception in the foot shock test (Menescal-de-Oliveira and Hoffmann, 1995).

Rostral Ventral Medulla (RVM). By the early 1980s, the RVM was known to be a major site of action of opioid and electrical stimulation-produced analgesia. The RVM contains the nucleus raphe magnus, nucleus reticularis gigantocellularis, nucleus reticularis magnocellularis pars alpha, and nucleus reticularis paragigantocellularis lateralis, and relays descending information modulating spinal nociceptive transmission (Gebhart and Randich, 1990; Willis and Westlund, 1997). There are numerous markers of muscarinic and nicotinic cholinergic transmission within the RVM (see Iwamoto, 1991). Microinjections of carbachol into the RVM of rats produced antinociception in the hot plate and tail flick tests that was antagonized by atropine (Brodie and Proudfit, 1984). Spinal α2 noradrenergic mechanisms appeared to be involved because the carbachol-induced antinociception was antagonized by intrathecal injections of yohimbine or phentolamine (Brodie and Proudfit, 1986). Acetylcholine increased the firing rates of most pinch-excited and biphasic (inhibited then excited) cells but inhibited most pinch-inhibited cells recorded extracellularly in the rat RVM (Hentall et al., 1993). An inhibitory cholinergic postsynaptic receptor interaction modulated the activity of a subpopulation of serotonergic neurons in the RVM (Pan and Williams, 1994).

Pedunculopontine Tegmental Nucleus (PPTg). The main source of cholinergic input to the RVM originates from cholinergic neurons situated within the PPTg, which extends 1.5 mm from the caudal substantia nigra to regions surrounding the superior cerebellar peduncle. The PPTg is composed of large, multipolar cholinergic neurons which project rostrally to thalamus and caudally to the RVM and whose dendrites are accessed by collaterals of the spinothalamic tract (Rye et al., 1987; Woolf, 1991). Thus the PPTg has significant connections with central regions known to receive and process pain-related information.

Nicotine Releases Acetylcholine. Microinjections of nanomole amounts of nicotine into the rat PPTg produced antinociception in the hot plate and tail flick tests that was unaccompanied by disruption of the corneal reflex, a foot placing reaction, the righting reflex, or negative geotaxis (Iwamoto, 1989). Nicotine-induced antinociception was antagonized by co-microinjections of mecamylamine, scopolamine, or pirenzepine, indicating that nicotinic antinociception had a muscarinic component. Microinjections of the muscarinic agonist (+)-*cis*-methyldioxolane into the PPTg produced antinociception that was blocked by antimuscarinic but not antinicotinic agents. Nicotinic antinociception was diminished in rats preinjected with hemicholinium-3 or (−)-vesamicol, drugs that interfere with acetylcholine synthesis, storage and/or release. This suggested that nicotine promoted acetylcholine release from presynaptic stores in the PPTg on to postsynaptic muscarinic cholinergic sites to inhibit nociception (Iwamoto, 1989, 1991). This conclusion was supported by findings showing that PPTg microinjections of the M2 muscarinic antagonist methoctramine produced antinociception (Iwamoto, 1989).

PPTg-to-RVM Pathway. Nicotine injections along the entire lengths of the PPTg and RVM were the most effective sites in rat brain eliciting antinociception (Iwamoto, 1991). Nicotine-produced antinociception was unaffected by naloxone. Antinociception produced by nicotine injections into the PPTg was blocked by inactivation of the RVM by procainamide, but not when nicotine was injected into the RVM and the PPTg was inactivated; it was therefore concluded that the "polarity" of this cholinergic pathway was "PPTg-to-RVM." PPTg lesions or hemicholinium-3 pretreatment of the RVM did not alter baseline nociceptive responses but did diminish both nicotine- and (+)-*cis*-methyldioxolane-induced antinociception produced at the PPTg. RVM microinjections of methoctramine produced antinociception in rats (Iwamoto, 1991; Spinella et al., 1997) that could be blocked by hemicholinium-3 (Iwamoto, 1991). These data suggested that the PPTg-to-RVM cholinergic pathway was tonically active but under autoinhibitory control (Iwamoto, 1991).

Spinal Mediation of Central Nicotinic Antinociception. Hot plate and tail flick nicotinic antinociception was produced by microinjections of 40 nmol of the nicotinic agonist, *N*-methylcarbachol, into either the PPTg or the RVM (Iwamoto and Marion, 1993a). Experiments involving intrathecal delivery of various receptor antagonists determined that the antinociception activated by nicotinic stimulation of the PPTg or RVM was mediated via the release of serotonin, norepinephrine, and acetylcholine onto 5-HT-1C/2 and 5-HT-3, α2, and M2 receptors in the lumbar spinal cord (Iwamoto and Marion, 1993a). These conclusions were supported by our finding that the antinociception produced by subcutaneous administration of 0.375 mg/kg of nicotine was blocked at the level of the RVM by hemicholinium and at the spinal level by intrathecal administration of α-2 adrenergic, serotonergic, and muscarinic cholinergic antagonists in rats (Rogers and Iwamoto, 1993). Thus muscarinic and nicotinic agents may modulate nociception at the spinal level by activating descending pain-inhibitory pathways originating in the RVM.

Nitric Oxide Mediation of Muscarinic Antinociception in the RVM.
The antinociception produced by microinjections of (+)-*cis*-methyldioxolane into the RVM was antagonized by preinjection of the RVM with either pirenzepine or the irreversible muscarinic receptor antagonist, 4-DAMP mustard (Iwamoto and Marion, 1994a). Administration of the nitric oxide synthase inhibitor L-N^G-nitroarginine into the RVM also antagonized (+)-*cis*-methyldioxolane-induced antinociception, and this antagonism was reversed by L-arginine, the precursor of nitric oxide. In addition, (+)-*cis*-methyldioxolane-induced antinociception was diminished by inhibiting guanylyl cyclase in the RVM. Membrane-permeable analogues of cyclic GMP produced antinociception when injected alone into the RVM. It was concluded that the antinociception produced by muscarinic stimulation of the RVM in the rat was mediated by an M1 receptor/L-arginine/nitric oxide/cyclic GMP cascade of events (Iwamoto and Marion, 1994a). The RVM was also implicated by the Gebhart laboratory as being a significant component of central cholinergic analgesic mechanisms. Stimulation of the nucleus reticularis gigantocellularis and nucleus gigantocellularis pars alpha in rats produced tail flick antinociception that was blocked by intrathecally administered muscarinic, serotonergic, and noradrenergic antagonists (Zhuo and Gebhart, 1990).

Other Supraspinal Sites of Cholinergic Antinociception

Carbachol produced antinociception in the tail flick test after microinjection into the PPTg, medial geniculate, habenular complex, amygdala, and various limbic structures (Klamt and Prado, 1991). The mechanisms of action of carbachol-produced antinociception were muscarinic, nicotinic, and opioid after injection into the habenular complex (Terenzi and Prado, 1990), nicotinic and α-adrenergic after injection into the dorsal periaqueductal gray (Oliveira and Prado, 1994), and nonopioid and muscarinic after injection into the amygdala

(Guimarães and Prado, 1994) or lateral reticular nucleus of the caudal medulla (Ossipov and Gebhart, 1986). (−)-Nicotine microinjected into the rat midbrain, pons, medulla, and fourth ventricle produced either antinociception or hyperalgesia depending upon site and dosage (Hamann and Martin, 1992; Parvini et al., 1993). Thus, although cholinergic agonists produced antinociception or hyperalgesia at numerous sites in brain, the mechanisms underlying these effects varied, depending on drug dose and the brain structure being stimulated.

SPINAL MECHANISMS OF CHOLINERGIC ANALGESIA

Intrathecal Drug Administration

Muscarinic Agents. Almost all known neurotransmitters, neuropeptides, and their receptors can be found in the spinal cord dorsal horn (Weihe, 1992; Coggeshall and Carlton, 1997). Intrathecal (within the spinal subarachnoid space) drug administration, developed for rats following implantation of a chronic cannula (Yaksh and Rudy, 1976) and mice following a percutaneous lumbar puncture injection (Hylden and Wilcox, 1980), opened up a new era of pain research. Intrathecally administered oxotremorine, carbachol, or acetylcholine plus physostigmine produced antinociception in rats using the tail flick, hot plate, and acetic acid writhing assays (Yaksh et al., 1985), which was antagonized by atropine but not by naloxone. Others subsequently demonstrated that carbachol, neostigmine, physostigmine, echothiophate, edrophonium, oxotremorine, arecoline, or pilocarpine produced antinociception after intrathecal administration in rats (Smith et al., 1989; Gillberg et al., 1989, 1990; Zhuo and Gebhart, 1991; Naguib and Yaksh, 1994, 1997; Abram and O'Connor, 1995; Abram and Winne, 1995) and sheep (Lothe et al., 1994; Bouaziz et al., 1995) in tests involving thermal, chemical, or mechanical nociceptive stimuli. These antinociceptive responses were blocked by atropine, hemicholinium-3, the M1 antagonist pirenzepine, the M2 antagonist AFDX 116, the M3 antagonist 4-DAMP, and the norepinephrine depletor DSP4, but not by naloxone or mecamylamine. Thus spinal cholinergic antinociception in rats depends on muscarinic and noradrenergic, but not opioid or nicotinic, mechanisms of action.

Adverse Effects of Intrathecal Muscarinic Agents. Above certain dosage levels, intrathecally administered carbachol produced motor impairment, transient agitation, hindlimb weakness, decreases in locomotion and rearing activity, and salivation, which were reversed by atropine, indicating a muscarinic mechanism of action (Gillberg et al., 1989, 1990; Naguib and Yaksh, 1994; Abram and O'Connor, 1995). However, histopathological examination revealed no neurotoxic reactions after 14 days of chronic intrathecal carbachol (Svensson et al., 1991).

Muscarinic Mechanisms of Spinal Cholinergic Analgesia

Monoamines. Intrathecal administration of (+)-*cis*-methyldioxolane produced hot plate and tail flick antinociception in rats without interfering with other motor reflex activity. This antinociception was blocked in a dose-related manner in rats pretreated intrathecally with M1, M2, α-2 adrenergic, 5-HT-1C/2, and 5-HT-3 receptor antagonists (Iwamoto and Marion, 1993b). The data indicated that (+)-*cis*-methyldioxolane activated local muscarinic, noradrenergic, and serotonergic circuits within the lumbar spinal cord to produce its antinociceptive effects.

Nitric Oxide. The antinociception produced by intrathecal (+)-*cis*-methyldioxolane was antagonized by intrathecally administered L-N^G-nitroarginine, an inhibitor of nitric oxide synthesis (Iwamoto and Marion, 1994b). This antagonism was reversed by coadministration of L- but not D-arginine. Intrathecal pretreatment with the guanylyl cyclase inhibitor methylene blue also antagonized (+)-*cis*-methyldioxolane-produced antinociception. Intrathecally administered dibutyryl cyclic GMP or 8-bromo cyclic GMP produced antinociception when given alone. These data indicated that the antinociception produced by muscarinic agonist administration into the lumbar spinal cord was mediated by antinociceptive actions of L-arginine, nitric oxide, and cyclic GMP (Iwamoto and Marion, 1994b). This view was consistent with data showing that the pronociceptive effect of spinal atropine was potentiated by inhibiting the nitric oxide/cyclic GMP pathway and diminished by enhancing nitric oxide production (Zhuo et al., 1993), by other reports indicating that antinociception produced by spinal clonidine in sheep was enhanced by intrathecal neostigmine and antagonized by inhibiting nitric oxide synthase (Lothe et al., 1994), and by in vitro studies showing that acetylcholine stimluated the release of nitric oxide from slices of rat spinal cord (Xu et al., 1996a,b). However, nitric oxide also has pronociceptive activity (see Discussion in Iwamoto and Marion, 1994b). Thus the foundation supporting the role of nitric oxide in cholinergic analgesia has not yet settled.

Nicotinic Mechanisms of Spinal Cholinergic Analgesia

Intrathecal Nicotinic Agonists in Rats. Although antinociception was produced in rats by intrathecally administered nicotine in two studies, the animals used were either anesthetized with pentobarbital or acutely transected at T_6 to T_8 (Aceto et al., 1986; Christensen and Smith, 1990). Most studies showed that nicotine, cytisine, and tetrahydroacridine were not antinociceptive after intrathecal administration in intact rats (Yaksh et al., 1985; Smith et al., 1989; Gillberg et al., 1990; Rogers and Iwamoto, 1993).

Adverse Effects of Intrathecal Nicotine in Rats. Drug-induced gnawing, vocalization, and hyperactivity were observed after intrathecal nicotine, tetrahydroacridine, and cytisine, and these effects were reversed by mecamylamine, indicating a spinal nicotinic mechanism (Gillberg et al., 1990). Intrathecal nicotine produced rapid increases in blood pressure and heart rate followed by behavioral agitation and a possible *nociceptive* response characterized by movement of the limbs, body twisting and turning, tail erection, and high-pitched squeaking (Khan et al., 1994a). The nicotinic receptors responsible for the nicotinic nociceptive response resided in the low-thoracic and lumbar regions of the spinal cord (Khan et al., 1994b). In contrast to brain, where more than one subtype of nicotinic binding site exists, only a single class of nicotinic binding site was revealed in spinal cord (Khan et al., 1994c). The nociceptive responses evoked by intrathecal nicotine and cytisine in rats were accompanied by increased spinal release of aspartic and glutamic acids (Khan et al., 1996). Intrathecal epibatidine also elicited pressor, positive chronotropic, and behavioral agitation responses in rate (Khan et al., 1997). Thus is appears that the nicotinic receptor in rat spinal cord is responsible for the nociceptive effects of nicotinic agonists, and that parenteral nicotine-induced antinociception arises from actions at a different nicotinic receptor in rat brain.

Species Differences in Response to Intrathecal Nicotinic Agonists.
In contrast to rats, the antinociceptive actions of nicotine and epibatidine were readily demonstrated in mice after intrathecal administration. This antinociception was antagonized by mecamylamine but not by naloxone (Damaj et al., 1994a,b, 1996b). In mice, intrathecal lobeline produced antinociception in the tail flick test (Damaj et al., 1997b), but in rats, intrathecal lobeline, which lacked effects of its own, blocked the nociceptive responses produced by intrathecal nicotine (Khan et al., 1994a). Species differences between mice and rats with respect to the molecular subtypes of nicotinic receptors present in the spinal cord may account for the differences in response to the antinociceptive effects of intrathecally administered nicotinic agonists.

Adrenergic and Opioid Interactions in Spinal Cholinergic Analgesia

With more than 50 messenger candidates present in the spinal cord dorsal horn (Wcihc, 1992), the potential for functional interaction during the neurotransmission of pain and analgesia is great. Pert (1987) and Hartvig et al. (1989) cited the earlier literature with respect to cholinergic interactions with the monoamine and endogenous opioid peptide systems within the brain. Investigations of the neurotransmitter interactions within the spinal cord are recent developments. Intrathecally administered clonidine produced dose-dependent antinociception in sheep, and increased acetylcholine levels in cerebrospinal fluid (Detweiler et al., 1993). In humans, epidurally administered clonidine increased cerebrospinal levels of acetylcholine at the peak of analgesia (Detweiler et al., 1993). Systemically administered opioids increased the concentration of norepinephrine and acetylcholine in microdialysates of the dorsal horn of sheep (Bouaziz et al., 1996). Painful stimulation increased the levels of norepinephrine and acetylcholine in the lumbar cerebrospinal fluid of sheep (Eisenach et al., 1996). Intrathecal administration of clonidine increased acetylcholine concentrations in spinal cord microdialysates of sheep (Klimscha et al., 1997). Intrathecally administered neostigmine enhanced the analgesia but not the respiratory depression induced by intravenous alfentanil in humans (Hood et al., 1997). Finally, morphine and neostigmine administered intrathecally just before spinal administration of bupivacaine showed similar analgesic effectiveness in patients undergoing vaginoplasty (Klamt et al., 1997). These data strongly support the hypothesis that spinal cholinergic and noradrenergic systems enhance the analgesic effects of the other, additively or synergistically, after intrathecal administration in animals and humans. Furthermore, the analgesic effects of systemically or intrathecally administered opioids are enhanced by administration of either clonidine or neostigmine.

CLINICAL CHOLINERGIC ANALGESIA

An increasing number of studies are examining the analgesic effect produced by solitary administration of cholinergic agents in humans. In a double-blind, placebo-controlled study, physostigmine produced significant but short-lived analgesia in postoperative patients without depressing ventilatory rate (Petersson et al., 1986). In a placebo-controlled study, 15 μg/kg of nicotine significantly increased pain latencies to a computer-controlled radiant heat stimulus (Perkins et al., 1994), and in another placebo-controlled, within-subjects counterbalanced study, 20 μg/kg of nicotine significantly elevated thermal pain detection latencies with no evidence of the development of acute tolerance (Perkins et al., 1995). Intrathecal neostigmine produced analgesia in an ice water immersion test without producing unexpected side effects in a recent Phase I clinical study (Hood et al., 1995). In a randomized blinded trial, intrathecal neostigmine produced significant postoperative analgesia (Lauretti et al., 1996). In a placebo-controlled, open-label, and dose-escalating design, intrathecal neostigmine produced 10 hr of post-cesarean section analgesia without causing adverse fetal effects (Krukowski et al., 1997). Finally, neostigmine administered at L4 to L5 afforded complete pain relief in two cancer patients (Klamt et al., 1996). These studies strengthen the credibility of the search for safer, more selective, cholinergic analgesics.

THE NEXT TEN YEARS

The concept of developing therapeutically useful cholinergic analgesics is a viable one. Because cholinergic analgesia is mediated by a central, nonopioid pain-suppression system and may not be associated with the development of tolerance, it is possible that nonaddicting analgesics will be developed that will be especially useful in the management of chronic pain in opioid-tolerant patients. A matrix of information on cholinergic sites and mechanisms of analgesia is now being rapidly filled. The section headings are animal and human; presynaptic and postsynaptic nicotinic agonists; presynaptic muscarinic antagonists and postsynaptic muscarinic agonists; supraspinal, spinal, and peripheral sites of analgesic action; nicotinic and muscarinic receptor molecular subtypes; and second and third messengers of signal transduction. The methods used to fill these sections should integrate current cellular and molecular biologic tehcniques with studies of nociception in the whole organism or signals associated with nociception in tissue preparations. However, this matrix must also include data on the side effects, adverse reactions, and drug toxicities induced by the cholinergic drugs. What is missing from this table? The problem of chronic pain should be approached directly by a systematic evaluation of cholinergic agents using the many models of neuropathic pain that have been developed (Kim et al., 1997). Subsequent reviews on cholinergic analgesics may well include several new cholinergic therapeutic agents.

ACKNOWLEDGMENTS

Supported in part by NIH grant NS-28847. This review is dedicated to my parents, Harry and Sayuri, and my Ph.D. advisor, Eddie Way.

REFERENCES

Abram SE, O'Connor TC (1995): Characteristics of the analgesic effects and drug-interactions of intrathecal carbachol in rats. Anesthesiology 83:844–849.

Abram SE, Winne RP (1995): Intrathecal acetylcholinesterase inhibitors produce analgesia that is synergistic with morphine and clonidine in rats. Anesth Analg 81: 501–507.

Aceto MD, Bagley RS, Dewey WL, Fu T-C, Martin BR (1986): The spinal cord as a major site for the antinociceptive action of nicotine in the rat. Neuropharmacol 25: 1031–1036.

Badio B, Daly JW (1994): Epibatidine, a potent analgesic and nicotinic agonist. Mol Pharmacol 45:563–569.

Badio B, Garraffo HM, Spande TF, Daly JW (1994). Epibatidine. discovery and definition as a potent analgesic and nicotinic agonist. Med Chem Res 4:440–448.

Badio B, Shi D, Garraffo M, Daly JW (1995): Antinociceptive effects of the alkaloid epibatidine: further studies on involvement of nicotinic receptors. Drug Devel Res 36:46–59.

Badio B, Garraffo HM, Plummer CV, Padgett WL, Daly JW (1997): Synthesis and nicotinic activity of epiboxidine: an isoxazole analogue of epibatidine. Eur J Pharmacol 321:189–195.

Bannon AW, Gunther KL, Decker MW (1995a): Is epibatidine really analgesic—dissociation of the activity, temperature and analgesic effects of ($\pm$)-epibatidine. Pharmacol Biochem Behav 51:693–698.

Bannon AW, Gunther KL, Decker MW, Arneric SP (1995b): The influence of Bay K 8644 treatment on (±)-epibatidine-induced analgesia. Brain Res 678:244–250.

Bannon AW, Decker MW, Holladay MW, Curzon P, Donnelly-Roberts D, Puttfarcken PS, Bitner RS, Diaz A, Dickenson AH, Porsolt RD, Williams M, Arneric SP (1998): Broad-spectrum, non-opioid analgesic activity by selective modulation of neuronal nicotinic acetylcholine receptors. Science 279:77–81.

Bartolini A, Ghelardini C, Fantetti L, Malcangio M, Malmberg-Aiello P, Giotti A (1992): Role of muscarinic receptor subtypes in central antinociception. Br J Pharmacol 105:77–82.

Benarroch EE, Low PA (1991): The acetylcholine-induced flare response in evaluation of small fiber dysfunction. Ann Neurol 29:590–595.

Bonhaus DW, Bley KR, Broka CA, Fontana DJ, Leung E, Lewis R, Shieh A, Wong EHF (1995): Characterization of the electrophysiological, biochemical and behavioral actions of epibatidine. J Pharmacol Exp Ther 272:1199–1203.

Bouaziz H, Tong C, Eisenach JC (1995): Postoperative analgesia from intrathecal neostigmine in sheep. Anesth Analg 80:1140–1144.

Bouaziz H, Tong C, Yoon Y, Hood DD, Eisenach JC (1996): Intravenous opioids stimulate norepinephrine and acetylcholine release in spinal cord dorsal horn. Anesthesiology 84:143–154.

Brodie MS, Proudfit HK (1984): Hypoalgesia induced by the local injection of carbachol into the nucleus raphe magnus. Brain Res 291:337–342.

Brodie MS, Proudfit HK (1986): Antinociception induced by local injections of carbachol into the nucleus raphe magnus in rats: alteration by intrathecal injection of monoaminergic antagonists. Brain Res 371:70–79.

Caggiula AR, Epstein LH, Perkins KA, Saylor S (1995): Different methods of assessing nicotine-induced antinociception may engage different neural mechanisms. Psychopharmacology 122:301–306.

Chen D, Patrick JW (1997): The α-bungarotoxin-binding nicotinic acetylcholine receptor from rat brain contains only the α7 subunit. J Biol Chem 272:24024–24029.

Chin CWY, Block RC, Wu WH, Zbuzek VK (1993): Modulation of nicotine-induced analgesia by calcium agonist and antagonist in adult rats. Psychopharmacology 110: 497–499.

Christensen M-K, Smith DF (1990): Antinociceptive effects of the stereoisomers of nicotine given intrathecally in spinal rats. J Neural Transm 80:189–194.

Coggeshall RE, Carlton SM (1997): Receptor localization in the mammalian dorsal horn and primary afferent neurons. Brain Res Rev 24:28–66.

Damaj MI (1997): Altered behavioral sensitivity of Ca^{2+}-modulating drugs after chronic nicotine administration in mice. Eur J Pharmacol 322:129–135.

Damaj MI, Martin BR (1993): Calcium agonists and antagonists of the dihydropyridine type: effect on nicotine-induced antinociception and hypomotility. Drug Alcohol Depend 32:73–79.

Damaj MI, Martin BR (1996): Tolerance to the antinociceptive effect of epibatidine after acute and chronic administration in mice. Eur J Pharmacol 300:51–57.

Damaj MI, Welch SP, Martin BR (1993): Involvement of calcium and L-type channels in nicotine-induced antinociception. J Pharmacol Exp Ther 266:1330–1338.

Damaj MI, Creasy KR, Grove AD, Rosecrans JA, Martin BR (1994a): Pharmacological effects of epibatidine optical enantiomers. Brain Res 664:34–40.

Damaj MI, Welch SP, Martin BR (1994b): Nicotine-induced antinociception in mice: role of G-proteins and adynylate cyclase. Pharmacol Biochem Behav 48:37–42.

Damaj MI, Creasy KR, Welch SP, Rosecrans JA, Aceto MD, Martin BR (1995): Comparative pharmacology of nicotine and ABT-418, a new nicotinic agonist. Psychopharmacology 120:483–490.

Damaj MI, Glassco W, Dukat M, May EL, Glennon RA, Martin BR (1996a): Pharmacology of novel nicotinic analogs. Drug Devel Res 38:177–187.

Damaj MI, Welch SP, Martin BR (1996b): Characterization and modulation of acute tolerance to nicotine in mice. J Pharmacol Exp Ther 277:454–461.

Damaj MI, Glassco W, Marks MJ, Slobe B, James JR, May EL, Rosecrans JA, Collins AC, Martin BR (1997a): Pharmacological investigation of (+)- and (−)-cis-2,3,3a,4,5,9b-hexahydro-1-methyl-1H-pyrrolo-[3,2-h]isoquinoline, a bridged-nicotine analog. J Pharmacol Exp Ther 282:1425–1434.

Damaj MI, Patrick GS, Creasy KR, Martin BR (1997b): Pharmacology of lobeline, a nicotinic receptor ligand. J Pharmacol Exp Ther 282:410–419.

Detweiler DJ, Eisenach JC, Tong C, Jackson C (1993): A cholinergic interaction in alpha2 adrenoceptor-mediated antinociception in sheep. J Pharmacol Exp Ther 265: 536–542.

Eisenach JC, Detweiler DJ, Tong C, D'Angelo R, Hood DD (1996): Cerebrospinal fluid norepinephrine and acetylcholine concentrations during acute pain. Anesth Analg 82: 621–626.

Gebhart GF, Randich A (1990): Brainstem modulation of nociception. In Klemm WR, Vertes RP (eds): *Brainstem Mechanisms of Behavior*. New York: John Wiley & Sons, pp. 315–352.

Ghelardini C, Malmberg-Aiello P, Giotti A, Malcangio M, Bartolini A (1990): Investigation into atropine-induced antinociception. Br J Pharmacol 101:49–54.

Ghelardini C, Galeotti N, Figini M, Imperato A, Nicolodi M, Sicuteri F, Gessa GL, Bartolini A (1996): The central cholinergic system has a role in the antinociception induced in rodents and guinea pigs by the antimigraine durg sumatriptan. J Pharmacol Exp Ther 279:884–890.

Ghelardini C, Galeotti N, Barlocco D, Bartolini A (1997a): Antinociceptive profile of the new nicotinic agonist DBO-83. Drug Devel Res 40:251–258.

Ghelardini C, Galeotti N, Gualtieri F, Bellucci C, Manetti D, Giotti A, Malmberg-Aiello P, Galli A, Bartollini A (1997b): Antinociceptive profile of 3-α-tropanyl-(2-Cl)-acid phenoxybutyrate (SM-21): a novel analgesic with a presynaptic cholinergic mechanism of action. J Pharmacol Exp Ther 282:430–439.

Ghelardini C, Galeotti N, Gualtieri F, Romanelli MN, Bartolini A (1997c): Antinociception induced by SM 32 depends on a central cholinergic mechanism. Pharmacol Res 35:141–147.

Ghelardini C, Gualtieri F, Romanelli MN, Angeli P, Pepeu G, Giovannini MG, Casamenti F, Malmberg-Aiello P, Giotti A, Bartolini A (1997d): Stereoselective increase in cholinergic transmission by R-(+)-hyoscyamine. Neuropharmacology 36:281–294.

Gillberg P-G, Gordh Jr. T, Hartvig P, Jansson I, Pettersson J, Post C (1989): Characterization of the antinociception induced by intrathecally administered carbachol. Pharmacol Toxicol 64:340–343.

Gillberg PG, Hartvig P, Gordh T, Sottile A, Jansson I, Archer T, Post C (1990): Behavioral effects after intrathecal administration of cholinergic receptor agonists in the rat. Psychopharmacology 100:464–469.

Grant GA, Al-Rabiee R, Xu XL, Zhang Y-P (1997): Critical interactions at the dimer interface of κ-bungarotoxin, a neuronal nicotinic acetylcholine receptor antagonist. Biochemistry 36:3353–3358.

Gualtieri F, Conti G, Dei S, Giovannoni MP, Nannucci F, Romanelli MN, Scapecchi S, Teodori E, Fanfani L, Ghelardini C, Giotti A, Bartolini A (1994): Presynaptic cholinergic modulators as potent cognition enhancers and analgesic drugs. 1. Tropic and 2-phenylpropionic acid esters. J Med Chem 37:1704–1711.

Guimarães APC, Prado WA (1994): Antinociceptive effects of carbachol microinjected into different portions of the mesencephalic periaqueductal gray matter of the rat. Brain Res 647:220–230.

Hamann SR, Martin WR (1992): Opioid and nicotinic analgesic and hyperalgesic loci in the rat brain stem. J Pharmacol Exp Ther 261:707–715.

Hartvig P, Gillberg PG, Gordh T, Post C (1989): Cholinergic mechanisms in pain and analgesia. Trends Pharmacol Sci 10(Suppl.):75–79.

Hentall ID, Andresen MJ, Taguchi K (1993): Serotonergic, cholinergic and nociceptive inhibition or excitation of raphe magnus neurons in barbiturate-anesthetized rats. Neuroscience 52:303–310.

Hood DD, Eisenach JC, Tuttle R (1995): Phase I safety assessment of intrathecal neostigmine methylsulfate in humans. Anesthesiology 82:331–343.

Hood DD, Mallak KA, James RL, Tuttle R, Eisenach JC (1997): Enhancement of analgesia from systemic opioid in humans by spinal cholinesterase inhibition. J Pharmacol Exp Ther 282:86–92.

Hylden JLK, Wilcox GL (1980): Intrathecal morphine in mice: a new technique. Eur J Pharmacol 67:313–316.

Iwamoto ET (1989): Antinociception after nicotine administration into the mesopontine tegmentum of rats: evidence for muscarinic actions. J Pharmacol Exp Ther 251:412–421.

Iwamoto ET (1991): Characterization of the antinociception induced by nicotine in the pedunculopontine tegmental nucleus and the nucleus raphé magnus. J Pharmacol Exp Ther 257:120–133.

Iwamoto ET, Marion L (1993a): Adrenergic, serotonergic and cholinergic components of nicotinic antinociception in rats. J Pharmacol Exp Ther 265:777–789.

Iwamoto ET, Marion L (1993b): Characterization of the antinociception produced by intrathecally administered muscarinic agonists in rats. J Pharmacol Exp Ther 266:329–338.

Iwamoto ET, Marion L (1994a): Pharmacological evidence that nitric oxide mediates the antinociception produced by muscarinic agonists in the rostral ventral medulla of rats. J Pharmacol Exp Ther 269:699–708.

Iwamoto ET, Marion L (1994b): Pharmacologic evidence that spinal muscarinic analgesia is mediated by an L-arginine/nitric oxide/cyclic GMP cascade in rats. J Pharmacol Exp Ther 271:601–608.

Katayama Y, Watkins LR, Becker DP, Hayes RL (1984): Non-opiate analgesia induced by carbachol microinjection into the pontine parabrachial region of the cat. Brain Res 296:263–283.

Khan IM, Taylor P, Yaksh TL (1994a): Cardiovascular and behavioral responses to nictotinic agents administered intrathecally. J Pharmacol Exp Ther 270:150–158.

Khan IM, Taylor P, Yaksh TL (1994b): Stimulatory pathways and sites of action of intrathecally administered nicotinic agents. J Pharmacol Exp Ther 271:1550–1557.

Khan IM, Yaksh TL, Taylor P (1994c): Ligand specificity of nicotinic acetylcholine receptors in rat spinal cord: studies with nicotine and cytisine. J Pharmacol Exp Ther 270:159–166.

Khan IM, Marsala M, Printz MP, Taylor P, Yaksh TL (1996): Intrathecal nicotinic agonist-elicited release of excitatory amino acids as measured by *in vivo* spinal microdialysis in rats. J Pharmacol Exp Ther 278:97–106.

Khan IM, Yaksh TL, Taylor P (1997): Epibatidine binding sites and activity in the spinal cord. Brain Res 753:269–282.

Kim KJ, Yoon YW, Chung JM (1997): Comparison of three rodent neuropathic pain models. Exp Brain Res 113:200–206.

Klamt JG, Prado WA (1991): Antinociception and behavioral changes induced by carbachol microinjected into identified sites of the rat brain. Brain Res 549:9–18.

Klamt JG, Reis MPD, Neto JB, Prado WA (1996): Analgesic effect of subarachnoid neostigmine in two patients with cancer pain. Pain 66:389–391.

Klamt JG, Slullitel A, Garcia IV, Prado WA (1997): Postoperative analgesic effect of intrathecal neostigmine and its influence on spinal anaesthesia. Anaesthesia 52:547–551.

Klimscha W, Tong C, Eisenach JC (1997): Intrathecal α2-adrenergic agonists stimulate acetylcholine and norepinephrine release from the spinal cord dorsal horn in sheep. Anesthesiology 87:110–116.

Krukowski JA, Hood DD, Eisenach JC, Mallak KA, Parker RL (1997): Intrathecal neostigmine for post-cesarean section analgesia: dose response. Anesth Analg 84:1269–1275.

Lauretti GR, Reis MP, Prado WA, Klamt JG (1996): Dose-response study of intrathecal morphine versus intrathecal neostigmine, their combination, or placebo for postoperative analgesia in patients undergoing anterior and posterior vaginoplasty. Anesth Analg 82:1182–1187.

Lindstrom J, Anand R, Peng X, Gerzanich V, Wang F, Li Y (1995): Neuronal nicotinic receptor subtypes. Ann NY Acad Sci 757:100–116.

Lothe A, Li P, Tong C, Yoon Y, Bouaziz H, Detweiler DJ, Eisenach JC (1994): Spinal cholinergic alpha-2-adrenergic interactions in analgesia and hemodynamic control —role of muscarinic receptor subtypes and nitric oxide. J Pharmacol Exp Ther 270:1301–1306.

McGehee DS, Role LW (1995): Physiological diversity of nicotinic acetylcholine receptors expressed by vertebrate neurons. Ann Rev Physiol 57:521–546.

McGehee DS, Heath MJS, Gelber S, Devay P, Role LW (1995): Nicotine enhancement of fast excitatory synaptic transmission in CNS by presynaptic receptors. Science 269:1692–1696.

Menescal-de-Oliveira L, Hoffmann A (1995): Temporal modulation of antinociception by reciprocal connections between the dorsomedial medulla and parabrachial region. Brain Res Bull 37:467–474.

Naguib M, Yaksh TL (1994): Antinociceptive effects of spinal cholinesterase inhibition and isobolographic analysis of the interaction with μ and α2 receptor systems. Anesthesiology 80:1338–1348.

Naguib M, Yaksh TL (1997): Characterization of muscarinic receptor subtypes that mediate antinociception in the rat spinal cord. Anesth Analg 85:847–853.

Olesen PH, Sauerberg P, Treppendahl S, Larsson O, Sheardown MJ, Suzdak PD, Mitch CH, Ward JS, Bymaster FP, Shannon HE, Swedberg MDB (1996): 3-(3-alkylthio-1,2,5-thiadiazol-4-yl)-1-azabicycles. Structure-activity relationships for antinociception mediated by central muscarinic receptors. Eur J Med Chem 31:221–230.

Oliveira MA, Prado WA (1994): Antinociception and behavioral manifestations induced by intracerebroventricular or intra-amygdaloid administration of cholinergic agonists in the rat. Pain 57:383–391.

Ossipov MH, Gebhart GF (1986): Opioid, cholinergic and α-adrenergic influences on the modulation of nociception from the lateral reticular nucleus of the rat. Brain Res 384:282–293.

Pan ZZ, Williams JT (1994): Muscarine hyperpolarizes a subpopulation of neurons by activating an M2 receptor in rat nucleus raphe magnus *in vitro*. J Neurosci 14:1332–1338.

Parvini S, Hamann SR, Martin WR (1993): Pharmacologic characteristics of a medullary hyperalgesic center. J Pharmacol Exp Ther 265:286–293.

Pavone F, Battaglia M, Sansone M (1993): Attenuation of cholinergic analgesia by nifedipine. Brain Res 623:308–310.

Perkins KA, Grobe JE, Stiller RL, Scierka A, Goettler J, Reynolds W, Jennings JR (1994): Effects of nicotine on thermal pain detection in humans. Exp Clin Psychopharmacol 2:95–106.

Perkins KA, Grobe JE, Mitchell SL, Goettler J, Caggiula A, Stiller RL, Scierka A (1995): Acute tolerance to nicotine in smokers: lack of dissipation within 2 hours. Psychopharmacology 118:164–170.

Pert A (1987): Cholinergic and catecholaminergic modulation of nociceptive reactions; interactions with opiates. In Gildenberg PL (series ed): *Pain and Headache*, Vol. 9, Akil A, Lewis JW (volume eds): *Neurotransmitters and Pain Control*. Basel: S. Karger, pp. 1–63.

Petersson J, Gordh TE, Hartvig P, Wiklund L (1986): A double-blind trial of the analgesic properties of physostigmine in postoperative patients. Acta Anaesthesiol Scand 30:283–288.

Rao TS, Correa LD, Reid RT, Lloyd GK (1996): Evaluation of antinociceptive effects of neuronal nicotinic acetylcholine receptor (NAChR) ligands in the rat tail-flick assay. Neuropharmacology 35:393–405.

Rogers DT, Iwamoto ET (1993): Multiple spinal mediators in parenteral nicotine-induced antinociception. J Pharmacol Exp Ther 267:341–349.

Rupniak NMJ, Patel S, Marwood R, Webb J, Traynor JR, Elliott J, Freedman SB, Fletcher SR, Hill RG (1994): Antinociceptive and toxic effects of (+)-epibatidine oxalate attributable to nicotinic agonist activity. Br J Pharmacol 113:1487–1493.

Rye DB, Saper CB, Lee HJ, Wainer BH (1987): Pedunculopontine tegmental nucleus of the rat: cytoarchitecture, cytochemistry, and some extrapyramidal connections of the mesopontine tegmentum. J Comp Neurol 259:483–528.

Seale TW, Nael R, Basmadjian G (1996): Inherited, selective hyporesponsiveness to the analgesic action of nicotine in mice. Neuroreport 8:191–195.

Shannon HE, Sheardown MJ, Bymaster FP, Calligaro DO, Delapp NW, Gidda J, Mitch CH, Sawyer BD, Stengel PW, Ward JS, Wong DT, Olesen PH, Suzdak PD, Sauerberg P, Swedberg MDB (1997): Pharmacology of butylthio[2.2.2] (LY297802/NNC11-1053): a novel analgesic with mixed muscarinic receptor agonist and antagonist activity. J Pharmacol Exp Ther 281:884–894.

Sheardown MJ, Shannon HE, Swedberg MDB, Suzdak PD, Bymaster FP, Olesen PH, Mitch CH, Ward JS, Sauerberg P (1997): M1 receptor agonist activity is not a requirement for muscarinic antinociception. J Pharmacol Exp Ther 281:868–875.

Smith MD, Yang X, Nha J-Y, Buccafusco JJ (1989): Antinociceptive effect of spinal cholinergic stimulation: interaction with substance P. Life Sci 45:1255–1261.

Spande TF, Garraffo HM, Edwards MW, Yeh HJC, Pannell L, Daly JW (1992): Epibatidine: a novel (chloropyridyl)azabicycloheptane with potent analgesic activity from an Ecuadoran poison frog. J Am Chem Soc 114:3475–3478.

Spinella M, Schaefer LA, Bodnar RJ (1997): Ventral medullary mediation of mesencephalic morphine analgesia by muscarinic and nicotinic cholinergic receptor antagonists in rats. Analgesia 3:119–130.

Stroud RM, McCarthy MP, Shuster M (1990): Nicotinic acetylcholine receptor superfamily of ligand-gated ion channels. Biochemistry 29:11009–11023.

Sullivan JP, Decker MW, Brioni JD, Donnelly-Roberts D, Anderson DJ, Bannon AW, Kang C-H, Adams P, Piattoni-Kaplan M, Buckley MJ, Gopalakrishnan M, Williams M, Arneric SP (1994): (±)-Epibatidine elicits a diversity of *in vitro* and *in vivo* effects mediated by nicotinic acetycholine receptors. J Pharmacol Exp Ther 271: 624–631.

Svensson BA, Sottile A, Gordh T (1991): Studies on the development of tolerance and potential spinal neurotoxicity after chronic intrathecal carbachol-antinociception in the rat. Acta Anaesth Scand 35:141–147.

Swedberg MDB, Sheardown MJ, Sauerberg P, Olesen PH, Suzdak PD, Hansen KT, Bymaster FP, Ward JS, Mitch CH, Calligaro DO, Delapp NW, Shannon HE (1997): Butylthio[2.2.2] (NNC 11-1053/LY297802): an orally active muscarinic agonist analgesic. J Pharmacol Exp Ther 281:876–883.

Terenzi MG, Prado WA (1990): Antinociception elicited by electrical or chemical stimulation of the rat habenular complex and its sensitivity to systemic antagonists. Brain Res 545:18–24.

Weihe E (1992): Neurochemical anatomy of the mammalian spinal cord: functional implications. Ann Anat 174:89–118.

Willis WD, Westlund KN (1997): Neuroanatomy of the pain system and of the pathways that modulate pain. J Clin Neurophysiol 14:2–31.

Wonnacott S (1997): Presynaptic nicotinic ACh receptors. Trends Neurosci 20:92–98.

Woolf NJ (1991): Cholinergic systems in mammalian brain and spinal cord. Prog Neurobiol 37:475–524.

Xu Z, Li P, Tong C, Figueroa J, Tobin JR, Eisenach JC (1996a): Location and characteristics of nitric oxide synthase in sheep spinal cord and its interaction with α2-adrenergic and cholinergic antinociception. Anesthesiology 84:890–899.

Xu Z, Tong C, Eisenach JC (1996b): Acetylcholine stimulates the release of nitric oxide from rat spinal cord. Anesthesiology 85:107–111.

Yaksh TL, Dirksen R, Harty GJ (1985): Antinociceptive effects of intrathecally injected cholinomimetic drugs in the rat and cat. Eur J Pharmacol 117:81–88.

Yaksh TL, Rudy TA (1976): Chronic catheterization of the spinal subarachnoid space. Physiol Behav 17:1031–1036.

Yang C-Y, Wu W-H, Zbuzek VK (1992): Antinociceptive effect of chronic nicotine and nociceptive effect of its withdrawal measured by hot-plate and tail-flick in rats. Psychopharmacology 106:417–420.

Zhuo M, Gebhart GF (1990): Spinal cholinergic and monoaminergic receptors mediate descending inhibition from the nuclei reticularis gigantocellularis and gigantocellularis pars alpha in the rat. Brain Res 535:67–78.

Zhuo M, Gebhart GF (1991): Tonic cholinergic inhibition of spinal mechanical transmission. Pain 46:211–222.

Zhuo M, Meller ST, Gebhart GF (1993): Endogenous nitric oxide is required for tonic cholinergic inhibition of spinal mechanical transmission. Pain 54:71–78.

CHAPTER 14

DOPAMINERGIC DRUGS AS ANALGESICS

KEITH B. J. FRANKLIN
McGill University
Montreal, Quebec, Canada

The sympathomimetic amines and cocaine were the first drugs with dopaminergic action to be identified as having analgesic activity. Though nineteenth-century travelers' reports that cocaine banished fatigue and discomfort might have suggested it could be used as an analgesic, the first mention in the literature appears to have been a 1911 case report of the use of cocaine as an analgesic in a human (Harrison cited in Pertovaara et al., 1988). The first experimental trial of a sympathomimetic stimulant did not occur until the 1940s and then it was the synthetic drug amphetamine that was tested. During World War II, there was considerable concern about the sedative effects of the opiates which were, at that time, the only powerful analgesic drugs available. For the treatment of wounded soldiers or civilians in the field, the sedative effects of opiates are a serious problem because they "... turn the walking wounded into litter cases" (Neal cited in Evans, 1967). Ivy et al. (1944) reported that dextroamphetamine enhanced the analgesic action of morphine and counteracted its depressive effects in humans. Later the same year, they reported that both *d*- and *l*-amphetamine raised the threshold for pain elicited by the electrical stimulation of tooth pulp (Burrill et al., 1944). In spite of these promising results, the use of amphetamine alone as an analgesic does not seem to have been contemplated, possibly because its stimulant effect was considered undesirable in civilian medicine. However, the morphine–amphetamine combination was attractive to anesthesiologists because it counteracts opiate-induced respiratory depression. The combination was recommended for use in obstetrics, where there was concern about depression of respiration in the baby when opiates were used for pain control in the mother during the later stages of labor. A retrospective comparison of an amphetamine–morphine combination with

---

Novel Aspects of Pain Management: Opioids and Beyond, Edited by Jana Sawynok and Alan Cowan
ISBN 0-471-180173 Copyright © 1999 by Wiley-Liss, Inc.

other types of medication in a sample of 7000 obstetric cases (Abel et al., 1951) found that the combination gave good analgesia and produced no significant respiratory depression in the infants. This paper was presented at a meeting and comments by members of the audience are interesting because they indicate that quite a number of anesthesiologists had used opioids in combination with sympathomimetic amines at this time. Though there appear to be no reports of serious problems with the use of these drugs in anesthesia, there are few subsequent reports of the clinical use of amphetamines as analgesics in the literature. Nevertheless, over the next 30 years several investigators confirmed in rats and in human subjects that amphetamine and other stimulant phenylethylamines produced analgesia and potentiated the analgesic effects of opiates (Nickerson and Goodman, 1947; Saxena and Gupta, 1957; Evans and Bergner, 1964; Evans, 1967; Ahmed et al., 1970; Webb et al., 1978). The treatment received favorable recommendations in the published studies, but never became widely used. A major double-blind clinical trial with dose–response data was carried out on 450 patients in the late 1970s. It concluded that the combination of 10 mg dextroamphetamine with morphine made morphine appear twice as potent, and that dextroamphetamine generally offset undesirable effects of morphine (Forrest et al., 1977). Methylphenidate has also been tested, with negative results when used as the sole analgesic in postoperative pain (Dodson and Fryer, 1980) but positive results when used as an adjuvant to opioids in pain due to advanced cancer (Bruera et al., 1987). Nevertheless, sympathomimetics still remain orphan drugs in the area of pain control, probably because they are perceived as having too high a potential for abuse. This belief is supported by experimental evidence that amphetamine potentiates the euphoric effect of morphine as well as analgesia (Jasinski and Preston, 1986).

Cocaine was used in a preparation of opiates for oral use—the "Brompton Cocktail." This contained variable amounts of morphine or diacetylmorphine with a fixed dose of cocaine (usually 10 mg) dissolved in alcohol, chloroform, water, and syrup (Twycross, 1979). However, the cocaine probably contributed little to the efficacy of the preparation, since an oral dose of 10 mg does not produce detectable physiological or subjective effects in humans (Resnik et al., 1977), and the cocktail was frequently accompanied by a dopamine antagonist to control nausea (Twycross, 1979). Clinical trials failed to show any benefit from the combination (Twycross, 1979; Kaiko et al., 1987), and the practice of including cocaine in the cocktail has been abandoned (Twycross, 1979).

DOPAMINERGIC ANALGESICS IN HUMAN EXPERIMENTS

In experimental tests with human subjects, dopaminergic drugs consistently produced analgesia, and potentiated opioid analgesia. Thus amphetamine (Webb et al., 1978) and intranasal cocaine (Yang et al., 1982) attenuated pain in the tourniquet test. A comparison of the effects of dextro, levo, and racemic amphetamine with aspirin, phenacetin, codeine, and placebo on pain elicited by electrical stimulation of the tooth pulp found that both the dextro and levo isomers elevated the threshold (Burrill et al., 1944). Five or 10 mg of dextro or racemic amphetamine was more effective than 30 mg of codeine, and 15 mg *d*-amphetamine was even more effective. The authors noted that the threshold raising effect of *l*-amphetamine decreased rapidly with successive administrations even if they were separated by several days. On the other hand, the effects of *d*-amphetamine seemed to remain constant over repeated tests. Positive results were also found with L-DOPA on the heat pain threshold (Battista and Wolff, 1973). In a clinical trial, Evans (1967) found that desoxyephedrine was about as effective as morphine in relieving pain after a hernia operation. He counted the number of cases in which pain was reduced by half by the analgesic and found that 10 mg of morphine relieved 69% of the patients and desoxyephedrine relieved 72%, but the combination produced relief in 96%.

Combining a sympathomimetic with an opioid significantly improves the analgesic effect of the opioid. This has been found for dextroamphetamine in experimental (Ivy et al., 1944; Nickerson and Goodman, 1947; Jasinski and Preston, 1986) and postsurgical (Forrest et al., 1977) pain. Potentiation of opioids is also seen with ephedrine, desoxyephedrine, and methylamphetamine (Saxena and Gupta, 1957; Evans, 1967; Tekol et al., 1994). The most detailed study was that of Forrest et al. (1977) who obtained dose–response curves for relief of postsurgical pain by morphine with 0, 5, or 10 mg *d*-amphetamine as supplemental medication. Morphine dose-dependently relieved pain, and pain relief was markedly increased by 5 and 10 mg *d*-amphetamine. The analgesic effect of a given dose of morphine could be matched by approximately half the dose of morphine plus 10 mg *d*-amphetamine. Ephedrine also approximately doubles the potency of morphine (Tekol et al., 1994).

ANALGESIC EFFECTS OF DOPAMINERGIC AGENTS IN ANIMALS

The early studies on analgesic effects of sympathomimetics in humans and animals preceded the discovery of the role dopamine in the behavioral stimulant effects of these drugs. Later studies in animals found that selective dopaminergic agonists produced effects similar to the sympathomimetic drugs, but the findings were difficult to interpret because the direction of effects was inconsistent in different studies. To add to the apparent inconsistency, the various studies also used different dose ranges and different species. It can be seen from Table 14.1 that most of the inconsistencies can be resolved by considering the pain tests used in these studies. The pain tests that are thought to be sensitive to forebrain-mediated analgesia, especially the hot plate test, formalin test, and postshock vocalization test, consistently detect an analgesic effect of both direct and indirect dopamine agonists (Table 14.1). They also detect the potentiating effect of dopamine agonists on analgesia induced by opioids (Tocco et al., 1985; Kauppila et al., 1992). In contrast, dopaminergic agonists

TABLE 14.1 The Sensitivity of Animal Pain Tests to the Analgesic Effects of Dopaminergic Drugs[a]

Pain Test	Drug	Analgesia	References
Hot plate	Amphetamine	yes	Major and Pleuvry, 1971; Little and Rees, 1974; Drago et al., 1984; Crisp et al., 1989 (Tocco et al., 1985)
	Cocaine	yes	Lin et al., 1989; Kauppila et al., 1992; Pertovaara and Hamalainen, 1994
	D2 agonists	yes	Dunai-Kovacs and Székely, 1977; Lin et al., 1981; Michael-Titus et al., 1990; Suaudeau and Costentin, 1995 (Dennis and Melzack, 1983)
	MDMA	yes	Crisp et al., 1989
Tail flick	Amphetamine	no	Dewey et al., 1970; Tocco and Maickel, 1984; Morgan and Franklin, 1990
	Cocaine	no/yes	Nott, 1968; Pertovaara et al., 1988 (Kauppila et al., 1992; Ushijima and Horita, 1993; Kiritsy-Roy et al., 1994; Pertovaara and Hamalainen, 1994)
	D2 agonists	no/yes	Tulunay et al., 1975; Dunai-Kovacs and Székely, 1977; Robertson et al., 1981; Ben-Sreti et al., 1983; Slikker, et al., 1984; Wesler and Frey, 1985 (Dennis and Melzack, 1983; Verma and Kulkarni, 1991)
	MDMA	no	Crisp et al., 1989
Formalin	Amphetamine	yes	Morgan and Franklin, 1991; Clarke and Franklin, 1992; Kauppila et al., 1992; Altier and Stewart, 1993; Abbott et al., 1995; Abbott and Guy, 1995
	Cocaine	yes	Lin et al., 1987; Lin et al., 1989; Kauppila et al., 1992
	D2 agonists	yes	Dennis and Melzack, 1983; Morgan and Franklin, 1991
Paw pressure	Amphetamine	yes	Gorlitz and Frey, 1972
	D2 agonists	yes	Dunai-Kovacs and Székely, 1977
Writhing	Amphetamine	yes	Major and Pleuvry, 1971; Tocco and Maickel, 1984; Frussa et al., 1996
	Cocaine	yes	Frussa et al., 1996
	D2 agonists	yes	Frussa et al., 1996
Vocalization	D2 agonists	yes	Paalzow and Paalzow, 1975, 1983; Carr, 1984

[a] The category "D2 agonists" refers to drugs acting directly on D2 receptors such as apomorphine, bromocriptine, quinpirole, and RU 24926. References to papers with findings inconsistent with the majority are shown in parentheses.

frequently have no effect in tests that measure the latency of the reflex withdrawal of the tail (Dunai-Kovacs and Székely, 1977; Tocco and Maickel, 1984; Pertovaara et al., 1988; Crisp et al., 1989; Morgan and Franklin, 1991) and are reported to antagonize the analgesic effects of opioids in these tests (Ahmed et al., 1970; Major and Pleuvry, 1971; Malec and Langwinski, 1981). A number of laboratories have compared different tests under similar conditions and found that the tail flick test is insensitive (Dunai-Kovacs and Székely, 1977; Crisp et al., 1989; Morgan and Franklin, 1990; Altier and Stewart, 1993) or less sensitive (Kauppila et al., 1992; Pertovaara and Hamalainen, 1994) to dopaminergic agonists than other tests. Overall, the formalin test seems to be the most consistently sensitive animal pain measure for detecting the analgesic effect of dopaminergic drugs (see Table 14.1).

Mechanisms of Dopamine Agonist Analgesia

The early studies of the effects of sympathomimetic drugs on pain and opioid analgesia were carried out in the context of the then-current knowledge of the adrenergic effects of these drugs. Amphetamine and cocaine are now known to increase the release of noradrenaline, dopamine, and serotonin in the brain but, because there have been no studies on the mechanism of sympathomimetic analgesia in humans, the probable mechanisms must be inferred from animal experiments. The evidence from animal experiments implicates dopamine as the primary mediator of the analgesic effect of these drugs.

Pharmacology of Dopaminergic Analgesics in the Formalin Test

The formalin test is the most consistent for detecting the analgesic effects of dopaminergic agents, and it is also the most consistent with regard to the mechanisms involved. Figure 14.1 shows dose–response curves for several direct and indirect dopamine agonists in this test. In addition to amphetamine and cocaine (see Table 14.1), we have found that formalin pain is attenuated by the selective catecholamine uptake inhibitor, nomifensine, in the range of doses that produces locomotor stimulation. It is unlikely that noradrenaline is responsible for the analgesic effect because the specific noradrenaline uptake inhibitor, desipramine, has only a minor analgesic effect (Lund et al., 1991) whereas nomifensine produces full analgesia at moderate doses (Fig. 14.1). The direct dopamine agonists that have been tested also produce analgesia at doses below those producing significant stereotyped behavior (Morgan and Franklin, 1991). Recently we have screened the mixed D3/D2 agonist 7-hydroxydipropylaminotetralin (7-OH-DPAT) in the formalin test. It also produces analgesia, but only at 0.6 mg/kg (Fig. 14.1). Below 0.1 mg/kg, 7-OH-DPAT binds specifically to D3 receptors but above 0.3 mg/kg it increasingly occupies D2 receptors (Levant et al., 1996). Thus the analgesic effect of dopamine agonists seems to be reliably associated with activity at D2 receptors. Furthermore, the analgesic effects of dopamine agonists are blocked by specific D2 antagonists

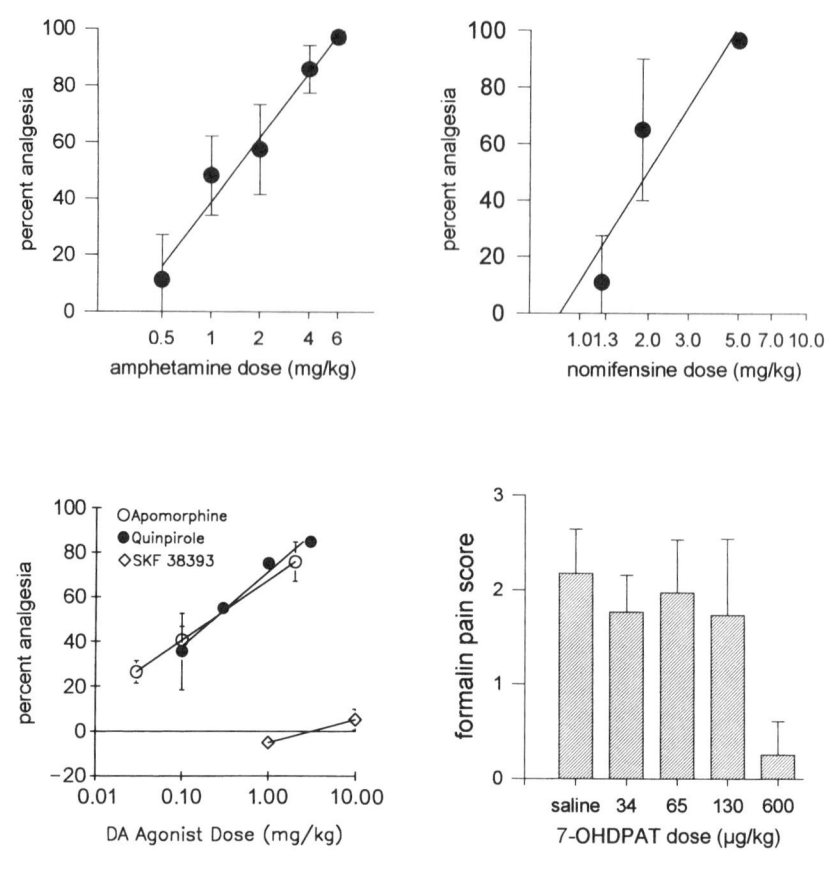

Figure 14.1 Dose–response relations for direct and indirect dopaminergic agonists in the formalin test. *Top left*: dextroamphetamine (replotted from Morgan and Franklin, 1991). *Top right*: nomifensine (Goto and Franklin, unpublished). *Lower left*: apomorphine, quinpirole, and SKF 38393 (Morgan and Franklin, 1991). *Lower right*: racemic 7-hydroxydipropylaminotetralin (Goto and Franklin, unpublished).

including pimozide (Morgan and Franklin, 1991), chlorpromazine (Shyu et al., 1992), eticlopride (Lin et al., 1989; Shyu et al., 1992), and alpha-flupenthixol (Morgan and Franklin, 1991). Amphetamine- and cocaine-induced analgesia in the formalin test are also blocked by the specific D1 antagonist SCH 23390. The D1 agonist, SKF 38393, does not produce analgesia (Morgan and Franklin, 1991).

The Role of the Ventral Striatum in Analgesia. The data discussed above suggest that analgesia produced by dopamine agonists is mediated by a D2 receptor mechanism in which D1 and D2 receptors interact (Carlson et al., 1987). The D2 receptors that mediate analgesia are probably located in forebrain dopamine terminal areas, most likely in the ventral striatum, because amphetamine-induced analgesia is blocked by 6-hydroxydopamine-induced lesions of the dopamine cells in the ventral tegmentum (Morgan and Franklin, 1990), or of their terminals in the ventral striatum (Clarke and Franklin, 1992). Consistent with this interpretation, analgesia is induced by direct injections of amphetamine into the ventral striatum, but not by injections in the medial prefrontal cortex (Altier and Stewart, 1993). Other treatments thought to stimulate the mesolimbic dopamine system also induce analgesia in the formalin test. Thus morphine microinjected into the ventral tegmental area (VTA) stimulates the release of forebrain dopamine (Leone et al., 1991) and produces analgesia (Franklin, 1989; Manning et al., 1994). The substance P analogue [pGlu5-Mephe8-MeGly9]SP(5-11) (DiMe-C7) injected into the VTA also stimulates dopamine release (Elliott et al., 1986) and attenuates the response to formalin (Altier and Stewart, 1993). Systemic injection of dopamine antagonists blocks the analgesic effect of morphine and DiMe-C7 microinjected into the VTA, and of amphetamine microinjected into the ventral striatum (Altier, 1997). This confirms that analgesia produced by stimulation of the mesolimbic dopamine system is truly dopamine mediated.

Spinal and Thalamic Mechanisms of Dopaminergic Analgesia.

In addition to ventral striatal mechanisms, there may be both thalamic and spinal components to dopaminergic analgesia. Cocaine inhibits responses of thalamic parafascicular and lateral central cells to high-intensity electrical stimulation, and this effect is blocked by dopamine antagonists (Shyu et al., 1992) [but see (Clatworthy and Barasi, 1987)]. The evidence that this effect is relevant to the analgesic action of dopaminergic drugs is that neurotoxin-induced lesions of the parafascicular nucleus attenuate the analgesic effect of cocaine in the formalin test (Shyu et al., 1992). Likewise, systemic cocaine selectively inhibits unit discharges in the spinal cord dorsal horn evoked by noxious stimulation of the hindpaw; this effect is blocked by dopamine antagonists, as well as by spinal cord transection (Kiritsy-Roy et al., 1994). Moreover, in one experiment in which cocaine did potentiate the antinociceptive effect of morphine in the tail flick test, spinal transection eliminated the potentiating effect of cocaine (Kauppila et al., 1992). Consistent with the idea that the effect of cocaine may be attributed to dopamine release in the spinal cord, dopamine delivered by intrathecal injection dose-dependently increases tail flick latencies in the lightly anesthetized rat (Liu et al., 1992). This effect is blocked by the D2 antagonist, sulpiride, but not by SCH 23390, methysergide, or naloxone. The antinociceptive effect of intrathecal dopamine is also blocked by the noradrenergic alpha-antagonist, phentolamine. These data suggest that descending projections of the diencephalic dopamine cell group (A11) to the spinal cord (Skagerberg and Lindvall, 1985) may interact with other spinal antinociceptive mechanisms. On the other hand, although the tail flick test rather directly reflects the responsiveness of dorsal horn neurons, it is relatively insensitive to dopaminergic analgesics. This indicates that dopaminergic drugs are not very efficacious in blocking transmission of nociceptive input in the dorsal horn. Thus it is likely that the role of spinal dopamine in analgesia demonstrated by the formalin test is minor.

Dopaminergic Analgesia in Tests of Pain with Noninjurious Stimuli. With measures other than the formalin test, information on the pharmacology and mechanisms of analgesia produced by dopaminergic drugs favors an important role for dopamine. In hot plate and tail flick tests, reserpine, the nonselective monoamine depletor, blocks the analgesic effects of amphetamines (Major and Pleuvry, 1971; Kubota et al., 1982), methylphenidate (Major and Pleuvry, 1971), and the amphetamine-like ingredient of khat—cathinone (Nencini et al., 1984). Similarly, the analgesic effects of the direct dopamine agonists apomorphine, RU 24926, and RU 24213 are blocked by haloperidol, sulpiride, or pimozide in the hot plate (Lin et al., 1981; Gonzales-Rios et al., 1986; Michael-Titus et al., 1990; Suaudeau and Costentin, 1995), tail flick (Verma and Kulkarni, 1991), paw pressure (Gorlitz and Frey, 1972), writhing (Gonzales-Rios et al., 1986), and shock-vocalization tests (Carr, 1984). As in the formalin test, the effects of dopaminergic agents are probably mediated by D2 receptors because RU 24926 and RU 24213 are D2 selective agonists and their analgesic effect was found to be blocked by D2 antagonists and not by SCH 23390 (Carr, 1984; Michael-Titus et al., 1990). On the other hand, the analgesia induced by methylamphetamine in the hot plate test has been reported to be dose-dependently increased by the catecholamine synthesis inhibitor, α-methyl-p-tyrosine, and blocked by the specific noradrenaline synthesis inhibitor, diethyldithiocarbamate (Major and Pleuvry, 1971). This finding is particularly puzzling because α-methyl-p-tyrosine is known to block the psychostimulant effects of amphetamines rapidly and completely by eliminating the cytoplasmic pool of catecholamines (Weissman et al., 1966; Franklin and Herberg, 1974).

The Role of Nondopaminergic Mechanisms. The role of other neurochemical mediators of analgesia in psychostimulant effects is problematic. The formalin test is not directly affected by opioid antagonists (North, 1978; Kocher, 1988) and, in the only test of naloxone against a psychostimulant, it failed to alter the analgesic effect of cocaine (Lin et al., 1989). In the hot plate, tail flick, and writhing tests the analgesic effects of amphetamine, apomorphine, or 3,4-methylenedioxyamphetamine were not blocked by naloxone or naltrexone (Drago et al., 1984; Gonzales-Rios et al., 1986; Crisp et al., 1989; Verma and Kulkarni, 1991). However, the analgesia produced by the D2 agonist RU 24926 and the stimulant cathinone are attenuated by naloxone (Nencini et al., 1984; Suaudeau and Costentin, 1995), and the effect of apomorphine is reported to be reduced in mice made tolerant to morphine (Michael-Titus et al., 1990). There is some evidence that serotonergic mechanisms may be involved, for in several tests the effects of dopaminergic drugs are attenuated by serotonergic antagonists or the synthesis inhibitor, p-chlorophenylalanine (Gorlitz and Frey, 1972; Kubota et al., 1982; Nencini et al., 1984; Crisp et al., 1989). However, the interaction between dopaminergic agonists and serotonin antagonists has not been evaluated in the formalin test, in which both classes of drug tend to reduce pain (Eide et al., 1987; Abbott and Young, 1988).

Dopaminergic Analgesia and Stress. Nencini et al. (1984) have commented on the problem of interpreting drug interactions in psychostimulant analgesia. They point out that psychostimulants, being powerful sympathomimetics, have effects similar to stressors such as foot shock or cold exposure, and may be able to induce analgesia indirectly by acting as stressors. Such analgesia could, therefore, exhibit the dependence on opioid and serotonergic transmission that has been shown for some types of stress-induced analgesia (Amit and Galina, 1986). The ability of stress produced by incidental aspects of an experimental test to modify the magnitude and neurochemistry of analgesia has been shown in the case of morphine-induced analgesia. It is well known that morphine's effect on the tail flick test is potentiated by situational stress (Appelbaum and Holtzman, 1984; 1985). This potentiation is mediated by the serotonergic neurons of the raphe magnus (Kelly and Franklin, 1984). The stress-induced release of sympathetic amines enhances brain uptake of the serotonin precursor L-tryptophan, thus presumably increasing the amount of serotonin available for release by morphine (Kelly and Franklin, 1985; Franklin and Kelly, 1986). In the absence of situational stress, the role of serotonin in the analgesic effect of morphine is greatly reduced or eliminated (Kelly and Franklin, 1984). Thus there is reason to suspect that, at least for the sympathomimetic amines, the neural systems identified as mediators of stress analgesia are likely to play a role in the analgesic effects of dopaminergic drugs.

Whether stress-analgesia mechanisms might underlie the analgesic effects of selective dopaminergic drugs, particularly those administered by direct injection into the brain, is uncertain. The evidence reviewed above suggests that the centrally mediated analgesic effects of these drugs depends on an action at the terminals of the mesolimbic dopamine system in the ventral striatum. Stimulation of dopamine D2 receptors in the ventral striatum is known to be rewarding, and these receptors are known to play an important role in drug self-administration and other motivated behaviors (Wise, 1987). Furthermore, the majority of centrally acting analgesics have abuse potential in humans, and show rewarding effects in animals that are mediated by the mesolimbic dopamine system (Franklin, 1989). From these ideas it has been argued that analgesia induced by dopamine agonists is linked to the rewarding effects of these drugs (Franklin, 1989).

The majority of stressors used experimentally are events such as electric shock, restraint, or cold, which are highly aversive. As a consequence, it is usually superficially assumed that stress and reward are antithetical. However, popular belief and the experimental literature suggest that mild to moderate stress may be associated with rewarding events as well as aversive events. Thus the actions of sympathomimetic amines are both stressful and rewarding. To rodents, a novel environment is stressful enough to produce stress potentiation of opioid analgesia (Kelly and Franklin, 1985) or even a mild stress analgesia

(Abbott et al., 1986) but also induces exploratory behavior and can act as a reward (Hebb, 1955). The curious behavior of humans who jump out of airplanes for fun is a dramatic illustration of the rewarding effects associated with stress.

At the neurochemical level, stress and reward mechanisms are also somewhat interlinked. Stress is an important activator of the VTA dopamine system, and stress induces release of dopamine in the prefrontal cortex and ventral striatum (Abercrombie et al., 1989; Imperato et al., 1992). Among the mediators of stress-induced dopamine release are opioid and substance P receptors in the ventral tegmental area (Deutch and Roth, 1990). It has recently been shown that opioid and substance P microinjected in the VTA can induce analgesia in the formalin test (Altier and Stewart, 1997b; Manning et al., 1994), whereas anti-opioid drugs microinjected in the VTA block both morphine- and stress-induced analgesia (Altier and Stewart, 1996; 1997a). Analgesia induced by foot shock stress can also be blocked by a substance P antagonist infused into the VTA (Altier, 1997).

CLINICAL POTENTIAL OF DOPAMINERGIC ANALGESICS

Behaviorally, dopamine release in the mesolimbic sites is associated with an increase in locomotor and exploratory activity (Kelly et al., 1975; Fink and Smith, 1980) and the execution of a goal-directed behavior (Gratton and Wise, 1994). It is thought that the function of this system is to "facilitate the generation of appropriate (goal directed) behavior, and to increase its vigour until the goal is obtained" (Scheel-Krüger and Willner, 1991). In contrast, the effect of pain on voluntary behavior is to diminish and restrict it. Thus our current understanding of the role of dopamine in behavior might predict the special value of dopaminergic agents as analgesics that was noted in the early experimental clinical trials. In contrast to the sedative opioid analgesics, which tend to promote passivity or sleep and interfere with constructive thought, the dopaminergic agents increase alertness and readiness to act though at the same time having some of the ability of the opioids to relieve suffering. It is interesting in this regard that there is growing interest in the use of dopaminergic agents to improve the functioning of patients whose capabilities are restricted by illness or sedative effects of analgesics (Bruera and Watanabe, 1994; Yee and Berde, 1994). With a growing population of elderly and infirm whose lives are adversely affected by chronic and debilitating conditions, it may be time for a serious re-examination of the potential clinical usefulness of the dopaminergic analgesics.

REFERENCES

Abbott FV, Franklin KBJ, Connell B (1986): The stress of a novel environment reduces formalin pain: possible role of serotonin. Eur J Pharmacol 126:141–144.

REFERENCES

Abbott FV, Guy ER (1995): Effects of morphine, pentobarbital and amphetamine on formalin-induced behaviours in infant rats: sedation versus specific suppression of pain. Pain 62:303–312.

Abbott FV, Young SN (1988): Effect of 5-hydroxytryptamine precursors on morphine analgesia in the formalin test. Pharmacol Biochem Behav 31:855–860.

Abbott FV, Franklin KBJ, Westbrook RF (1995): The formalin test: scoring properties of the first and second phases of the pain response in rats. Pain 60:91–102.

Abel S, Ball ZB, Harris SG (1951): The advantages to mother and infant of amphetamine in obstetrical analgesia. Am J Obst Gynecol 62:15–25.

Abercrombie ED, Keefe KA, DiFrischia DS, Zigmond MJ (1989): Differential effect of stress on in vivo dopamine release in striatum, nucleus accumbens, and medial frontal cortex. J Neurochem 52:1655–1658.

Ahmed SS, Abraham GJS, Assari M (1970): Dose dependent modification of codeine analgesia by d-amphetamine in albino rats. Arch Int Pharmacodyn Ther 184:240–244.

Altier N (1997): An analysis of the role of midbrain dopamine systems in the suppression of tonic pain. Doctoral Thesis Concordia University, Montreal, pp. 1–203.

Altier N, Stewart J (1993): Intra-VTA infusions of the substance P analogue, DiMe-C7, and intra-accumbens infusions of amphetamine induce analgesia in the formalin test for tonic pain. Brain Res 628:279–285.

Altier N, Stewart J (1996): Opioid receptors in the ventral tegmental area contribute to stress-induced analgesia in the formalin test for tonic pain. Brain Res 718:203–206.

Altier N, Stewart J (1997a): Neuropeptide FF in the VTA blocks the analgesia effects of both VTA-morphine and exposure to stress. Brain Res 758:250–254.

Altier N, Stewart J (1997b): Tachykinin NK-1 and NK-3 selective agonists induce analgesia in the formalin test for tonic pain following intra-VTA or intra-accumbens microinfusions. Behav Brain Res 89:151–165.

Amit Z, Galina ZH (1986): Stress-induced analgesia: adaptive pain suppression. Psychol Rev 66:1091–1120.

Appelbaum BD, Holtzman SG (1984): Characterization of stress-induced potentiation of opioid effects in the rat. J Pharmacol Exp Ther 231:555–565.

Appelbaum BD, Holtzman SG (1985): Restraint stress enhances morphine-induced analgesia in the rat without changing apparent affinity of receptor. Life Sci 36:1069–1074.

Battista AF, Wolff BB (1973): Levadopa and induced pain response: a study of patients with Parkinsonian and pain syndromes. Arch Int Med 132:70–74.

Ben-Sreti MM, Gonzales JP, Sewell RDE (1983): Differential effects of SKF 38393 and LY 141865 on nociception and morphine analgesia. Life Sci 33(Suppl. 1):665–668.

Bruera E, Watanabe S (1994): Psychostimulants as adjuvant analgesics. J Pain Symp Manag 9:412–415.

Bruera E, Chadwick S, Brenneis C, Hanson J, MacDonald RN (1987): Methylphenidate associated with narcotics for the treatment of cancer pain. Cancer Treatment Rep 71:67–70.

Burrill DY, Goetzl FR, Ivy AC (1944): The pain threshold raising effects of amphetamine. J Dent Res 23:337–344.

Carlson JH, Bergstrom DA, Walters JR (1987): Stimulation of both D1 and D2 dopamine receptors appears necessary for full expression of post-synaptic effects of dopamine agonists. A neurophysiological study. Brain Res 400:205–218.

Carr KD (1984): Dopaminergic mechanisms in the supraspinal modulation of pain. Eur Neuropsychopharmacol (Suppl. 2):S223.

Clarke PBS, Franklin KBJ (1992): Infusions of 6-hydroxydopamine into the nucleus accumbens abolish the analgesic effect of amphetamine but not of morphine in the formalin test. Brain Res 580:106–110.

Clatworthy A, Barasi S (1987): Intrathecally administered apomorphine or LY171555 reduces nociceptive responses recorded from ventrobasal thalamic neurones in urethane anaesthetised rats. Neurosci Lett 75:308–312.

Crisp T, Stafinsky JL, Boja JW, Schechter MD (1989): The antinociceptive effects of 3,4,-methylenedioxymethamphetamine (MDMA) in the rat. Pharmacol Biochem Behav 34:497–501.

Dennis SG, Melzack R (1983): Effects of cholinergic and dopaminergic agents on morphine analgesia measured by three pain tests. Exp Neurol 81:167–176.

Deutch AY, Roth RH (1990): The determinants of stress-induced activation of the prefrontal cortical dopamine system. Prog Brain Res 85:367–402.

Dewey WL, Harris LS, Howes JF, Nuite JA (1970): The effect of various neurohumoral modulators on the activity of morphine and the narcotic anatgonists in the tail-flick and phenylquinone tests. J Pharmacol Exp Ther 175:435–442.

Dodson ME, Fryer JM (1980): Postoperative effects of methylphenidate. Br J Anaesth 52:1265–1270.

Drago F, Caccamo G, Continella G, Scapagnini U (1984): Amphetamine-induced analgesia does not involve brain opioids. Eur J Pharmacol 101:267–269.

Dunai-Kovacs Z, Székely JI (1977): Effect of apomorphine on the antinociceptive activity of morphine. Psychopharmacology 53:65–72.

Eide PK, Berge OG, Hunskaar S (1987): Test-dependent changes in nociception after administration of the putative serotonin antagonist metitepin in mice. Neuropharmacology 26:1121–1126.

Elliott PJ, Alpert JE, Bannon MJ, Iversen SD (1986): Selective activation of the mesolimbic and mesocortical dopamine metabolism in rat brain by infusion of a stable substance P analogue into the ventral temental area. Brain Res 363:145–147.

Evans WO (1967): The effect of stimulant drugs on opiate induced analgesia. Arch Biol Med Exp 4:144–149.

Evans WO, Bergner DP (1964): A comparison of the analgesic potencies of morphine, pentazocine, and a mixture of methamphetamine and pentazocine in the rat. J New Drugs 4:82–85.

Fink JS, Smith GP (1980): Relationships between selective denervation of dopamine terminal fields in the anterior forebrain and behavioral responses to amphetamine and apomorphine. Brain Res 201:107–127.

Forrest WHJ, Brown BW, Brown CR, Defalque R, Gold M, Gordon HE, James KE, Katz J, Mahler DL, Schroff P, Teutsch G (1977): Dextroamphetamine with morphine for the treatment of postoperative pain. New Engl J Med 296:712–715.

Franklin KBJ (1989): Analgesia and the neural substrate of reward. Neurosci Biobehav Rev 35:157–163.

Franklin KBJ, Herberg LJ (1974): Self-stimulation and catecholamines: drug induced mobilization of the 'reserve'-pool re-estabishes responding in catecholamine depleted rats. Brain Res 67:429–437.

Franklin KBJ, Kelly SJ (1986): Sympathetic control of tryptophan uptake and morphine analgesia in stressed rats. Eur J Pharmacol 126:145–150.

Frussa R, Rocha JBT, Conceicao IM, Mello CF, Pereira ME (1996): Effects of dopaminergic agents on visceral pain measured by the mouse writhing test. Arch Int Pharmacodyn Ther 331:74–93.

Gonzales-Rios F, Vlaiculescu A, Ben Natan L, Protais P, Costentin J (1986): Dissociated effects of apomorphine on various nociceptive responses in mice. J Neural Transm 67:87–103.

Gorlitz B-D, Frey H-H (1972): Central monoamines and antinociceptive drug action. Eur J Pharmacol 20:171–180.

Gratton A, Wise RA (1994): Drug- and behavior-associated changes in dopamine-related electrochemical signals during intravenous cocaine self-administration in rats. J Neurosci 14:4130–4146.

Hebb DO (1955): Drives and the CNS (Conceptual nervous system). Psychol Rev 62:243–254.

Imperato A, Angelucci L, Casolini P, Zocchi A, Puglisi-Allegra S (1992): Repeated stressful experiences differently affect dopamine release during and following stress. Brain Res 577:194–199.

Ivy AC, Goetzl FR, Burrill DY (1944): Morphine-dextroamphetamine analgesia. War Med 6:67–71.

Jasinski DR, Preston K (1986): Evaluation of mixtures of morphine and D-amphetamine for subjective and physiological effects. Drug Alcohol Depend 17:1–13.

Kaiko RF, Kanner R, Foley KM, Wallenstein SL, Canel AM, Rogers AG, Houde RW (1987): Cocaine and morphine interaction in acute and chronic cancer pain. Pain 31:35–45.

Kauppila T, Mecke E, Pertovaara A (1992): Enhancement of morphine-induced analgesia and attenuation of morphine-induced side-effects by cocaine in rats. Pharmacol Toxicol 71:173–178.

Kelly SJ, Franklin KBJ (1984): Electrolytic raphe magnus lesions block analgesia induced by a stress-morphine interaction but not analgesia induced by morphine alone. Neurosci Lett 52:147–152.

Kelly SJ, Franklin KBJ (1985): An increase in tryptophan may be a general mechanism for the effect of stress on sensitivity to pain. Neuropharmacol 24:1019–1025.

Kelly PH, Seviour PW, Iversen SD (1975): Amphetamine and apomorphine responses in the rat following 6-OHDA lesions of the nucleus accumbens septi and corpus striatum. Brain Res 94:507–522.

Kiritsy-Roy JA, Shyu BC, Danneman PJ, Morrow TJ, Belczynski C, Casey, KL (1994): Spinal antinociception mediated by a cocaine-sensitive dopaminergic supraspinal mechanism. Brain Res 644:109–116.

Kocher L (1988): Systemic naloxone does not affect pain-related behavior in the formalin test in rat. Physiol Behav 43:265–268.

Kubota K, Matsuoka Y, Sakuma M, Satoh S, Uruno T, Sunagane N (1982): Characteristic of analgesia induced by noncatecholic phenylethylamines in mice. Life Sci 31: 1221–1224.

Leone P, Pocock D, Wise RA (1991): Morphine-dopamine interaction: ventral tegmental morphine increases nucleus accumbens dopamine release. Pharmacol Biochem Behav 39:469–472.

Levant B, Bancroft GN, Selkirk CM (1996): In vivo occupancy of D2 dopamine receptors by 7-OH-DPAT. Synapse 24:60–64.

Lin MT, Wu JJ, Chandra A, Tsay BL (1981): Activation of striatal dopamine receptors induces pain inhibition in rats. J Neural Transm 51:213–222.

Lin Y, Morrow TJ, Casey KL (1987): Cocaine: mechanisms of CNS analgesic action in the rat. Soc Neurosci Abs 13:1588.

Lin Y, Morrow TJ, Kiritsy-Roy JA, Cass Terry L, Casey KL (1989): Cocaine: evidence for supraspinal, dopamine-mediated, non-opiate analgesia. Brain Res 479:306–312.

Little HJ, Rees JMH (1974): Tolerance development to the antinociceptive actions of morphine, amphetamine, physostigmine and 2-aminoindane in the mouse. Experientia 30:930–932.

Liu QS, Qiao JT, Dafny N (1992): D2 dopamine receptor involvement in spinal dopamine-produced antinociception. Life Sci 51:1485–1492.

Lund A, Mjellem-Joly N, Hole K (1991): Chronic administration of desipramine and zimelidine changes the behavioural response in the formalin test in rats. Neuropharmacol 30:481–487.

Major CT, Pleuvry BJ (1971): Effects of α-methyl-p-tyrosine, p-chlorophenyalanine L-β(3,4-dihydroxyphenyl)alanine, 5-hydroxytryptophan and diethldithiocarbamate on the analgesic activity of morphine and methylamphetamine in the mouse. Br J Pharmacol 42:512–521.

Malec D, Langwinski R (1981): Central action of narcotic analgesics. VIII. The effect of dopaminergic stimulants on the action of analgesics in rats. Pol J Pharmacol Pharm 33:273–282.

Manning BH, Morgan MJ, Franklin KBJ (1994): Morphine analgesia in the formalin test: evidence for forebrain and midbrain sites of action. Neurosci 63:289–294.

Michael-Titus A, Bousselmame R, Costentin J (1990): Stimulation of dopamine D2 receptors induces an analgesia involving an opioidergic but non enkephalinergic link. Eur J Pharmacol 187:201–207.

Morgan MJ, Franklin KBJ (1990): 6-hydroxydopamine lesions of the ventral tegmentum abolish D-amphetamine and morphine analgesia in the formalin test but not in the tail flick test. Brain Res 519:144–149.

Morgan MJ, Franklin KBJ (1991): Dopamine receptor subtypes and formalin test analgesia. Pharmacol Biochem Behav 40:317–322.

Nencini P, Ahmed AM, Anania MC, Moscucci M, Paroli E (1984): Prolonged analgesia induced by cathinone. Pharmacol 29:269–281.

Nickerson M, Goodman LS (1947): Synergistic isonipecaine-amphetamine analgesia. Fed Proc 6:360–361.

North MA (1978): Naloxone reversal of morphine analgesia but failure to alter reactivity to pain in the formalin test. Life Sci 22:295–302.

Nott MW (1968): Potentiation of morphine analgesia by cocaine in mice. Eur J Pharmacol 5:93–99.

Paalzow G, Paalzow L (1975): Enhancement of apomorphine-induced inhibition of vocalization after-discharge response by theophylline. Life Sci 17:1145–1151.

Paalzow GHM, Paalzow LK (1983): Opposing effects of apomorphine on pain in rats. Evaluation of the dose-response curve. Eur J Pharmacol 88:27–35.

Pertovaara A, Hamalainen MM (1994): Spinal potentiation and supraspinal additivity in the antinociceptive interaction between systemically administered alpha 2-adrenoceptor agonist and cocaine in the rat. Anesth Analg 79:261–266.

Pertovaara A, Belczynski CR, Morrow TJ, Casey KL (1988): The effect of systemic cocaine on spinal nociceptive reflex activity in the rat. Brain Res 438:286–290.

Resnik RB, Kestenbaum RS, Schwartz LK (1977): Acute systemic effects of cocaine in man: A controlled study by intranasal and intravenous routes. Science 195:696–698.

Robertson J, Weston R, Lewis MJ, Barasi S (1981): Evidence for the potentiation of the antinociceptive action of morphine by bromocriptine. Neuropharmacol 20:1029–1032.

Saxena PN, Gupta GP (1957): Analgesic potentiating effects of ephedrine and methamphetamine. J Indian Med Prof 4:1553.

Scheel-Krüger J, Willner P (1991): The mesolimbic system: principles of operation. In Willner P, Scheel-Krüger J (eds): *The Mesolimbic Dopamine System: From Motivation to Action*. Chichester, UK: John Wiley & Sons, pp. 559–597.

Shyu BC, Kiritsy-Roy JA, Morrow TJ, Casey KL (1992): Neurophysiological, pharmacological and behavioral evidence for medial thalamic mediation of cocaine-induced dopaminergic analgesia. Brain Res 572:216–223.

Skagerberg G, Lindvall O (1985): Organization of diencephalic dopamine neurones projecting to the spinal cord in the rat. Brain Res 342:340–351.

Slikker W, Jr., Brocco MJ, Killam KF, Jr. (1984): Reinstatement of responding maintained by cocaine or thiamylal. J Pharmacol Exp Ther 228:43–52.

Suaudeau C, Costentin J (1995): Analgesic effect of the direct D2 dopamine receptor agonist RU 24926 and cross tolerance with morphine. Fund Clin Pharmacol 9:147–152.

Tekol Y, Tercan E, Esmaoglu A (1994): Ephedrine enhances analgesic effect of morphine. Acta Anaesthesiol Scand 38:396–397.

Tocco DR, Maickel RP (1984): Analgesic activities of amphetamine isomers. Arch Int Pharmacodyn Ther 268:25–31.

Tocco DR, Spratto GR, Maickel RP (1985): Differential analgetic actions of amphetamine enantiomers in the mouse: a drug-drug interaction study. Arch Int Pharmacodyn Ther 278:261–272.

Tulunay FC, Sparber SB, Takemori AE (1975): The effect of dopaminergic stimulation and blockade on the nociceptive and antinociceptive responses of mice. Eur J Pharmacol 33:65–70.

Twycross RG (1979): Effect of cocaine in the brompton cocktail. In Bonica J, Liebeskind JC, Albe-Fessard D (eds): *Advances in Pain Research and Therapy*. New York: Raven Press, pp. 927–932.

Ushijima I, Horita A (1993): Cocaine: evidence for NMDA- and opioid-mediated antinociception in the tail-flick test. Pharmacol Biochem Behav 44:365–370.

Verma A, Kulkarni SK (1991): Alpha 2-adrenoceptor- and D2-dopamine receptor-mediated analgesic response of B-HT 920. J Pharm Pharmacol 43:131–133.

Webb SS, Smith GM, Evans WO, Webb NC (1978): Toward the development of a potent, nonsedating, oral analgesic. Psychopharmacology 60:25–28.

Weissman A, Koe BK, Tenen SS (1966): Antiamphetamine effects following inhibition of tyrosine hydroxylase. J Pharmacol Exp Ther 151:339–352.

Wesler LS, Frey AH (1985): Differential apomorphine effects. Behav Neurosci 99:776–777.

Wise RA (1987): The role of reward pathways in the development of drug dependence. Pharmacol Ther 35:227–263.

Yang JC, Clark WC, Dooley JC, Mignogna FV (1982): Effect of intranasal cocaine on experimental pain in man. Anesth Analg 61:358–361.

Yee JD, Berde CB (1994): Dextroamphetamine or methylphenidate as adjuvants to opioid analgesia for adolescents with cancer. J Pain Symp Manag 9:122–125.

CHAPTER 15

TRICYCLIC AND OTHER ANTIDEPRESSANTS AS ANALGESICS

A. ESCHALIER, D. ARDID, and C. DUBRAY
Equipe NPPUA
Université d'Auvergne
Clermont-Ferrand, France

The potential value of antidepressants (ADs) in the treatment of chronic pain syndromes was noted as early as 1960 by Paoli et al., who observed an analgesic effect of imipramine in 14 of 21 patients mainly treated for neurogenic pain. Lance and Curran (1964) performed the first placebo-controlled trial with amitriptyline in tension headache. They concluded that the AD was of value and that its effect was independent of any antidepressive action, and suggested that the benefit could result from vasodilatation. Several ($n = 13$) subsequent controlled studies were performed between 1966 and 1980 in patients suffering from various chronic pain syndromes. The first controlled study in peripheral neuropathic pain (diabetic neuropathy) was published by Turkington in 1980. Since this date, several controlled clinical studies of AD effects in chronic pain patients have been published. Simultaneously, there have been at least 30 traditional narrative reviews on ADs and pain, and many animal experiments. Interest in these medications parallels a considerable clinical use even though no ADs (e.g., in the United Kingdom), or just a few of them (e.g., two in France) have a product license for this particular indication. Callies and Popkin (1987) demonstrated that among 216 patients hospitalized on adult medical-surgical services of Minnesota Hospital (Minneapolis), 30% received ADs (amitriptyline, doxepin, imipramine) for the treatment of pain. Antidepressants were initiated during hospitalization in 66% of cases for treatment of pain and in 36% for treatment of depression. A survey carried out in 44% of Italian oncological centers showed that 43% of the subjects treated for cancer-related pain received ADs (Magni et al., 1987). Thus, even though some discrepancies exist (Goodkin and Guillion, 1989; Richardson and Williams, 1993), the pro-

---

Novel Aspects of Pain Management: Opioids and Beyond, Edited by Jana Sawynok and Alan Cowan
ISBN 0-471-180173 Copyright © 1999 by Wiley-Liss, Inc.

longed and widespread use of these drugs throughout the world suggests their utility, justifying this chapter in a comprehensive book on the pharmacology of pain.

The following two issues are developed in this chapter: (1) A synthesis of clinical and experimental evidence for the efficacy of ADs as analgesics (Table 15.1). This analysis is based on two recent meta-analyses of controlled clinical studies (Onghena and Van Houdenhove, 1992; McQuay et al., 1996) and an extensive review of animal studies found by searching Medline (1970–1997). (2) A survey of present hypotheses on their mechanisms of action in terms of (*a*) site of action and (*b*) interactions with neurochemical systems involved in pain transmission or modulation.

EFFICACY OF ANTIDEPRESSANTS

Clinical Data

Chronic Nonmalignant Pain. The two published meta-analyses have presented data on the use of ADs in chronic nonmalignant pain in general (Onghena and Van Houdenhove, 1992) and in neuropathic pain specifically (McQuay et al., 1996). These studies involved a large number of patients (1740 and 886, respectively), and the overall results of the two studies were similar: ADs have an analgesic effect compared with placebo. According to Onghena and Van Houdenhove (1992), "the average of chronic pain patients who received an antidepressant treatment had less pain than 74% of the chronic pain patients who received a placebo." A median of 58% of the patients reported at least 50% pain reduction. The efficacy of ADs was better in neurogenic pain [the mean effect size (ES) ranges from 0.7 ± 0 (central pain) to 1.7 ± 0 (diabetic neuropathy)] than in rheumatological pain (ES = 0.37 ± 0.19). Considering headaches, this parameter ranged from 0.82 ± 0.26 (migraine) to 1.11 ± 0.15 (tension headache). Among the 46 drug-placebo comparisons, for 39 studies analyzed, amitriptyline was the most frequently used ($n = 15$) compared to doxepin ($n = 6$), imipramine ($n = 6$), mianserin ($n = 4$), and clomipramine ($n = 3$). Specific serotonin re-uptake inhibitors (SSRIs) were used in only six comparisons. The highest ES was obtained for doxepin (0.96 ± 0.30), but the variability was greater than for amitriptyline (0.73 ± 0.15). When drugs of differing chemical structures were compared, ES for tricyclic drugs (0.69 ± 0.10) was significantly higher than for heterocyclic drugs (0.36 ± 0.17). Other data concerning the monoaminergic mechanism of action of ADs are considered below.

The review of McQuay et al. (1996) focused on neuropathic pain and included 21 controlled studies. "Compared with placebo, of 100 patients with neuropathic pain who are given ADs, 30 will obtain more than 50% pain relief . . . ." Outcomes considered in this study were different from those used in the previous meta-analysis; the odds ratio was measured to determine the

TABLE 15.1 Antidepressants Used in Clinical and Experimental Studies on Pain

Antidepressive Agent	Chemical Structure	Preferential Monoamine Effect
Amitriptyline	TCA	Mixed
Citalopram	Original	SSRI
Clomipramine	TCA	SSRI (metabolite: SNRI)
Desipramine	TCA	SNRI
Doxepine	TCA	Mixed
Femoxetine	Original	SSRI
Fluvoxamine	Original	SSRI
Fluoxetine	Original	SSRI
Imipramine	TCA	Mixed
Indalpine	Original (retired)	SSRI
Iprindole	TCA	Mixed*
Maprotiline	Tetrac	SNRI
Metapramine	TCA	SNRI
Mianserin	Tetrac	SNRI (α_2 antagonist)
Minalcipran	Original	Mixed
Moclobemide	Original	MAOI (type A)
Nefazodone	Original	Mixed (5-HT2A antagonist)
Nortriptyline	TCA	SNRI
Paroxetine	Original	SSRI
Phenelzine	Original	MAOI
Protriptyline	TCA	SNRI
Sertraline	Original	SSRI
Trazodone	Original	SSRI
Trimipramine	TCA	Mixed
Viloxazine	Original	SNRI (Beta agonist)
Zimelidine	Original (retired)	SSRI

TCA = tricyclic antidepressant, tetrac = tetracyclic antidepressant, original = nontricyclic or non-tetracyclic antidepressant, SSRI = specific serotonin re-uptake inhibitor, SNRI = specific noradrenaline re-uptake inhibitor, * = weak re-uptake inhibitor, MAOI = monoamine oxidase inhibitor.

benefit of treatment compared with placebo and the number-needed-to-treat (NNT) to appreciate the degree of efficacy or side effect induction compared with placebo. In six of 13 placebo-controlled reports in diabetic neuropathy, the odds ratios showed significant benefit compared with placebo with, for all 13 reports, a NNT of 3. However, marked differences were observed among the nine different ADs used: for example, NNT for eight combined tricyclics was 3.2, but 5 for paroxetine and 15.3 for fluoxetine (where the odds ratio fails to show a significant effect versus placebo). NNT was 2.3 in two of the three studies in postherpetic neuralgia, 2.8 in two atypical facial pain studies, and 1.7 in one of the three studies in central pain.

These two meta-analyses led to similar conclusions in terms of the efficacy of ADs. (1) ADs are effective for chronic benign pain relief but their overall effect is only partial; (2) neuropathic pain of peripheral or central origin is particularly sensitive to these effects; (3) tricyclic antidepressant drugs (TCAs) are more effective than SSRIs; (4) the analgesic benefit of ADs appears without significant change in mood. Some other interesting points emerged. Many additional factors in these studies (duration of pain, sample homogeneity, within- or between-subject designs, physician ratings vs. patient self-ratings, variation in the proportion of placebo responders, which in some cases reached 75%) were variable, and some of these factors may influence the magnitude of effect of ADs. They must be taken into account in further clinical studies. The comparison with another meta-analysis performed on anticonvulsants in pain management (McQuay et al., 1995) shows that the combined NNT for benefit in diabetic neuropathy was similar for ADs (3) and anticonvulsants (2.5); the NNT for minor or adverse effects was also similar. McQuay et al. (1996) estimated that these systematic reviews "show little to choose between ADs and anticonvulsants."

Cancer Pain. The use of ADs is generally justified by the discovery of a neuropathic component in cancer pain. However, although ADs have been used over a long period (Walsh, 1983; Kocher, 1984), this use is not based on well-conducted controlled clinical trials. A comparative trial of clomipramine and placebo, in only eight patients, failed to show any difference (Beaumont and Seldrup, 1980).

Acute Pain. Only a few papers have been published with ADs in acute postoperative pain or in evoked pain in painfree human subjects. With postoperative pain, two controlled studies performed with tricyclics observed negative effects (Portenoy et al., 1984; Levine et al., 1986), but a significant analgesia was obtained with clomipramine (Nobili et al., 1987). Seven double-blind placebo-controlled studies have examined experimental pain in healthy volunteers, after acute administration of ADs. The results obtained were equivocal. Negative results obtained in both postoperative and experimental pain paradigms, and the limited degree of analgesia when this was obtained suggest that the action of ADs on acute pain is not substantial, providing no evidence for their use in clinical conditions of acute pain.

Experimental Data

Since the first work performed in animals (Sethy et al., 1970), 90 studies have investigated the effects of ADs in several pain conditions in animals. A variety of ADs have been used (Fig. 15.1A). Most of the studies involved standard acute nociceptive pain tests; only a few ($n = 9$ studies) involved persistent pain models. Thermal stimuli were most frequently used, as is often the case in animal research on the pharmacology of pain, followed by chemical, electrical,

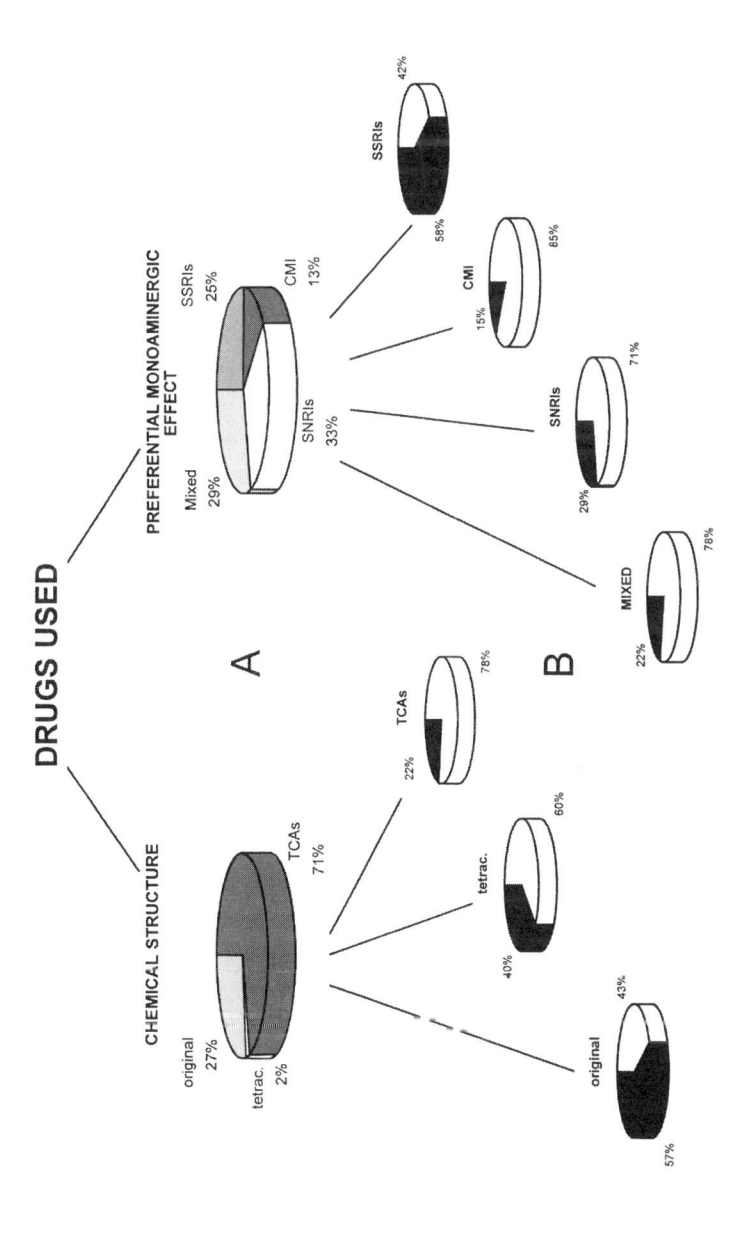

Figure 15.1 Influence of chemical structure and preferential monoaminergic effect on the antinociceptive efficacy of acutely administered ADs in animals. (A) Proportion of ADs used according to their chemical structure and preferential monoaminergic effect. (B) Percent efficacy of ADs, by chemical structure and preferential monoaminergic effect (white = antinociceptive effect; black = no effect). TCAs = tricyclic antidepressants, tetrac. = tetracyclic antidepressants, original = nontricyclic or nontetracyclic antidepressants, SSRIs = specific serotonin re-uptake inhibitors, SNRIs = specific noradrenaline reuptake inhibitors, CMI = clomipramine.

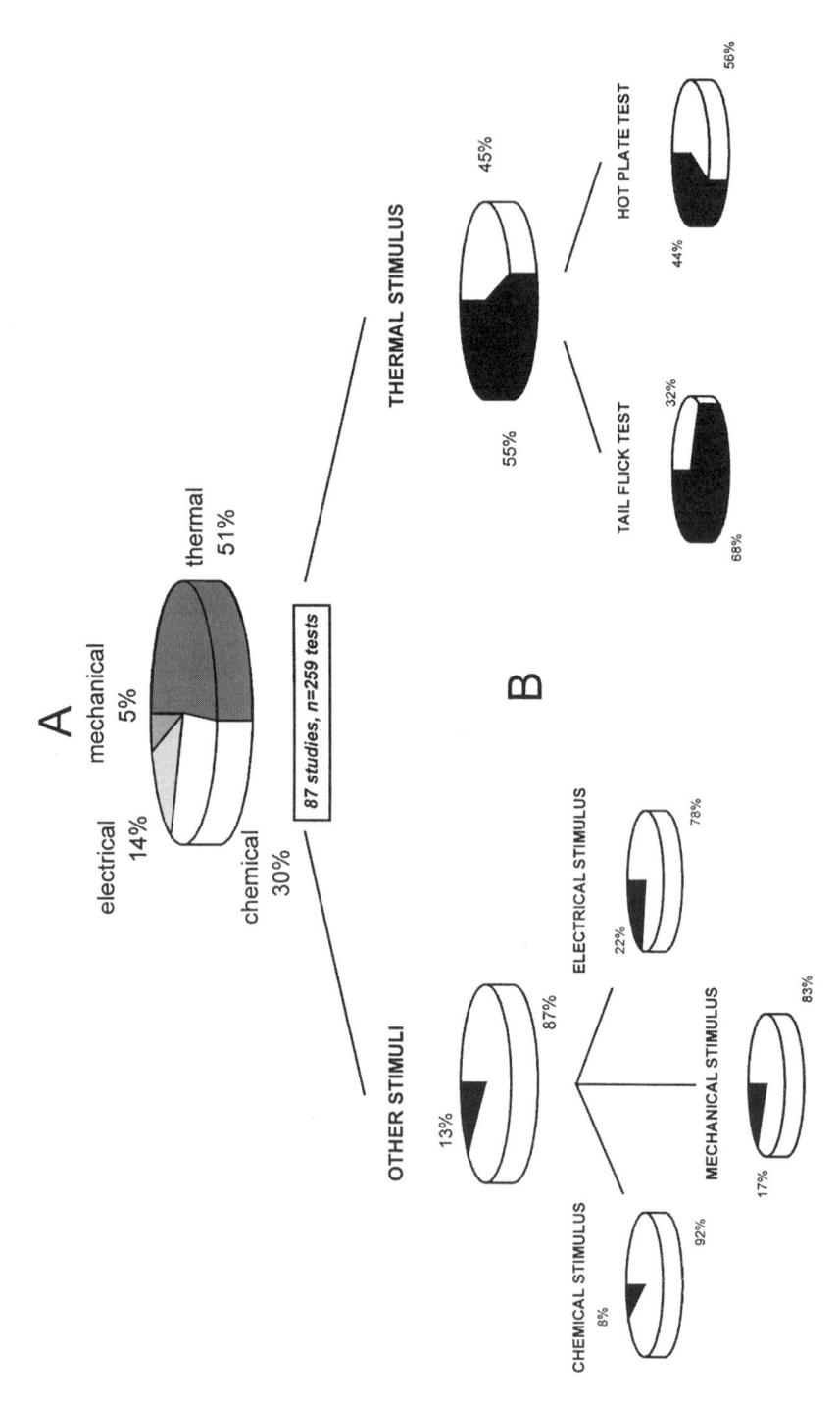

Figure 15.2 Influence of the type of acute pain stimulus used on the effect of acute administration of ADs in animals. (A) Proportion of each kind of noxious stimulus. (B) Percent efficacy according to different stimuli (white = antinociceptive effect; black = no effect).

and mechanical stimuli (Fig. 15.2A). Systemic drug administration was most often used (82%), compared to central (17%) and local (1%) injections. Acute administration was typical (87%), with a high proportion of intraperitoneal injections (66%) and lesser use of subcutaneous (19%), intravenous (9%), or oral (6%) routes. Some studies (16%) used repeated injections with different protocols, using daily or twice-daily injections or injections every half-life time. Finally, the range of the systemic doses used was relatively large; ranging from 0.125 mg/kg intravenously to 100 mg/kg subcutaneously.

The majority (66%) of these studies concluded that ADs can have an antinociceptive effect. However, some differences were observed depending on the nature of the stimulus used (Fig. 15.2B) and the chemical structure (Fig. 15.1B). Differences exist when results are compared according to the preferential monoaminergic profile of the various ADs (Fig. 15.1B), a point discussed below.

The patterns of administration seem also to be of importance. When repeated administrations were used, ADs were more effective than after an acute administration. In particular, TCAs were consistently effective in the few studies using both repeated administration and persistent models of pain, such as polyarthritis and nerve injury (Butler et al., 1985; Abad et al., 1989; Seltzer et al., 1989; Ardid and Guilbaud, 1992; Courteix et al., 1994).

With regard to the different routes of administration, the intravenous route gave better results (91% analgesic effects) compared to intraperitoneal, subcutaneous, and peroral, with 67, 54, and 50% of positive effects, respectively. Supraspinal injections gave better results than intrathecal injections for which the data are contradictory. These issues are discussed below.

Although these studies indicate that ADs are often effective in animal pain tests, they also suggest that attention to particular design features may enhance the ability of animal studies to provide more specific information about the circumstances under which ADs are most effective. The use of chronic pain models with chronic injection paradigms appears to be the best way to obtain consistent results, and this is particularly important for studying the mechanisms of analgesic action of ADs.

MECHANISM OF ACTION

One important view of the mechanism of therapeutic benefit of ADs involves their antidepressive effect. It is likely that ADs were originally used in chronic pain to relieve concomitant depression and improve patient complaints (Kraemlinger et al., 1983; Turkington, 1980). However, several clinical observations suggest that ADs have an independent analgesic effect (Eschalier, 1990). The two previously mentioned meta-analyses confirm this point, indicating that mood changes are not necessary for the analgesic benefit of ADs but may play a significant role in alleviating the distress of the pain experience.

Sites of Action

The psychotropic action of ADs and the insensitivity of neuropathic pain to peripheral analgesics both suggest the hypothesis of a predominantly central effect. However, we also discuss the hypothesis of a peripheral site of action.

Peripheral Site of Action of Antidepressants. The sodium channel-blocking effects of some TCAs and the possible peripheral effect on neuronal discharges of class Ib antiarrhythmic drugs (see ref. in Jett et al., 1997) used to treat neuropathic pain in humans (Galer, 1995), would suggest a possible interaction of ADs on ion influx and nerve transmission. However, electrophysiological studies using models of nerve injury are needed, similar to those with antiarrhythmic drugs, before concluding that ADs have an effect on peripheral nerves.

Several animal studies have used models of subacute and chronic articular inflammation to test the effect of ADs on the inflammatory process, even though inflammatory pain has not been a major clinical target for these medications. Using the classical model of carrageenan-induced inflammatory pain, Ardid et al. (1991) showed that clomipramine, which was ineffective in altering pain thresholds after intraplantar administration, possessed antinociceptive activity and increased edema after systemic injection. This result, which tends to exclude any peripheral mechanism, disagrees with other data that show a reduction of both acute and chronic experimental inflammation (Arrigoni-Martelli et al., 1967; Anstee, 1979; Butler et al. 1985; Opavsky et al., 1993; Bianchi et al., 1994) and a reduction of prostaglandin E_2-like activity in the exudate (Bianchi et al., 1995) or prostaglandin synthetase activity (Krupp and Wesp, 1975).

Central Site of Action of Antidepressants. Several clinical and experimental results argue for a central effect of these drugs. Indalpine and desipramine have been shown to produce an analgesic effect on the RIII reflex, a method that explores in humans the central effects of analgesics (Willer et al., 1982; Coquoz et al., 1993).

Similarly, arguments from animal studies suggest the involvement of such a site of action. (1) In general, ADs are effective in tests sensitive to central analgesics (e.g., hot plate; paw pressure in normal animals). (2) The effect of intravenously administered clomipramine is significantly decreased after lesions of the dorsolateral funiculus (DLF), which conducts inhibitory bulbospinal pathways (Ardid et al., 1995). (3) Supraspinal injection of ADs gave 90% positive results in 11 tests using this route of administration. The last two arguments for a central effect suggest that ADs may act supraspinally by activating descending inhibitory bulbospinal pathways. However, a spinal effect cannot be ruled out. Half of the 32 tests using intrathecally administered ADs showed positive effects, although they were mostly performed with poorly sensitive acute thermal pain tests. The demonstration of a systematic effect of different ADs when administered intrathecally in persistent neuropathic pain models (Eschalier et al., 1994) suggests that chronic pain-induced spinal neuronal changes could provide a substrate for a spinal effect.

Although the nature of the drug used and the type of the induced pain may influence the site of action of the ADs (e.g. Coquoz et al., 1993; Dirksen et al., 1994; Mestre et al., 1997), it appears that in the context of human persistent pain, ADs mainly act spinally and supraspinally, through an activation of inhibitory bulbospinal pathways.

Neurochemical Mechanisms

Even before the experimental demonstration of the inhibitory effect of lesions of the DLF on the antinociceptive action of clomipramine, the activation by ADs of monoaminergic bulbospinal pathways through their monoamine re-uptake blocking effect (Glowinski and Axelrod, 1964; Segawa and Kuruma, 1968) was the most often invoked mechanism for the analgesic action of ADs. However, other hypotheses have also been suggested.

Monoaminergic Mechanism. This hypothesis was first based on serotonin, with the principal mechanism involved believed to be inhibition of serotonin re-uptake; however, both clinical and animal studies invalidate such a mechanism. The two meta-analyses suggest a lower efficacy of SSRIs compared to mixed noradrenaline and serotonin re-uptake inhibitors in clinical studies. A similar picture emerged from animal studies, for acutely administered SSRIs and mixed ADs were effective in 42 and 78% of tests, respectively. Regarding a noradrenergic mechanism, clinical data are equivocal. Onghena and Van Houdenhove (1992) concluded that specific noradrenaline re-uptake inhibitors are less effective than mixed ADs, and no more effective than SSRIs. Max (1994) showed a similar efficacy of the mixed AD, amitriptyline, and the specific noradrenaline re-uptake inhibitor, desipramine, which was greater than the modest efficacy of the SSRI, fluoxetine, in patients with neuropathic pain. The same results were obtained in animal studies in which 71% of tests showed an antinociceptive effect of noradrenergic ADs. However, use of acute pain models and single administration procedures in many of these tests may limit their comparison to clinical uses.

This predominance of mixed ADs in clinical use is in line with the known interactions between serotonin and noradrenaline in the modulation of pain (Post and Archer, 1990). They have been very clearly analyzed by Sawynok and Reid (1996) at the spinal level where the two monoamines produce a synergistic interaction. However, a more definitive argument would involve the demonstration that the inhibition of these monoaminergic systems reduces the analgesic effect of mixed ADs. No such clinical data are available and only a few animal studies have studied this point. *p*-Chlorophenylalanine (an inhibitor of serotonin synthesis) and serotonin receptor antagonists inhibit the analgesic effect of mixed ADs such as amitriptyline or imipramine (De Felipe et al., 1986; Valverde et al., 1994; Sierralta et al., 1995); of the preferential inhibitor of serotonin re-uptake, clomipramine (Eschalier et al., 1981; Sacerdote et al., 1987; Valverde et al., 1994); and of noradrenergic ADs such as desipramine, nortriptyline, and desmethylclomipramine (Valverde et al., 1994). Similarly, α-methyl-*p*-tyrosine (a competitive inhibitor of tyrosine hydroxylase) inhibited the effect of the three groups of ADs when acutely administered intraperitoneally in mice (Valverde et al., 1994). Finally, yohimbine, an α_2-adrenoceptor antagonist, suppresses the antinociceptive effect of clomipramine (Eschalier et al., 1994), consistent with a similar interaction between this antagonist or phentolamine and serotonin (Sawynok and Reid, 1992). The findings tend to demonstrate that intact serotonin and noradrenaline systems are required to obtain an antinociceptive effect with acutely administered ADs. However, further studies of the monoaminergic hypothesis are needed, particularly experiments using chronic administration of ADs, in animal models of persistent pain or in conditions of clinical use. This need is emphasized by the demonstration of differential effects of acute and repeated treatments by ADs on noradrenergic and serotonergic neuronal activity (e.g., Blier et al., 1990; Baldessarini, 1996).

Opioidergic Mechanisms. The main evidence for an opioidergic component of action is that the antinociceptive effect of ADs in animals can be inhibited by naloxone, an opioid antagonist (Biegon and Samuel, 1979; Eschalier et al., 1981; Ardid and Guilbaud, 1992). This finding has been confirmed in humans; the analgesic effect of indalpine in healthy volunteers was reversed by naloxone (Willer et al., 1982). However, several studies failed to find any inhibition by naloxone of the antinociceptive effect of ADs (e.g., Ogren and Holm, 1980; Bergman et al., 1991; Schreiber et al., 1996). Further evidences come from animal studies. The levels of met- and leu-enkephalin are increased in some rat central nervous system regions after daily administration of various ADs (De Felipe et al., 1985; Hamon et al., 1987). Antidepressants are able to displace radiolabeled opioid receptor ligands from their binding sites and, after repeated administration, to modify opioid receptor density (Somoza et al., 1981; Isenberg and Cicero, 1984; Hamon et al., 1987). Antidepressants can also enhance morphine antinociception after a single administration, but repeated treatment with clomipramine or imipramine attenuates the effect of morphine analgesia (see refs. in Fialip et al., 1989). In humans, ADs potentiate (Levine et al., 1986; Gordon et al., 1993), fail to modify (Levine et al., 1986; Max et al., 1992; Kerrick et al., 1993), or antagonize (Gordon et al., 1994) postoperative opioid analgesia.

All of these data suggest an interaction between ADs and opioid systems, the nature of which remains to be elucidated. However, the low affinity (IC_{50} about 10^{-5} *M*) of ADs for opioid receptors (Isenberg and Cicero, 1984) does not suggest a direct effect on these receptors. Thus an indirect involvement via a monoaminergic linkage, may be involved.

Other Potential Mechanisms

Involvement of Other Pharmacological Properties of Tricyclic Antidepressants in Their Analgesic Activity. Because tricyclic drugs are more efficacious than SSRIs in clinical and experimental studies of pain relief, other biochemical actions of these "dirty" drugs which are not characteristic of SSRIs may be involved in the mechanism of their analgesic action.

SEDATIVE EFFECT. TCAs act as antagonists at α_1-adrenergic and H_1 histaminergic receptors and hence can induce sedation. This property has been considered as the main explanation for the antinociceptive effect of ADs by some authors (e.g., Kocher, 1976; Meyers, 1985). In their meta-analysis, Onghena and Van Houdenhove (1992) concluded that neither more highly sedative drugs, nor higher drug doses (related to more sedation) were more effective in decreasing pain. However, α_1-adrenoceptor antagonism might participate in the efficacy of ADs in neurogenic pain involving a sympathetic component.

QUINIDINE-LIKE EFFECT. Another specific property of TCAs is their quinidine-like effect, that is, an inhibition of sodium channels. In fact, a comparable analgesic effect was obtained with ADs and anticonvulsants, other sodium channel blockers (McQuay et al., 1995, 1996). This ionic mechanism (also found for class Ib antiarrhythmic drugs used in neuropathic pain management) has been proposed by Jett et al. (1997) as a hypothesis for the antinociceptive effect of desipramine. It should be noted that this hypothesis is presently based only on an analogy, that TCAs show similarities with drugs known to be sodium channel blockers and have better efficacy than drugs (SSRI) devoid of this property.

ANTICHOLINERGIC PROPERTIES. This effect of TCAs appears to conflict with their analgesic property, for cholinergic activity rather than anticholinergic activity contributes to antinociception (e.g. Naguib and Yaksh, 1994; Hood et al., 1995; Beilin et al., 1997).

Interaction between Antidepressants and Noxious Transmission

ANTIDEPRESSANTS AND EXCITATORY AMINO ACIDS. This hypothesis is based on several observations: (1) structural similarities between TCAs and classical NMDA (*N*-methyl-D-aspartate) receptor antagonists such as MK801 have been described (Iwamoto and Marion, 1994); (2) TCAs bind to the NMDA receptor complex with an IC_{50} around 10^{-6} M (Reynolds and Miller, 1988; Sills and Loo, 1989); (3) chronic treatment of mice with ADs of all major classes alter NMDA receptor ligand binding in cortex (e.g., Skolnick et al., 1996); (4) some ADs may act as antagonists of NMDA receptors (Svensson et al., 1994; Wilkinson et al., 1994) and reduce NMDA-induced spinal hyperalgesia (Mjellem et al., 1993; Eisenach and Gebhart, 1995). All these data suggest that ADs may thus induce antinociception by inhibiting glutamatergic transmission at the spinal level; however, the molecular mechanisms of this action remain to be elucidated.

ANTIDEPRESSANTS AND NEUROKININS. Intrathecally administered imipramine shows a dose-dependent inhibitory effect on substance P-induced nociceptive behavior. However, this effect is observed at tissue concentrations of the antidepressant too low to involve neurokinin NK1-receptors (Imahita and Shimizu, 1992). Peripherally, clomipramine, but not fluoxetine, reduced substance P production in carrageenan-induced inflammatory exudate, which was considered by the authors as the mechanism that underlies the anti-inflammatory effect of this drug (Bianchi et al., 1995).

ANTIDEPRESSANTS AND CALCIUM CHANNELS. Some ADs can inhibit calcium uptake (Lavoie et al., 1994; Beauchamp et al., 1995). A synergistic interaction between ADs and calcium channel blockers (e.g., nifedipine, nicardipine) has been described in animal pain tests (Antkiewicz-Michaluk et al., 1991; Muthal and Chopde, 1993). However, several authors suggest that this calcium channel inhibition is not involved in the effects of TCAs (Lavoie et al., 1994; Beauchamp et al., 1995; Wananukul et al., 1996). Finally, Antkiewicz-Michaluk et al. (1991) propose an interesting inverse correlation between cortical [^{3}H]nitrendipine binding site density and the efficacy in the hot plate test after chronic administration of ADs. Imipramine failed to induce any change in the density of cortical binding sites but induced analgesia; citalopram and chlorprothixene produced hyperalgesia and an elevation of the density of cortical [^{3}H]nitrendipine binding sites.

Other Effects of Antidepressants. Other adaptations to repeated antidepressant treatment have been described (effects on γ-aminobutyric acid (GABA) receptors, desensitization of D_2 dopamine autoreceptors, interaction with adenosine or cyclic-AMP dependent phosphorylation systems) (see Baldessarini, 1996). Their potential involvement in the antinociceptive effect of ADs remains to be elucidated.

In summary, clinical studies and recent meta-analyses confirm the therapeutic value of ADs historically used in the management of chronic pain syndromes. This property is independent of mood improvement and particularly marked in neurogenic pain. Both clinical and experimental data suggest better efficacy of mixed serotonin and noradrenaline re-uptake inhibitors, which, up until now, possessed a tricyclic chemical structure. Concerning their mechanism of action, evidence exists for a predominant central (spinal and supraspinal) rather than peripheral effect. Although a monoaminergic mechanism is the most often discussed, other hypotheses (e.g., opioidergic, quinidine-like effect, interaction with glutaminergic transmission) have been proposed. However, further clinical and experimental research is needed to definitively evaluate these hypotheses. Clinical studies in patients with neurogenic pain syndromes and animal experiments, using chronic (particularly neurogenic) pain models after repeated administration of antidepressants, which are too rarely done, may be particularly important in these evaluations.

To conclude, it is essential to keep in mind the fact that the value of ADs, and particularly TCAs, in chronic pain management is limited by both their partial efficacy and their side effects. For this reason, further well-performed research is needed (1) to determine the efficacy of new non-TCAs that inhibit both re-uptake of noradrenaline and serotonin and are devoid of anticholinergic, antihistaminergic, and α_1 adrenoceptor blocking effects (e.g., venlafaxine, nefazodone, minalcipran), and (2) to clarify the mechanism of action of TCAs in order to create efficacious new compounds.

REFERENCES

Abad F, Feria M, Boada J (1989): Chronic amitriptyline decreases autotomy following dorsal rhizotomy in rats. Neurosci Lett 99:187–190.

Anstee J (1979): Animal pharmacological studies on the effect of imipramine on pain. Pharmacol Med 1:78–79.

Antkiewicz-Michaluk L, Romanska I, Michaluk J, Vetulani J (1991): Role of calcium channels in effects of antidepressant drugs on responsiveness to pain. Psychopharmacology 105:269–274.

Ardid D, Guilbaud G (1992): Antinociceptive effects of acute and "chronic" injections of tricyclic antidepressant drugs in a new model of mononeuropathy in rats. Pain 49:253–256.

Ardid D, Eschalier A, Lavarenne J (1991): Evidence for a central but not a peripheral analgesic effect of clomipramine in rats. Pain 45:95–100.

Ardid D, Jourdan D, Mestre C, Villanueva L, Le Bars D, Eschalier A (1995): Involvement of bulbospinal pathways in the antinociceptive effect of clomipramine in the rat. Brain Res 695:253–256.

Arrigoni-Martelli E, Toth E, Segre AD, Corsico N (1967): Mechanism of inhibition of experimental inflammation by antidepressant drugs. Eur J Pharmacol 2:229–233.

Baldessarini RJ (1996): Drugs and the treatment of psychiatric disorders. In Hardman JG, Limbird LE, Molinoff PB, Ruddon RW, Gilman AG (eds): Goodman and Gilman's *The Pharmacological Basis of Therapeutics*. New York: McGraw-Hill, pp. 431–459.

Beauchamp G, Lavoie PA, Elie R (1995): Differential effect of desipramine and 2-hydroxydesipramine on depolarization-induced calcium uptake in synaptosomes from rat limbic sites. Can J Physiol Pharmacol 73:619–623.

Beaumont G, Seldrup JL (1980): Comparative trial of clomipramine and placebo in the treatment of terminal pain. J Int Med Res 8:67–69.

Beilin B, Nemirovsky AY, Zeidel A, Maibord E, Zelman V, Katz RL (1997): Systemic physostigmine increases the antinociceptive effect of spinal morphine. Pain 70:217–221.

Bergman DA, Wynn RL, Alvarez L, Asher K, Thut PD (1991): Imipramine-fentanyl antinociception in a rabbit tooth pulp model. Life Sci 49:1279–1288.

Bianchi M, Sacerdote P, Panerai AE (1994): Clomipramine differently affects inflammatory edema and pain in the rat. Pharmacol Biochem Behav 48:1037–1040.

Bianchi M, Rossoni G, Sacerdote P, Panerai AE, Berti F (1995): Effects of chlomipramine and fluoxetine on subcutaneous carrageenin-induced inflammation in the rat. Inflamm Res 44:466–469.

Biegon A, Samuel D (1979): Interaction of tricyclic antidepressants with opiate receptors. Biochem Pharmacol 29:460–462.

Blier P, de Montigny C, Chaput Y (1990): A role for the serotonin system in the mechanism of action of antidepressant treatments: preclinical evidence. J Clin Psychiatry 51:14–20.

Butler SH, Weil-Fugazza J, Godefroy F, Besson JM (1985): Reduction of arthritis and pain behaviour following chronic administration of amitriptyline or imipramine in rats with adjuvant-induced arthritis. Pain 23:159–175.

Callies AL, Popkin MK (1987): Antidepressant treatment of medical-surgical in patients by nonpsychiatric physicians. Arch Gen Psychiatry 44:157–160.

Coquoz D, Porchet HC, Dayer P (1993): Central analgesic effects of desipramine, fluvoxamine and moclobemide after single oral dosing: a study in healthy volunteers. Clin Pharmacol Ther 54:339–344.

Courteix C, Bardin M, Chantelauze C, Lavarenne J, Eschalier A (1994): A study of the sensitivity of the diabetes-induced pain model in rats to a range of analgesics. Pain 57:153–160.

De Felipe MDC, De Ceballos ML, Gil C, Fuentes JA (1985): Chronic antidepressant treatment increases enkephalin levels in n. accumbens and striatum of the rat. Eur J Pharmacol 112:119–122.

De Felipe MDC, De Ceballos ML, Fuentes JA (1986): Hypoalgesia induced by antidepressants in mice : a case for opioids and serotonin. Eur J Pharmacol 125:193–199.

Dirksen R, Van Diejen D, Van Luijtelaar EL, Booij LH (1994): Site- and test-dependent antinociceptive efficiency of amitriptyline in rats. Pharmacol Biochem Behav 47:21–26.

Eisenach JC, Gebhart GF (1995): Intrathecal amitriptyline acts as an N-methyl-D-aspartate receptor antagonist in the presence of inflammatory hyperalgesia in rats. Anesthesiology 83:1046–1054.

Eschalier A (1990): Antidepressants and pain management. In Besson JM, (ed): *Serotonin and Pain*. Amsterdam: Elsevier, pp. 305–325.

Eschalier A, Montastruc JL, Devoize JL, Rigal F, Gaillard-Plaza G, Pechadre JC (1981): Influence of naloxone and methysergide on the analgesic effect of clomipramine in rats. Eur J Pharmacol 74:1–7.

Eschalier A, Mestre C, Dubray C, Ardid D (1994): Why are antidepressants effective as pain relief? CNS Drugs 2:261–267.

Fialip J, Marty H, Makambila MC, Civiale MA, Eschalier A (1989): Patterns of administration of antidepressants in animals: II. Relevance in a study of the influence of clomipramine on morphine analgesia in mice. J Pharmacol Exp Ther 248:747–751.

Galer BS (1995): Neuropathic pain of peripheral origin: Advances in pharmacologic treatment. Neurology 45:17–25.

Glowinski J, Axelrod J (1964): Inhibition of uptake of tritiated noradrenaline in the intact rat brain by imipramine and structurally related compounds. Nature 204:1318–1319.

Goodkin K, Guillion CM (1989): Antidepressants for the relief of chronic pain: do they work? Ann Behav Med 11:83–101.

Gordon NC, Heller PH, Gear RW, Levine JD (1993): Temporal factors in the enhancement of morphine analgesia by desipramine. Pain 53:273–276.

Gordon NC, Heller PH, Gear RW, Levine JD (1994): Interactions between fluoxetine and opiate analgesia for postoperative dental pain. Pain 58:85–88.

Hamon M, Gozlan H, Bourgoin S, Benoliel JJ, Mauborgne A, Taquet H, Cesselin F, Mico JA (1987): Opioid receptors and neuropeptides in the CNS in rats treated chronically with amoxapine or amitriptyline. Neuropharmacol 26:531–539.

Hood DD, Eisenach JC, Tuttle R (1995): Phase I safety assessment of intrathecal neostigmine in humans. Anesthesiology 82:331–343.

Imahita T, Shimizu T (1992): Imipramine inhibits intrathecal substance P-induced behavior and blocks spinal cord substance P receptors in mice. Brain Res 581:59–66.

Isenberg K, Cicero TC (1984): Possible involvement of opiate receptors in the pharmacological profiles of antidepressant compounds. Eur J Pharmacol 103:57–63.

Iwamoto ET, Marion L (1994): Pharmacological evidence that nitric oxide mediates the antinociception produced by muscarinic agonists in the rostral ventral medulla of rats. J Pharmacol Exp Ther 269:699–708.

Jett MF, McGuirk J, Waligora D, Hunter JC (1997): The effects of mexiletine, desipramine and fluoxetine in rat models involving central sensitization. Pain 69:161–169.

Kerrick JM, Fine PG, Lipman AG, Love G (1993): Low-dose amitriptyline as an adjunct to opioids for postoperative orthopedic pain: a placebo-controlled trial. Pain 52:325–330.

Kocher R (1976): Use of psychotropic drugs for the treatment of chronic severe pain. In Bonica JJ and Albe-Fressard (eds): *Advances in Pain Research and Therapy*, Vol. 1. New York: Raven Press, pp. 579–582.

Kocher R (1984): The use of psychotropic drugs in the treatment of cancer pain. Recent Results Cancer Res 89:118–126.

Kraemlinger KG, Swanson DN, Maruta T (1983): Are patients with chronic pain depressed? Am J Psychiatry 140.747–749.

Krupp P, Wesp M (1975): Inhibition of prostaglandin synthetase by psychotropic drugs. Experientia 31:330–331.

Lance JW, Curran DA (1964): Treatment of chronic tension headache. Lancet I:1234–1239.

Lavoie PA, Beauchamp G, Elie R (1994): Absence of stereoselectivity of some tricyclic antidepressants for the inhibition of depolarization-induced calcium uptake in rat cingulate cortex synaptosomes. J Psychiatry Neurosci 19:208–212.

Levine JD, Gordon NC, Smith R, McBryde R (1986): Desipramine enhances opiate postoperative analgesia. Pain 27:45–49.

Magni G, Arsie D, De Leo D (1987): Antidepressants in the treatment of cancer pain. A survey in Italy. Pain 29:347–353.

Max MB (1994): Antidepressants as analgesics. In Fields HL, Liebeskind JC (eds): *Progress in Pain Research and Management*, Vol. 1. Seattle: IASP Press, pp. 229–246.

Max MB, Zeigler D, Shoaf SE, Craig E, Benjamin J, Li SH, Buzzanelli C, Perez M, Ghosh BC (1992): Effects of a single oral dose of desipramine on postoperative morphine analgesia. J Pain Symptom Manag 7:454–462.

McQuay H, Carroll D, Jadad AR, Wiffen P, Moore A (1995): Anticonvulsant drugs for management of pain: a systematic review. Br Med J 311:1047–1052.

McQuay HJ, Tramer M, Nye BA, Carroll D, Wiffen PJ, Moore RA (1996): A systematic review of antidepressants in neuropathic pain. Pain 68:217–227.

Mestre C, Hernandez A, Eschalier A, Pelissier T (1997): Effects of clomipramine and desipramine on a C-fiber reflex in rats. Eur J Pharmacol 335:1–8.

Meyers C (1985): L'associaton mélitrancène-flupentixol: bistouri chimique ou outil d'estompage de la douleur chronique. Méd Hygiène 43:630–634.

Mjellem N, Lund A, Hole K (1993): Reduction of NMDA-induced behaviour after acute and chronic administration of desipramine in mice. Neuropharmacology 32:591–595.

Muthal AV, Chopde CT (1993): Modification of tricyclic antidepressant analgesia by calcium channel blockers. Indian J Physiol Pharmacol 37:238–240.

Naguib M and Yaksh TL (1994): Antinociceptive effects of spinal cholinesterase inhibition and isobolographic analysis of the interaction with μ and α_2 receptor systems. Anesthesiology 80:1338–1348.

Nobili R, Corli O, Romandi C, Bracco S, Panerai AE (1987): Clomipramine and baclofen in voluntary abortion analgesia: a placebo controlled study. Pain(Suppl 4):S48.

Ogren SO, Holm AC (1980): Test-specific effects of the 5-HT re-uptake inhibitors alaprociate and zimelidine on pain sensitivity and morphine analgesia. J Neural Transm 392:135–140.

Onghena P, Van Houdenhove B (1992): Antidepressant-induced analgesia in chronic non-malignant pain: a meta-analysis of 39 placebo-controlled studies. Pain 49:205–219.

Opavsky J, Kvapilova P, Jezdinsky J (1993): Antinociceptive and antiedematous effects of the combination of antidepressant drug and calcium channel blockers on the rat model of inflammation. Homeostasis 34:219–220.

Paoli F, Farcourt G, Cossa P (1960): Note préliminaire sur l'action de l'imipramine dans les états douloureux. Rev Neurol 102:503–504.

Portenoy RK, Rapscak S, Kanner W (1984): Letter to editor. Pain 144:566–569.

Post C, Archer T (1990): Interactions between 5-HT and noradrenaline in analgesia. In Besson JM (ed): *Serotonin and Pain*. Amsterdam: Elsevier, pp. 153–173.

Reynolds IJ, Miller RJ (1988): Tricyclic antidepressants block N-methyl-D-aspartate receptors: similarities to the action of zinc. Br J Pharmacol 95:95–102.

Richardson W, Williams AC (1993): Meta-analysis of antidepressant-induced analgesia in chronic pain: comment (letter comment). Pain 52:247–249.

Sacerdote P, Brini A, Mantegazza P, Panerai AE (1987): A role of serotonin and beta-endorphin in the analgesia induced by some tricyclic antidepressant drugs. Pharmacol Biochem Behav 26:153–158.

Sawynok J, Reid A (1992): Noradrenergic mediation of spinal antinociception by 5-hydroxytryptamine: characterization of receptor subtypes. Eur J Pharmacol 223: 49–56.

Sawynok J, Reid A (1996): Interaction of descending serotonergic system with other neurotransmitters in the modulation of nociception. Behav Brain Res 73:63–68.

Schreiber S, Backer MM, Yanai J, Pick CG (1996): The antinociceptive effect of fluvoxamine. Eur Neuropsychopharmacol 6:281–284.

Segawa T, Kuruma IK (1968): The influence of drugs on the uptake of 5-hydroxytryptamine by nerve-ending particles of rabbit brain stem. J Pharm Pharmacol 20:320–322.

Seltzer Z, Tal M, Sharav Y (1989): Autotomy behavior in rats following peripheral deafferentation is suppressed by daily injections of amitriptyline, diazepam and saline. Pain 37:245–250.

Sethy VH, Pradhan RJ, Mandrekar SS, Shetu UK (1970): Role of catecholamines in morphine and meperidine analgesia. Indian J Med Res 58:1453–1458.

Sierralta F, Pinardi G, Miranda HF (1995): Effect of p-chlorophenylalanine and alpha-methyltyrosine on the antinociceptive effect of antidepressant drugs. Pharmacol Toxicol 77:276–280.

Sills MA, Loo PS (1989): Tricyclic antidepressants and dextromethorphan bind with higher affinity to the phencyclidine receptor in the absence of magnesium and L-glutamate. Mol Pharm 36:160–165.

Skolnick P, Layer RT, Popik P, Nowak G, Paul IA, Trullas R (1996): Adaptation of N-methyl-D-aspartate (NMDA) receptors following antidepressant treatment: implications for the pharmacotherapy of depression. Pharmacopsychiatry 29:23–26.

Somoza E, Galindo A, Bazan E, Guillamon A, Valencia A, Fuentes JA (1981): Antidepressants inhibit enkephalin binding to synaptosome-enriched fractions of rat brain. Neuropsychobiology 7:297–301.

Svensson BE, Werkman TR, Rogawski MA (1994): Alaproclate effects on voltage-dependent K+ channels and NMDA receptors: studies in cultured rat hippocampal neurons and fibroblast cells transformed with Kv1.2 K+ channel cDNA. Neuropharmacology 33:795–804.

Turkington RW (1980): Depression masquerading as diabetic neuropathy. J Am Med Assoc 243:1147–1150.

Valverde O, Mico JA, Maldonado R, Mellado M, Gibert-Rahola J (1994): Participation of opioid and monoaminergic mechanisms on the antinociceptive effect induced by tricyclic antidepressants in two behavioural pain tests in mice. Prog Neuro-Psychopharmacol Biol Psychiat 18:1073–1092.

Walsh TD (1983): Antidepressants in chronic pain. Clin Neuropharmacol 6:271–295.

Wananukul W, Keyler DE, Pentel PR (1996): Effect of calcium chloride and 4-aminopyridine therapy on desipramine toxicity in rats. J Toxicol Clin Toxicol 34: 499–506.

Wilkinson A, Courtney M, Westlind-Danielsson A, Hallnemo G, Akerman KE (1994): Alaproclade acts as a potent, reversible and noncompetitive antagonist of the NMDA receptor coupled ion flow. J Pharmacol Exp Ther 271:1314–1319.

Willer JC, Roby A, Gerard A, Maulet C (1982): Electrophysiological evidence for a possible serotonergic involvement in some endogenous opiate activity in humans. Eur J Pharmacol 78:117–120.

CHAPTER 16

VOLTAGE-GATED ION CHANNEL MODULATORS

JOHN C. HUNTER
Roche Bioscience
Palo Alto, California

Voltage-gated ion channels play a fundamental role in the control of neuronal excitability throughout the peripheral and central nervous systems. The principal types of voltage-gated ion channel performing this essential function, sodium, calcium, and potassium, in each case represent one or more large, multigene families encoding a variety of subtypes with diverse biophysical and pharmacological properties and are expressed in a tissue- and often cell-dependent manner (for reviews see Catterall, 1992, 1995; Pongs, 1992; Kallen et al., 1993; Reuter, 1996). The selective expression of specific combinations of channel subtypes or subunits plays a fundamental role in determining the heterogeneity and functional specialization of many types of cells, particularly neurons. The relative importance of voltage-gated ion channels to normal cell physiology is illustrated by the number of diseases, some quite debilitating and even fatal, that are caused by defects in ion channel function (Ackerman and Clapham, 1997).

Alterations in voltage-gated ion channel expression and/or function can have a profound influence on the firing properties of primary afferent as well as central neurons and, consequently, may contribute to many types of chronic, abnormal pain syndromes. Such changes have been suggested, for example, to contribute to the ongoing, abnormal repetitive discharge from ectopic sites established within primary afferent neurons following injury (reviewed by Devor, 1994). The barrage of spontaneous and/or evoked afferent impulse traffic then precipitates a process of central sensitization involving increased neuronal excitability and synaptic reorganization within the spinal dorsal horn (Devor, 1994; Woolf and Doubell, 1994). Such alterations in peripheral and central

---

Novel Aspects of Pain Management: Opioids and Beyond, Edited by Jana Sawynok and Alan Cowan
ISBN 0-471-180173 Copyright © 1999 by Wiley-Liss, Inc.

neuronal function are believed to underlie the paresthesias and pain associated with either nerve or soft tissue injury.

A prominent role for voltage-gated ion channels in the pathophysiology of an injured neuron is supported by the clinical effectiveness of agents that act primarily through a common, use-dependent block of sodium channels, that is, local anesthetics, antiarrhythmics, and anticonvulsants (Catterall, 1987), in the treatment of many types of chronic and, in particular, neuropathic pains (Backonja, 1994; Tanelian and Victory, 1995). However, membrane events that play a role in the redistribution of sodium channels clearly can also cause alterations in the localization and distribution of other membrane-bound voltage-gated ion channels, particularly calcium and potassium channels, that could contribute to the establishment and maintenance of the neuronal hyperexcitability (Devor, 1994). Modulation of the function or distribution of these additional channels, therefore, also has the potential for providing novel agents for the treatment of chronic pain.

SODIUM CHANNELS

In excitable tissue such as nerve and muscle, voltage-gated sodium channels (VGSCs), located in the plasma membrane, permit entry of sodium ions into the cell causing depolarization and generation of the action potential (Catterall, 1992; Kallen et al., 1993). This control of membrane excitability is mediated by the tissue-dependent expression of distinct genes encoding individual VGSC subtypes that have been distinguished on the basis of primary structure but can also be differentiated by their biophysical properties and sensitivity to the neurotoxin tetrodotoxin (TTX). Most VGSCs are characterized by rapid inactivation kinetics and low, nanomolar sensitivity to TTX: rat brain types I, IIA and III, skeletal muscle type I (μI) (Catterall, 1992; Kallen et al., 1993) and the recently described novel channels, sodium channel protein 6 (SCP6; Schaller et al., 1995), the closely homologous peripheral nerve 4 (PN4; Dietrich et al., 1998) and peripheral nerve 1 (PN1; Sangameswaran et al., 1997; Toledo-Aral et al., 1997); the last-named appears to be the rodent orthologue of the human neuroendocrine channel. However, more persistent sodium currents with slower inactivation kinetics have also been described, specifically in heart and sensory ganglia. The cardiac channel (H1; Catterall, 1992; Kallen et al., 1993) exhibits low, micromolar (1–5 μM) sensitivity to TTX, whereas the recently described novel channel cloned from rat dorsal root ganglion (DRG), termed either peripheral nerve 3 (PN3; Sangameswaran et al., 1996) or sensory nerve specific (SNS; Akopian et al., 1996), is TTX-resistant ($\sim$100 μM).

In many chronic pain syndromes, especially of neuropathic origin, a major contributing factor to the initiation and maintenance of the ectopic, repetitive firing capability of primary afferent fibers following injury appears to be a redistribution of sodium channels along injured or regenerating axons resulting in an abnormal accumulation and increased membrane density of sodium channels at focal sites of injury, that is, neuroma end bulbs or at sites of demyelination (Devor et al., 1993; England et al., 1996a). This membrane remodeling contributes to a lower threshold for action potential generation at these sites and, consequently, precipitates ectopic impulse generation in a chronically injured nerve (Wall and Devor, 1983; Matzner and Devor, 1994; Devor, 1994). Mathematical modeling by Devor and colleagues led to the proposal that the changes in membrane hyperexcitability could be solely accounted for by the increase in sodium channel density (Matzner and Devor, 1992). Consistent with this hypothesis has been the observation that interruption of fast axonal transport decreases ectopic impulse generation in injured peripheral nerves without blocking nerve conduction (Devor and Govrin-Lippmann, 1983). Alterations in either the level of expression or distribution of sodium channels within the injured nerve therefore have a major influence on the pathophysiology of pain associated with this type of trauma. This concept is supported by numerous pharmacological studies involving the use of sodium channel modulating agents in animal models and in the clinic.

Local Anesthetics

Although local anesthetics have traditionally been used to abolish pain by blocking nerve conduction, an expanded role of local anesthetics as analgesics per se is now accepted as an effective form of treatment for many chronic and, to a much lesser extent, acute pain conditions (Backonja, 1994; Tanelian and Victory, 1995).

In acute pain, the use of local anesthetics has been restricted primarily due to equivocal efficacy (Cassuto et al., 1985; Birch et al., 1987) and safety concerns over potential central nervous system (CNS) and cardiac toxicity that may be precipitated by the need to achieve target plasma concentrations rapidly in order to produce an adequate analgesic effect during the postoperative period. However, there is an emerging appreciation for the ability of these agents to provide preemptive analgesia at low, nontoxic, systemic concentrations in order to limit any potential hypersensitivity reaction to surgery (Woolf and Chong, 1993). Local anesthetics have been shown to be effective in the treatment of cancer pain (Ellemann et al., 1989; Brose and Cousins, 1991; Bruera et al., 1992) and in many chronic, nonmalignant pain states including adiposis dolorosa (Atkinson, 1982; Petersen and Kastrup, 1987) and migraine headaches (Kaube et al., 1994; Maizels et al., 1996). However, despite reports of successful treatment, the universal impression has been that local anesthetics have questionable efficacy and marginal safety and are therefore not generally regarded as a serious analgesic alternative for these types of pain.

This can be sharply contrasted with the potential of these agents as effective therapies for a variety of chronic neuropathic pain syndromes, particularly because many of these conditions are unresponsive to treatment with standard opioids and nonsteroidal anti-inflammatory drugs (Backonja, 1994; Tanelian and Victory, 1995). However, although there are many clinical studies and case reports on the analgesic effectiveness of local anesthetics, only a comparatively small number involve randomized, single- or double-blind, placebo-controlled trials (see review by Kingery, 1997). The types of chronic neuropathic pain syndromes reported to be successfully treated by local anesthetics include painful diabetic polyneuropathy (Kastrup et al., 1987; Dejgard et al., 1988; Bach et al., 1990), neuralgic pain (Lindstrom and Lindblom, 1987; Rowbotham et al., 1991, 1995; Marchettini et al., 1992), lumbar radiculopathies (Nagaro et al., 1995; Ferrante et al., 1996), and peripheral nerve injury (Tanelian and Brose, 1991; Chabal et al., 1992a,b; Galer et al., 1996). In addition to some of the conditions listed above, two retrospective studies of large patient groups found local anesthetics provided partial to good relief of pain associated with reflex sympathetic dystrophy (Edwards et al., 1985; Galer et al., 1993). As a general rule, it would appear that these agents are more effective against neuropathic pain originating in the peripheral nervous system than in the CNS. Central pain conditions following stroke, thalamic lesions, and multiple sclerosis have responded to local anesthetics but with a much more mixed degree of success when compared to the peripheral neuropathies (Awerbuch and Sandyk, 1990; Backonja and Gombar, 1992; Edmondson et al., 1993).

Of the local anesthetics investigated, by far the most prevalent agent used is intravenous lidocaine which, in addition to the routine acute effect, has been reported to produce pain relief, in some cases for several days, an effect that far outlasts drug elimination from the plasma (Petersen et al., 1986; Arner et al., 1990; Bach et al., 1990). The mechanism(s) related to this phenomenon is (are) presently unknown. Other local anesthetics that have been used include flecainide (Sinnott et al., 1991) and the oral agents tocainide (Lindstrom and Lindblom, 1987) and mexiletine, the type Ib antiarrhythymic agent (Dejgard et al., 1988; Chabal et al., 1992a). Mexiletine, in particular, has been used relatively successfully either as a monotherapy or sequentially following an initial lidocaine infusion. Indeed, intravenous lidocaine has been advocated increasingly as a diagnostic aid for the presence of pain associated with nerve injury (Marchettini et al., 1992), and as a predictor of potential analgesic efficacy of oral local anesthetic agents such as mexiletine for follow up therapy (Tanelian and Brose, 1991; Galer et al., 1996).

However, despite producing varying degrees of relief in many different types of chronic pain, the full analgesic potential of these agents has been frequently limited by the onset of numerous adverse side effects. Many of these clinical signs are CNS-related and thus lead to restricted patient tolerability and, therefore, restricted use over a long-term period. Side effects commonly reported include nausea and emesis, dizziness and lightheadedness, somnolence, ataxia, and tinnitus. Cardiotoxicity can also be problematic, particularly in the elderly population (Covino and Wildsmith, 1998).

In animal models of neuropathic pain, the local anesthetics appear to have a profile similar to that reported clinically. In the two most rigorously tested animal models available, the chronic constriction injury to the sciatic nerve (CCI) (Bennett and Xie, 1988) and the spinal nerve (L5/L6) ligation model

(Kim and Chung, 1992), local anesthetics are effective against both mechanical and thermal hyperalgesia and tactile and cold allodynia but with differential sensitivity and limited efficacy (Abram and Yaksh, 1994; Hedley et al., 1995; Koch et al., 1996; Gogas et al., 1997; Jett et al., 1997). In most cases, a ceiling to the degree of analgesic effect was observed, this being almost always the result of the appearance of side effects, that is, sedation and loss of righting reflex and, at high doses, convulsions, that limited further escalation of the dose. In another model representative of facilitated processing of sensory information, the formalin test, lidocaine (Abram and Yaksh, 1994) and mexiletine (Jett et al., 1997) attenuated both phases of the behavioral response. Interestingly, at much higher doses than those observed to diminish the hyperesthetic state following a peripheral nerve injury, lidocaine and mexiletine are ineffective against an acute, high threshold thermal noxious stimulus in the rat tail flick test (Hedley et al., 1995). Such a profile might be considered to be consistent with the predicted use-dependent nature of the sodium channel block produced by these agents. Moreover, a critical aspect of this analgesic action is the ability, at these low subanesthetic concentrations, to block spontaneous and/or evoked afferent activity (impulse initiation) without affecting nerve conduction (impulse propagation) (Chabal et al., 1989; Devor et al., 1992; Matzner and Devor, 1994). Consequently, these agents are able to target injured nerves on the basis of their high frequency, repetitive firing characteristics while having minimal impact on normal, somatosensory (i.e., nociceptive) neuronal function.

As a therapeutic class, local anesthetics are therefore capable of achieving a reasonable degree of relief in the treatment of many intractable pain states. However, optimal clinical performance is restricted by the prevalence of side effects, many of which are CNS related, that in most cases lead to a significant reduction in patient tolerability and ultimately withdrawal/transferral to other forms of treatment or, in the more extreme cases, surgery.

Anticonvulsants

In 1885, Trousseau noted that the paroxysmal component of trigeminal neuralgia was remarkably similar to epilepsy and termed it "epileptiform neuralgia" (for review see Swerdlow, 1984). This early observation was then followed by successful trials of novel anticonvulsant therapies as they became available, including diphenylhydantoin (or phenytoin) (Bergouignan, 1942) and carbamazepine (Blom, 1962). Anticonvulsant drugs have subsequently remained amongst the more commonly used pharmacological interventions for the treatment of chronic pain (Swerdlow, 1984; McQuay et al., 1995).

It has been a common perception, possibly influenced by these early reports, that drugs of this class provide effective and sustained relief *only* when there is a paroxysmal, lancinating component to the pain, for example, trigeminal neuralgia (Campbell et al., 1966; Killian and Fromm, 1968). Although neuralgic pain remains a primary indication, review of the literature finds that carbamazepine and, to a more variable extent, phenytoin can also be effective analgesics in other types of painful, peripheral neuropathies such as diabetic neuropathy (Rull et al., 1969; Saudek et al., 1977; Chadda and Mathur, 1978). In central pain, however, carbamazepine does not appear to be significantly better than placebo (Leijon and Boivie, 1989). Moreover, in many of the studies involving peripheral nerve injury, the general clinical impression was that pain relief was almost always obtained concomitantly with numerous adverse side effects (Campbell et al., 1966; Killian and Fromm, 1968; Rull et al., 1969) and/or limitations in efficacy (Killian and Fromm, 1968; Saudek et al., 1977). The adverse side effect profile of these anticonvulsants can be severe and frequently includes CNS effects such as dizziness, ataxia, lightheadedness, somnolence, and alterations in mood. Hepatic dysfunction and leukopenia have also been reported to occur with carbamazepine.

The questionable analgesic efficacy of phenytoin and, to a lesser extent, carbamazepine, at doses not associated with side effects, is also a consistent observation in most experimental animal models of peripheral nerve injury (Koch et al., 1996) and inflammation (Nakamura-Craig and Follenfant, 1995). Because the use-dependent block of sodium channels produced by both drugs is analogous to that obtained with the local anesthetics, it has been proposed that these inconsistencies may be related to the manner in which these drugs bind to the sodium channel (Kuo and Bean, 1994; Kuo et al., 1997). Relative to the local anesthetics, both drugs (but particularly phenytoin) require a sustained membrane depolarization in order to bind with optimal affinity to the fast inactivated state of the sodium channel. Such a state of sustained depolarization may be achieved only during abnormal neuronal discharges of the intensity and duration often associated with certain types of epilepsy but not peripheral nerve injury (Kuo and Bean, 1994; Kuo et al., 1997).

Recent years have seen the emergence of several novel anti-epileptic agents, exemplified by lamotrigine (Lamictal®; Fitton and Goa, 1995), that may also have utility in the treatment of chronic pain but with an improved therapeutic window over the established drugs. Lamotrigine produces a voltage- and frequency-dependent block of sodium channels leading to stabilization of neuronal membrane excitability. Subsequent alterations in the presynaptic release of the excitatory amino acids, glutamate and aspartate, have been suggested to contribute to the anticonvulsant action and may therefore also play a role in an analgesic effect (Leach et al., 1986; Cheung et al., 1992).

Lamotrigine has been tested in only a limited number of clinical studies but has been reported to show a promising analgesic effect. In a controlled trial of trigeminal neuralgia patients refractory to carbamazepine and phenytoin, lamotrigine provided pain relief but at doses accompanied by adverse, predominantly CNS, experiences (Zakrzewska et al., 1997). In an open label case series of patients with diabetic neuropathy (Eisenberg et al., 1996), and either postherpetic neuralgia, causalgia, or phantom limb pain (Harbison et al., 1997), lamotrigine also provided effective pain relief but with minimal, significant adverse side effects. In rodents, lamotrigine has been tested in models of both neuropathic and inflammatory pain with equivocal success. In rat sciatic nerve injury models, lamotrigine produced a reversal of cold allodynia but was ineffective against tactile allodynia (Hunter et al., 1997). In two inflammatory pain models, lamotrigine reversed both prostaglandin E_2 and streptozotocin-induced mechanical hyperalgesia (Nakamura-Craig and Follenfant, 1995). Lamotrigine, however, had a negligible effect against acute, high-threshold noxious stimuli; that is, it was inactive in the rat tail immersion test at 52°C (Hunter et al., 1997). This would imply a selective interaction with pathways associated with pathophysiological events rather than with normal sensory nociceptive function, which would be consistent with its use-dependent block of sodium channels.

The overall profile of newer anti-epileptic drugs such as lamotrigine suggest, therefore, that these agents could provide an effective alternative to current therapies, including the established anticonvulsants carbamazepine and phenytoin, for neuropathic pain. An additional advantage of these drugs is the potential for an improved margin of safety, despite the possible need for higher doses than those required for anti-convulsant activity.

Peripheral Neuron-Specific Sodium Channels

Several lines of evidence suggest that sodium channels located in the peripheral, sensory neuron may play an important role, not only in the initial injury discharge, but also in spontaneous, ongoing, and stimulus-evoked pain and dysesthesias characteristic of many types of peripheral neuropathies. Targeting these peripheral channels, therefore, may provide a novel opportunity for producing an analgesic with an improved therapeutic window.

In clinical studies, lidocaine applied topically to either the skin (Rowbotham et al., 1995), the region of the nerve supplying the painful foci (Arner et al., 1990; Gracely et al., 1992; Koltzenburg et al., 1994) or the neuroma (Chabal et al., 1992b), produces complete relief of spontaneous, ongoing, and stimulus-evoked pain. Moreover, in animal models of inflammatory and neuropathic pain, respectively, local application of bupivacaine produces a reversal of mechanical hyperalgesia (Fletcher et al., 1997) and allodynia (Yoon et al., 1996). Following sciatic nerve transection in an anesthetized rat, either systemic (Chabal et al., 1989; Devor et al., 1992) or perineuromal (Matzner and Devor, 1994) application of subanesthetic doses of lidocaine silences the ectopic discharge recorded from the nerve-end neuroma. Similarly, systemic administration of QX-314, the quaternarized derivative of lidocaine, reduces ectopic neuronal activity emanating from the neuroma and DRG at doses considerably below those required to affect spinal dorsal horn neuron hyperexcitability (Omana-Zapata et al., 1997a). In conscious animals, QX-314, at doses shown not to penetrate the CNS, produced an anti-allodynic effect in the CCI model on days 3–5 of chronic twice-daily dosing that was comparable to the near-maximal effect of acutely administered lidocaine (Hunter et al., 1995). These studies would suggest, therefore, that in chronic pain of inflammatory or neuropathic origin where there is nociceptor-modulated central sensitization, sustained blockade of peripheral sodium channels may cause wind-down of neuronal hyperexcitability and subsequently produce analgesia.

A potential novel approach, therefore, has been to target individual VGSC sub-types that may be either specific to sensory, nociceptive neurons (Akopian et al., 1996; Sangameswaran et al., 1996) or selectively regulated (Waxman et al., 1994) in response to a peripheral nerve injury. DRG neurons are a heterogeneous population of cells expressing multiple sodium channel genes and both the rapidly inactivating, TTX-sensitive (TTX-S I_{Na}) and the more slowly inactivating, TTX-resistant (TTX-R I_{Na}) sodium currents (Roy and Narahashi, 1992; Elliott and Elliott, 1993; Ogata and Tatebayashi, 1993). The relative proportions of these sodium currents in individual DRG neurons determine the wide range of firing behaviors and, consequently, functional properties of these cells. TTX-S currents are the predominant I_{Na} in all types of DRG cells at all stages of development and have been found to be the main, if not sole, I_{Na} associated with the large-diameter, fast-conducting, myelinated Aβ fibers (Roy and Narahashi, 1992; Elliott and Elliott, 1993; Rizzo et al., 1994). However, it has not yet been established which sodium channels are the predominant mediators of TTX-S I_{Na}, as several α-subunits are known to be expressed in DRG neurons: brain types I, IIA, and III, glial, and atypical (Black et al., 1996; Sangameswaran et al., 1996), PN1/hNE (Sangameswaran et al., 1997; Toledo-Aral et al., 1997) and SCP6/PN4 (Schaller et al., 1995; Dietrich et al., 1998). In comparison, in the adult DRG, TTX-R I_{Na} appears to have a more restricted distribution, appearing predominantly in a subpopulation of small-diameter, unmyelinated, capsaicin-sensitive neurons, otherwise referred to as C fibers or nociceptors (Roy and Narahashi, 1992; Elliott and Elliott, 1993; Arbuckle and Docherty, 1995). The slow inactivation and rapid repriming properties of TTX-R I_{Na} appear particularly well suited to sustained firing at the depolarized potentials characteristic of an injured peripheral nerve (Elliott and Elliott, 1993; Elliott, 1997). Moreover, to date, only the PN3/SNS α-subunit has been identified, displaying these distinct kinetics, resistance to TTX and discrete localization (Akopian et al., 1996; Sangameswaran et al., 1996).

At present it is not clear what the relative contributions of TTX-S and TTX-R sodium channels are toward either normal, sensory nociceptive function or altered processing of sensory input into the spinal dorsal horn following a peripheral nerve or tissue injury. In response to transection of the sciatic nerve, TTX has been shown to eliminate ectopic nerve activity recorded from the neuroma or DRG following either topical application directly onto the surface of the neuroma (Matzner and Devor, 1994) or via systemic administration (Omana-Zapata et al., 1997b). Moreover, DRG cell bodies expressing both TTX-S and TTX-R under normal conditions appear to exhibit a shift in kinetics to a predominantly, rapidly activating and inactivating TTX-S I_{Na} following axotomy (Rizzo et al., 1995). This phenotypic switch has been attributed to changes in the level of mRNA expression of specific sodium channels with an upregulation in brain type III (Waxman et al., 1994) and a downregulation in PN3/SNS (Dib-Hajj et al., 1996).

By comparison, the selective expression of TTX-R I_{Na} and, coincidentally, PN3/SNS, in a specific subpopulation of capsaicin-sensitive, primary afferent neurons suggests that this channel may also be of particular importance in the regulation of sensory, nociceptive function. Stimulation of unmyelinated, C-fiber afferent input into the spinal dorsal horn is not blocked by TTX (Jeftinija, 1994). In addition, the more rapid repriming kinetics of TTX-R I_{Na}, indicative of a rapid recovery from inactivation, suggest that cells expressing a large proportion of TTX-R sodium channels should be ideally suited to sustain repetitive firing of the peripheral neuron in response to injury; that is, they will be slowly adapting in response to a persistent, depolarizing stimulus (Elliott and Elliott, 1993). Consistent with this notion, modulation of TTX-R I_{Na} by a number of naturally occurring hyperalgesic substances, for example, PGE_2, adenosine and serotonin, has been suggested to be a mechanism that could underlie the subsequent increase in excitability and sensitization of sensory neurons mediated by these agents following a peripheral nerve or tissue injury (England et al., 1996b; Gold et al., 1996a, Cardenas et al., 1997). Furthermore, in a rat model of neuropathic pain, a redistribution of PN3/SNS protein has been shown to occur leading to intraneural channel accumulation just proximal to the site of injury (Novakovic et al., 1998). The onset and subsequent reversal of PN3/SNS channel redistribution appeared to correlate closely with temporal changes in behavioral thermal hyperalgesia and, morphologically, with the damage and recovery of primary afferent fibers following this type of nerve ligation (Coggeshall et al., 1993).

It remains to be determined whether selective blockade of PN3/SNS or, alternatively, any of the TTX-S channels in peripheral sensory neurons, will produce either an improvement in analgesic efficacy or the therapeutic window over currently available non-subtype selective agents. However, the discrete localization of PN3/SNS may be an important factor in the safety profile of drugs targeted at this channel. The more widespread distribution of the TTX-S channels identified in DRG neurons would imply that, although selective blockade of some of these channels might produce analgesia, it might possibly also affect additional motor/efferent function in a number of peripheral tissues and in the CNS.

CALCIUM CHANNELS

Voltage-gated calcium channels (VGCCs) play an important role in the regulation of many cellular and subcellular functions throughout the peripheral and central nervous systems. Calcium influx through neuronal VGCCs contributes to membrane depolarization in many excitable cells and plays a critical role in the presynaptic regulation of neurotransmitter release, second messenger signal transduction pathways, and gene transcription (for reviews see Hofmann et al.,

1994; Catterall, 1995; Miljanich and Ramachandran, 1995; Reuter, 1996). Multiple isoforms of neuronal VGCCs have been identified and distinguished on the basis of unique, primary structural features of each α_1 subunit and distinct biophysical properties. Low-voltage-activated channels, designated T-type, mediate transient calcium currents and high voltage activated channels, designated L-, N-, P-, Q-, and R-, mediate calcium currents with varying rates of inactivation depending on the composition of subunits. However, many of these VGCC subtypes are best distinguished pharmacologically, by agents that selectivity block channel function (Miljanich and Ramachandran, 1995; Reuter, 1996). For L-type channels these agents can be subdivided on the basis of chemical class into the dihydropyridines (e.g., nifedipine, nimodipine), phenylalkylamines (e.g., verapamil), and benzothiazepines (e.g., diltiazem). The N-type channel can be distinguished from other VGCCs by selective sensitivity to the ω-conotoxins GVIA and MVIIA, members of a family of polypeptides isolated from the venom of several species of the marine snail, *Conus*. P- and Q-type channels are relatively insensitive to either the dihydropyridines or conotoxins but can be distinguished on the basis of sensitivity to low (P-type) and high (Q-type) concentrations of the peptide ω-agatoxin IVA, a toxin from the funnel web spider *Agelenopsis aperta* (Miljanich and Ramachandran, 1995; Reuter, 1996).

Several lines of evidence have implicated calcium channels in the processing of acute, nociceptive information and in the pathogenesis of chronic pain. DRG cells differentially express various types of calcium current (I_{Ca}) including L-, N-, P/Q- and T-type I_{Ca} (Mintz et al., 1992; Scroggs and Fox, 1992; Cardenas et al., 1995). L- and N-type currents are expressed by all sizes of DRG cells, although their relative contribution to overall I_{Ca} appears highest in small diameter, capsaicin-sensitive, cells with the characteristics of nociceptors (Scroggs and Fox, 1992; Cardenas et al., 1995). In contrast, P- (Mintz et al., 1992) and T-type (Scroggs and Fox, 1992; Cardenas et al., 1995) currents, although present in some small-diameter cells, appear to be preferentially expressed by medium- and large-diameter, capsaicin-insensitive neurons with the overall biophysical and morphological properties consistent with Aβ fibers or non-nociceptors. In the spinal cord, L-type channels are present in the dorsal horn with a density comparable to many brain areas (Gandhi and Jones, 1988). In contrast, N-type channels appear to have a much more discrete localization with highest densities found in the superficial laminae I and II (Kerr et al., 1988; Gohil et al., 1994), the termination field of the small-diameter, primary afferent neurons. All VGCCs, however, have a widespread distribution throughout the peripheral and central nervous systems.

Although more than one type of VGCC has been identified in nociceptive pathways, the N-type VGCC has emerged as the predominant calcium channel involved in the processing of sensory, nociceptive information, particularly at the spinal level. The N-type selective inhibitors, ω-conopeptide GVIA and MVIIA, as well as numerous synthetic homologues, are antinociceptive in several animal models of acute and chronic pain (Malmberg and Yaksh,

1994, 1995). ω-Conotoxin GVIA and SNX-111, a synthetic homologue of ω-conopeptide MVIIA, produce a modest antinociceptive effect against an acute, high-threshold, thermal stimulus in the rat tail flick (Wei et al., 1996) and hot plate test (Malmberg and Yaksh, 1994, 1995), respectively. In addition to this direct antinociceptive effect, ω-conotoxin GVIA potentiates the antinociceptive response to both morphine and the α_2-agonist clonidine in the tail flick test (Wei et al., 1996). SNX-111 and various N-type selective synthetic derivatives, when administered by either acute or continuous intrathecal infusion, inhibited both the early (acute) and late (tonic) phases of flinching behavior following an intraplantar injection of formalin in the rat (Malmberg and Yaksh, 1994, 1995; Bowersox et al., 1996). In these studies, the conopeptides also produced a range of general behaviors and motor effects but at doses usually in excess of those producing antinociception and may thus be related to a nonspecific, non-N-type blocking effect. In an electrophysiological study of dorsal horn neuron activity in situ, ω-conotoxin GVIA reduced both phases of the formalin response in a manner comparable to the behavioral studies (Diaz and Dickenson, 1997). ω-Conotoxin GVIA has also been shown to reduce the excitability of dorsal horn neurons receiving either nociceptive or innocuous mechanosensory input from the knee joint, both under normal conditions and in the presence of inflammation induced by either carrageenan or kaolin (Neugebauer et al., 1996). In the rat spinal nerve (L5/L6) ligation model of neuropathic pain, SNX-111 and a close analogue, [leu10]-ω-conotoxin MVIIA (SNX-239), via continuous intrathecal administration over 7 days, reversed tactile allodynia (Chaplan et al., 1994; Bowersox et al., 1996). However, when administered intravenously or by regional application to the nerve, neither agent was effective (Chaplan et al., 1994). In rats with a CCI sciatic nerve injury, bolus administration of SNX-111 and SNX-124 (a synthetic homologue of ω-conopeptide GVIA), applied directly to the site of injury via chronically implanted perineural cannulae, reduced thermal hyperalgesia and mechano-allodynia but not mechanical hyperalgesia (Xiao and Bennett, 1995).

SNX-111 is currently undergoing clinical trials for the treatment of chronic malignant and nonmalignant pain. In an open label feasibility study of 31 patients, SNX-111, administered intrathecally, has been reported to produce partial to complete pain relief in a patient population previously found to be opioid-resistant (Brose et al., 1996). The pain syndromes included cancer and AIDS pain, phantom limb pain, postherpetic neuralgia, spinal cord injury, and thalamic pain. The most commonly reported side effects were (in order of prevalence): nausea, dizziness and lightheadednesss, headache, constipation, confusion, and nystagmus. Orthostatic hypotension without reflex tachycardia has also been noted within the analgesic dose range (Bowersox and Luther, 1994).

It would appear from both the preclinical and clinical data that although N-type VGCC antagonists, like SNX-111, may be analgesic, they may also have a relatively narrow therapeutic window. As with some of the sodium channel blockers, many of the side effects are CNS related and are likely due to the widespread localization of N-type calcium channels in the peripheral and central nervous systems. However, a peripheral VGCC N-type isoform with some distinct structural and functional characteristics was recently discovered in the superior cervical ganglion (Lin et al., 1997). If this discovery indicates the existence of additional N-channel subtypes that may be selectively expressed in, for example, sensory systems, then it may provide the opportunity for drug targeting in the search for analgesics with an improved side-effect profile.

In comparison to the N-type VGCC, evidence in support of an antinociceptive effect mediated through a selective block of the L-type VGCC has been more limited and controversial. In the rodent hot plate or tail flick test of acute, thermal nociception, L-type VGCC antagonists, when administered alone, do not display any significant antinociception (Miranda et al., 1992; Omote et al., 1993; Hodoglugil et al., 1996). However, many of these agents potentiate the antinociception produced in these tests by either morphine or clonidine (Omote et al., 1993; Hodoglugil et al., 1996; Wei et al., 1996). In a postoperative pain study in patients, nifedipine, administered sublingually, potentiated the analgesic effect of epidural morphine (Pereira et al., 1993). Furthermore, nimodipine has enhanced opiate analgesia in cancer patients (Santillan et al., 1994), although this evidence has been challenged (Roca et al., 1996). In contrast to the effect on the opioid system, L-type antagonists attenuate the acute antinociceptive response to a variety of cholinomimetic agents (nicotine, epibatidine, oxotremorine, physostigmine) acting through either nicotinic or muscarinic receptors (Damaj et al., 1993; Pavone et al., 1993; Bannon et al., 1995).

L-type VGCC antagonists have been found to be intrinsically antinociceptive when administered systemically under conditions of both acute inflammation in the acetic acid induced abdominal constriction test (Miranda et al., 1992) and in the formalin model of acute, persistent nociception (Coderre and Melzack, 1992; Miranda et al., 1992). However, the latter observations are controversial, as both behavioral (Malmberg and Yaksh, 1994) and electrophysiological (Diaz and Dickenson, 1997) studies have found intraspinal administration of L-type antagonists to be ineffective in the formalin test. Furthermore, in models of peripheral nerve injury, L-type antagonists appear universally ineffective at modulating either the spontaneous discharge recorded from a sciatic neuroma (Matzner and Devor, 1994) or the tactile allodynic behavioral response to tight ligation of spinal nerves L5 and L6 (Chaplan et al., 1994).

In contrast to the N- and L-types of VGCC, very little information is available on the potential involvement of other VGCCs in the control of nociceptive transmission. The P/Q type channel blocker, ω-agatoxin IVA, appears to have no effect in acute tests of nociception such as rat hot plate (Malmberg and Yaksh, 1994). However, behavioral and electrophysiological studies have demonstrated ω-agatoxin IVA selective attenuation of the late, tonic phase in the formalin test of acute, persistent nociception. This suggests a potential role for the P/Q channel in facilitated, rather than acute, processing of nociceptive information in the spinal cord (Malmberg and Yaksh, 1994; Diaz and Dickenson,

1997). ω-Agatoxin IVA, however, had no effect on tactile allodynia in a peripheral neuropathy model (Chaplan et al., 1994).

In conclusion, in primarily animal models of neuropathic pain and inflammation, N-type channel blockers appear capable of producing effective analgesia at a spinal level but may have to operate within a relatively narrow therapeutic window. It will therefore be interesting to observe clinically whether direct, intrathecal application of a drug, like SNX-111, to the potential target site of action in the spinal cord, at doses sufficient to cause a sustained analgesic effect, will enable a suitable therapeutic window to be achieved. The therapeutic potential of L-type VGCC antagonists appears to be extremely limited but may find use as a combination therapy with morphine. The P-type VGCC may also have potential, but from a future perspective, for this will depend largely on the development of selective, nontoxin antagonists for this type of channel.

POTASSIUM CHANNELS

In contrast to the evidence in support of sodium and calcium channels, comparatively little is known about potassium channels as a potential target for the development of novel analgesics. This might be considered surprising because the role of potassium channels in the control of membrane excitability is as well established as that of the other types of voltage-gated channels (Pongs, 1992; Catterall, 1995; Kaczorowski et al., 1996; Isomoto et al., 1997). Potassium channel activation in the cell membrane allows potassium ions to move out of the cell, causing membrane repolarization and after-hyperpolarization, and therefore plays an integral role in setting the firing rhythm of the cell. Consequently, potassium currents (I_K) have a major impact on spike repolarization and interspike interval as well as burst adaptation. Several members of the potassium channel family have been identified and can be differentiated on the basis of voltage dependency, kinetics, calcium dependency, and pharmacology (Cook, 1988; Rudy, 1988; Pongs, 1992; Catterall, 1995; Kaczorowski et al., 1996). The main types of voltage-sensitive potassium channels include those mediating a transient, rapidly inactivating A-type current $I_{K(A)}$ and a family of delayed rectifiers mediating currents characterized by delayed activation and slowed inactivation, $I_{K(V)}$, although several variants of each have been identified (Pongs, 1992). The major Ca^{2+}-activated potassium channel is a voltage-dependent, large conductance channel termed maxi K or BK (Kaczorowski et al., 1996). Finally, there is a superfamily of voltage-insensitive, inwardly rectifying potassium channels mediating a series of inward currents activated either by hyperpolarization (K_{IR}) or regulated by a variety of G-protein-coupled inhibitory neurotransmitter receptors (K_G), ATP (K_{ATP}) or sodium (K_{Na}) (Isomoto et al., 1997).

Cutaneous primary afferent neurons heterogeneously express both transient and sustained voltage-gated potassium currents, as well as the major Ca^{2+}-dependent BK current, each identified on the basis of distinct biophysical and pharmacological features. In adult DRG neurons, an A-type current (I_A) sensitive to 4-aminopyridine (4-AP) and tetraethylammonium (TEA) is preferentially expressed in the small diameter, capsaicin-sensitive cells referred to as nociceptors (Akins and McCleskey, 1993; Pearce and Duchen, 1994; Gold et al., 1996b). However, additional A-type currents have also been reported from adult DRG neurons that display either slower inactivation kinetics or insensitivity to TEA when compared to the predominant I_A (Gold et al., 1996b). Interestingly, the TEA insensitive $I_{K(Af)}$ was found to be exclusively expressed by large-diameter DRG cells that would correspond to Aβ fibers or non-nociceptors (Gold et al., 1996b). At least three types of sustained, delayed rectifier $I_{K(V)}$ and a Ca^{2+}-activated BK current have also been recorded from DRG cells. Although each of these currents is found in all categories of DRG neurons, most have a higher frequency of expression in the small-diameter, capsaicin-sensitive, nociceptors (Akins and McCleskey, 1993; Gold et al., 1996b). In addition to the voltage-sensitive currents, two types of voltage-insensitive, inwardly rectifying currents have been described in DRG neurons (Scroggs et al., 1994). I_H and I_{IR}, appear to be preferentially expressed by large- and medium-diameter cells, respectively, which were insensitive to capsaicin and regarded to be non-nociceptors (Scroggs et al., 1994; Cardenas et al., 1995).

The preferential expression of specific categories of potassium currents in subpopulations of DRG neurons may be important from several perspectives. It suggests that certain types of voltage-sensitive potassium channels could play an important role in the functional diversity of primary afferent neurons, particularly adaptive responses to nerve or tissue injury. This was illustrated by the increase in either the spontaneous firing of active fibers or in the recruitment of quiescent fibers caused by the voltage-sensitive potassium channel blockers TEA and, to a more variable extent, 4-AP, in a sciatic (Matzner and Devor, 1994) or saphenous (Burchiel and Russell, 1985) neuroma. In a rat saphenous nerve-skin in vitro preparation, 4-AP and TEA also induced bursting discharges in all fiber types (e.g., C, Aδ, and Aβ) of cutaneous primary afferent neurons by an action at or near the action potential generator region at the nerve terminal (Kirchhoff et al., 1992). In conscious animals, however, evidence for the involvement of voltage-sensitive potassium channels in the transmission of nociceptive information has been limited to a few studies of acute nociception.

TEA and 4-AP have been shown to block the antinociceptive effect of the GABA$_B$ agonist, baclofen, but appear ineffective against either μ-opioid or α$_2$-agonist antinociception (Ocana and Baeyens, 1993; Ocana et al., 1996). Interestingly, this contrasts with modulation of K$_{ATP}$, the voltage- and calcium-insensitive potassium channel regulated by ATP. Thus K$_{ATP}$ channel activation and inhibition have been shown to be ineffective at modulating baclofen mediated antinociception (Ocana et al., 1996). In contrast, although not antinociceptive *per se*, K$_{ATP}$ channel openers potentiate, and inhibitors block, the central antinociceptive effect of μ- and δ-opioid agonists (Wild et al., 1991; Ocana and Baeyens, 1993; Ocana et al., 1995, 1996) and the α$_2$-adrenoceptor agonist, clonidine (Ocana et al., 1996). However, although potentiation of morphine is consistently observed, not all μ-opioid agonists are similarly affected (Ocana et al., 1995; Raffa and Martinez, 1995). The K_{ATP} channel opener, cromakalim, failed to potentiate the antinociceptive properties of the κ-opioid agonist U-50,488. In the mouse tail flick test, the antinociceptive response to the tricyclic antidepressants clomipramine and amitriptyline was blocked by an antisense oligodeoxynucleotide to the mouse $K_v1.1$ delayed rectifier (Galeotti et al., 1997).

Voltage-gated potassium channels, therefore, function to limit neuronal excitability by regulating action potential threshold and accommodation. Modulation of these channels by agents that selectively increase potassium conductance therefore could play an important role in the control of baseline rhythmogenesis (impulse initiation) and burst firing in a chronically injured axon. However, the relative importance of the voltage-gated potassium channel family to primary afferent neuronal function and, consequently, to acute and facilitated processing of nociceptive information at a peripheral and spinal level still remains a largely unexplored area owing to the lack of potent and/or selective channel activators. Potassium channels will therefore remain an unknown quantity for the treatment of pain until sufficient clinical experience is obtained with potassium channel openers and a general opinion is formed as to whether they have analgesic potential.

FUTURE PERSPECTIVE

Modulation of voltage-gated ion channels or at least blockade of sodium channels, has been an area where moderate success has been achieved at producing effective relief in a number of chronic pain conditions. However, in many instances, the drug has had to be withdrawn from the patient before the full analgesic potential was realized owing to the onset of many, often severe side effects. The main issue for the future, therefore, is not simply to maintain or improve analgesic efficacy but also to improve markedly the therapeutic window. On initial investigation, for sodium, calcium, and potassium channels, there would appear to be no shortage of potential targets in order to attempt to achieve this goal. However, a major limitation becomes immediately apparent in that many of these subtypes have a ubiquitous distribution throughout the peripheral and central nervous systems. This would suggest, therefore, that there is a very real potential of side effects continuing to limit therapeutic potential. An intriguing possibility to circumvent this potential scenario is the recent opportunity of specific localization of the target to those tissues associated with, in particular, peripheral nociceptive pathways, for example, the TTX-resistant sodium channel PN3/SNS. Such a profile suggests that a selective inhibitor of such a channel might therefore produce analgesia and be relatively devoid of autonomic and motor side effects. It is also possible that, although the widespread distribution of other channels might not afford selective analgesic action, some of these channels may be targeted on the basis of their biophysical properties and, consequently, their contribution to the abnormal, repetitive firing behavior of peripheral and central neurons following injury. Thus the specialized pathophysiology of injured sensory neurons may provide a chance of selectivity over other neuronal types not affected by the injury.

In conclusion, it is worth re-emphasizing that whatever future generation ion channel selective blocker or activator is obtained it will need to retain at least as good, if not better, analgesic efficacy than the present generation but with a marked improvement in the therapeutic window to be successful in the treatment of chronic pain conditions of most etiologies.

REFERENCES

Abram SE, Yaksh TL (1994): Systemic lidocaine blocks nerve injury-induced hyperalgesia and nociceptor-driven spinal sensitization in the rat. Anesthesiology 80: 383–391.

Ackerman MJ, Clapham DE (1997): Ion channels-basic science and clinical disease. New Engl J Med 336:1575–1586.

Akins PT, McCleskey EW (1993): Characterization of potassium currents in adult rat sensory neurons and modulation by opioids and cyclic AMP. Neuroscience 56: 759–769.

Akopian AN, Sivilotti L, Wood JN (1996): A tetrodotoxin-resistant voltage-gated sodium channel expressed by sensory neurons. Nature 379:257–262.

Arbuckle JB, Docherty RJ (1995): Expression of tetrodotoxin-resistant sodium channels in capsaicin-sensitive dorsal root ganglion neurons of adult rats. Neurosci Lett 185: 70–73.

Arner S, Lindblom U, Meyerson BA, Molander C (1990): Prolonged relief of neuralgia after regional anesthetic blocks. A call for further experimental and systematic clinical studies. Pain 43:287–297.

Atkinson RL (1982): Intravenous lidocaine for the treatment of intractable pain of adiposis dolorosa. Intl J Obesity 6:351–357.

Awerbuch GI, Sandyk R (1990): Mexiletine for thalamic pain syndrome. Intl J Neurosci 55:129–133.

Bach FW, Jensen TS, Kastrup J, Stigsby B, Dejgard A (1990): The effect of intravenous lidocaine on nociceptive processing in diabetic neuropathy. Pain 40:29–34.

Backonja MM (1994): Local anesthetics as adjuvant analgesics. J Pain Symp Manag 9:491–499.

Backonja M, Gombar KA (1992): Response of central pain syndromes to intravenous lidocaine. J Pain Symp Manag 7:172–178.

Bannon AW, Gunther KL, Decker MW, Arneric SP (1995): The influence of Bay K 8644 treatment on ($+/-$):-epibatidine-induced analgesia. Brain Res 678:244–250.

Bennett GJ, Xie YK (1988): A peripheral mononeuropathy in rat that produces disorders of pain sensation like those seen in man. Pain 33:87–107.

Bergouignan M (1942): Cures heureuses de nevralgies faciales essentielles par le phenyl-hydentoinate de soude. Rev Laryngol Otol Rhinol 63:34–41.

Birch K, Jorgensen J, Chraemmer-Jorgensen B, Kehlet H (1987): Effect of i.v. lignocaine on pain and the endocrine metabolic responses after surgery. Br J Anaesth 59: 721–724.

Black JA, Dib-Hajj S, McNabola K, Jeste S, Rizzo MA, Kocsis JD, Waxman SG (1996): Spinal sensory neurons express multiple sodium channel α-subunit mRNAs. Mol Brain Res 43:117–131.

Blom S (1962): Trigeminal neuralgia: its treatment with a new anticonvulsant drug (G-32883). Lancet 1:839–840.

Bowersox SS, Luther RR (1994): SNX-111. N-type voltage-sensitive calcium channel antagonist. Drugs of the Future 19:128–130.

Bowersox SS, Gadbois T, Singh T, Pettus M, Wang YX, Luther RR (1996): Selective N-type neuronal voltage-sensitive calcium channel blocker, SNX-111, produces spinal antinociception in rat models of acute, persistent and neuropathic pain. J Pharmacol Exp Ther 279:1243–1249.

Brose WG, Cousins MJ (1991): Subcutaneous lidocaine for treatment of neuropathic cancer pain. Pain 45:145–148.

Brose WG, Pfeiffer BL, Hassenbusch SJ, Burchiel KJ, Byas-Smith M, Krames E, McGuire D, Tich N, Luther RR (1996): Analgesia produced by SNX-111 in patients with morphine-resistant pain. In *Abstracts 15th Annual Scientific Meeting of the American Pain Society*, Washington, DC, p. A122.

Bruera E, Ripamonti C, Brenneis C, Macmillan K, Hanson J (1992): A randomized double-blind crossover trial of intravenous lidocaine in the treatment of neuropathic cancer pain. J Pain Symp Manag 7:138–140.

Burchiel KJ, Russell LC (1985): Effects of potassium channel-blocking agents on spontaneous discharges from neuromas in rats. J Neurosurg 63:246–249.

Campbell FG, Graham JG, Zilkha KJ (1966): Clinical trial of carbamazepine (Tegretol) in trigeminal neuralgia. J Neurol Neurosurg Psychiatry 29:265–267.

Cardenas CG, Del Mar LP, Scroggs RS (1995): Variation in serotonergic inhibition of calcium channel currents in four types of rat sensory neurons differentiated by membrane properties. J Neurophysiol 74:1870–1879.

Cardenas CG, Del Mar LP, Scroggs RS (1997): 5HT$_4$ receptors couple positively to tetrodotoxin insensitive sodium channels in a subpopulation of capsaicin-sensitive rat sensory neurons. J Neurosci 17:7181–7189.

Cassuto J, Wallin G, Hogstrom S, Faxen A, Rimback G (1985): Inhibition of postoperative pain by continuous low-dose intravenous infusion of lidocaine. Anesth Analg 64:971–974.

Catterall WA (1987): Common modes of drug action on Na$^+$ channels: Local anesthetics, antiarrhythmics and anticonvulsants. Trends in Pharmacol Sci 8:57–65.

Catterall WA (1992): Cellular and molecular biology of voltage-gated sodium channels. Physiol Rev 72:S15–S48.

Catterall WA (1995): Structure and function of voltage-gated ion channels. Ann Rev Biochem 64:493–531.

Chabal C, Russell LC, Burchiel KJ (1989): The effect of intravenous lidocaine, tocainide, and mexiletine on spontaneously active fibers originating in rat sciatic neuromas. Pain 38:333–338.

Chabal C, Jacobson L, Mariano A, Chaney E, Britell CW (1992a): The use of oral mexiletine for the treatment of pain after peripheral nerve injury. Anesthesiology 76: 513–517.

Chabal C, Jacobson L, Russell LC, Burchiel KJ (1992b): Pain response to perineuromal injection of normal saline, epinephrine, and lidocaine in humans. Pain 49:9–12.

Chadda VS, Mathur MS (1978): Double blind study of the effects of diphenylhydantoin sodium on diabetic neuropathy. J Assoc Phys India 26:403–406.

Chaplan SR, Pogrel JW, Yaksh TL (1994): Role of voltage-dependent calcium channel subtypes in experimental tactile allodynia. J Pharmacol Exp Ther 269:1117–1123.

Cheung H, Kamp D, Harris E (1992): An in vitro investigation of the action of lamotrigine on neuronal voltage-activated sodium channels. Epilepsy Res 13:107–112.

Coderre TJ, Melzack R (1992): The role of NMDA receptor-operated calcium channels in persistent nociception after formalin-induced tissue injury. J Neurosci 12:3671–3675.

Coggeshall RE, Dougherty PM, Pover CM, Carlton SM (1993): Is large myelinated fiber loss associated with hyperalgesia in a model of experimental peripheral neuropathy in the rat? Pain 52:233–242.

Cook NS (1988): The pharmacology of potassium channels and their therapeutic potential. Trends Pharmacol Sci 9:21–28.

Covino BG, Wildsmith JAW (1998): Clinical pharmacology of local anesthetic agents. In Cousins MJ, Bridenbaugh PO (eds): *Neural Blockade In Clinical Anesthesia and Management of Pain*, 3rd ed. Philadelphia: Lippincott-Raven, pp. 97–128.

Damaj MI, Welch SP, Martin BR (1993): Involvement of calcium and L-type channels in nicotine-induced antinociception. J Pharmacol Exp Ther 266:1330–1338.

Dejgard A, Petersen P, Kastrup J (1988): Mexiletine for treatment of chronic painful diabetic neuropathy. Lancet 1:9–11.

Devor M (1994): The pathophysiology of damaged peripheral nerves. In Wall PD, Melzack R (eds): *Textbook of Pain*, 3rd ed. Edinburgh: Churchill Livingstone, pp. 79–100.

Devor M, Govrin-Lippmann R (1983): Axoplasmic transport block reduces ectopic impulse generation in injured peripheral nerves. Pain 16:73–85.

Devor M, Wall PD, Catalan N (1992): Systemic lidocaine silences ectopic neuroma and DRG discharge without blocking nerve conduction. Pain 48:261–268.

Devor M, Govrin-Lippmann R, Angelides K (1993): Na+ channel immunolocalization in peripheral mammalian axons and changes following nerve injury and neuroma formation. J Neurosci 13:1976–1992.

Diaz A, Dickenson AH (1997): Blockade of spinal N- and P-type, but not L-type, calcium channels inhibits the excitability of rat dorsal horn neurones produced by subcutaneous formalin inflammation. Pain 69:93–100.

Dib-Hajj S, Black JA, Felts P, Waxman SG (1996): Down-regulation of transcripts for Na channel alpha-SNS in spinal sensory neurons following axotomy. Proc Natl Acad Sci (USA) 93:14950–14954.

Dietrich PS, McGivern JG, Delgado SG, Koch BD, Rabert DK, Ilnicka M, Eglen RM, Hunter JC, Sangameswaran L (1998): Functional analysis of a voltage-gated sodium channel and its splice variant from rat dorsal root ganglia. J Neurochem 70:2262–2272.

Edmondson EA, Simpson RK Jr, Stubler DK, Beric A (1993): Systemic lidocaine therapy for poststroke pain. Southern Med J 86:1093–1096.

Edwards WT, Habib F, Burney RG, Begin G (1985): Intravenous lidocaine in the management of various chronic pain states. A review of 211 cases. Reg Anesth 10:1–6.

Eisenberg E, Alon N, Yarnitsky D, Ishay A, Daoud D (1996): Lamotrigine for the treatment of painful diabetic neuropathy. In *Abstracts 8th World Congress on Pain*, Vancouver, Canada, p. 372.

Ellemann K, Sjogren P, Banning AM, Jensen TS, Smith T, Geertsen P (1989): Trial of intravenous lidocaine on painful neuropathy in cancer patients. Clin J Pain 5:291–294.

Elliott JR (1997): Slow Na^+ channel inactivation and bursting discharge in a simple model axon: implications for neuropathic pain. Brain Res 754:221–226.

Elliott AA, Elliott JR (1993): Characterization of TTX-sensitive and TTX-resistant sodium currents in small cells from adult rat dorsal root ganglia. J Physiol 463:39–56.

England JD, Happel LT, Kline DG, Gamboni F, Thouron CL, Liu ZP, Levinson SR (1996a): Sodium channel accumulation in humans with painful neuromas. Neurology 47:272–276.

England S, Bevan S, Docherty RJ (1996b): PGE_2 modulates the tetrodotoxin-resistant sodium current in neonatal rat dorsal root ganglion neurones via the cyclic AMP-protein kinase A cascade. J Physiol 495:429–440.

Ferrante FM, Paggioli J, Cherukuri S, Arthur GR (1996): The analgesic response to intravenous lidocaine in the treatment of neuropathic pain. Anesth Analg 82:91–97.

Fitton A, Goa KL (1995): Lamotrigine. An update of its pharmacology and therapeutic use in epilepsy. Drugs 50:691–713.

Fletcher D, Le Corre P, Guilbaud G, Le Verge R (1997): Antinociceptive effect of bupivacaine encapsulated in poly(D,L):-lactide-co-glycolide microspheres in the acute inflammatory pain model of carrageenin-injected rats. Anesth Analg 84:90–94.

Galeotti N, Ghelardini C, Capaccioli S, Quattrone A, Nicolin A, Bartolini A (1997): Blockade of clomipramine and amitriptyline analgesia by an antisense oligonucleotide to mKv1.1, a mouse Shaker-like K^+ channel. Eur J Pharmacol 330:15–25.

Galer BS, Miller KV, Rowbotham MC (1993): Response to intravenous lidocaine infusion differs based on clinical diagnosis and site of nervous system injury. Neurology 43:1233–1235.

Galer BS, Harle J, Rowbotham MC (1996): Response to intravenous lidocaine infusion predicts subsequent response to oral mexiletine: a prospective study. J Pain Symp Manag 12:161–167.

Gandhi VC, Jones DJ (1988): Identification and characterization of [^{3}H]nitrendipine binding sites in rat spinal cord. J Pharmacol Exp Ther 247:473–480.

Gogas KG, Jacobson LO, Waligora D, Martin B, Hunter JC (1997): The cold bath assay: a simple and reliable method to assess cold allodynia in neuropathic animals. Analgesia 3:111–118.

Gohil K, Bell JR, Ramachandran J, Miljanich GP (1994): Neuroanatomical distribution of receptors for a novel voltage-sensitive calcium-channel antagonist, SNX-230 (omega-conopeptide MVIIC). Brain Res 653:258–266.

Gold MS, Reichling DB, Shuster MJ, Levine JD (1996a): Hyperalgesic agents increase a tetrodotoxin-resistant Na+ current in nociceptors. Proc Natl Acad Sci (USA) 93: 1108–1112.

Gold MS, Shuster MJ, Levine JD (1996b): Characterization of six voltage-gated K+ currents in adult rat sensory neurons. J Neurophysiol 75:2629–2646.

Gracely RH, Lynch SA, Bennett GJ (1992): Painful neuropathy: altered central processing maintained dynamically by peripheral input. Pain 51:175–194.

Harbison J, Dennehy F, Keating D (1997): Lamotrigine for pain with hyperalgesia. Irish Med J 90:56.

Hedley LR, Martin B, Waterbury LD, Clarke DE, Hunter JC (1995): A comparison of the action of mexiletine and morphine in rodent models of acute and chronic pain. Proc West Pharmacol Soc 38:103–104.

Hodoglugil U, Guney HZ, Savran B, Guzey C, Gorgun CZ, Zengil H (1996): Temporal variation in the interaction between calcium channel blockers and morphine-induced analgesia. Chronobiol Intl 13:227–234.

Hofmann F, Biel M, Flockerzi V (1994): Molecular basis for Ca^{2+} channel diversity. Ann Rev Neurosci 17:399–418.

Hunter JC, Martin B, Lewis R, Smith L, Fontana DJ, Lee C-H (1995): The contribution of peripheral sensory neuronal input towards the maintenance of neuropathic pain. Soc Neurosci Abstr 21:1411.

Hunter JC, Gogas KR, Hedley LR, Jacobson LO, Kassotakis L, Thompson J, Fontana DJ (1997): The effect of novel anti-epileptic drugs in rat experimental models of acute and chronic pain. Eur J Pharmacol 324:153–160.

Isomoto S, Kondo C, Kurachi Y (1997): Inwardly rectifying potassium channels: their molecular heterogeneity and function. Jap J Physiol 47:11–39.

Jeftinija S (1994): The role of tetrodotoxin-resistant sodium channels of small primary afferent fibers. Brain Res 639:125–134.

Jett MF, McGuirk J, Waligora D, Hunter JC (1997): The effects of mexiletine, desipramine and fluoxetine in rat models involving central sensitization. Pain 69:161–169.

Kaczorowski GJ, Knaus HG, Leonard RJ, McManus OB, Garcia ML (1996): High-conductance calcium-activated potassium channels; structure, pharmacology, and function. J Bioenerg Biomembr 28:255–267.

Kallen RG, Cohen SA, Barchi RL (1993): Structure, function and expression of voltage-dependent sodium channels. Mol Neurobiol 7:383–428.

Kastrup J, Petersen P, Dejgard A, Angelo HR, Hilsted J (1987): Intravenous lidocaine infusion—a new treatment of chronic painful diabetic neuropathy? Pain 28:69–75.

Kaube H, Hoskin KL, Goadsby PJ (1994): Lignocaine and headache: an electrophysiological study in the cat with supporting clinical observations in man. J Neurol 241:415–420.

Kerr LM, Filloux F, Olivera BM, Jackson H, Wamsley JK (1988): Autoradiographic localization of calcium channels with [^{125}I]omega-conotoxin in rat brain. Eur J Pharmacol 146:181–183.

Killian JM, Fromm GH (1968): Carbamazepine in the treatment of neuralgia. Use of side-effects. Arch Neurol 19:129–136.

Kim SH, Chung JM (1992): An experimental model for peripheral neuropathy produced by segmental spinal nerve ligation in the rat. Pain 50:355–363.

Kingery WS (1997): A critical review of controlled clinical trials for peripheral neuropathic pain and complex regional pain syndromes. Pain 73:123–139.

Kirchhoff C, Leah JD, Jung S, Reeh PW (1992): Excitation of cutaneous sensory nerve endings in the rat by 4-aminopyridine and tetraethylammonium. J Neurophysiol 67:125–131.

Koch BD, Faurot GF, McGuirk JR, Clarke DE, Hunter JC (1996): Modulation of mechano-hyperalgesia by clinically effective analgesics in rats with a peripheral mononeuropathy. Analgesia 2:157–164.

Koltzenburg M, Torebjork HE, Wahren LK (1994): Nociceptor modulated central sensitization causes mechanical hyperalgesia in acute chemogenic and chronic neuropathic pain. Brain 117:579–591.

Kuo C-C, Bean BP (1994): Slow binding of phenytoin to inactivated sodium channels in rat hippocampal neurons. Mol Pharmacol 46:716–725.

Kuo CC, Chen RS, Lu L, Chen RC (1997): Carbamazepine inhibition of neuronal Na^+ currents: quantitative distinction from phenytoin and possible therapeutic implications. Mol Pharmacol 51:1077–1083.

Leach MJ, Marden CM, Miller AA (1986): Pharmacological studies on lamotrigine, a novel potential antiepileptic drug. II. Neurochemical studies on the mechanism of action. Epilepsia 27:490–497.

Leijon G, Boivie J (1989): Central post-stroke pain—a controlled trial of amitriptyline and carbamazepine. Pain 36:27–36.

Lin Z, Haus S, Edgerton J, Lipscombe D (1997): Identification of functionally distinct isoforms of the N-type Ca^{2+} channel in rat sympathetic ganglia and brain. Neuron 18:153–166.

Lindstrom P, Lindblom U (1987): The analgesic effect of tocainide in trigeminal neuralgia. Pain 28:45–50.

Maizels M, Scott B, Cohen W, Chen W (1996): Intranasal lidocaine for treatment of migraine: a randomized, double-blind, controlled trial. JAMA 276:319–321.

Malmberg AB, Yaksh TL (1994): Voltage-sensitive calcium channels in spinal nociceptive processing: blockade of N- and P-type channels inhibits formalin-induced nociception. J Neurosci 14:4882–4890.

Malmberg AB, Yaksh TL (1995): Effect of continuous intrathecal infusion of omega-conopeptides, N-type calcium-channel blockers, on behavior and antinociception in the formalin and hot-plate tests in rats. Pain 60:83–90.

Marchettini P, Lacerenza M, Marangoni C, Pellegata G, Sotgiu ML, Smirne S (1992): Lidocaine test in neuralgia. Pain 48:377–382.

Matzner O, Devor M (1992): Na^+ conductance and the threshold for repetitive neuronal firing. Brain Res 597:92–98.

Matzner O, Devor M (1994): Hyperexcitability at sites of nerve injury depends on voltage-sensitive Na^+ channels. J Neurophysiol 72:349–359.

McQuay H, Carroll D, Jadad AR, Wiffen P, Moore A (1995): Anticonvulsant drugs for the management of pain: a systematic review. Br Med J 311:1047–1052.

Miljanich GP, Ramachandran J (1995): Antagonists of neuronal calcium channels: structure, function, and therapeutic implications. Ann Rev Pharmacol Toxicol 35:707–734.

Mintz IM, Adams ME, Bean BP (1992): P-type calcium channels in rat central and peripheral neurons. Neuron 9:85–95.

Miranda HF, Bustamante D, Kramer V, Pelissier T, Saavedra H, Paeile C, Fernandez E, Pinardi G (1992): Antinociceptive effects of Ca^{2+} channel blockers. Eur J Pharmacol 217:137–141.

Nagaro T, Shimizu C, Inoue H, Fujitani T, Adachi N, Amakawa K, Kimura S, Arai T, Watanabe T, Oka S (1995): The efficacy of intravenous lidocaine on various types of neuropathic pain. Jap J Anesth 44:862–867.

Nakamura-Craig M, Follenfant RL (1995): Effect of lamotrigine in the acute and chronic hyperalgesia induced by PGE_2 and in the chronic hyperalgesia in rats with streptozotocin-induced diabetes. Pain 63:33–37.

Neugebauer V, Vanegas H, Nebe J, Rumenapp P, Schaible HG (1996): Effects of N- and L-type calcium channel antagonists on the responses of nociceptive spinal cord neurons to mechanical stimulation of the normal and the inflamed knee joint. J Neurophysiol 76:3740–3749.

Novakovic SD, Tzoumaka E, McGivern JG, Haraguichi M, Sangameswaran L, Gogas KR, Eglen RM, Hunter JC (1998): Distribution of the tetrodotoxin-resistant sodium channel, PN3, in rat sensory neurons in normal and neuropathic conditions. J Neurosci 18:2174–2187.

Ocana M, Baeyens JM (1993): Differential effects of K^+ channel blockers on antinociception induced by alpha 2-adrenoceptor, $GABA_B$ and kappa-opioid receptor agonists. Br J Pharmacol 110:1049–1054.

Ocana M, Del Pozo E, Barrios M, Baeyens JM (1995): Subgroups among mu-opioid receptor agonists distinguished by ATP-sensitive K^+ channel-acting drugs. Br J Pharmacol 114:1296–1302.

Ocana M, Barrios M, Baeyens JM (1996): Cromakalim differentially enhances antinociception induced by agonists of $alpha_2$ adrenoceptors, gamma-aminobutyric $acid_B$, mu and kappa opioid receptors. J Pharmacol Exp Ther 276:1136–1142.

Ogata N, Tatebayashi H (1993): Kinetic analysis of two types of Na^+ channels in rat dorsal root ganglia. J Physiol 466:9–37.

Omana-Zapata I, Khabbaz MA, Hunter JC, Bley KR (1997a): QX-314 inhibits ectopic nerve activity associated with neuropathic pain. Brain Res 771:228–237.

Omana-Zapata I, Khabbaz MA, Hunter JC, Clarke DE, Bley KR (1997b): Tetrodotoxin inhibits neuropathic ectopic activity in neuromas, dorsal root ganglia and dorsal horn neurons. Pain 72:41–49.

Omote K, Sonoda H, Kawamata M, Iwasaki H, Namiki A (1993): Potentiation of antinociceptive effects of morphine by calcium-channel blockers at the level of the spinal cord. Anesthesiology 79:746–752.

Pavone F, Battaglia M, Sansone M (1993): Attenuation of cholinergic analgesia by nifedipine. Brain Res 623:308–310.

Pearce RJ, Duchen MR (1994): Differential expression of membrane currents in dissociated mouse primary sensory neurons. Neuroscience 63:1041–1056.

Pereira IT, Prado WA, Dos Reis MP (1993): Enhancement of the epidural morphine-induced analgesia by systemic nifedipine. Pain 53:341–345.

Petersen P, Kastrup J (1987): Dercum's disease (adiposis dolorosa). Treatment of the severe pain with intravenous lidocaine. Pain 28:77–80.

Petersen P, Kastrup J, Zeeberg I, Boysen G (1986): Chronic pain treatment with intravenous lidocaine. Neurol Res 8:189–190.

Pongs O (1992): Molecular biology of voltage-dependent potassium channels. Physiol Rev 72:S69–S88.

Raffa RB, Martinez RP (1995): The 'glibenclamide-shift' of centrally-acting antinociceptive agents in mice. Brain Res 677:277–282.

Reuter H (1996): Diversity and function of presynaptic calcium channels in the brain. Curr Opinion Neurobiol 6:331–337.

Rizzo MA, Kocsis JD, Waxman SG (1994): Slow sodium conductances of dorsal root ganglion neurons: intraneuronal homogeneity and interneuronal heterogeneity. J Neurophysiol 72:2796–2815.

Rizzo MA, Kocsis JD, Waxman SG (1995): Selective loss of slow and enhancement of fast Na+ currents in cutaneous afferent dorsal root ganglion neurones following axotomy. Neurobiol Disease 2:87–96.

Roca G, Aguilar JL, Gomar C, Mazo V, Costa J, Vidal F (1996): Nimodipine fails to enhance the analgesic effect of slow release morphine in the early phases of cancer pain treatment. Pain 68:239–243.

Rowbotham MC, Reisner-Keller LA, Fields HL (1991): Both intravenous lidocaine and morphine reduce the pain of postherpetic neuralgia. Neurology 41:1024–1028.

Rowbotham MC, Davies PS, Fields HL (1995): Topical lidocaine gel relieves postherpetic neuralgia. Ann Neurol 37:246–253.

Roy ML, Narahashi T (1992): Differential properties of tetrodotoxin-sensitive and tetrodotoxin-resistant sodium channels in rat dorsal root ganglion neurons. J Neurosci 12:2104–2111.

Rudy B (1988): Diversity and ubiquity of K channels. Neuroscience 25:729–749.

Rull J, Quibrera R, Gonzalez-Millan H, Lozano Castenada O (1969): Symptomatic treatment of peripheral diabetic neuropathy with carbamazepine: double-blind crossover study. Diabetologia 5:215–220.

Sangameswaran L, Delgado SG, Fish LM, Koch BD, Jakeman LB, Stewart GR, Sze P, Hunter JC, Eglen RM, Herman RC (1996): Structure and function of a novel voltage-gated, tetrodotoxin-resistant sodium channel specific to sensory neurons. J Biol Chem 271:5953–5956.

Sangameswaran L, Fish LM, Koch BD, Rabert DK, Delgado SG, Ilnicka M, Jakeman LB, Novakovic S, Wong K, Sze P, Tzoumaka E, Stewart GR, Herman RC, Chan H, Eglen RM, Hunter JC (1997): A novel tetrodotoxin-sensitive, voltage-gated sodium channel expressed in rat and human dorsal root ganglia. J Biol Chem 272:14805–14809.

Santillan R, Maestre JM, Hurle MA, Florez J (1994): Enhancement of opiate analgesia by nimodipine in cancer patients chronically treated with morphine: a preliminary report. Pain 58:129–132.

Saudek CD, Werns S, Reidenberg MM (1977): Phenytoin in the treatment of diabetic symmetrical polyneuropathy. Clin Pharmacol Ther 22:196–199.

Schaller KL, Krzemien DM, Yarowsky PJ, Krueger BK, Caldwell JH (1995): A novel, abundant sodium channel expressed in neurons and glia. J Neurosci 15:3231–3242.

Scroggs RS, Fox AP (1992): Calcium current variation between acutely isolated adult rat dorsal root ganglion neurons of different size. J Physiol 445:639–658.

Scroggs RS, Todorovic SM, Anderson EG, Fox AP (1994): Variation in IH, IIR, and ILEAK between acutely isolated adult rat dorsal root ganglion neurons of different size. J Neurophysiol 71:271–279.

Sinnott C, Edmonds P, Cropley I, Hanks G, Dunlop RJ, Hockley JM, Tate T, Turner P (1991): Flecainide in cancer nerve pain. Lancet 337:1347.

Swerdlow M (1984): Anticonvulsant drugs and chronic pain. Clin Neuropharmacol 7:51–82.

Tanelian DL, Brose WG (1991): Neuropathic pain can be relieved by drugs that are use-dependent sodium channel blockers: lidocaine, carbamazepine, and mexiletine. Anesthesiology 74:949–951.

Tanelian DL, Victory RA (1995): Sodium channel-blocking agents: Their use in neuropathic pain conditions. Pain Forum 4:75–80.

Toledo-Aral JJ, Moss BL, He ZJ, Koszowski AG, Whisenand T, Levinson SR, Wolf JJ, Silos-Santiago I, Halegoua S, Mandel G (1997): Identification of PN1, a predominant voltage-dependent sodium channel expressed principally in peripheral neurons. Proc Natl Acad Sci (USA) 94:1527–1532.

Wall PD, Devor M (1983): Sensory afferent impulses originate from dorsal root ganglia as well as from the periphery in normal and nerve injured rats. Pain 17:321–339.

Waxman SG, Kocsis JD, Black JA (1994): Type III sodium channel mRNA is expressed in embryonic but not adult spinal sensory neurons, and is reexpressed following axotomy. J Neurophysiol 72:466–470.

Wei ZY, Karim F, Roerig SC (1996): Spinal morphine/clonidine antinociceptive synergism: involvement of G proteins and N-type voltage-dependent calcium channels. J Pharmacol Exp Ther 278:1392–1407.

Wild KD, Vanderah T, Mosberg HI, Porreca F (1991): Opioid delta receptor subtypes are associated with different potassium channels. Eur J Pharmacol 193:135–136.

Woolf CJ, Chong MS (1993): Preemptive analgesia-treating postoperative pain by preventing the establishment of central sensitization. Anesth Analg 77:362–379.

Woolf CJ, Doubell TP (1994): The pathophysiology of chronic pain—increased sensitivity to low threshold Aβ-fibre inputs. Curr Opinion Neurobiol 4:525–534.

Xiao WH, Bennett GJ (1995): Synthetic omega-conopeptides applied to the site of nerve injury suppress neuropathic pains in rats. J Pharmacol Exp Ther 274:666–672.

Yoon YW, Na HS, Chung JM (1996): Contributions of injured and intact afferents to neuropathic pain in an experimental rat model. Pain 64:27–36.

Zakrzewska JM, Chaudhry Z, Nurmikko TJ, Patton DW, Mullens EL (1997): Lamotrigine (Lamictal) in refractory trigeminal neuralgia: results from a double-blind placebo controlled crossover trial. Pain 73:223–230.

CHAPTER 17

SPINAL DRUG INTERACTIONS

JAMES C. EISENACH
Wake Forest University School of Medicine
Winston-Salem, North Carolina

G. F. GEBHART
University of Iowa College of Medicine
Iowa City, Iowa

Opioids administered by the spinal route are widely used in the management of pain. In addition to their intended analgesic effect, opioids also can produce unwanted pruritus, nausea and vomiting, urinary retention, hypotension, and respiratory depression following spinal administration, as well as analgesic tolerance on chronic spinal administration. In addition to opioids, other drug classes (e.g., α_2-adrenoceptor and cholinergic agonists, local anesthetics, *N*-methyl-D-aspartate (NMDA) receptor antagonists) are also given spinally, but they too are associated with undesirable effects. Accordingly, concomitant use of opioid and nonopioid drugs, each at reduced dosage, offer the potential for optimizing pain control while minimizing unwanted side effects. This strategy is based on presumed differences in mechanism and/or site (e.g., presynaptic vs. postsynaptic) of action between opioid and non-opioid drugs. We discuss below the means by which spinal drug interactions are studied and review results from both nonhuman animal and human studies.

ANTAGONISM, ADDITIVITY, AND SYNERGY

When drugs are given simultaneously, their effects may be antagonistic (subadditive), additive, or synergistic (supraadditive). Subadditive effects are expressed as less than the sum of effects produced by either agent alone, additive effects represent the simple sum of effects produced by either agent alone, and supraadditive effects are greater than the sum of effects produced by either

---

Novel Aspects of Pain Management: Opioids and Beyond, Edited by Jana Sawynok and Alan Cowan
ISBN 0-471-180173 Copyright © 1999 by Wiley-Liss, Inc.

agent alone (see below and Figure 17.1). To restate the rationale given above, the therapeutic objective of combined drug therapy is analgesic synergy and reduced side effects. A variety of models have been developed to study drug interactions (see Gessner, 1974; Wessinger, 1986; Berenbaum, 1989; Tallarida et al., 1989; Gennings et al., 1990; Tallarida, 1992).

A common way in which drug interactions have been studied involves demonstration of a statistically significant increase in drug effect produced by co-administration of an inactive dose of a second drug. This approach, however, is of limited value because it assumes linear dose–response functions and only one dose of each drug is typically tested. A more powerful model takes both dose and effect into account. Such models permit quantitative evaluation of the magnitude of drug interaction. One way in which this is done is to determine the dose–response function of a drug in the absence and then in the presence of a fixed dose of a second drug. A synergistic interaction is concluded by a significant leftward shift or change in the slope of the dose–response function of the first drug in the presence of the second drug. Although this "dose-addition" model appears to be intuitively straightforward, it is not mechanism-free, is based on the assumption of a linear shift in the dose–response function, and most important, is applied without predefined criteria for establishing a drug interaction as synergistic.

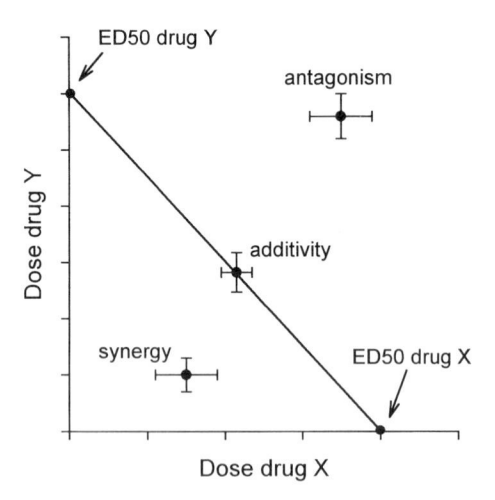

Figure 17.1 Illustration of a theoretical isobologram. The experimentally determined analgesic effective dose 50s (ED_{50}s) for drugs Y and X are indicated on the Y and X axes, respectively. The line connecting these ED_{50} drug doses indicates the line of additivity of analgesic drug effect. When given in combination (at the respective times of peak effect of each drug), a significantly greater analgesic potency of a ratio of doses of drugs Y and X will fall below the line of additivity and represent a supra-additive effect or synergism; an experimentally determined interaction that lies above the line of additivity represents antagonism (see Berenbaum, 1989; Tallarida, 1992 for details).

The most powerful model for evaluation of drug interactions is the isobolographic method (e.g., Berenbaum, 1989; Tallarida, 1992). This method involves comparison of doses of each drug alone with those of the drugs in fixed dose-ratio combinations to produce a given effect (e.g., analgesia) along dose–response functions of the drugs given alone or in combination. The isobolographic analysis makes no assumptions about mechanism of drug action or the shape of dose–response functions. Most importantly, it has been proven mathematically valid, defines a priori the criteria for assessing the quality of drug interactions (antagonistic, additive, or synergistic), and provides a convenient graphic representation of the drug interaction. Because drug interactions may differ at different dose ratios of a pair of drugs, isobolographic analyses with several dose-ratio combinations best define the nature of the drug interaction. Figure 17.1 illustrates a theoretical isobologram.

Because of the ability to evaluate unambiguously drug interactions using the isobolographic model, the overview of spinal drug interactions below focuses on studies in nonhuman animals that have employed this model. This model, however, is less readily applicable to studies of drug interactions in humans, emphasizing the importance of isobolographic analyses in nonhuman animal studies when results are extended to human medicine.

SPINAL DRUG INTERACTIONS: NONHUMAN STUDIES

A wide variety of drug interactions have been studied in nonhuman animal studies (e.g., see Solomon and Gebhart, 1994; Yaksh and Malmberg, 1994 for recent overviews). Many of the earlier studies employed dose-addition models to study interactions and most studied acute nociceptive input (e.g., thermal stimulation of the tail or hindpaw in rodents). More recently, isobolographic methods have been employed and models of tonic and visceral nociceptive input have been studied. It is beyond the scope of this chapter to review all of the published literature; the following illustrates what we consider to be some of the potentially more clinically relevant spinal drug interaction studies.

As summarized in Table 17.1, multiple spinal drug interactions have been studied. The representative studies presented in Table 17.1 do not include those in which the isobolographic method was not employed (see Solomon and Gebhart, 1994; Yaksh and Malmberg, 1994 for additional examples).

Opioid–Local Anesthetic Interactions

Spinal administration of either opioids or local anesthetics is commonly employed in humans (see below). Because the mechanism of action of drugs in these classes differ, their combined use is attractive. An early report (Akerman et al., 1988) suggested that combined intrathecal administration of morphine with lidocaine or bupivacaine produced antinociceptive effects on thermal tests in rats that were more rapid in onset, longer in duration, and greater in peak

TABLE 17.1 Representative Synergistic Spinal Drug Interaction Studies in the Rat[a]

Agonists	Test[b]	Reference
Mu–delta opioids	Thermal	Malmberg and Yaksh, 1992
Morphine–α_2-adrenoceptor agonists	Thermal	Monasky et al., 1990
	Thermal	Ossipov et al., 1990a,b
	Neuropathic	Ossipov et al., 1997
	Formalin	Przesmycki et al., 1997
	Thermal, mechanical	Sherman et al., 1988
Morphine–local anesthetics	Thermal, visceral	Maves and Gebhart, 1992
	Thermal	Penning and Yaksh, 1992
Morphine–NSAIDs	Formalin	Malmberg and Yaksh, 1993

[a] All studies employed the isobolographic model.
[b] Most nociceptive tests used acute thermal (tail flick or paw withdrawal) stimuli, but tonic neuropathic (spinal nerve ligation) and chemical (formalin) tests have also been studied.

effect than when any of the three agents were administered at the same doses alone. Two isobolographic studies (Maves and Gebhart, 1992; Penning and Yaksh, 1992) extended these results to confirm a synergism between morphine and lidocaine or bupivacaine. In the study by Maves and Gebhart (1992), the intrathecal administration of morphine with lidocaine (at their respective times of peak effect) revealed significant synergy in both acute thermal and acute visceral nociceptive tests at dosages that did not affect motor function. Interestingly, the visceral nociceptive responses to colorectal distension displayed statistically greater synergism than did the somatic nociceptive response to thermal stimulation of the hindpaw. Penning and Yaksh (1992) similarly studied the spinal interaction between morphine and local anesthetics, reporting synergy in both acute thermal and acute mechanical nociceptive tests. In addition, they documented that the co-administration of bupivacaine did not alter the clearance of morphine from the intrathecal space.

The clinical implications of these outcomes are clearly important. Intrathecal/epidural opioids and local anesthetics have been combined in the management of visceral pain in postoperative, obstetric, and oncologic patients (e.g. Cullen et al., 1985; Hjortso et al., 1986; Logas et al., 1987; Chestnut et al., 1988). Summarizing a series of clinical studies, Kehlet (1998) concludes that the "stress response" to major surgical procedures is best minimized by a combination of spinal opioids and local anesthetics.

Opioid–α-Adrenoceptor Interactions

A variety of studies have supported the interactions between spinal opioids and α-adrenoceptor agonists as synergistic. As with local anesthetics, the α_2-

adrenoceptor agonist clonidine has been used in humans for pain management (see Eisenach et al., 1995 for overview) and the interaction between spinal opioids and clonidine (and other α_2-adrenoceptor agonists) is both rational and clinically important.

There have been several nonisobolographic studies in mice or monkeys suggesting that drug combinations of morphine with α-adrenoceptor agonists is greater than additive. Hylden and Wilcox (1983) produced nociceptive behaviors in mice by intrathecal injection of substance P (which produces a caudally directed biting and scratching) and reported a synergistic interaction between norepinephrine and morphine. In the monkey, Yaksh and Reddy (1981) reported greater than additive effects by combinations of spinal morphine and α-adrenoceptor agonists (ST-91, norepinephrine, or clonidine) in a shock-titration paradigm. In addition to spinal interactions with morphine, the prototypical μ-opioid receptor preferring agonist, a spinal interaction between the α_2-adrenoceptor agonist clonidine and the δ-opioid receptor agonist DPDPE was established in an isobolographic analysis in mice to be synergistic (Roerig and Fujimoto, 1989).

In tests using acute noxious stimulation in rats, convincing evidence for synergistic interactions between α-adrenoceptor agonists and morphine or fentanyl have been reported. Sherman et al. (1988) reported that combined intrathecal administration of oxymetazoline and morphine was synergistic in tail flick and paw pressure tests. Monasky et al. (1990) documented greater than additive effects of spinal morphine and the α_2-adrenoceptor agonist ST-91. These authors also found that the clearance of morphine from the intrathecal space was not affected by ST-91. In an interesting series of experiments, Ossipov et al. (1990a,b) reported that the interaction between morphine and clonidine (when given systemically in rats) was generally additive, whereas synergistic interactions between clonidine or medetomidine and morphine or fentanyl were found in the thermal tail flick test when drugs were administered spinally. Similarly, models of tonic nociceptive inputs reveal spinal synergy between morphine and clonidine; Przesmycki et al. (1997), using the formalin model, and Ossipov et al. (1997), using a model of neuropathic pain, both report robust antinociceptive synergy between these two drugs.

Overall, the results of both nonisobolographic and isobolographic analyses of spinal opioid and α adrenoceptor agonist interactions reveal a clear synergistic interaction. Primary afferent fiber terminals in the spinal cord, presumably nociceptors, contain both opioid and α_2-adrenoreceptors, as do spinal neurons postsynaptic to primary afferent input. However, opioids and α_2-adrenoceptor agonists do not interact at α_2-adrenoceptor or opioid receptors, respectively, verifying that although the site(s) of drug action may be similar in terms of location, they are effected at separate receptors. Interestingly, there is evidence that μ-opioid receptor agonists and α_2-adrenoceptor agonists exhibit cross-tolerance at the spinal level (e.g. Solomon and Gebhart, 1988). Accordingly, the combination of currently available opioids with clonidine for long-term pain management may not offer a significant therapeutic advantage in terms of development of analgesic tolerance, but may be very appropriate for shorter-term pain management.

Opioid–NMDA Receptor Antagonist and NSAID Interactions

The role of spinal NMDA receptors in the development and maintenance of hyperalgesic/allodynic states has been well established. Recent evidence suggests that hyperalgesia and analgesic tolerance to morphine may have in common intracellular events that link them (see Mao et al., 1995 for review). Trujillo and Akil (1991) and Marek et al. (1991) reported that morphine tolerance and dependence in the rat could be significantly attenuated by the NMDA receptor antagonist MK-801. Subsequently, other investigators were able to show that both competitive and noncompetitive NMDA receptor antagonists were able to attenuate or reverse analgesic tolerance to morphine (Tiseo and Inturissi, 1993; Elliott et al., 1994; Bilski et al., 1996; Lutfy et al., 1996).

The acute interaction between spinal morphine and NMDA receptor antagonists in nontolerant animals has not been similarly examined, but a clinical study suggests a potential interesting and useful interaction. Wong et al. (1996) reported that epidural administration of a subanalgesic dose of ketamine (10 mg), in combination with morphine (0.5 mg), produced a "strong analgesic effect" in a population of patients undergoing major joint replacement. They suggested that ketamine potentiates the analgesic effects of morphine, especially when administered as a pretreatment. They found that the requirement for postoperative pain relief by morphine was reduced, and suggest that pretreatment of patients with epidural ketamine, followed by combined injections of morphine and ketamine, could be a promising analgesic regimen. Isobolographic studies in nonhuman animals have yet to be reported, but obviously should be undertaken to evaluate this interaction.

Opioids and nonsteroidal anti-inflammatory drugs (NSAIDs) are commonly employed for pain management, often in combination. It is generally held that the antinociceptive effects of opioids are principally central in origin and those of NSAIDs are peripheral. A recent investigation however, of the spinal interaction between ketorolac and morphine in the formalin test has revealed a synergistic interaction (Malmberg and Yaksh, 1993). Because mechanisms of action of these classes of drugs are dissimilar, and presumably include effects on transmitter release from spinal nociceptive terminals, the reported interaction warrants further study.

MECHANISTIC INSIGHTS

The foregoing suggests useful, synergistic interactions between opioids and local anesthetics, α_2-adrenoceptor agonists, and NMDA receptor antagonists. Not reviewed above are potentially useful opioid–opioid interactions. For example, Malmberg and Yaksh (1992) established synergistic analgesic interactions between the δ-opioid receptor agonist DPDPE and the μ-opioid receptor agonists morphine, DAMGO, and PL017. At present, there are no δ-opioid receptor agonists available clinically, but this interaction could prove to be useful in providing enhanced analgesia with reduced potential for development of analgesic tolerance.

Most of the studies in nonhuman animals have employed acute nociceptive stimuli, typically thermal. Although the results of such studies using nociceptive input provide robust and statistically reliable results supporting synergistic drug interactions, the circumstances under which spinal administration of drugs are used in humans typically involve tonic or chronic nociceptive inputs. A few studies (e.g., Malmberg and Yaksh, 1993; Ossipov et al., 1997) have employed more tonic nociceptive or neuropathic inputs and similarly document synergistic interactions between opioids and NSAIDs and α_2-adrenoceptors, respectively. Interestingly, Yaksh and Malmberg (1994) note that analgesic synergy is most reliably observed in nonhuman animals when either or both of the drugs tested interact presynaptically with C-fiber terminals in the spinal cord, and that synergistic interactions are less robust or nonexistent with drugs believed to have only modest presynaptic effects. Accordingly, opioids, because they act presynaptically to reduce neurotransmitter release from nociceptive terminals in the spinal cord, are a logical choice for spinal administration and pain management. As indicated above, α_2-adrenoceptors are also located on primary afferent terminals in the spinal dorsal horn, but it is generally believed that their principal action is postsynaptic to both primary afferent input and descending, bulbospinal noradrenergic fibers. Accordingly, the interaction between opioids and α_2-adrenoceptor agonists may be advantageous because the site of action differs, but is potentially complicated by the likelihood that, at postsynaptic sites, the intracellular mechanisms by which their effects are produced involve the same intracellular messenger systems (i.e., can exhibit cross-tolerance). Local anesthetics produce effects by a mechanism distinct from those effected at G protein-coupled receptors and their interaction is documented as clearly synergistic and also useful clinically. Relatively little information is available about the analgesic synergy between opioids and NSAIDs or NMDA receptor antagonists, but what little information that does exists suggests a useful synergy. Both NMDA receptor antagonists and NSAIDs possess mechanisms of action unrelated to opioids, although recent reports suggest an interesting interaction at the intracellular level between opioids and NMDA receptor antagonists (see Mao et al., 1995 and citations above).

CLINICAL EXAMPLES AND IMPLICATIONS OF SPINAL DRUG INTERACTIONS

Treatment of mild clinical pain is typically achieved with relatively small doses of single agents, most commonly of the NSAID class. In most cases, this results in effective analgesia with few or no adverse events. In contrast, treatment of moderate to severe pain is typically achieved with relatively large doses of multiple agents, most commonly combinations of NSAIDs, opioids, and for neuropathic pain, drugs of a variety of other classes (local anesthetics, anticonvulsants, antidepressants). In many cases, this results in only partially effective analgesia with many and occasionally life-threatening adverse events.

The reasons for the discrepancies between treatment of mild and of severe pain are multiple. Mild pain is usually of an acute, peripheral nature, often involves an inflammatory state, and as such is amenable to NSAID therapy. Severe pain exceeds the ability of low-efficacy compounds such as NSAIDs to address, and may involve altered physiology and pharmacology in the central nervous system. Because potent, high-efficacy analgesics have very narrow therapeutic ratios, single agent therapy often leads to unacceptable side effects.

The above addresses systemically administered drugs, although it parallels experience with spinal (epidural and intrathecal) drug administration. Drugs are administered spinally for four major indications: anesthesia, analgesia, chemotherapy, and in the treatment of local infections. Drug interactions for the latter two indications are not discussed in this chapter.

There are two major reasons to combine drugs intraspinally for anesthesia and analgesia: to reduce toxicity from a single agent and to achieve an effect that is not possible with a single agent. These are, of course, often related because the dose of a single agent necessary for the wanted effect may produce unacceptable adverse events. The remainder of this chapter describes settings in which spinal drug combinations are deemed necessary because of some problem, and the results of studies of drug combinations to overcome this problem.

Spinal Anesthesia

Intrathecal injection of local anesthetics results in surgical anesthesia, as well as sympathetic blockade, resulting in hypotension. Clinically available local anesthetics have a duration of action from 30 to 180 min after intrathecal injection. Thus the two clinical problems are local anesthetic-induced hypotension and inadequate duration of action. Although it is clear that adding a small dose of opioid reduces the dose of local anesthetic required for surgical anesthesia by a small amount, this is, in most cases, clinically indistinguishable from a small increase in local anesthetic alone, and opioids are not typically used with the goal of prolonging spinal anesthesia.

Intrathecal injection of local anesthetics results in hypotension, presumably reflecting reductions in sympathetic outflow by axonal block of spinal nerve roots and/or synaptic failure of excitatory inputs into preganglionic sympathetic neurons in the intermediolateral (IML) cell columns. Although this is typically counteracted by systemic administration of a sympathomimetic agent, such as ephedrine, it may be diminished by interactions with other drugs administered intrathecally.

For many years, epinephrine has been added to local anesthetics for intrathecal administration, primarily to prolong anesthesia (see below). However, the dose administered (0.2 mg) is sufficiently great to result in cardiovascular stimulation following systemic absorption (Bonica et al., 1971). Clonidine has also been added to intrathecal local anesthetics to prolong anesthesia. This specific α_2-adrenoceptor agonist might be expected to exacerbate hypotension by its sympatholytic effects in the IML and in the brainstem. However, with the high degree of sympatholysis resulting from intrathecal local anesthetics in doses necessary for spinal anesthesia, the effect of clonidine appears to be minimal, as it results in no, or only minor increases in the incidence of hypotension during spinal anesthesia (Klimscha et al., 1995).

Neostigmine, a cholinesterase inhibitor, produces analgesia after intrathecal injection by enhancing cholinergic receptor stimulation by acetylcholine. Preganglionic sympathetic neurons are activated by local or intrathecal injection of cholinergic agonists or cholinesterase inhibitors, resulting in increased blood pressure and heart rate (Sundaram et al., 1989). Intrathecal injection of neostigmine diminishes hypotension from intrathecal local anesthetics in rats, sheep, and humans (Klamt et al., 1997). This, of course, argues against a complete axonal blockade of efferent activity by local anesthetics, such that partial blockade can be overcome by cellular stimulation within the spinal cord by neostigmine. The latter hypothesis is supported by studies in rats that demonstrate reduction in sympathetic efferent nerve activity by intrathecal injection of the local anesthetic bupivacaine, increases in sympathetic activity after intrathecal neostigmine, and no charge in sympathetic activity after intrathecal injection of their combination.

Although opioid receptors are present on IML cells and activation of such receptors in this region inhibits sympathetic activity, intrathecal injection of opioids has not been shown to alter hypotension during spinal anesthesia.

The second problem with spinal anesthesia is duration, because local anesthetics are usually injected through a needle as a single bolus for surgery. Two approaches have been used to prolong the duration of spinal anesthesia. First, systemic administration of opioid or α_2-adrenoceptor agonist analgesics has been demonstrated to prolong spinal anesthesia by approximately 25% (Sarantopoulos and Fassoulaki, 1994). Although the mechanism for this effect is unknown, it is speculated to be due in part to peripheral actions of these analgesics, resulting in decreased afferent nerve depolarization. It is thought that association and dissociation of local anesthetics from their site(s) of action on Na^+ channels occurs primarily during depolarization, so reduced afferent nerve firing could retard dissociation of local anesthetic from its site of channel blockade.

Another approach to prolong the duration of spinal anesthesia is to alter local pharmacokinetics of local anesthetics. Glucose is commonly added to local anesthetics for intrathecal injection to yield a solution hyperbaric compared to cerebrospinal fluid. Addition of glucose, coupled with alterations in patient position after intrathecal injection of local anesthetics, can have a profound effect on distribution of anesthesia. Its effect on duration, however, is considerably smaller and more variable. Although literature reports conflict, it appears to prolong duration of anesthesia by <25%.

Co-injection of vasoconstrictors could also reduce removal of intrathecally administered local anesthetics from their sites of action and thereby prolong spinal anesthesia. Both clonidine and epinephrine produce a dose-dependent increase in the duration of surgical anesthesia resulting from intrathecal bupivacaine (Eisenach et al., 1996). Although there are few good dose–response studies available, it would appear that no further prolongation occurs in doses of epinephrine exceeding 200 μg and in doses of clonidine exceeding 150 μg. Prolongation of bupivacaine anesthesia appears to be greater with clonidine (50–75%) than with epinephrine (0–25%).

The interaction between epinephrine and local anesthetics on duration of spinal anesthesia differs with the local anesthetic, and this is speculated to reflect differing actions of the local anesthetics themselves on spinal cord blood flow. Tetracaine increases spinal cord blood blow (and perhaps hastens its own removal), an effect abolished by epinephrine, and epinephrine increases the duration of tetracaine spinal anesthesia by as much as 100% (Kozody et al., 1985). In contrast, bupivacaine and lidocaine alone reduce spinal cord blood flow, an effect that is not significantly altered by epinephrine, and epinephrine has minimal effects (0–25%) on duration of spinal anesthesia from these agents.

Epidural Anesthesia

Epidural injection of local anesthetics in adequate doses results in surgical anesthesia accompanied, like spinal anesthesia, with hypotension. One problem with spinal anesthesia, inadequate duration, is usually not encountered with epidural anesthesia for surgery because epidural injections are typically performed through a catheter, through which re-injections can be made. Thus although epinephrine, opioids, and clonidine can prolong the duration of epidural anesthesia, this is not of major benefit in the operating room. The case is different with epidural analgesia for obstetrics (however, see below). Epidural anesthesia has two problems that spinal anesthesia does not: a higher frequency of breakthrough discomfort or pain during surgery, and toxicity from systemic absorption of the large doses of local anesthetics necessary for surgical epidural anesthesia.

Pain during surgery with epidural anesthesia is typically treated by systemic injection of opioids and/or epidural injection of more local anesthetic. However, the incidence of pain has been described by many to be reduced by addition of opioids and clonidine epidurally. Because both of these agents produce analgesia after systemic injection, it is unclear whether this reflects a local interaction in the epidural space or systemic absorption of drug. Similarly, reports in the veterinary literature suggest an increased success rate when α_2-adrenoceptor agonists or opioids are added to local anesthetics, although there has been little investigation into the mechanism or nature of this interaction (Grubb et al., 1993).

Major morbidity from local anesthetic injection, seizures, and cardiac dysrhythmias, leading to cardiac arrest, most commonly occur with accidental intravenous injection through a catheter inserted into an epidural vein. However, plasma concentrations of local anesthetics after epidural injection of doses necessary for anesthesia for abdominal operations approximate toxicity, and it is not uncommon to see evidence of central nervous system excitation (jitteriness, anxiety, dysphoria) during epidural anesthesia. For this reason, opioids are sometimes added to reduce local anesthetic dose by approximately 25%. Because opioids do not provide surgical anesthesia alone, this interaction is technically synergistic.

Epinephrine and clonidine have been added to local anesthetics in order to reduce systemic absorption after epidural administration. Plasma concentrations of lidocaine are reduced after epidural co-administration of epinephrine, but not clonidine (Nishikawa and Dohi, 1990). Because lidocaine is metabolized in the liver, and because clonidine reduces hepatic blood flow, it has been argued that failure of clonidine to reduce lidocaine concentrations in plasma could reflect a balance of reduced absorption from the epidural space by clonidine-induced vasoconstriction and decreased elimination by clonidine-induced reductions in hepatic blood flow.

Spinal Analgesia

Spinal analgesia is provided as a single injection through a needle in women in labor and postoperative patients and by repeated or continuous infusion through a catheter for chronic pain. Problems and drug interactions differ considerably between these two situations.

Initiation of analgesia for women in labor is now commonly performed by insertion of a spinal needle through an epidural needle, injection of drugs intrathecally, then insertion of an epidural catheter for later use. Intrathecal injection of fentanyl, 10–40 μg, or sufentanil, 2–8 μg, results in rapid onset, complete pain relief, lasting approximately 90 min in women in early labor, and 30–60 min in women in late labor. These opioids also produce pruritus, nausea, and respiratory depression with an incidence of 80, 20, and 0.02%, respectively (Honet et al., 1992).

Because the major clinical problem in this setting is duration, not efficacy, most of the clinical research has focused on drug interactions on duration of analgesia. Thus addition of morphine, 100–200 μg, to fentanyl or sufentanil was investigated. Although this resulted in prolonged (>6 hr) pruritus and severe nausea, morphine did not prolong the duration of fentanyl or sufentanil analgesia (Grieco et al., 1993). This may reflect the need for surgical anesthesia for late labor and delivery, which clearly is not provided by opioids.

Local anesthetics, epinephrine, clonidine, and neostigmine have been added to opioids for spinal analgesia. Few dose–response studies have been performed, and no formal, isobolographic interactions have been examined. The focus of most studies has been on duration of analgesia. Bupivacaine, 2.5 mg, prolongs analgesia from intrathecal fentanyl or sufentanil by approximately 30% (to 120 min) while increasing the likelihood of hypotension and minor motor blockade. Addition of both bupivacaine, 2.5 mg, and epinephrine, 200 μg, further increases duration of fentanyl or sufentanil analgesia by 10% (to 180 min) (Campbell et al., 1997). Similarly, clonidine, 25–50 μg, prolongs sufentanil analgesia (to 120 min) and clonidine plus bupivacaine prolongs sufentanil analgesia more, to 240 min.

Intrathecal injection of neostigmine in doses up to those producing nausea (20 μg) does not provide pain relief to women in labor. To investigate its interaction with sufentanil, a sequential up–down methodology was employed, as originally described by Dixon and Massey (1983). In this method, women received, in a two-phase study, either intrathecal saline or a fixed dose (10 μg) of neostigmine plus sufentanil. If they had completed analgesia within 10 min lasting at least 60 min, the next woman received a larger dose. By this method, we demonstrated an ED_{50} of 4.4 μg for intrathecal sufentanil for women in early labor. This was significantly reduced to 3.0 μg by neostigmine, representing a synergistic interaction.

The focus of spinal drug interaction studies for single injections in postoperative patients has been primarily on interactions with morphine, because the other opioids produce brief (<4–6 hr) analgesia. Epinephrine has little effect on duration or intensity of intrathecal morphine analgesia in postoperative patients. Similarly, although there are exceptions, most reports demonstrate a minimal effect of clonidine on the duration of intrathecal morphine analgesia in these patients. This is perhaps not surprising, because neither clonidine nor epinephrine exerts a prolonged effect after intrathecal administration.

Problems with continuous spinal analgesia for chronic pain relate to efficacy and side effects, because duration is unimportant with a continuous infusion. Opioids, typically morphine, are the first drugs usually administered in this setting. Efficacy may be lost because of the development of tolerance, leading to escalation of dose into dose-limiting side effects, or because of the presence of poorly opioid sensitive pain, often described clinically as neuropathic pain.

Only local anesthetics and clonidine have been studied systematically for their interactions with opioids for continuous intrathecal analgesia for chronic pain. Other agents (e.g., ketamine, CPP, somatostatin, calcitonin, adenosine, and $MgSO_4$) have been reported anecdotally or in small series, usually alone. It is clear that efficacy can be regained or enhanced by addition of local anesthetics or clonidine to intrathecal opioids in these patients; however, formal interaction or mechanistic studies have not been performed.

Epidural Analgesia

Different problems, and hence different emphases, characterize drug interaction studies with epidural analgesia in obstetric, postoperative, and chronic pain patients. In obstetrics both bolus and infusion interaction studies have been performed. In the bolus studies, both duration and efficacy have been studied. Addition of epidural fentanyl results in a dose-dependent reduction in the bupivacaine dose required for adequate analgesia during labor (Polley et al., 1996). Only one isobolographic study has examined the interaction between opioids and local anesthetics in labor. In that study, dose–responses were obtained for intrathecal sufentanil (via the combined spinal–epidural technique described above), epidural bupivacaine, and their combination (Abouleish et al., 1994). There was a clear enhancement by one agent of the other, which was statistically additive. Similar results have been obtained after continuous infusion.

Other studies have examined epidural drug interactions for duration of analgesia in women in labor. Thus addition of fentanyl, 50 µg, epinephrine, 50 µg, or clonidine, 75 µg, increases by 50–100% the duration of analgesia from epidural bupivacaine, 25 mg (Eisenach et al., 1996). The addition of both fentanyl, 50 µg, and epinephrine, 50 µg (or clonidine, 75 µg), to bupivacaine results in an even greater increase of 100–200% in duration.

The major problems with epidural analgesia in obstetrics are hypotension and motor blockade following local anesthetic injection. Addition of opioid has been shown to reduce the dose of local anesthetic required, leading to a reduction in the degree of motor blockade. Opioids do not reduce the incidence of hypotension in these studies, however. Both epinephrine and clonidine increase the incidence and degree of motor blockade from epidural local anesthetics, whereas only clonidine increases the incidence of hypotension (Eisenach et al., 1996). Again, formal interaction studies have not been performed concerning these side effects.

The problems with epidural analgesia in postoperative patients are similar to those in obstetrics. Epidural injection of local anesthetics alone results in hypotension and motor blockade, opioids alone result in nausea, sedation, and rare respiratory depression, and α_2-adrenoceptor agonists alone result in incomplete or brief analgesia, sedation, and hypotension. A large number of studies have addressed these drugs in combinations, either after bolus or continuous infusion.

Surprisingly, the literature concerning epidural local anesthetic–opioid combinations in postoperative patients does not clearly demonstrate a synergistic interaction. Thus several studies that compare epidural infusions of fentanyl or sufentanil alone to these agents with various doses of bupivacaine fail to demonstrate improved analgesia or reduced opioid dose, even with bupivacaine doses large enough to lead to hypotension (Salomaki et al., 1995). Some studies do demonstrate opioid dose reduction by addition of bupivacaine, but the effect is minor and inconsistent compared to the results in obstetrics. Although this can, in some cases, be explained by epidural injection of inadequate volumes of solution or injection too distant from the dermatomal site of postsurgical pain, these factors are not always present in the negative studies.

In contrast, clonidine clearly prolongs the duration of epidural fentanyl analgesia in postoperative patients after a bolus, and diminishes by 20–50% fentanyl dose required by continuous postoperative epidural infusion (Rostaing et al., 1991). This interaction is not due to altered systemic absorption, because plasma fentanyl concentrations following epidural injection are not affected by addition of clonidine. One isobolographic study of bolus epidural fentanyl and clonidine following surgery has been performed (Eisenach et al., 1994). In this study, the ED50 of the combination, although numerically less than the theoretical additive doses required, did not statistically differ from additivity. Although both opioids and clonidine produce sedation, studies of their combination fail to demonstrate enhanced sedation when they are combined. In one study examining respiratory depression by continuous measurement of oxyhemoglobin saturation by pulse oximetry, addition of clonidine reduced the mild respiratory depression induced by continuous epidural sufentanil. No formal interaction studies between opioids and clonidine concerning side effects have been performed.

The problems with epidurally administered analgesics in the treatment of chronic pain do not differ significantly from those with intrathecal administration discussed above. Despite reasonably widespread use and common application of multi-drug therapy, there are few descriptions of drug interactions in this patient population and no formal interaction studies. The most commonly discussed problem is reduced efficacy of epidural opioids in patients with neuropathic pain. A variety of adjuvants have been described, including local anesthetics, somatostatin, and clonidine, but only clonidine has been shown to be effective. In that study, epidural clonidine or saline was added to morphine in patients with cancer and severe pain, and clonidine successfully improved pain relief in more than 50% of patients, compared to only 5% with saline placebo (Eisenach et al., 1995).

SUMMARY

The interest in drug interactions following spinal administration comes from problems unique to the route of administration (epidural vs. intrathecal), method of injection (bolus vs. infusion), and patient population (obstetric vs. postoperative vs. chronic pain). The most commonly studied combination, local anesthetic plus opioid, demonstrates frequently, but in some situations not consistently, a synergism. In most cases, combination of clonidine and local anesthetics or opioids results in synergism of the desired effect, either duration or efficacy. Although it is clear that such drug combinations are commonly used and effective, their precise interactions for efficacy and for adverse effects remain poorly understood in humans.

REFERENCES

Abouleish A, Camann W, Holden D, Emami A, Eisenach J, Yun E, Datta S (1994): Antinociceptive interaction between intrathecal sufentanil and epidural bupivacaine: additivity or synergism? Anesthesiology 81:A1144.

Akerman B, Arwestrom E, Post C (1988): Local anesthetics potentiate spinal morphine antinociception. Anesth Analg 67:943–948.

Berenbaum MC (1989): What is synergy? Pharmacol Rev 41:93–142.

Bilsky EJ, Inturrisi CE, Sadee W, Hruby VJ, Porreca F (1996): Competitive and noncompetitive NMDA antagonists block the development of antinociceptive tolerance to morphine, but not to selective mu or delta opioid agonists in mice. Pain 68: 229–237.

Bonica JJ, Akamatsu TJ, Berges PU, Morikawa K, Kennedy WF Jr (1971): Circulatory effects of peridural block: II. Effects of epinephrine. Anesthesiology 34:514–522.

Campbell DC, Banner R, Crone LA, Gore-Hickman W, Yip RW (1997): Addition of epinephrine to intrathecal bupivacaine and sufentanil for ambulatory labor analgesia. Anesthesiology 86:525–531.

Chestnut DH, Owen CL, Bates JN, Ostman LG, Choi WW, Geiger MW (1988): Continuous infusion epidural analgesia during labor: a randomized double-blind comparison of 0.0625% bupivacaine/0.0002% fentanyl *versus* 0.125% bupivacaine. Anesthesiology 68:754–759.

Cullen ML, Staren ED, El-Ganzouri A, Logas WG, Ivankovich AD, Economou SG (1985): Continuous epidural infusion for analgesia after major abdominal operations: a randomized prospective double-blind study. Surgery 98:718–728.

Dixon WJ, Massey FJ (1983): *Introduction to Statistical Analysis*. 4th ed. New York: McGraw-Hill, pp. 428–439.

Eisenach JC, D'Angelo R, Taylor C, Hood DD (1994): An isobolographic study of epidural clonidine and fentanyl after cesarean section. Anesth Analg 79:285–290.

Eisenach JC, DuPen S, Dubois M, Miguel R, Allin D, Epidural Clonidine Study Group (1995): Epidural clonidine analgesia for intractable cancer pain. Pain 61:391–399.

Eisenach JC, De Kock M, Klimscha W (1996): α_2-Adrenergic agonists for regional anesthesia—A clinical review of clonidine (1984–1995). Anesthesiology 85:655–674.

Elliott K, Minami N, Kolesnikov YA, Pasternak GW, Inturrisi CE (1994): The NMDA receptor antagonists, LY274614 and MK-801, and nitric oxide synthase inhibitor, NG-nitro-L-arginine, attenuate analgesic tolerance to the mu-opioid morphine but not kappa opioids. Pain 56:69–75.

Gennings C, Carter WH, Campbell ED, Staniswalis JG, Martin TJ, Martin BR, White KL (1990): Isobolographic characterization of drug interactions incorporating biological variability. J Pharmacol Exp Ther 252:208–217.

Gessner, PK (1974): The isobolographic method applied to drug interactions. In Morselli PL, Garattini S, Cohen SN (eds): *Drug Interactions*. New York: Raven Press, pp. 349–362.

Grieco WM, Norris MC, Leighton BL, Arkoosh VA, Huffnagle HJ, Honet JE, Costello D (1993): Intrathecal sufentanil labor analgesia: The effects of adding morphine or epinephrine. Anesth Analg 77:1149–1154.

Grubb TL, Riebold TW, Huber MJ (1993): Evaluation of lidocaine, xylazine, and a combination of lidocaine and xylazine for epidural analgesia in llamas. J Am Vet Med Assoc 203:1441–1444.

Hjortso NC, Lund C, Mogensen T, Bigler D, Kehlet H (1986): Epidural morphine improves pain relief and maintains sensory analgesia during continuous epidural bupivacaine after abdominal surgery. Anesth Analg 65:1033–1036.

Honet JE, Arkoosh VA, Norris MC, Huffnagle HJ, Silverman NS, Leighton BL (1992): Comparison among intrathecal fentanyl, meperidine, and sufentanil for labor analgesia. Anesth Analg 75:734–739.

Hylden JLK, Wilcox GL (1983): Pharmacological characterization of substance P-induced nociception in mice: modulation by opioid and noradrenergic agonists at the spinal level. J Pharmacol Exp Ther 226:398–404.

Kehlet H (1998): Modification of responses to surgery and anesthesia by neural blockade: clinical implications. In Cousins MJ, Bridenbaugh PO (eds): *Neural Blockade in Clinical Anesthesia and Management of Pain.* Philadelphia: Lippincott, pp. 129–175.

Klamt JG, Slullitel A, Garcia V, Prado WA (1997): Postoperative analgesic effect of intrathecal neostigmine and its influence on spinal anaesthesia. Anaesthesia 52:547–551.

Klimscha W, Chiari A, Krafft P, Plattner O, Taslimi R, Mayer N, Weinstabl C, Schneider B, Zimpfer M (1995): Hemodynamic and analgesic effects of clonidine added repetitively to continuous epidural and spinal blocks. Anesth Analg 80:322–327.

Kozody R, Palahniuk RJ, Cumming MO (1985): Spinal cord blood flow following subarachnoid tetracaine. Can Anaesth Soc J 32:23–29.

Logas WG, El-Baz N, El-Ganzouri A, Cullen M, Staren E, Faber P, Ivankovich AD (1987): Continuous thoracic epidural analgesia for postoperative pain relief following thoracotomy: a randomized prospective study. Anesthesiology 67:787–791.

Lutfy K, Shen KZ, Woodward RM, Weber E (1996): Inhibition of morphine tolerance by NMDA receptor antagonists in the formalin test. Brain Res 731:171–181.

Malmberg AB, Yaksh TL (1992): Isobolographic and dose-response analyses of the interactions between intrathecal mu and delta agonists: effects of naltrindole and its benzofuran analog (NTB). J Pharmacol Exp Ther 263:264–275.

Malmberg AB, Yaksh TL (1993): Pharmacology of the spinal action of ketorolac, morphine, ST-91, U50488H, and L-PIA on the formalin test and an isobolographic analysis of the NSAID interaction. Anesthesiology 79:270–281.

Mao J, Price DD, Mayer DJ (1995): Experimental mononeuropathy reduces the antinociceptive effects of morphine: implications for common intracellular mechanisms involved in morphine tolerance and neuropathic pain. Pain 61:353–364.

Marek P, Ben-Eliyahu S, Gold M, Liebeskind JC (1991): Excitatory amino acid antagonists (kynurenic acid and MK-801) attenuate the development of morphine tolerance in the rat. Brain Res 547:77–81.

Maves TJ, Gebhart GF (1992): Antinociceptive synergy between intrathecal morphine and lidocaine during visceral and somatic nociception in the rat. Anesthesiology 76:91–99.

Monasky MS, Zinsmeister AR, Stevens CW, Yaksh TL (1990): Interaction of intrathecal morphine and ST-91 on antinociception in the rat: dose-response analysis, antagonism and clearance. J Pharmacol Exp Ther 254:383–392.

Nishikawa T and Dohi S (1990): Clinical evaluation of clonidine added to lidocaine solution for epidural anesthesia. Anesthesiology 73:853–859.

Ossipov MH, Harris S, Lloyd P, Messineo E (1990a): An isobolographic analysis of the antinociceptive effect of systemically administered combinations of clonidine and opiates. J Pharmacol Exp Ther 255:1107–1116.

Ossipov MH, Harris S, Lloyd P, Messineo E, Lin B-S, Bagley J (1990b): Antinociceptive interaction between opioids and medetomidine: systemic additivity and spinal synergy. Anesthesiology 73:1227–1235.

Ossipov MH, Lopez Y, Bian D, Nichols ML, Porreca F (1997): Synergistic antinociceptive interactions of morphine and clonidine in rats with nerve-ligation injury. Anesthesiology 86:1–9.

Penning JP, Yaksh TL (1992): Interaction of intrathecal morphine with bupivacaine and lidocaine in the rat. Anesthesiology 77:1186–1200.

Polley LS, Columb MO, Lyons G, Nair SA (1996): The effect of epidural fentanyl on the minimum local analgesic concentration of epidural chloroprocaine in labor. Anesth Analg 83:987–990.

Przesmycki K, Dzieciuch JA, Czuczwar SJ, Kleinrok Z (1997): Isobolographic analysis of interaction between intrathecal morphine and clonidine in the formalin test in rats. Eur J Pharmacol 337:11–17.

Roerig SC, Fujimoto JM (1989): Multiplicative interaction between intrathecally and intracerebroventricularly administered mu opioid agonists but limited interactions between delta and kappa agonists for antinociception in mice. J Pharmacol Exp Ther 249:762–768.

Rostaing S, Bonnet F, Levron JC, Vodinh J, Pluskwa F, Saada M (1991): Effect of epidural clonidine on analgesia and pharmacokinetics of epidural fentanyl in postoperative patients. Anesthesiology 75:420–425.

Salomaki TE, Laitinen JO, Vainionpaa V, Nuutinen LS (1995): 0.1% Bupivacaine does not reduce the requirement for epidural fentanyl infusion after major abdominal surgery. Reg Anesth 20:435–443.

Sarantopoulos C, Fassoulaki A (1994): Systemic opioids enhance the spread of sensory analgesia produced by intrathecal lidocaine. Anesth Analg 79:94–97.

Sherman SE, Loomis CW, Milne B, Cervenko FW (1988): Intrathecal oxymetazoline produces analgesia via spinal α-adrenoceptors and potentiates spinal morphine. Eur J Pharmacol 148:371–380.

Solomon RE, Gebhart GF (1988): Intrathecal morphine and clonidine: antinociceptive tolerance and cross-tolerance and effects on blood pressure. J Pharmacol Exp Ther 245:444–454.

Solomon RE, Gebhart GF (1994): Synergistic antinociceptive interactions among drugs administered to the spinal cord. Anesth Analg 78:1164–1172.

Sundaram K, Murugaian J, Krieger A, Sapru H (1989): Microinjections of cholinergic agonists into the intermediolateral cell column of the spinal cord at T_1-T_3 increase heart rate and contractility. Brain Res 503:22–31.

Tallarida RJ (1992): Statistical analysis of drug combinations for synergism [published erratum appears in Pain 1993 Jun 53(3):365] [review]. Pain 49:93–97.

Tallarida RJ, Porreca F, Cowan A (1989): Statistical analysis of drug-drug and site-site interactions with isobolograms. Life Sci 45:947–961.

Tiseo PJ, Inturrisi CE (1993): Attenuation and reversal of morphine tolerance by the competitive N-methyl-D-aspartate receptor antagonist, LY274614. J Pharmacol Exp Ther 264:1090–1096.

Trujillo KA, Akil H (1991): Inhibition of morphine tolerance and dependence by the NMDA receptor antagonist MK-801. Science 251:85–87.

Wessinger WD (1986): Approaches to the study of drug interactions in behavioral pharmacology. Neurosci Biobehav Rev 10:103–113.

Wong CS, Liaw WJ, Tung CS, Su YF, Ho ST (1996): Ketamine potentiates analgesic effect of morphine in postoperative epidural pain control. Reg Anesth 21:534–541.

Yaksh TL, Malmberg AB (1994): Interaction of spinal modulatory receptor systems. In Fields HL, Liebeskind JC (eds): *Progress in Pain Research and Management*. Seattle: IASP Press, pp. 151–171.

Yaksh TL, Reddy SVR (1981): Studies in the primate on the analgesic effects associated with intrathecal actions of opiates, alpha-adrenergic agonists and baclofen. Anesthesiology 54:451–467.

INDEX

ABT-594, 271–272
Acetaminophen, 82–83
Acetylcholine
　nicotinic receptors and, 270–273
　spinal cholinergic analgesia, 277–278
Acute pain
　animal models, 23–26
　anesthetics and, 323
　antidepressants and, 306, 311
　neurophysiology of, *see*
　　Neurophysiology of acute and chronic pain
Adenosine
　A_1 receptors, 231, 239
　A_2 receptors, 231, 239
　A_3 receptors, 231–232
　analogues, 230
　epidural analgesia, 356
　function of, generally, 29
　indirectly acting agents, 232
　pain perception and, 229
　serotonin receptors and, 216
Adenosine 3′,5′-cyclic monophosphate (cAMP)
　NSAID pharmacology and, 83
　prostanoid antagonists and, 99–100
　purines, effect on, 230, 235
　vanilloid antagonists and, 124
Adenosine triphosphate (ATP)
　ATP receptors, pain transmission, 229–230, 233
　function of, generally, 5–6
　purines and, 229, 236
Adenylate cyclase, 98
a-adrenoceptors, opioid interaction with, 348–349

β-adrenorecptor agonist, 205
AFDX 116, 275
Afferent nerves, 6–7
Alfentanil, 278
Allosteric sites, EAAs and, 162–163
4-aminopyridine (4-AP), 334
Alpha-2 adrenergic agonists
　antinociceptive actions
　　in human pain states, 192–194
　　overview, 188–191
　functioning coupling of, 181
　nociception, spinal adrenoceptors, 181–182
　nonantinociceptive actions, 191–192
　overview, 179–181
　spinal adrenoceptors
　　antinociceptive effects of, 181–184
　　overview
　subtypes, 180
Alpha-flupenthixol, 292
Alphaxalone, 255
Amino acids, 12
5′-amino-5′-deoxyadenosine (NH_2dAD), 232
Aminophylline, 232
4-aminopyridine (4-AP), 334
Amitriptyline, 311–312
AMPA, 168
Amphetamines, 287–289, 291–292
Amygdala, 274–275
Analgesia
　epidural, 356–358
　spinal, 355–356
Analgesic agents, peripherally acting
　cytokines, peripheral hyperalgesia and, 103–104

363

364 INDEX

Analgesic agents (*Continued*)
  kinin and kinin receptors, in hyperalgesia, 100–103
  nerve growth factor
    hyperalgesia, role in, 104–107
    inhibitors, 107
  prostanoid antagonists
    overview, 96–98
    receptor specificity, 98
    stimulus specificity, 98–100
Analgesics
  alpha-2 adrenergic agonists, 179–195
  animal models, 24
  antidepressants, 303–315
  cholinergic agonists, 265–279
  dopaminergic drugs, 287–296
  excitatory amino acid (EAA) antagonists, 162–163
  purines, 229–239
  vanilloids, 117–126
Analogues, *see specific types of analgesics*
Anesthesia
  epidural, 354–355
  local, *see* Local anesthesia
  spinal, 352–354
Animal models
  acute pain, 23–26
  incisional pain, 31
  neuropathic pain, 34–36
  nociceptive stimulus, 22–23
  persistent pain, 26–30, 159–160
  visceral pain, 31–34
Ankylosing spondylitis, 74
Antagonists, *see specific types of analgesics*
Anti-inflammatory drugs, 323
Antibodies, serotonin receptors and, 204
Anticonvulsants, 325–327
Antidepressants (AD), *see* Tricyclic antidepressants (TCAs)
  administration of, 309
  effects of, generally, 314–315
  efficacy of
    acute pain, 306
    cancer pain, 306
    chronic nonmalignant pain, 304–306
  experimental data, 306–309

function of, generally, 29
mechanism of action
  central site, 310–311
  peripheral site, 310
neurochemical mechanisms
  monoaminergic mechanism, 311–312
  opioidergic mechanisms, 312
  potential mechanisms, generally, 313
  noxious transmission, interaction with, 313–315
overview, 303–304
Antiepileptics, 29
Antihistamine, 232
Antihyperalgesic manipulation, 50
Antinociception
  alpha-2 adrenergic agonists
    overview, 186
    peripheral actions, 189
    spinal actions, 189, 191
    supraspinal actions, 191
  antidepressants and, 314
  calcium channels and, 332
  capsaicin-induced, 125
  central nicotinic, spinal mediation, 274
  cholinergic analgesia, 267
  epibatidine, 268–269
  morphine, 312
  muscarinic in RVM, nitric oxide mediation, 274
  nicotinic cholinergic analgesia, 270–271
  purines and, 234–237
  spinal cholinergic analgesia, 276
Antinociceptive manipulation, 50
Arachidonic acid, 5
Arecoline, 267, 275
Arthritis, 73–74, 146, 215
Asimadoline, 34
Aspartate, anticonvulsants and, 326
Aspirin, 289
Atropine, 272, 275
Autoradiography, 58, 158, 207

Baclofen, 252, 255–258
Barbiturates, 252, 254
Bay K 8644, 270

INDEX   365

Benzodiazepines, 252–254
Benzothiazepines, 330
Bicuculline, 252, 255–256
Blood-brain barrier, 237
Bombesin (BOM), 7–8, 13
Bradykinin, 4–5, 98–101
Brain-derived neurotrophic factor (BDNF), 106
Brain, neurophysiology, *see specific brain regions*
Brompton Cocktail, 288
B_2 receptors, 101
Bulbospinal system, 204
κ-bungarotoxin, 271
Bupivacaine
  effect of, generally, 327
  epidural analgesia, 356–357
  local anesthesia, 347
  spinal anesthesia, 353–354
Butylthio[2,2,2], 267

Caffeine, analgesic properties of, 238
Calcitonin, 356
Calcitonin gene-related peptide (CGRP)
  in GABAergic system, 251
  overview, 5, 7–8, 13, 105
  serotonin receptors and, 218
Calcium channel blockers, 314
Calcium channels, 314, 329–333
Cancer pain, 288, 306, 358
Capsaicin
  serotonin receptors and, 218
  therapeutic efficacy in humans, 117–120
Capsazepine, 122, 126
Carbachol, 274–275
Carbamazepine, 325–326
Cardiac pain, 232–233, 237
Cardiac toxicity, 323
Catecholamines, 294
Catecholamine uptake inhibitor, 291
Central nervous system (CNS)
  calcium channels and, 331
  serotonin and, 203
  sodium channels and, 323–324, 326
Cerebrospinal fluid (CSF), 158, 237
Chlordiazepoxide, 254
p-chlorophenylalanine, 294, 311
Chlorpromazine, 292

Chlorprothixene, 314
Cholecystokinin (CCK), 7–8, 60–61
Cholinergic agonists
  background, 265–267
  clinical analgesia, 278
  future directions for, 278–279
  muscarinic mechanisms, research strategies, 267–268
  nicotinic mechanisms
    epibatidine, 268–269
    research strategies, 269–272
  spinal mechanisms
    adrenergic and opioid interactions, 277–278
    muscarinic mechanisms, 276
    nicotinic mechanisms, 276–277
    overview, 275
  supraspinal mechanisms, 272–275
Chronic constriction injury (CCI), 63–64, 324–325, 331
Chronic inflammatory disorders, 73–83
Chronic pain
  antidepressants and, 303, 315
  GABA changes in, 250–252
  local anesthesia, 356
  neurophysiology of, *see* Neurophysiology of acute and chronic pain
  nonmalignant, 304–306, 323
  spinal analgesia, 355
Chronic pain syndromes, sodium channels and, 322–323
Cicaprost, 99
Citalopram, 314
Clomipramine, 312, 314
Clonidine
  alpha-2 adrenergic agonists and, 184, 186, 193
  animal models, 34
  calcium channels and, 335
  epidural analgesia, 357–358
  serotonin receptors and, 217
  spinal analgesia
    cholinergic, 278
    generally, 356
  spinal anesthesia, 353, 355
  spinal drug interactions, 349, 353, 355
C-mechanoreceptors, 2
CNQX, 159

Cocaine, 288–289, 291–293
C-polymodal nociceptor, 4
Cold plate procedure, 36
Colorectal distension test, 31, 34
Corticotropin-releasing factor (CRF), 7
Corynanthine, 184
CPP, 356
Cromakalim, 335
Cyclooxygenase (COX), 5, 74, 76, 81
N^6-cyclopentyladenosine (CPA), 231
Cytisine, 276–277
Cytokines, peripheral hyperalgesia and, 103–104

DAMGO, 52–59, 62, 351
4-DAMP, 274–275
Dental pain, 145–146
Depression, 303
Desensitization, capsaicin-induced, 123–124
Desipramine, 291, 310–312
Desmethylclomipramine, 312
Desoxyephedrine, 289
Dexamethasone, 74
Dexmedetomidine, 184, 186, 191, 193
Dextroamphetamine, 288
Dextromethorphan, 30, 36, 75, 159
5,7 Dihydroxytryptamine (5, 7-DHT), 208
Diabetic neuropathy, 324, 326
Diclofenac, 74
Dihydropyridines, 330
Diltiazem, 330
DiMe-C7, 293
L-DOPA, 289
Dopamine, 271
Dopaminergic drugs
  animal studies
    formalin test, pharmacology of, 291–296
    mechanisms, 291
    overview, 289–291
  clinical potential of, 296
  human experiments, 288–289
  nondopaminergic mechanisms, 294–295
  overview, 287–288
  pain tests, noninjurious stimuli, 294
  spinal mechanisms, 293–294
  stress and, 295–296
  thalamic mechanisms, 293–294
Dorsal horn, effects on
  alpha-2 adrenergic antagonists, 191
  cholinergic agonists, 249
  dopaminergic drugs, 293
  glutamate, 157–158, 163
  serotonin receptors and, 204, 207, 210, 213, 216–217
Dorsal parabrachial region, 272
Dorsal root ganglion (DRG)
  calcium channels and, 330
  function of, generally, 7–8, 13
  opioids, effect on, 54–55
  purines and, 235
  serotonin receptors and, 217
  sodium channels and, 322, 328
Dose-addition models, 346–347
Double-blind studies, 278, 288, 324
DPDPE, 52–53, 55, 58–59, 349, 351
Drug interactions, evaluation of, 346–347
DSP4, 275
Dynorphin (DYN), 7–8, 61–64

Echothiophate, 275
Edrophonium, 275
Endorphin (END), 7
β-endorphin, 57
Enkephalin (ENK), 7–8, 204
EP_2 receptors, 98, 100
EP_3 receptors, 98–99
Ephedrine, 289
Epibatidine
  adverse effects, 269
  calcium channels and, 332
  discovery and early characterization of, 268
  nicotinic receptors and, 270, 277
  pharmacology, 268–269
Epiboxidine, 269
Epilepsy, 326
Epinephrine, 354, 356–357
Epipedobates tricolor, 268
Eticlopride, 292
Evoked response, 11
Excitatory amino acids (EAAs)
  antagonists, *see* Excitatory amino acid (EAA) antagonists

anticonvulsants and, 326
antidepressants and, 313–314
receptors, 74
Excitatory amino acid (EAA) antagonists
anticonvulsants and, 326
glutamate, role in nociception, 157–159
ionotropic glutamate receptor antagonists
clinical utilization of, 159–160
interaction with metabotropic glutamate receptors, 168
motor deficits and side effects of, 161–162
metabotropic glutamate receptors, nociception and, 163–167
NMDA receptor complex, allosteric sites and analgesic combinations, 162–163
Excitatory postsynaptic potential (EPSP), 12, 137
Experimental pain, excitatory amino acid (EAA) antagonists and, 160–161

Fentanyl, 58, 357
Flecainide, 324
Fluoxetine, 311, 314
Foot shock test, 272
Formalin test
adenosine receptors, 231
animal models, 26–28
dopaminergic agents, 289, 291–296
serotonin receptors, 213
sodium channels, 325

GABA$_A$ receptors
agonists, 253
antagonism, 255
modulators, 253–255
overview, 252
GABA$_B$ receptors, mechanisms, 255–258
Gabapentin, 257
Galanin (GAL), 7
γ-aminobutyric acid (GABA)
antagonists, 29
antidepressants and, 314
chronic pain models, 250–252
derivatives, 257
function of, 13–14

future directions, 257–258
nicotinic receptors and, 271
pain pathways, presence, localization and function of, 249–250
pharmacological aspects
GABA$_A$, 253–254
GABA$_B$, 255–257
receptors, 252
serotonin receptors and, 214
Glucocorticosteroids, 74
Glutamate
anticonvulsants and, 326
function of, generally, 12
nicotinic receptors and, 271
in nociception, 157–159, 192
Glycine, 13
GMP, spinal cholinergic analgesia, 276
Gout, 74
G proteins, 83, 252
Gray matter, serotonin receptors and, 207
Guanylyl cyclase, 274

HEK 293 cells, 122
Hemicholinium, 274
Hemicholinium-3, 275
Histamine, 106, 232
HOE 140, 101
Hot plate test, 23, 331
Hot plate test
cholinergic agents, 253, 255–256
dopaminergic analgesics, 289, 294
Human immunodeficiency virus (HIV), 76–77
5-hydroxytryptamine (5HT), 106–107
function of, generally, 5
serotonin receptors and, 203–205, 208, 211–212
5-HT$_{1A}$ receptors, 205, 207, 209, 212–213
5-HT$_{1B}$ receptors, 205, 207, 209, 212–213
5-HT$_{2A}$ receptors, 208, 213
5-HT$_3$, 205, 214–216
5-HT$_5$, 205
7-Hydroxy-dipropyl-amino tetralin, 291
8-Hydroxy-dipropyl-amino tetralin, 212–213
Hyperalgesia, 50, 100–104
Hypoalgesia, 105

Ibuprofen, 80–82
Imipramine, 312
In situ hybridization, 54, 98
Incisional pain, 31
Indalpine, 310
Indoleamine, 212, 217
Inflammatory pain, 60, 256, 310, 327
Inhibitory cytokines, 104
Interferon B, 75
Interleukins (Ils), 75, 77, 102–104, 107
International Association for the Study of Pain (IASP), 50
Intrathecal morphine, 64
Ionotropic glutamate receptor (iGluRs) antagonists
  clinical utilization of, 159–160
  interaction with metabotropic glutamate receptors, 168
  motor deficits and, 161–162
  role in nociception, 158
  side effects of, 161–162

Joint replacement, 359
Juvenile arthritis, 73–74

Kallidin, 100
Ketamine, 50, 159, 356
Ketanserin, 213, 232
Kininogen, 100
Kinin and kinin receptors, in hyperalgesia, 100–103
Knee surgery, 59

Lamotrigine, 326–327
Lesions, thalamic, 324
Lidocaine
  effects of, generally, 324–325, 327
  as local anesthetic, 347–348
Lipoxygenase, 5
Lissauer's tract, 8
Lobeline, 277
Local anesthesia
  opioids, interaction with, 347–348
  sodium channels, 323–325
  spinal, 353
Lornoxicam, 77–80
Lumbar radiculopathies, 324

Magnesium, 159

Magnesium Sulfate (MgSO$_4$), 356
Mast cells, 5, 232
Mecamylamine, 272, 275
Mechanoreceptors, 2–3
Medetomidine, 349
Memantine, 30, 36, 159
Mesolimbic dopamine system, 295
Methylamphetamine, 289
Methyllycaconitine, 270
Methylphenidate, 288
Metabotropic glutamate receptors (mGluRs), nociception and, 163–167
N-methyl-D-aspartate receptors, *see* NMDA
Mexiletine, 324
Midazolam, 254
Migraine headache, 147, 211
MK-801, 64, 162
Monoamines, spinal cholinergic analgesia, 276
Monoarthritis, 256
Morphine
  alpha-2 adrenergic antagonists and, 193
  animal models, 34, 36
  antidepressants and, 312
  calcium channels and, 331
  cholinergic agonists and, 272
  dopaminergic drugs and, 287–288, 295
  opioids and, 50, 54, 57, 59, 63–64
  spinal drug interactions, 347–348, 350
Morphine-amphetamine combination, 287–288
Motor deficits, 161–162
Multiple sclerosis, 324
Muscarinic agents, intrathecal drug administration, 275

Nabumetone, 81
Naloxone, 272, 275, 312
Naltrindole (NTI), 50
Neostigmine, 275, 353, 355–356
Nerve growth factor (NGF)
  hyperalgesia, role in, 104–107
  inhibitors, 107
Nerve inactivation, capsaicin-induced, 123–124

Nerve injury, sodium channels and, 324, 329
5'-N-ethylcarboxamidoadenosine (NECA), 234
Neuralgic pain, 324–325
Neurokinin A, 13
Neurokinin antagonists
  NK$_1$ and NK$_2$ receptor antagonists, 139–147
  nonpeptide tachykinin receptor antagonists, 138–139
  tachykinins, role in nociception, 136–138
Neurokinin (NK) receptors, 30. *see also* NK$_1$ and NK$_2$ receptor antagonists
Neurokinins, antidepressants and, 314
Neuronal response, in spinal cord, 10–11
Neuropathic pain
  alpha-2 adrenergic antagonists and, 193–194
  animal models, 34–36, 324–325, 333
  anticonvulsants and, 327
  antidepressants and, 311, 314
  local anesthetics and, 323–324
  neurokinin antagonists, 146–147
  opioids and, 60–61
  purines and, 233, 237
  spinal drug interactions, 349
Neuropathy
  CCK levels, 60–61
  peripheral nerve signaling, 7
Neurophysiology of acute and chronic pain
  dorsal root ganglia, 7–8
  nociceptors, 3–6
  peripheral nerve signaling mechanisms, 6–7
  peripheral receptor signaling, 1–5
  spinal cord signaling mechanisms, 8–13
Neurosteroids, 255
Neurotoxicity, capsaicin-induced, 124–125
Nicardipine, 314
Nicotine, 267, 276, 332
Nicotinic acetylcholine receptor antagonist (ABT-594), 36
Nicotinic cholinergic analgesia
  ABT-594, 271–272

antinociception, 271
cross-tolerance, 269–270
nicotinic receptor subtypes, 270–271
signal transducers, 270
stereoenantiomers, 269
structure-activity relationships, 269
Nifedipine, 314, 330
Nimodipine, 330
Nitric oxide, 274, 276
NK$_1$ and NK$_2$ receptor antagonists
  animal assays, 141–144
  clinical potential of, 144–147
  electrophysiological studies, 139–141
  immunocytochemical assays, 144
NMDA
  antagonists, 159–161
  purines and, 235
  receptor antagonists, 30–31, 36–37, 75, 350, 352
  receptors
    antidepressants, 313
    EAA antagonists and, 162–163
    function of, generally, 12
    NSAID pharmacology, 74
    opioids and, 64
  spinal drug interactions, 345, 350
Nociception, *see specific types of analgesics*
Nociceptive stimulus, 22–23
Nociceptors
  activation, chemicals contributing to, 4–6
  overview, 3–4
Nomifensine, 291
Nonpeptide tachykinin receptor antagonists, 138–139
Nonsteroidal anti-inflammatory drugs (NSAIDs)
  combination therapy, 13–15
  function of, generally, 29
  future directions, 83–84
  novel effects
    acetaminophen, 82–83
    ibuprofen, 80–82
    lornoxicam, 77–80
    pravadoline, 80
    salicylate, 75–76
  pharmacology of, 73–84
  spinal drug interactions, 350, 352

Noradrenaline (NA), 233, 291, 294
Noradrenaline re-uptake inhibitors, 314
Norepinephrine, 271, 277–278, 349
Nortriptyline, 312
NRM neurons, 53–54
NSAIDS, see Nonsteroidal anti-inflammatory drugs (NSAIDs)
Nuvanil, 125

Obstetrics
　dopaminergic drugs in, 287–288
　epidural analgesia, 356–357
　spinal analgesia, 355–356
Olvanil, 125
Ondansetron, 216
Opiates, 288
Opioid peptide systems, 277
Opioids
　activity in pain states
　　overview, 49–51
　　peripheral sites, 55–60
　　spinal sites, 54–55
　　supraspinal sites, 51–54
　cholinergic analgesia and, 267
　dopaminergic drugs and, 288
　epidural
　　analgesia, 357–358
　　anesthesia, 354–355
　function of, generally, 13, 22
　neurochemical changes in chronic pain states
　　inflammatory pain, 60
　　neuropathic pain, 60–62
　stressors and, 295–296
Ossification, 79
Osteoarthritis (OA), 73
Oxotremorine, 267, 275, 332
Oxymetazoline, 349

Pain, see specific types of pain
　defined, 50
　perception, 140–141
Paw incision test, 31
Pedunculopontine tegmental nucleus (PPTg), 273–274
Pentobarbitone, 254
Peripheral nerve injury
　altered analgesic responsiveness, 62–63
　anticonvulsants and, 326
Peripheral nerve signaling mechanisms
　afferent nerves, 6–7
　neuropathy, peripheral changes occurring in, 7
Peripheral neuron-specific sodium channels, 327–329
Peripheral opioids, 55–56
Peripheral receptor signaling
　mechanoreceptors, 2–3
　nociceptors, 3–5
　sensory receptors, 1–2
　thermoreceptors, 3
Persistent pain
　animal models, 26–30
　antidepressants and, 306
　excitatory amino acid antagonists for, 157–168
Pharmacology
　animal studies, 29–30
　dopaminergic drugs, 291–296
　nonsteroidal anti-inflammatory drugs, 73–84
　serotonin receptors, 211–216
　of spinal cord, 12
Phenacetin, 289
Phenoxybenzamine, 181
Phenylalkylamines, 330
R-phenylisopropyladenosine (R-PIA), 234–235
Phenytoin, 326
Physostigmine, 275, 332
Picrotoxin, 255
Pilocarpine, 267, 275
Pimozide, 292
Pirenzepine, 275
PL017, 351
Placebo-controlled studies, 278, 324
Platelet-derived growth factor (PDGF), 77
PN3/SNS, 329, 335
Postoperative pain, 192–193, 289, 306, 356–359
Postshock vocalization test, 289
Potassium channels, 333–335
PPTg, see Pedunculopontine tegmental nucleus (PPTg)
PPTg-to-RVM cholinergic pathway, 273
Pravadoline, 80

Prazosin, 184, 186
Pronociception
  ATP receptors, 233
  caffeine and, 238
Prostacyclins, 99
Prostaglandin (PG) synthesis, 75, 77–78
Prostanoid antagonists
  overview, 96–98
  receptor specificity, 98
  stimulus specificity, 98–100
Protein kinase C (PKC), 64, 101, 168
Psoriatic arthritis, 74
Purines
  caffeine, analgesic properties of, 238
  overview, 229–230
  peripheral effects on
    adenosine A_1 receptors, 231
    adenosine A_2 receptors, 231
    adenosine A_3 receptors, 231–232
    algogenic actions in humans, 232–233
    ATP receptors, 233
    indirectly acting adenosine agents, 232
  P_{2X}, 239
  spinal effects
    adenosine, 234–237
    adenosine analogues, 234–237
    ATP, ATP analogues, and antagonists, 236
    indirectly acting adenosine agents, 235–236
  therapeutic implications, 238–239

QX-314, 327

Randall-Sellito test, 75
Raphe complex, 204
Rat studies, *see specific types of analgesia*
  arthritis, adjuvant-induced, 75–80
  formalin test, 26–28
  nicotinic agonists in, 276–277
  paw incision test, 31, 35
Rauwolscine, 184
Receptors, *see specific types of receptors*
Reflex sympathetic dystrophy, 324
Resiniferatoxin (RTX), capsaicin and, 119, 121–122

Rhesus monkey, analgesics research study, 24–25
Rheumatoid arthritis (RA), 74, 77–78, 80, 146
Ritanserin, 213
mRNA, 56, 211
Rostral ventral medulla (RVM), 272–273
RT-PCR, 210
RU 24213, 294
RU 24926, 294
RU 24969, 213

Salicylate, 75–76
SCH 23390, 292, 294
Sedation, alpha-2 adrenergic agonists and, 191–192
Sensory fiber activation, vanilloids and, 120–121
Sensory receptors, 1–2
Serotonin
  bulbospinal system, 204–205
  effect on receptors
    central receptors, heterogeneity, 205
    generally, 5, 203–204
    in spinal cord, 207–211
    in trigeminal complex, 211
  nicotinic receptors and, 271
  nociception
    mechanisms involved in, 216–218
    overview, 213–214
    pharmacological control of, 211–216
Serotonin reuptake inhibitors (SSRIs), 304, 311
Signal transduction, 270, 329
Silver staining technique, 56
SKF 38393, 292
Slowly adapting receptors, 2
SM-21, 268
SM-32, 268
SNX-111, 331, 333
Sodium channels
  anticonvulsants, 325–327
  local anesthetics, 323–325
  overview, 322–323
  peripheral neuron-specific, 327–329
Somatostatin (SOM), 7–8, 13, 204, 356

Spinal cord
  adenosine, effects on, 234–237
  calcium channels and, 332–333
  dopaminergic analgesia, 293–294
  pharmacology of, 12–13
  serotonin receptors in
    cells expressing, 208–211
    generally, 207–208
  signaling mechanisms, central
    neuronal organization, 8–9
    neuronal responses, 10–11
    pharmacology, of spinal cord, 12–13
Spinal drug interactions
  antagonism, additivity, and synergy, 345–347
  clinical examples and implications
    epidural analgesia, 356–358
    epidural anesthesia, 354–355
    generally, 351–352
    spinal analgesia, 355–356
    spinal anesthesia, 352–354
  mechanistic insights, 350–351
  nonhuman studies
    opioid-*a*-adrenoreceptor interactions, 348–350
    opioid-local anesthetic interactions, 347–348
    opioid-NMDA receptor antagonist and NSAID interactions, 350
Spinal laminae, 8–10
Spinal opioids, 54–55
Spiperone, 213
ST-91, 184, 349
Stereoenantiomers, 269
Stress, dopaminergic analgesia and, 295–296
Stress response, 348
Stroke, 324
Substance P
  animal models, 5, 7–8, 13
  antidepressants and, 314
  arthritis and, 146
  kinins and kinin receptors, 105
  neurokinin antagonists and, 135–138
  opioids and, 54, 57
  purines and, 232, 235
  serotonin receptors and, 204, 216, 218
Sufentanil, 356–357

Sumatriptan, 268
Supraspinal opioids, 51–54
Sympathetic nervous system, 233
Sympathomimetic drugs, 289, 291
Synergy, analgesic, 346, 348, 350–351

T cells, 77
Tachykinins, role in nociception
  animal assays, 138
  electrophysiological studies
    in vitro, 136–137
    in vivo, 137–138
Tactile allodynia, 63
Tail flick/dip tests, 23, 63, 294, 331, 335
Tetracaine, 354
Tetraethylammonium (TEA), 334
Tetrahydroacridine, 276–277
Tetrodotoxin (TTX), 322, 328–329
Tetrodotoxin-resistant (TTX-R) sodium channels, 100, 335
Thermal hyperalgesia, 63
Thermoreceptors, 3
Thiopentone, 254
THIP, 253
Thyrotropin-releasing hormone, 204
Tolerance, nicotinic cholinergic analgesia, 269–270
Tourniquet test, 288–289
Tramadol, 34
Tricyclic antidepressants (TCAs), efficacy of
  anticholinergic properties of, 313
  generally, 305–306, 310, 315
  noxious transmission, interaction with excitatory amino acids, 313–314
  quinidine-like effect, 313
  sedative effect, 313
Trigeminal complex, serotonin receptors, 211
Trigeminal neuralgia, 325
trkA receptor, 105
Tropisetron, 216, 218
L-tryptophan, 295
Tumor necrosis factor (TNF), 75–76, 103, 107

Vanilloids, as analgesics
Vasoactive intestinal polypeptide (VIP), 7–8, 13

Vasoconstrictors, 354
Ventral striatum, role in analgesia, 292–293, 295
Ventral tegmental area (VTA), 293
Verapamil, 330
Visceral pain, animal models, 31–34
Voltage-gated calcium channels (VGCC), 329–331
Voltage-gated ion channels
  alterations in, 321–322
  calcium channels, 329–333
  function of, generally, 321
  future directions, 335–336
  potassium channels, 333–335
  sodium channels
    anticonvulsants, 325–327
    local anesthetics, 323–325
    overview, 322–323
    peripheral neuron-specific, 327–329
Voltage-gated potassium channels, 335
Voltage-gated sodium channels (VGSCs), 322

Yohimbine
  alpha-2 adrenergic antagonists and, 183–184, 186
  antidepressants and, 312
  serotonin receptors and, 217

Ziconotide, 36